Mechanisms of
CLINICAL SIGNS

In Memoriam
Doctor John Morgan 27.9.1930–14.7.2014
Surgeon, gentleman, teacher and friend.

'I shall not see his like again'

Mechanisms of CLINICAL SIGNS

2nd Edition

Mark Dennis MBBS (Honours)
Cardiology Advance Trainee /Intensive Care Trainee,
Royal Prince Alfred Hospital, Clinical Lecturer, Sydney Medical School,
University of Sydney, NSW, Australia

William Talbot Bowen MBBS, MD
Emergency Medicine Physician, Board Eligible
Louisiana State University Health Sciences Center
New Orleans, LA, United States

Lucy Cho BA, MBBS, MIPH
General Practice Registrar
Appletree Family Practice
Newcastle, NSW, Australia

ELSEVIER

ELSEVIER

Elsevier Australia, ACN 001 002 357
(a division of Reed International Books Australia Pty Ltd)
Tower 1, 475 Victoria Avenue, Chatswood, NSW 2067

> **Notice**
> This publication has been carefully reviewed and checked to ensure that the content is as accurate and current as possible at time of publication. We would recommend, however, that the reader verify any procedures, treatments, drug dosages or legal content described in this book. Neither the author, the contributors, nor the publisher assume any liability for injury and/or damage to persons or property arising from any error in or omission from this publication.

National Library of Australia Cataloguing-in-Publication Data

Dennis, Mark, 1978- author.
Mechanisms of clinical signs / Mark Dennis, William Talbot Bowen, Lucy Cho.
Second edition.
9780729542371 (paperback)
Symptoms—Handbooks, manuals, etc.
Diagnosis—Handbooks, manuals, etc.
Bowen, William Talbot, author.
Cho, Lucy, author.

616.075

Content Strategist: Larissa Norrie
Senior Content Development Specialist: Neli Bryant and Lauren Santos
Senior Project Manager: Karthikeyan Murthy
Edited by Katie Millar
Proofread by Annabel Adair
Illustrations by Toppan Best-set Premedia Limited and Alan Laver
Design by Tania Gomes
Index by Robert Swanson
Typeset by Toppan Best-set Premedia Limited
Printed by CTPS, China

Contents

Chapter 1
Musculoskeletal Signs   1

Chapter 2
Respiratory Signs   77

Contents

Contents

Contents by Condition

Foreword

In the 21st-century world of advanced imaging and other diagnostic techniques, it is tempting to consign clinical signs from careful physical examination to the 'dustbin of history'. This would be a terrible error. Not only are physical signs and their accurate interpretation of primary importance in resource-poor environments, they are also necessary to allow clinicians to triage appropriate further high-technology investigations and to appropriately question those results when they do not tally with the physical signs obtained. These are vital skills for every medical student and qualified practitioner.

Some physical signs are very difficult, such as JVP interpretation in the obese patient or hearing the abdominal bruit in the young hypertensive patient with renal artery stenosis. Some signs are easy to elicit but too easily forgotten, such as the 'tell-tale' radio-femoral delay of aortic coarctation. A careful understanding of the mechanisms of clinical signs not only adds to the intellectual satisfaction of understanding disease pathophysiology, but also provides the key learning reinforcement to appreciate the value of a thorough and caring physical examination.

This book is well organised; there are systems-based chapters (such as musculoskeletal, respiratory etc.) and then short sub-sections on common signs, arranged in alphabetical order. Almost each sign is illustrated by a photograph, a figure and/or a relevant diagram. The large font and clearly drawn diagrams render this a very easy-to-read and comprehensible tour-de-force of medical education. Readers will use it as a specific reference for particular questions, or as a book to read from cover-to-cover, to optimise their ability to interpret signs and to practise maximally effective 'laying on of hands'. To my knowledge, there is no other book quite like it.

This is the second edition of *Mechanisms of Clinical Signs* and it remains a clear and thorough reference covering the major aspects of clinically apparent manifestations of human disease. The second edition contains additional features of interest and importance such as audio and video files, as well as easy-to-follow 'flow diagrams' and highlighted 'Clinical Pearls'.

This textbook will be a joy for medical trainees both at medical school and at postgraduate level. Even seasoned clinicians will enjoy learning more about the mechanisms behind many of the clinical signs that they elicit on a frequent basis. As practised by our medical forebears, clinical history and physical examination remain the underpinnings of accurate diagnosis and our ability to serve our patients well. This book provides a wonderful resource to those wishing to become more complete physicians.

David S Celermajer AO MB BS PhD DSc FRACP

Preface

Much has changed in the three years since the release of the first edition of this book. Accurate physical exam interpretation remains pertinent to medical decision making in an age of readily available advanced diagnostic tests. The authors are grateful for and heartened by the feedback from students and junior and senior clinicians alike who have found the first edition valuable in patient care.

Reader feedback has driven the updates and improvements to the second edition. The same focus remains – understanding the mechanisms of clinical signs in medicine. There is a fine line between too much content and oversimplification – the authors have strengthened some entries and simplified others. Several new clinical signs have been added to the text. Many new photographs, illustrations and flow diagrams are available to improve understanding. Finally, in this technological age, it would be remiss if a textbook was not enhanced by the use of online material. Audio and video files, demonstrating and/or explaining signs, are available to the reader.

The evidence base for each clinical sign has been re-examined. The predictive value for a sign has been reviewed and revised where possible. Signs of particular clinical value have been highlighted under the heading 'Clinical Pearl'.

In many ways modern medicine has become more algorithmic or guideline focused. The accurate retrieval and interpretation of bedside patient information via the history and physical exam remains the art and science of medicine and the foundation upon which all good clinical decisions are made.

Acknowledgements

The authors would like to thank their families and friends for their unwavering support: it takes a village. Finally, to all the medical students who continue to ask 'why' and who have, with more senior clinician guidance, provided direction for improvements of the text – thank you.

Reviewers

Chapter 2 Respiratory Signs:
Dr Keith Wong MBBS(Hons)
MMed(Clin Epi) PhD FRACP
Research Fellow, Sleep and Circadian Research Group, Woolcock Institute of Medical
Research; Staff Specialist, Department of Respiratory and Sleep Medicine, Royal Prince
Alfred Hospital, University of Sydney
Professor Ivan Young PhD FRACP
Clinical Professor, Central Clinical School (Medicine), University of Sydney; Department of
Respiratory Medicine, Royal Prince Alfred Hospital

Chapter 3 Cardiovascular Signs:
Dr Rajesh Puranik MBBS PhD FRACP
Consultant Cardiologist, Royal Prince Alfred Hospital, NHMRC/NHF Postdoctoral
Fellow, University of Sydney

Chapter 4 Haematological and Oncological Signs:
Professor Douglas Joshua MD
Professor of Internal Medicine, University of Sydney; Head of Institute of Haematology,
Royal Prince Alfred Hospital

Chapter 5 Neurological Signs:
Dr John Carmody MB BCh MRCPI FRACP
Staff Specialist Neurologist, Hon. Clinical Senior Lecturer, University of Wollongong
Associate Professor Leo Davies MD MB BS FRACP
Sub-Dean and Head of Assessment, Sydney Medical School, University of Sydney;
Australian & New Zealand Association of Neurologists; Australian Association of
Neurologists

Chapter 6 Gastroenterological Signs:
Associate Professor Meng C Ngu MBBS(Hons) BMedSc(Hons) PhD FRACP
Clinical Associate Professor, University of Sydney; Consultant Gastroenterologist

Chapter 7 Endocrinological Signs:
Professor Stephen Twigg MBBS (Hons-I) PhD FRACP
Professor in Medicine, Central Clinical School and the Bosch Institute, University of
Sydney; Senior Staff Specialist in Endocrinology, Royal Prince Alfred Hospital

---

Awais Saleem Babri (MBBS, PGDipSc, PhD, GradCertEdu)
School of Biomedical Sciences, The University of Queensland, Qld, Australia

Timothy Billington PhD
Lecturer Medical Sciences and Medical Education, School of Medicine, University of
Wollongong, NSW, Australia

Wai Ping (Alicia) Chan MBBS FRACP PhD FCSANX

Shiv Chitturi FRACP
Staff Specialist, Canberra Hospital, ACT, Australia

Simon Dimmitt MBBS, BMedSc(Hons), FRACP, FCSANZ
Clinical Professor of Medicine, University of Western Australia

Ulrich Orda Staatsexamen Medizin (D), PhD (D), Facharzt fuer Innere Medizin (D),
Allgemeinmedizin (D), Notfallmedizin (D), FACRRM / GEM
Director of Emergency Mount Isa Hospital, Director of Clinical Training North West
Hospital and Health Service, Qld, Australia; Associate Professor James Cook University/
Mount Isa Institute for Rural and Remote Medicine, Qld, Australia

Zoë Raos MBChB FRACP
Gastroenterologist and General Physician, North Shore Hospital – Waitemata District Health Board, Auckland, New Zealand

Philip Robinson B Med Sc, MB BS, MD, PhD FRACP
Paediatric Respiratory Physician, Royal Children's Hospital, Vic, Australia

Milana Votrubec MB BS MA MM ME USyd FRACGP FFPMANZCA
Senior Clinical Tutor University of Sydney and Notre Dame, NSW, Australia

Abbreviations

5-HT	5-hydroxytryptamine (serotonin)	CREST	calcinosis cutis, Raynaud's phenomenon, (o)esophageal dysfunction, sclerodactyly, telangiectasia syndrome
ACA	anterior cerebral artery		
ACE	angiotensin-converting enzyme	CRH	corticotrophin-releasing hormone
ACL	anterior cruciate ligament		
ACTH	adrenocorticotropic hormone	CRVO	central retinal vein occlusion
ADP	adenosine diphosphate	CS	cavernous sinus
ADH	antidiuretic hormone, or vasopressin	CSA	central sleep apnoea
		CSF	cerebrospinal fluid
AIDS	acquired immune deficiency syndrome	CT	computerised tomography
		CV	cortical veins
AION	anterior ischaemic optic neuropathy	CVP	central venous pressure
		DAS	dorsal acoustic stria
AN	acanthosis nigricans	DHEA-S	dehydroepiandrosterone sulfate
AP	anterioposterior		
AR	aortic regurgitation	DIP	distal interphalangeal joint
ARDS	acute respiratory distress syndrome	DI	diabetes insipidus
		DM	diabetes mellitus
ASD	atrial septal defect	DRE	digital rectal examination
AV	arterio-venous	DVT	deep vein thrombosis
AV (node)	atrioventricular (node)	EBV	Epstein–Barr virus
AVM	arteriovenous malformation	EGFR	epidermal growth factor receptor
BMI	body mass index		
BPH	benign prostatic hypertrophy	EMH	extramedullary haematopoiesis
BPPV	benign paroxysmal positional vertigo	ENAC	epithelial sodium (Na) channel
CCK	cholecystokinin	EOM	extraocular muscle
CG	ciliary ganglion	EW	Edinger–Westphal nucleus
CGL	chronic granulocytic leukaemia	FABER	flexion abduction external rotation
CGRP	calcitonin gene-related peptide	FGFR	fibroblast growth factor receptor
CHF	congestive heart failure	FSH	follicle-stimulating hormone
CI	confidence interval		
CLL	chronic lymphocytic leukaemia	G6PD	glucose-6-phosphate dehydrogenase
CMC	carpometacarpal	GABA	gamma-aminobutyric acid
cMOAT	canalicular multispecific organic anion transporter	GAS	group A streptococcus
		GBS	Guillain–Barré syndrome
CMT	Charcot–Marie–Tooth (disease)	GH	growth hormone
		GI	gastrointestinal
CMV	cytomegalovirus	GnRH	gonadotrophin-releasing hormone
COPD	chronic obstructive pulmonary disease		
		GORD	gastro-oesophageal reflux disease
CNS	central nervous system		
CRAO	central retinal artery occlusion	GPe	globus pallidus pars externa
		GPi	globus pallidus pars interns

Gs	guanine nucleotide-binding protein that couples to TSH receptor
GV	great vein of Galen
Hb	haemoglobin
HbSC	sickle cell haemoglobin C
hCG	human chorionic gonadotropin
HIV	human immunodeficiency virus
HLA	human leukocyte antigen
HOCM	hypertrophic obstructive cardiomyopathy
HPOA	hypertrophic pulmonary osteoarthropathy
HPV	human papilloma virus
HSV	herpes simplex virus
IAS	intermediate acoustic stria
IBD	inflammatory bowel disease
ICA	internal carotid artery
ICV	internal cerebral vein
IFN	interferon
IGF-1	insulin-like growth factor-1
IJ	internal jugular vein
IL	interleukin
INC	interstitial nucleus of Cajal
INO	internuclear ophthalmoplegia
IO	inferior oblique (muscle or subnucleus)
IR	inferior rectus (muscle or subnucleus)
ISS	inferior sagittal sinus
IVC	inferior vena cava
JVP	jugular venous pressure
LA	left atrial
LBBB	left bundle branch block
LGN	lateral geniculate nucleus
LH	luteinising hormone
LPS	lipopolysaccharides
LR	lateral rectus (muscle)
LR	likelihood ratio
LR	livedo reticularis
LS	lateral sinus
LTB$_4$	leukotriene B$_4$
LV	left ventricular
MAOI	monoamine oxidase inhibitor
MCA	middle cerebral artery
MCPJ	metacarpophalangeal joint
MD	muscular dystrophy
MDMA	methylenedioxymethamphetamine (Ecstasy)
MDPK	myotonic dystrophy protein kinase
MEN	multiple endocrine neoplasia
MLF	medial longitudinal fasciculus
MMP	matrix metalloproteinase
MPTP	1-methyl-4-phenyl-1,2,3,6-tetrahydropyridine (toxicity)
MR	medial rectus (muscle)
MRF	midbrain reticular formation
MRI	magnetic resonance imaging
mRNA	messenger ribonucleic acid
MSH	melanocyte-stimulating hormone
MTP	metatarsophalangeal
MV	mitral valve
NAA	N-acetyl-L-aspartate
NF-κB	nuclear factor kappa-light-chain-enhancer of activated B cells
NHL	non-Hodgkin lymphoma
NLD	necrobiosis lipodica diabeticorum
NO	nitric oxide
NPV	negative predictive value
OCP	oral contraceptive pill
OSA	obstructive sleep apnoea
PAI-1	plasminogen activator inhibitor-1
PC	posterior commissure
PCA	posterior cerebral artery
PComm	posterior communicating artery
PCOS	polycystic ovarian syndrome
PCP	phencyclidine (toxicity)
PCWP	pulmonary capillary wedge pressure
PDA	patent ductus arteriosus
PDGF	platelet-derived growth factor
PFO	patent foramen ovale
PGE	prostaglandin E
PGI$_2$	prostaglandin I$_2$
PGH	prostaglandin H
PICA	posterior inferior cerebellar artery
PIP	proximal interphalangeal joint

PLR	positive likelihood ratio	SNc	substantia nigra pars compacta
PND	paroxysmal nocturnal dyspnoea	SNr	substantia nigra pars reticulate
PPRF	paramedian pontine reticular formation	SO	superior oblique (muscle)
PPV	positive predictive value	SPS	stiff-person syndrome
POMC	pro-opiomelanocortin	SR	superior rectus (muscle or subnucleus)
PR (interval)	measured from the beginning of the P wave to the beginning of the QRS complex	SS	sigmoid sinus
		SS	straight sinus
		SSS	superior sagittal sinus
PR	pulmonary regurgitation	SSRI	selective serotonin reuptake inhibitor
PS	petrosal sinus		
PSA	prostate-specific antigen	STN	subthalamic nucleus
PSP	progressive supranuclear palsy	SVC	superior vena cava
		T_3	triiodothyronine (thyroid hormone)
PTH	parathyroid hormone		
PTH-rp	parathyroid hormone-related protein	T_4	thyroxine (thyroid hormone)
PTN	pretectal nucleus	TB	tuberculosis
RA	rheumatoid arthritis	TF	tissue factor
RA	right atrial	TGF-β	transforming growth factor-beta
RAA(S)	renin–angiotensin–aldosterone (system)	TH	torcular Herophili
RANK	receptor activator of nuclear factor kappa	Th-1	helper T cell type 1
		TIA	transient ischaemic attack
RAPD	relative afferent pupillary defect	TNF	tumour necrosis factor
RAR	rapidly adapting receptor	TRH	thyrotrophin-releasing hormone
RBBB	right bundle branch block	TS	transverse sinus
RBC	red blood cell	TSH	thyroid stimulating hormone
riMLF	rostral interstitial medial longitudinal fasciculus	TSHR	thyroid stimulating hormone receptor
RN	red nucleus		
RNA	ribonucleic acid	TTP	thrombotic thrombocytopenic purpura
RR	relative risk or risk ratio		
RTA	renal tubule acidosis	URTI	upper respiratory tract infection
RV	right ventricular		
SA (node)	sinoatrial (node)	V2 (receptor)	arginine vasopressin receptor 2
SC	superior colliculus		
SCA	superior cerebellar arteries	VAS	ventral acoustic stria
SCC	squamous cell carcinoma	VEGF	vascular endothelial growth factor
SCFE	slipped capital femoral epiphysis		
		VIP	vasoactive intestinal peptide
SLAP	superior labrum anterior posterior	VL	ventral lateral
		VSD	ventricular septal defect
SLE	systemic lupus erythematosus	vWF	von Willebrand factor
		VZV	varicella zoster virus

Sign Value

Eliciting or identifying a clinical sign is a requisite skill in medicine – however, it is merely the beginning of the story. More importantly, a good clinician understands a sign's predictive value, evidence base and role in diagnostic evaluation. The presence or absence of a clinical sign offers a data point, allowing us to refine the probability of the disease of interest as the differential diagnosis (i.e. the process of risk stratification).

In the *Sign Value* section, the reader will find a brief précis of the evidence base for the given sign, including (where available), sensitivity, specificity, positive or negative predictive values and/or likelihood ratios. With a positive LR (sign is present) or negative LR (sign is absent) value, one can determine the post-test probability of disease, using the following equation (a component of Bayesian Theory):

$$\text{Pre-test probability} \times \text{likelihood ratio} = \text{post-test probability}$$

Example:
A 20-year-old, immunocompetent, male student presents to his local Emergency Department, complaining of severe headache. The junior doctor assessing him notes that he appears toxic, is febrile and has a non-blanching purpuric rash and non-focal neurological signs. The doctor specifically identifies the absence of Kernig's sign. The entire clinical scenario is suspicious for bacterial meningitis due to *Neisseria meningitides,* complicated by meningococcaemia. This patient has a very high pre-test probability of bacterial meningitis. The absence of Kernig's sign (–LR 1.0) does not affect the probability of meningitis being present.

Very high pre-test probability $\times 1.0 =$ *very high post-test probability*

It is critical to understand the predictive value of the presence or absence of a clinical sign. The junior clinician should not be swayed by the absence of Kernig's sign. This patient requires emergent administration of IV antibiotics, lumbar puncture and public health notification. CT imaging prior to lumbar puncture may be considered in certain clinical scenarios.

The sensible clinician will judiciously consider examination findings and/or diagnostic tests and how they affect the probability of the diagnosis and management plan.

CHAPTER 1

MUSCULOSKELETAL SIGNS

Anterior drawer test

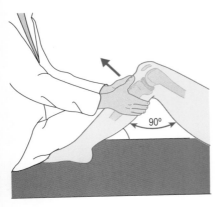

FIGURE 1.1
Anterior drawer test for anterior cruciate ligament injury

Description

With the patient lying supine, the knee at 90° flexion and the foot immobilised by the examiner, the proximal third of the tibia is pulled towards the examiner. In a positive test, there is anterior (forward) movement of the tibia without an abrupt stop.[1]

Condition/s associated with

• Anterior cruciate ligament (ACL) injury

Mechanism/s

The ACL arises from the anterior aspect of the tibial plateau and inserts into the medial aspect of the lateral femoral condyle. It limits anterior movement of the tibia upon the femur. Loss of continuity of the ACL permits inappropriate anterior movement of the tibia and thus knee joint instability.

Sign value

A literature review of six studies reported a sensitivity of 27–88%, specificity of 91–99%, positive LR of 11.5 and negative LR of 0.5.[2] A literature review by Solomon DH et al. of nine studies reported a sensitivity of 9–93% and specificity of 23–100%.[1]

A positive anterior drawer sign (+LR 11.5)[2] is strong evidence of ACL injury. A negative anterior drawer sign cannot reliably exclude ACL injury (sensitivity 27–88%; –LR 0.5).[2] When significant clinical suspicion persists, despite a negative anterior drawer sign, further diagnostic considerations are necessary (e.g. interval re-examination, MRI, arthroscopy).

Apley's grind test

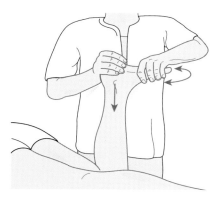

FIGURE 1.2
Apley's grind test

Description

With the patient lying prone and the knee at 90° flexion, the lower leg is passively internally and externally rotated while axial pressure is applied to the lower leg. The test is considered positive if tenderness is elicited.

Condition/s associated with

• Meniscal injury

Mechanism/s

Direct mechanical force upon the injured meniscus elicits tenderness.

Sign value

A review by Hegedus EJ et al. reported a pooled sensitivity of 60.7% and specificity of 70.2% with an odds ratio of 3.4.[3] Significant heterogeneity in the data limits its accuracy. Overall, Apley's grind test has limited diagnostic utility, limited supporting data and, in the acute setting, the manoeuvre produces severe pain.[4]

McMurray's grind test has more robust supporting data.

Apley's scratch test

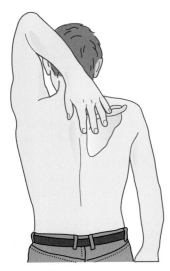

FIGURE 1.3
One of three manoeuvres of Apley's scratch test

Based on Woodward T, Best TM, The painful shoulder: part 1, clinical evaluation. Am Fam Phys *2000; 61(10): 3079–3088.*

Description

Apley's scratch test is a general range of movement assessment of the shoulder joint (i.e. glenohumeral, acromioclavicular, sternoclavicular and scapulothoracic joints). The patient is instructed to touch the unaffected shoulder anteriorly and posteriorly (behind their head), and touch the inferior scapula posteriorly (behind their back). Tenderness and/or limited range of movement while performing these movements is considered an abnormal test.[5]

Condition/s associated with

Common

- Rotator cuff muscle injury
- Labral tear
- Anterior shoulder dislocation
- Bicipital tendonitis
- Adhesive capsulitis (frozen shoulder)
- Acromioclavicular joint injury

Mechanism/s

The shoulder joint is a complex structure. Its components include the humeral head, glenoid fossa, acromion, clavicle, scapula and surrounding soft tissue structures. Under normal circumstances the shoulder joint is capable of a vast range of movement. Apley's scratch test assesses glenohumeral abduction, adduction, flexion, extension, internal rotation and external rotation. Tenderness or limited range of movement suggests injury to one or more components of the shoulder joint.

Sign value

Apley's scratch test is a useful component of the general shoulder exam but has limited utility for a specific diagnosis. The position of the shoulder at which tenderness or limited range of movement occurs should be noted. In the patient with an abnormal Apley's scratch test, further diagnostic manoeuvres should be performed to narrow the differential diagnosis.

Apparent leg length inequality (functional leg length)

1

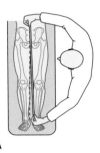 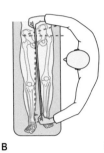 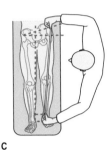

A B C

FIGURE 1.4
Measurement of leg lengths
A The apparent leg length is the distance from the umbilicus to the medial malleolus;
B pelvic rotation causing an apparent leg length discrepancy; **C** the true leg length is the distance from the anterior superior iliac spine to the medial malleolus.
Based on Firestein GS, Budd RC, Harris ED et al., Kelley's Textbook of Rheumatology, *8th edn, Philadelphia: WB Saunders, 2008: Fig 42-24.*

Description

A disparity between the relative distance from the umbilicus to the medial malleolus of each leg.[6] By definition it implies asymmetry of the lower extremities in the absence of a bony abnormality. (See 'True leg length inequality' in this chapter.)

Condition/s associated with

- Altered foot mechanics
- Adaptive shortening of soft tissues
- Joint contractures
- Ligamentous laxity
- Axial malalignments

Mechanism/s

An apparent or functional leg length inequality may occur at any point from the pelvis to the foot.[6]

Ligamentous laxity

The ligaments on one side (e.g. in the hip joint) may be more flexible or longer than their counterparts, making the femur sit lower in the joint capsule.

Joint contracture

A joint contracture impairs full range of movement. If the knee joint is contracted in a flexed position, the length of the affected side will be less than the opposite leg during maximal attempted extension.

Altered foot mechanics

Excessive pronation of the foot eventuates in and/or may be accompanied by a decreased arch height compared to the 'normal' foot, resulting in a functionally shorter limb.[6]

Sign value

The distance (anywhere from 3–22 mm) at which apparent leg length inequality results in a clinically significant effect is controversial.[6] The test should be interpreted in relation to the patient's history and full gait assessment.

Apprehension test

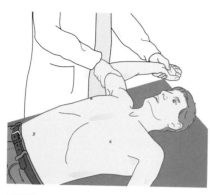

FIGURE 1.5
Apprehension test
The arm is abducted and placed in an externally rotated position. Note the right arm of the examiner is providing anterior traction on the humerus, pulling the posterior part of the humeral head forward. The same test can be done from the back, with the patient sitting up and the examiner pushing forward on the posterior head of the humerus.

Description

The apprehension test is an assessment of glenohumeral joint instability. With the patient sitting or lying supine, the shoulder is placed into 90° abduction, 90° external rotation and 90° elbow flexion. The examiner applies pressure to the posterior aspect of the proximal humerus and attempts to move the humeral head anteriorly (see Figure 1.5). The test is positive if the patient experiences *apprehension* due to impending subluxation or dislocation of the glenohumeral joint.[7]

Condition/s associated with

More common – traumatic

- Recurrent glenohumeral joint subluxation or dislocation

- Rotator cuff muscle injury
- Glenoid labrum injury
- Glenoid defect (e.g. Bankart's fracture)
- Humeral head defect (e.g. Hill–Sachs fracture)

Less common – atraumatic

- Connective tissue disorder: Ehlers–Danlos syndrome, Marfan's syndrome
- Congenital absence of glenoid

Mechanism/s

Glenohumeral joint instability is caused by dysfunction of the bony and/or soft tissue structures that maintain joint stability: glenoid, humeral head, joint capsule, capsuloligamentous or glenohumeral ligaments, labrum, and rotator cuff muscles. The shoulder joint is susceptible to instability due to its inherent mobility and complex soft tissue structures responsible for stability.

In the apprehension test, the joint is placed into a position vulnerable to instability. It is the typical position precipitating traumatic anterior shoulder dislocation. For this reason, a significant number of healthy patients will experience apprehension during this manoeuvre.

Sign value

T'Jonck et al. reported a sensitivity of 88.0%, specificity of 50%, positive likelihood ratio of 1.8 and negative likelihood ratio of 0.23.[8]

The apprehension test for glenohumeral joint instability is a moderately useful screening test. Based on available data, the test has limited utility to rule in the diagnosis. It is not used in the setting of acute anterior shoulder dislocation.

Apprehension–relocation test (Fowler's sign)

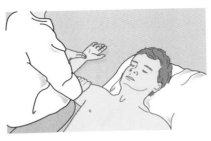

FIGURE 1.6
Apprehension–relocation (Fowler) test
Note that pressure is applied anteriorly to
the proximal humerus.

Description

The apprehension–relocation test is an
assessment of glenohumeral joint
instability. The relocation manoeuvre
is typically performed following the
apprehension test (See 'Apprehension
test'). With the patient sitting or lying
supine, the shoulder is placed into 90°
abduction, 90° external rotation and
90° elbow flexion. The examiner
applies pressure to the anterior aspect
of the proximal humerus and attempts
to move the humeral head posteriorly.
The test is positive if the patient
experiences relief of apprehension (i.e.
no longer feels impending shoulder
dislocation).

Condition/s associated with

- Recurrent glenohumeral joint
  subluxation or dislocation
- Rotator cuff muscle injury
- Glenoid labrum injury
- Glenoid defect (e.g. Bankart's
  fracture)
- Humeral head defect (e.g. Hill–
  Sachs fracture)

Less common – atraumatic

- Connective tissue disorder:
  Ehlers–Danlos syndrome, Marfan's
  syndrome
- Congenital absence of glenoid

Mechanism/s

The underlying anatomy and causes of
glenohumeral joint instability are
outlined under 'Apprehension test' and
apply here. In the apprehension–
relocation test, symptomatic relief is
due to restoration of the normal
anatomical relationship of the humeral
head in the glenohumeral joint.

Sign value

T'Jonck et al. reported a sensitivity of
85%, specificity of 87%, positive
likelihood ratio of 6.5 and negative
likelihood ratio of 0.18.[8] Lo et al.
reported sensitivity of 32% and
specificity of 100%.[9] Speer et al.
reported a sensitivity of 68% and
specificity of 100%.[10]

The apprehension–relocation test is
a useful screening manoeuvre for
anterior glenohumeral joint instability.
It appears to be more specific than the
'apprehension' test alone.

Bouchard's and Heberden's nodes

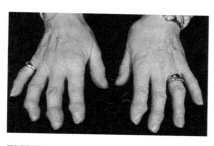

FIGURE 1.7
Prominent Heberden's nodes

Based on Ferri FF, Ferri's Clinical Advisor, *Philadelphia: Elsevier, 2011: Fig 1-223.*

Description

Bouchard's nodes are bony outgrowths or nodules found over the *proximal* interphalangeal joints of the hands.

Heberden's nodes are similar but located over the *distal* interphalangeal joints.

Condition/s associated with

- Osteoarthritis
- Familial

Mechanism/s

A number of studies have implicated *bony osteophyte growth* as the principal cause of Heberden's and Bouchard's nodes.[11] Other contributing factors or theories include:

- genetic predisposition
- endochrondral ossification of hypertrophied cartilage as a result of chronic osteoarthritic changes[12]
- traction spurs growing in tendons in response to excessive tension and repetitive strain.[13]

Sign value

Bouchard's or Heberden's nodes are a classical sign of interphalangeal osteoarthritis[13,14] and are associated with generalised osteoarthritis.[15,16] The presence of Bouchard's and/or Heberden's nodes is predictive of the radiographic changes of osteoarthritis.[17]

Boutonnière deformity

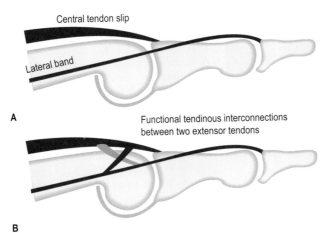

FIGURE 1.8
Digital extensor mechanism
A The proximal interphalangeal joint is extended by the central tendon slip (an extension of the hand's dorsal extensor tendon); **B** the *X* is a functional representation of the fibrous interconnections between the two systems.
Based on DeLee JC, Drez D, Miller MD, DeLee and Drez's Orthopaedic Sports Medicine, 3rd edn, Philadelphia: Saunders, 2009: Fig 20B2-27.

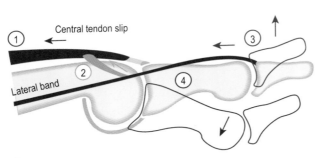

1. Central tendon slip pulls off bone
2. Retracted central tendon slip pulls on lateral band
3. The lateral band, in turn, hyper-extends the DIP joint
4. With no central tendon connection the PIP joint flexes, completing the full boutonnière deformity

FIGURE 1.9
Pathoanatomy of boutonnière deformity
The sequence is: rupture of the central tendon slip, which then simultaneously pulls on the lateral bands, pulling the DIP joint into hyper-extension and the PIP into flexion.
Based on DeLee JC, Drez D, Miller MD, DeLee and Drez's Orthopaedic Sports Medicine, 3rd edn, Philadelphia: Saunders, 2009: Fig 20B2-28.

Description

Used to describe a deformity of the resting finger in which the proximal interphalangeal (PIP) joint is flexed and the distal interphalangeal (DIP) joint is hyperextended.

Condition/s associated with

- Inflammatory arthropathy (e.g. rheumatoid arthritis)
- Central slip extensor tendon injury

Mechanism/s

Disruption or avulsion of the *central slip extensor tendon* and volar migration of the lateral bands of the extensor tendon mechanism result in PIP flexion and DIP extension. The sign derives its name from the appearance of the central tendon slip, which was thought to resemble a buttonhole, or *boutonnière* in French, when torn.

The central tendon slip attaches to the dorsal aspect of the middle phalanx. Its main function is to maintain PIP extension and stabilise the extensor tendon apparatus. If the central tendon is disrupted or avulsed (torn off the base of the middle phalanx), the actions of the lateral bands and flexor digitorum profundus are unopposed, resulting in resting PIP flexion and DIP hyperextension.

Inflammatory arthropathy (e.g. rheumatoid arthritis)

Pannus in the PIP joint (which may be present in rheumatoid arthritis) can damage the central slip tendon.[18] Chronic inflammation and synovitis of the joint may result in persistent PIP flexion and gradual elongation of the central slip tendon. Subsequent volar migration of the lateral bands results in the characteristic deformity.[19-22]

Trauma

Forced flexion of an extended PIP joint, crush injury or penetrating injury may result in avulsion of the central tendon slip. Typically, the degree of deformity increases in the days following the injury. Acutely, the deformity may be subtle.

Sign value

A boutonnière deformity is classically associated with rheumatoid arthritis occurring in up to 50% of patients with the disease.

In a patient with blunt or penetrating trauma, the presence of a boutonnière deformity should be considered evidence of a central slip extensor tendon injury.

Bulge/wipe/stroke test

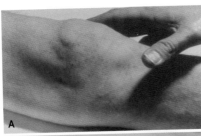
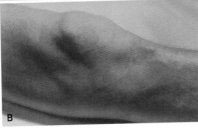

FIGURE 1.10
Demonstration of the bulge test for a small synovial knee effusion
The medial aspect of the knee has been stroked to move the synovial fluid from this area (shaded depressed area in **A**); **B** shows a bulge in the previously depressed area after the lateral aspect of the knee has been tapped.
Based on Firestein GS, Budd RC, Harris ED et al., Kelley's Textbook of Rheumatology, 8th edn, Philadelphia: WB Saunders, 2008: Figs 35-9A and B.

Description

The bulge, wipe or stroke test is used to assess for knee joint effusion. With the patient supine and their knee extended, the examiner 'swipes' the medial aspect of the knee joint to displace fluid into the superolateral aspect of the synovial compartment, and then swipes the lateral side looking for a visible fluid shift. The test is positive if the examiner sees a wave of fluid.

Condition/s associated with

Any condition causing a knee effusion.

More common

- Osteoarthritis
- Rheumatoid arthritis
- Haemoarthrosis – trauma, coagulopathy
- Gout
- Infection – septic arthritis, gonococcal arthritis, transient synovitis

Less common

- Pseudogout (calcium pyrophosphate deposition disease)
- Tumour

Mechanism/s

Mechanical manipulation of excess fluid in the synovial joint capsule results in visible fluid shift. The wipe or bulge test displaces synovial fluid from one part of the synovial joint to another, thus suggesting the presence of a joint effusion as the cause of knee swelling.

Sign value

Limited evidence has been gathered on the value of this test as an individual sign. Some authors report that this test may pick up on *as little as 4–8 mL of swelling.*[23] An effusion in the absence of acute traumatic injury or systemic disease is most commonly due to osteoarthritis.[24]

Gogus F et al.[25] reported the wipe test as having a sensitivity of 11–33% and specificity of 66–92% for identifying the presence of a knee effusion. Emphasis should be placed upon identifying a joint effusion in the setting of septic arthritis, an orthopaedic emergency.

Butterfly rash (malar rash)

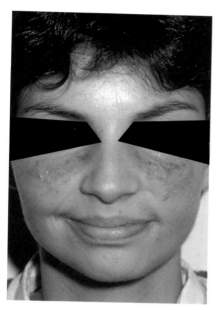

FIGURE 1.11
Malar rash of SLE

Reproduced, with permission, from Goldman L, Ausiello D, Cecil Medicine, 23rd edn, Philadelphia: Saunders, 2007: Fig 287-3.

Description

A red or purple, macular, mildly scaly rash that is seen over the bridge of the nose and cheeks. The shape of the rash can somewhat resemble a butterfly. The rash spares the nasolabial folds, which helps distinguish it from other rashes (e.g. rosacea). It is also photosensitive.

Condition/s associated with

Common

- Systemic lupus erythematosus (SLE)
- Drug-induced lupus erythematosus
- Dermatomyositis

Mechanism/s

The exact mechanism is unclear. However, like the underlying disorder in SLE, it is thought to result from an autoimmune reaction caused by genetic, environmental and immunological factors.

Factors shown to be involved include:[26]

- A genetic predisposition to ineffective or deficient complement, leading to a failure to clear immune complexes of apoptotic cells, which in turn increases the chance of the development of autoimmunity.

- Sunlight has been shown to damage and/or induce apoptosis of keratinocyte proteins in the epidermis and can stimulate autoantibody production. Sunlight may also increase the chance of keratinocytes being destroyed by complement and antibody-dependent mechanisms.

- Altered cellular and humoral immunity reactions have been seen in studies reviewing cutaneous manifestations of lupus.

It is likely that a combination of these factors leads to immune deposition in the skin, damage, oedema and the characteristic malar rash.

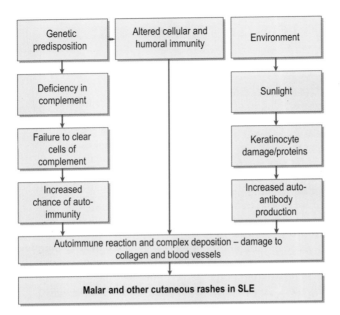

FIGURE 1.12
Mechanism of malar rash

Sign value

The malar rash is seen in approximately 40% of patients with SLE.[26] Its absence does not exclude the diagnosis.

Calcinosis/calcinosis cutis

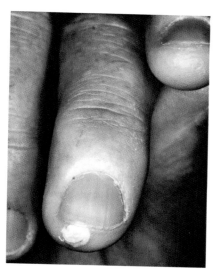

FIGURE 1.13
Calcinosis
Hard, whitish nodules of the digit representing dystrophic calcinosis in this patient with dermatomyositis.
Reproduced, with permission, from James WD, Berger T, Elston D, Andrews' Diseases of the Skin: Clinical Dermatology, 11th edn, Philadelphia: Saunders, 2011: Fig 26-12.

Description

Calcinosis refers to the formation or deposition of calcium in soft tissue. *Calcinosis cutis* more specifically refers to calcium deposits in the skin.

Condition/s associated with

Conditions associated with calcinosis may be classified as dystrophic, metastatic, tumour-related, iatrogenic or idiopathic.

- Dystrophic calcinosis
  » Scleroderma
  » Dermatomyositis
  » SLE

- Systemic sclerosis
- Burns
- Metastatic
  » Due to hypercalcaemia or hyperphosphataemia of any cause
  » Chronic renal failure – most common
  » Excess vitamin D
  » Primary hyperparathyroidism – rare
  » Paraneoplastic hypercalcaemia
  » Destructive bone disease (e.g. Paget's disease)
- Iatrogenic
  » Calcium gluconate injections
  » Tumour lysis syndrome

Mechanism/s

Dystrophic calcinosis

Dystrophic calcinosis occurs when *crystals of calcium phosphate or hydroxyapatite* are deposited in the skin *secondary to inflammation, tissue damage and degeneration.*[27] Calcium and phosphate levels are usually *normal.* Proposed mechanisms include:

- High local levels of alkaline phosphatase break down a pyrophosphate that normally inhibits calcification.[28]
- Tissue breakdown may lead to denatured proteins that bind to phosphate. These phosphate–protein compounds may react with calcium and thus provide a nidus for calcification.[29]

Metastatic calcinosis

Abnormal calcium or phosphate metabolism with high levels of either or both is present. Excess calcium and/

or phosphate allows for the formation and precipitation of calcium salts.

In chronic renal failure a number of mechanisms lead to altered phosphate and calcium metabolism:

- Decreased renal excretion of phosphate leads to hyperphosphataemia.
- Hyperphosphataemia results in a compensatory rise in parathyroid hormone (PTH) in an attempt to excrete phosphate. The rise in PTH results in an increase in phosphate absorption from the gut and also mobilises calcium from the bones, resulting in more calcium being available to precipitate with phosphate.
- Vitamin D deficiency owing to renal failure worsens initial hypocalcaemia and, therefore, further stimulates secondary hyperparathyroidism.

Iatrogenic

Intravenous administration of calcium or phosphate may cause local extravasation and precipitation of hydroxyapatite in surrounding tissue. Inflammation of the surrounding tissue secondary to the injection may also cause calcium and protein release, contributing to precipitation.

Idiopathic

Occurs in the absence of tissue injury or systemic metabolic disturbance.

Sign value

There is very limited evidence on this sign and it is rarely seen in isolation. If identified, further investigation is warranted.

Charcot foot

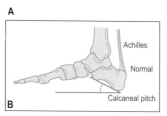
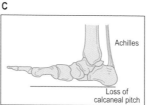

FIGURE 1.14
Charcot foot
A, B The classic rocker-bottom Charcot foot, with collapse and then reversal of the longitudinal arch; **C** loss of the normal calcaneal pitch, or angle relative to the floor, in patients with Charcot collapse of the arch.

Reproduced, with permission, from Mann JA, Ross SD, Chou LB, Chapter 9: Foot and ankle surgery. In: Skinner HB, Current Diagnosis & Treatment in Orthopedics, *4th edn, Fig 9-8. Available: http://proxy14.use.hcn.com.au/content.aspx?aID=2321540 [10 Mar 2011].*

Description

A progressive destructive arthropathy of the ankle and foot.[30] In its early stages, it may present as unilateral foot oedema following minor trauma. In advanced disease, significant destruction of bones and joints may occur (particularly in the midfoot), resulting in collapse of the plantar arch and development of 'rocker–bottom foot'.

Condition/s associated with

Conditions resulting in sensory neuropathy:

- Diabetes mellitus – most common
- Syphilis – original description by Charcot

Mechanism/s

In *neurotraumatic theory*, peripheral neuropathy caused by diabetes leads to decreased pain sensation and impaired proprioception. Thus, if an acute injury occurs (e.g. microfracture, subluxation or fracture), the patient feels little or no pain and does not 'guard' the foot when mobilising. This leads to a destructive cycle of continued loading on the injured foot and progressive damage.[31]

Under the *inflammatory theory*, when the same local insult occurs (microfracture, subluxation or fracture), inflammatory cytokines are released, including TNF-α and interleukin-1β. These two cytokines have been shown to increase activation of RANK ligand, which in turn increases the transcription factor NF-κB. The net result of this is *stimulation of the maturation of osteoclasts*, which further eat away at bone. This predisposes the patient to engage in another vicious cycle of further fractures, inflammation, abnormal weight loading and osteolysis.[31]

Other contributing factors include:

- Sympathetic denervation in distal limbs leads to increased peripheral blood flow – hyperaemia and more inflammation.[32]

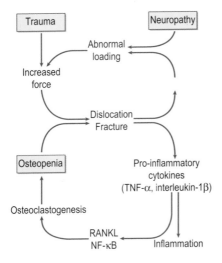

FIGURE 1.15
Inflammatory and neurotraumatic
mechanisms of Charcot foot

*Based on Jeffcoate WJ, Game F, Cavanagh PR,
Lancet 2005; 366: 2058–2061.*

- Pre-existing osteopaenia has been seen in both type 1 and type 2 diabetes via a number of mechanisms,[32] and this predisposes the diabetic patient to microfracture.
- Abnormal loading mechanics.

Sign value

Patients with Charcot foot are at higher risk of diabetic foot ulcers (affecting up to 50% of patients)[33,34] and amputation.[32]

Crepitus

Description

Grating, crunching, popping or crackling sounds heard and/or felt over joints during passive range of motion examination.

Condition/s associated with

- Arthropathy
  - » Osteoarthritis
  - » Rheumatoid arthritis
- Trauma
  - » Cartilaginous injury – meniscal injury, labral injury
  - » Ligamentous injury – anterior cruciate ligament
  - » Fracture

General mechanism/s

Crepitus of the joints is caused when *two rough surfaces grind against one another.*

Rheumatoid/osteoarthritis

In both rheumatoid arthritis and osteoarthritis arthritis, degeneration of the articular cartilage of the joint surfaces occurs, creating erosions and irregularity. Two rough surfaces moving against each other produce crepitus.

In rheumatoid arthritis, the autoimmune response and subsequent inflammation, cytokine release and pannus formation cause destruction of cartilage.

In osteoarthritis, repetitive strain with loss of glycosaminoglycans and activation of matrix metalloproteinases (MMPs) is principally responsible for damage.

Sign value

Altman R et al. reported crepitus had a sensitivity of 89%, specificity of 58%, positive likelihood ratio of 3.0 and negative likelihood ratio of 0.2 for predicting osteoarthritis of the knee.[35] Crepitus is common in patients with osteoarthritis. Crepitus alone has limited diagnostic value, due to its presence in other common disease states.

Dropped arm test

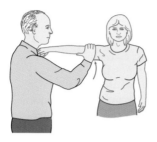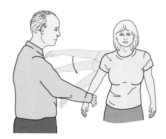

FIGURE 1.16
Dropped arm test

*Based on Multimedia Group LLC, Occupation Orthopedics. Available: http://www.eorthopod.com/
eorthopodV2/index.php?ID=7244790ddace6ee8ea5da6f0a57f8b45&disp_type=topic_detail&area
=6&topic_id=4357b9903d317fcb3ff32f72b24cb6b6 [28 Feb 2011].*

Description

With the patient upright, the examiner passively moves the patient's arm to 90° of abduction. Then the patient is asked to slowly lower the arm to the anatomical position. A positive test occurs if the patient is unable to perform the action due to pain or if the arm just 'drops' to the side.

Condition/s associated with

- Rotator cuff muscle injury (e.g. supraspinatus muscle)
- Subacromial impingement
- Neurogenic weakness
- Suprascapular nerve palsy
- Axillary nerve palsy
- C5 radiculopathy

Mechanism/s

Abduction of the arm from 0° to 90° is dependent upon the supraspinatus and deltoid muscles. The supraspinatus is responsible for the first 15° of motion. The deltoid muscle is responsible for movement beyond 15°.[36] Therefore, if a rotator cuff tear (e.g. supraspinatus muscle tear) or subacromial impingement is present, the ability of the arm to maintain abduction is impaired.

Sign value

Murrell GAC et al. and Dinnes J et al. reported a sensitivity of 10% and specificity of 98%, and a calculated positive likelihood ratio greater than 10 for rotator muscle tear.[37,38] Park HB et al. reported a sensitivity of 27%, specificity of 88%, positive likelihood ratio of 2.3 and negative likelihood ratio of 0.8 for subacromial impingement.[39]

When positive, the dropped arm test significantly increases the probability of rotator cuff muscle tear (supraspinatus muscle tear) or subacromial impingement. A negative test does not reliably exclude the diagnosis.

Finkelstein's test

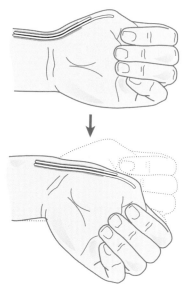

Description

The examiner applies force at the patient's thumb metacarpal, placing the wrist into forced ulnar deviation. Tenderness with the manoeuvre at the radial aspect of the wrist (at the abductor pollicis longus tendon or extensor pollicis brevis tendon) is considered a positive test result.

Condition/s associated with

• De Quervain's tenosynovitis

Mechanism/s

De Quervain's tenosynovitis is an inflammatory condition of the contents of the 1st extensor synovial compartment: abductor pollicis longus and extensor pollicis brevis tendons.

Repetitive strain injury or inflammatory disorders cause inflammation that, in turn, causes swelling over the radial aspect of the wrist. This narrows the space through which the abductor pollicis longus and extensor pollicis brevis pass on their way to the hand. When performing this manoeuvre, the abductor pollicis longus and extensor pollicis brevis tendons are moved into the narrowed compartment and stretched, causing pain.[40]

Sign value

There is limited data on the evidence for Finkelstein's test in diagnosing De Quervain's tenosynovitis. De Quervain's tenosynovitis is a clinical diagnosis.

Gottron's papules

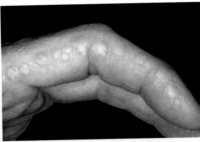
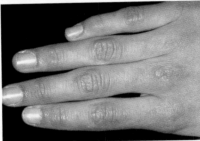

FIGURE 1.18
Gottron's papules
Found over bony prominences: fingers, elbows and knees. The lesions are slightly elevated, violaceous papules with slight scale.

Reproduced, with permission, from Habif TP, Clinical Dermatology, 5th edn, Philadelphia: Mosby, 2009: Figs 17-20, 17-21.

Description

Violaceous (violet-coloured) papular rash on the dorsal aspect of the interphalangeal joints.[41]

Condition/s associated with

- Dermatomyositis

Mechanism/s

One histological study[42] demonstrated lymphocytic infiltration, epidermal atrophy and vacuoles in the basal layer of the skin, in addition to other findings. The mechanism is unknown.

Sign value

Gottron's papules are said to be pathognomonic for dermatomyositis; however, they are not present in all patients with the disease.[43]

Hawkins' impingement test

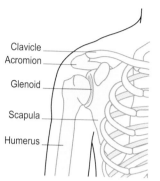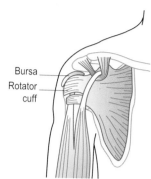

FIGURE 1.19
Hawkins' test anatomy

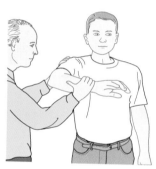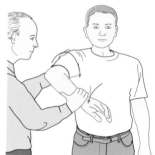

FIGURE 1.20
Hawkins' test

Description

With the patient upright, shoulder and elbow both flexed 90°, the examiner internally rotates the shoulder joint. The sign is positive if tenderness is elicited (see Figure 1.20).

Condition/s associated with

- Rotator cuff muscle impingement – supraspinatus, teres minor, infraspinatus muscles
- Rotator cuff tendonitis

Mechanism/s

The tendons of the rotator cuff muscles pass through a narrow space between the acromion process of the scapula, bursa and the head of the humerus. Hawkins' impingement test exacerbates narrowing in the coracoacromial space and will worsen pre-existing impingement of the tendons and muscles when present. This manoeuvre will also elicit tenderness when rotator cuff tendonitis is present, due to mechanical forces or compression on the injured tendon or muscle.[44]

Sign value

Calis M et al. reported a sensitivity of 92% and a specificity of 26–44% for identifying rotator cuff tendonitis.[45] Macdonald PB et al. reported a sensitivity of 83% and a specificity of 51% for NLR of 0.3 for rotator cuff tear.[46]

Given these results, a positive test is of little value to the examiner. A negative test has moderate utility.

Heliotrope rash

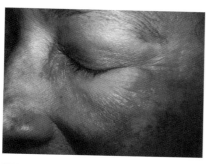

FIGURE 1.21
Heliotrope eruption seen in dermatomyositis

Reproduced, with permission, from Firestein GS, Budd RC, Harris ED et al., Kelley's Textbook of Rheumatology, 8th edn, Philadelphia: WB Saunders, 2008: Fig 47-10.

Description
Usually described as a macular, confluent, purple or violaceous rash over both eyelids and periorbital tissue. It can present with or without oedema.

Condition/s associated with
- Dermatomyositis
- Paraneoplastic syndrome

Mechanism/s
The mechanism is unknown but thought to be autoimmune in origin. Skin lesions demonstrate perivascular CD4 positive T-cell infiltration in the dermis.[47]

Sign value
Despite limited data, the heliotrope rash is highly characteristic of dermatomyositis and should trigger further diagnostic evaluation.

Kyphosis

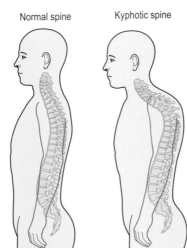

Normal spine   Kyphotic spine

FIGURE 1.22
The normal and kyphotic spines
Note the prominent convexity of the
kyphotic spine.

Description

Abnormally pronounced convex
curvature of the thoracic spine as seen
from the side. Kyphosis may be visible
from any direction when severe. Often
referred to in elderly females as the
'dowager's hump'.

Condition/s associated with

More common

- Osteoporosis/degenerative joint
  disease
- Traumatic – vertebral body fracture

Less common

- Ankylosing spondylitis
- Congenital
- Scheuermann kyphosis

Mechanism/s

Narrowing of the anterior aspect of the
vertebral body is common in most
forms of kyphosis.

Osteoporosis/degenerative joint disease

In degenerative or osteoporotic
kyphosis, poor posture, mechanical
straining and osteoporosis result in
degeneration and/or compression
fractures of the vertebrae. There is a
relative loss of height of the anterior
aspect of the vertebral body, leading to
increased thoracic kyphosis.

Congenital kyphosis

Congenital kyphosis results from either
a *failure of formation* or a *failure of
segmentation* of the vertebral body
elements.[48] In failure of segmentation,
the anterior part of the vertebral body
fails to separate from the vertebral body
below, resulting in anterior fusion of
the anterior aspect of the vertebrae.
The posterior aspect continues to grow,
resulting in kyphosis.[48]

Scheuermann kyphosis

Scheuermann kyphosis is a form of
adolescent kyphosis. The mechanism
behind Scheuermann kyphosis is
multifactorial,[49] including:

- herniation of vertebral disc material
  into the vertebral body, causing
  decreased vertebral height and
  increased pressure anteriorly,
  leading to abnormal growth and
  wedging of the vertebrae
- a thickened anterior ligament
- abnormal collagen matrix.

Sign value

Kyphosis in paediatric patients may be suggestive of congenital kyphosis, which can have serious complications and lead to significant disability if left untreated. Acute worsening in the degree of kyphosis in an elderly patient should prompt consideration of pathological fracture.

1

Lachman's test

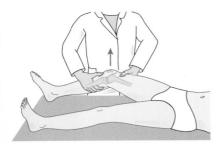

FIGURE 1.23
Lachman's test of the anterior cruciate ligament (ACL)
With 20–30° knee flexion, the tibia is moved forward on the femur to test the integrity of the ACL.

Description

The patient lies supine with the knee at 20–30° flexion. The examiner immobilises the femur just above the knee with one hand and attempts to pull the proximal tibia anteriorly with the other hand; the thumb is placed upon the tibial tuberosity. The test is positive if there is anterior movement of the tibia without an abrupt stop.

Condition/s associated with

- Anterior cruciate ligament (ACL) injury

Mechanism/s

The ACL arises from the anterior aspect of the tibial plateau and inserts into the medial aspect of the lateral femoral condyle. It limits anterior movement of the tibia on the femur. If the ACL is intact, the tibia should not have significant forward movement; if it is ruptured, there will be inappropriate anterior movement of the tibia and knee joint instability.

Sign value

A review by McGee of five studies reported a sensitivity of 48–96%, a specificity of 90–99%, a positive likelihood ratio of 17.0 and a negative likelihood ratio of 0.2.[2]

A positive Lachman's test is strongly predictive of ACL injury (+LR 17.0).[2] In a patient with a high clinical suspicion of ACL injury despite a negative Lachman's test (−LR 0.2),[2] further evaluation is necessary (e.g. interval re-examination, MRI). In general, Lachman's test is considered the best examination manoeuvre for ACL injury when compared with the anterior drawer sign and pivot-shift test.[50]

Livedo reticularis

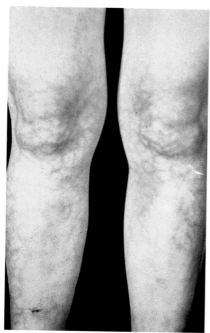

FIGURE 1.24
Livedo reticularis – a net-like pattern, often erythematous or violaceous in colour

Reproduced, with permission, from Floege J et al., Comprehensive Clinical Nephrology, 4th edn, Philadelphia: Saunders, 2010: Fig 64-13.

Less common

- Secondary LR
  Present in numerous disorders including:
  - Hypercoagulable state
    » Antiphospholipid syndrome
    » Cryoglobulinaemia
    » Multiple myeloma
    » DVT
  - Microangiopathy/microangiopathic haemolytic anaemia (MAHA)
    » Thrombotic/thrombocytopenic purpura (TTP)
    » Haemolytic uraemic syndrome
    » Disseminated intravascular coagulation
  - Vasculitis/arteriopathy
    » Snedden's syndrome
    » Calciphylaxis
  - Connective tissue disorders (e.g. SLE, dermatomyositis)
  - Embolisation (e.g. cholesterol embolisation syndrome)
  - Drug side effect
    » Amantadine
    » Quinine

Description

A macular, bluish/purple discolouration of the skin that has a lacy or net-like appearance.

Condition/s associated with

More common

- Primary or idiopathic livedo reticularis (LR)
- Hypothermia
- Elderly

General mechanism/s

Arterioles arising from the dermis divide to form a capillary bed. These capillaries then drain into the venules of the venous plexus. Livedo reticularis results from *increased visibility of the venules of the skin. Venodilatation of superficial venules* and *deoxygenation of blood* in the plexus are two main factors.[51]

In general, venodilatation is caused by altered autonomic nervous system function, circulating factors that cause venodilatation or in response to local hypoxia. Venodilatation results in engorged venules, making them larger and thus easier to see through the skin.

Deoxygenation is principally caused by decreased cutaneous perfusion,[51] which can be the result of decreased arteriolar inflow or decreased venous outflow. These are caused by:

- *decreased arteriolar inflow* – vasospasm due to cold, autonomic nervous system activity, arterial thrombosis or increased blood viscosity
- *decreased venous outflow* – venous thrombosis, increased blood viscosity.

Primary or idiopathic livedo reticularis

LR without the presence of underlying disease is associated with spontaneous arteriolar vasospasm, which decreases oxygenated blood inflow, causing tissue hypoxia and increased deoxygenation of venous blood.[52]

Hypothermia (autonomic nervous system)

The normal physiological response to hypothermia is arteriolar vasospasm. This decreases arteriolar blood flow, local tissue hypoxia and venous plexus dilation.

Elderly

The previous mechanisms apply to elderly patients, but with the added element of *thinning of the skin* that occurs with old age. This delicate and relatively translucent skin makes it more likely that the venous plexus will be visible.

Anti-phospholipid syndrome

Anti-phospholipid syndrome is associated with arterial and venous thrombosis, resulting in increased tissue hypoxia and venule dilation (due to venous stasis).

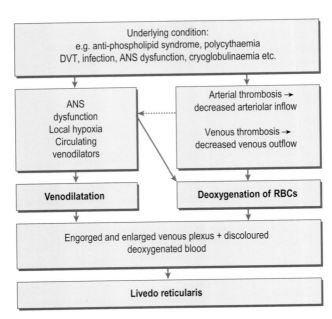

FIGURE 1.25
Mechanism of livedo reticularis

Cryoglobulinaemia

Cryoglobulins are proteins that become insoluble and precipitate when the temperature drops. Increasing viscosity results in stasis and tissue hypoxia. In addition, cryoglobulinaemia is associated with microvascular thrombosis.

Sign value

Primary or idiopathic LR is a diagnosis of exclusion; a secondary cause should be sought.

- LR has been shown to have a significant relationship with anti-phospholipid syndrome, with up to 40% of patients presenting with LR as the first sign.[53]
- Livedo reticularis in a patient with SLE is associated with the development of neuropsychiatric symptoms.

McMurray's test

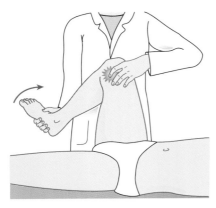

FIGURE 1.26
McMurray's test

Description

This test begins with the patient lying supine and knee flexed to 90°. The *medial meniscus* is palpated with one hand on the posteromedial edge of the joint, while the other hand holds the ankle and performs *external rotation*. The *lateral meniscus* is assessed with one hand over the posterolateral aspect of the joint while the leg is *internally rotated*. The test is positive if 'clunking' is felt as the meniscal fragment is moved against the femur.

Condition/s associated with

• Meniscal injury

Mechanism/s

By extending the flexed knee while applying external or internal rotation of the leg, the femoral condyle is moved over the tibia and meniscus. Crepitus will be present when the femur moves over the torn meniscal fragment.

Sign value

In a review of two studies McGee et al. reported a sensitivity of 17–29%, a specificity of 96–98%, a positive likelihood ratio of 8.0 and a negative likelihood ratio of 0.2 for detecting meniscal injury.[2] In a meta-analysis Scholten RJPM et al. reported a sensitivity of 10–63% and specificity of 57–98%.[54]

In the setting of acute knee joint injury this manoeuvre is often very painful in many knee joint disorders. These patients are often instructed to rest, ice, elevate and immobilise the affected knee, and return at a later date for repeat examination.

Neer's impingement test

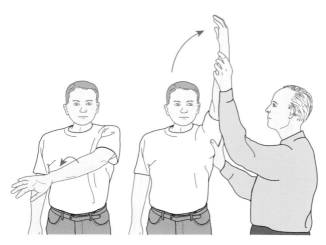

FIGURE 1.27
Neer's impingement test

Description

The patient's shoulder is placed into 90° flexion and internal rotation, with the elbow in full extension. The examiner then stabilises the scapula with one hand and passively moves the shoulder joint to 180° flexion with the other hand. If tenderness is elicited at the anterolateral aspect of the shoulder joint, the test is positive.

Condition/s associated with

- Rotator cuff impingement/ tendonitis
  - » Supraspinatus
  - » Infraspinatus
- Subacromial bursitis

Mechanism/s

The supraspinatus tendon and infraspinatus tendon transverse a narrow passage between the acromion, coracoacromial ligament and the humeral head before they insert into the proximal humerus. Narrowing of this space due to abnormalities of the acromion, acquired weakness in the posterior rotator cuff muscles (supraspinatus, infraspinatus, teres minor), or muscle hypertrophy in overuse, may cause impingement and inflammation.

In Neer's test, passive shoulder flexion from 90° to 180° exacerbates underlying narrowing of the passage made up by the acromion, coracoacromial ligament and humeral head, resulting in compression of its contents (i.e. the supraspinatus and infraspinatus tendons).

Sign value

Calis et al. reported a sensitivity of 88.7%, a specificity of 30.5%, a positive predictive value of 75.9% and a negative predictive value of 52.3%.[45] Macdonald et al. reported a sensitivity of 75%, a specificity of 47.5%, a positive predictive value of 36% and a negative predictive value of 82.9% for the test to identify patients with subacromial bursitis. The same study reported a sensitivity of 83.3%, a specificity of 50.8%, a positive predictive value of 40.0% and a negative predictive value of 88.6% for the test to identify patients with rotator cuff tendon impingement.[46]

Neer's impingement test is somewhat useful to exclude rotator cuff tendon impingement with a negative test. The test has limited potential to identify patients with rotator cuff impingement, because many painful shoulder conditions may result in a 'positive' test.

Patellar apprehension test

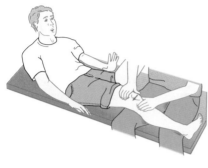

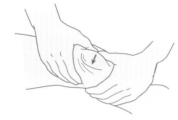

FIGURE 1.28

Patellar apprehension test
The patient experiences a sensation of the patella dislocating as a lateral force is applied to the medial edge of the patella with the knee slightly flexed.

Reprinted, with permission, from DeLee JC, Drez D, Miller MD, DeLee and Drez's Orthopaedic Sports Medicine, 3rd edn, Philadelphia: Saunders, 2009: Fig 22C1-5.

Condition/s associated with

- Patellofemoral instability

Mechanism/s

The patella normally rests in the patellofemoral groove, sliding up and down through this groove during knee flexion and extension. It is kept in place by the quadriceps tendon and patellar ligament, as well as other supporting structures. If these structures are damaged the patella is susceptible to lateral instability.

By displacing the patella laterally during attempted active knee extension, the examiner is deliberately attempting to displace the patella out of the groove to assess for patellofemoral instability.

Sign value

There is limited evidence supporting the use of this test. One small study reported a sensitivity of 39%.[55]

Description

With the patient supine and knee slightly flexed (20–30°), the examiner applies pressure, attempting to displace the patella laterally, while the patient is instructed to straighten the knee. The test is positive if apprehension is elicited due to impending lateral patella instability/dislocation or tenderness.

Patellar tap

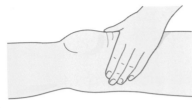

A

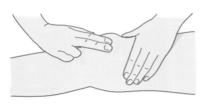

B

FIGURE 1.29
Patellar tap
Note that the left hand squeezes the
suprapatellar pouch (**A**), while the other
'taps' the patella (**B**).

Description
With the patient lying supine with the
leg extended, pressure is applied over
the suprapatellar pouch, displacing
synovial fluid forward towards the
patella. With the other hand the patella
is pushed or tapped downwards. A
palpable click as the patella hits the
underlying bone is a positive test.
Occasionally the patella will also
'bounce' back up to the examiner's
fingers.

Condition/s associated with
Any condition causing a knee effusion:

More common
- Osteoarthritis
- Rheumatoid arthritis
- Haemarthrosis – trauma,
  coagulopathy

- Gout
- Infection – septic arthritis,
  gonococcal arthritis, transient
  synovitis

Less common
- Pseudogout (calcium pyrophosphate
  deposition disease)
- Tumour

Mechanism/s
In the setting of a moderate-to-large
joint effusion, the patella is displaced
anteriorly relative to the distal femur at
the knee joint. Application of pressure
to the suprapatellar pouch accentuates
anterior patellar displacement. When
pushed or 'tapped', the patella can be
felt to float down through the fluid and
collide against the distal femur. In a
normal knee, the patella and femur are
in close contact and therefore cannot
be made to click together.

Sign value
Gogus et al. reported a sensitivity of
0–55% with specificity of 46–92%,
depending on the clinician completing
the examination.[25] A larger study by
Kastelein et al., looking at effusions in
traumatic knee injury, reported a
sensitivity of 83%, a specificity of
49%, a positive likelihood ratio of 1.6
and a negative likelihood ratio of 0.3.[56]
The same study indicated that,
although the bulge test may be able to
detect a smaller effusion, the patellar
test is more likely to be associated with
a clinically important effusion.

The available data, limited by
heterogeneity, suggests limited utility
of the patellar tap. Emphasis should be
placed upon the suspected aetiology of
a joint effusion, such as septic arthritis
(an orthopaedic emergency).

Patrick's test (FABER test)

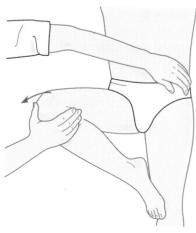

FIGURE 1.30
FABER test

Description

With the patient lying supine, the knee is flexed to 90° and the foot placed on the opposite knee. The flexed knee is then pushed down by the examiner to produce external rotation of the affected hip. If tenderness is elicited in the area of the buttocks, the test is considered positive for sacroiliitis, whereas tenderness in the groin suggests hip joint pathology.

FABER is a mnemonic for the movements of the hip during the test (i.e. **F**lexion, **Ab**duction, **E**xternal **R**otation).

Condition/s associated with

Any cause of sacroiliitis including, but not limited to:

More common

- Osteoarthritis/degenerative joint disease
- Trauma

Less common

- HLA–B27 spondyloarthropathy
  » Ankylosing spondylitis
  » Psoriatic arthritis
  » Reactive arthritis
  » Enteropathic arthritis (associated with inflammatory bowel disease)
- Infectious sacroiliitis

Mechanism/s

Manipulation of the hip with flexion, abduction and external rotation results in distraction of the inflamed sacroiliac joint,[57] thereby eliciting tenderness.

Sign value

Limited sound methodological studies exist for the FABER test.[58] Individual studies, however, have reported a sensitivity of 69–77%[58-60] and a specificity of 100%.[59]

Phalen's sign

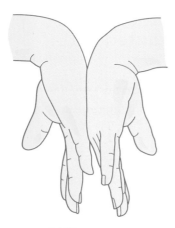

FIGURE 1.31
Hand placement in Phalen's test

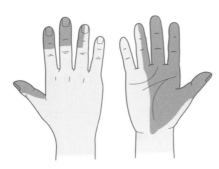

FIGURE 1.32
Median nerve distribution of paraesthesias
in the hand

Description

The patient puts their wrists into a
position of 90° flexion and presses them
into one another for 1 minute. The
presence of paraesthesias and/or
numbness in the distribution of the
median nerve is a positive test.

Condition/s associated with

- Carpal tunnel syndrome (the most
  common causes of median nerve
  palsy)

Mechanism/s

In carpal tunnel syndrome, crowding
within the carpal tunnel or repetitive
strain injury results in chronic
inflammation of the median nerve.
When the wrist is flexed, the flexor
retinaculum, which acts as a pulley on
the digital flexor tendons, pulls them
down onto the median nerve[61] and
acutely increases pressure on the nerve.
This manoeuvre increases pressure
within the carpal tunnel, further
irritating the nerve, thus worsening
neuropathic sensory abnormalities.

Sign value

D'Arcy et al. reported a wide range of
a sensitivity of 10–91%, a specificity
of 33–76%, a positive likelihood ratio
of 1.1–2.1 and a negative likelihood
ratio of 0.3–1.0.[62]

Phalen's test has limited value in the
diagnosis of carpal tunnel syndrome. A
negative test alone does not reliably
exclude the diagnosis.

Proximal weakness/proximal myopathy

Description

Proximal myopathy is a muscle disorder which results in proximal muscle group weakness (e.g. **shoulder**: pectoralis major, deltoid, biceps; **hip**: gluteal, quadriceps, iliopsoas, adductor). Proximal weakness is rapidly assessed by asking the patient to rise from a seated position and/or perform the motion of hanging washing on a clothesline. A complete assessment of power should be performed.

Condition/s associated with

- Inflammatory myopathy
  - » Polymyositis
  - » Dermatomyositis
- Endocrine myopathy
  - » Hyperthyroidism – see Chapter 7, 'Endocrinological signs'
  - » Hypothyroidism – see Chapter 7, 'Endocrinological signs'
  - » Hyperparathyroidism – see Chapter 7, 'Endocrinological signs'
- Systemic disorders
  - » Systemic lupus erythematosus (SLE)
  - » Rheumatoid arthritis
- Genetic
  - » Myotonic dystrophy
  - » Spinal muscular atrophy
- Other
  - » Myasthenia gravis
  - » Polymyalgia rheumatica

TABLE 1.1
Mechanisms of inflammatory myopathies

Disease	Mechanism
Polymyositis	T-cell (in particular CD8) and macrophage destruction of muscle fibres
Dermatomyositis	Complement and antibody destruction of microvasculature; the deposition of complement and antibody complexes leads to inflammation and destruction of muscle fibres and hence weakness

Mechanism/s

Inflammatory myopathies

Inflammatory myopathies result in immunologically mediated inflammation and destruction of skeletal muscle, causing weakness (Table 1.1).

Systemic disorders

Proximal myopathy may present in a number of systemic rheumatological disorders such as SLE and RA. It is thought that circulating antibody complexes, deposited in tissues and/or targeted at muscles, damage muscle fibres, resulting in weakness.

Sign value

Patients with gradual-onset progressive symmetric proximal muscle weakness should be evaluated for a myopathy.

Psoriatic nails/psoriatic nail dystrophy

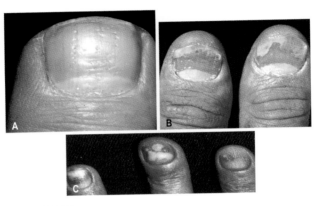

FIGURE 1.33
Nail dystrophic changes
A Nail pitting; **B** onycholysis; **C** severe destructive change with nail loss and pustule formation.

Reproduced, with permission, from Firestein GS, Budd RC, Harris ED et al., Kelley's Textbook of Rheumatology, 8th edn, Philadelphia: WB Saunders, 2008: Fig 72-3.

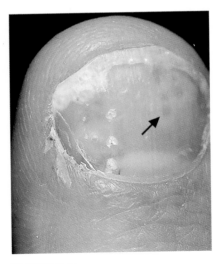

FIGURE 1.34
'Oil drops' under the nail

Reproduced, with permission, from Habif TP, Clinical Dermatology, 5th edn, Philadelphia: Mosby, 2009: Fig 8-23.

Description

Psoriatic nail changes refer to a number of different abnormalities seen in the nails rather than just one sign. Changes include:[63]

- Pitting of the nail plate
- Subungual hyperkeratosis under the nail plate
- Onycholysis (nail lifting) and changes in nail shape
- 'Oil drops' and 'salmon patches'
- Splinter haemorrhages

Condition/s associated with

- Psoriasis
- Psoriatic arthritis

Mechanism/s

The mechanism is poorly understood. It is likely that a combination of genetic, immunological and chronic inflammatory changes lead to psoriatic nail changes.

Psoriasis is thought to be a disease of abnormal immunology in which an atypical T-cell response occurs, part of which results in an aberrant proliferation of T cells which migrate to the skin and activate and release various cytokines (e.g. IFN-γ, TNF-α and IL-2). These cytokines induce changes in keratinocytes and are also associated with the development of the characteristic psoriatic skin lesions.[64]

Nail pitting

Nail pitting is the result of multifocal abnormal nail growth. The nail matrix is made up of keratinocytes, which generate the keratin that results in production of the nail plate. As new cells are produced, the older cells are pushed forwards and 'grow' the nail.

In psoriatic nails, there are parakeratotic cells that disrupt normal keratinisation and nail production. These abnormal cells group together and then get sloughed off as the nail grows, leaving a depression in the nail plate.[63,65]

Subungual keratosis

Excessive proliferation of keratinocytes under the nail plate leads to the accumulation of keratotic cells. This often leads to a raised and thickened nail plate.[64]

Oil drops

Thought to be caused by the accumulation of neutrophils that become visible through the nail plate.

Salmon patches

Focal hyperkeratosis of the nail bed and altered vascularisation.[63]

Splinter haemorrhages

See Chapter 3, 'Cardiovascular signs'.

Sign value

Studies report psoriatic nail changes may be present in up to 15–50% of cases of psoriasis and have a lifetime prevalence of 80–90%.[66,67] Several studies report a higher incidence of psoriatic nail changes (75–86%) in patients with psoriatic arthritis.[68-71]

Raynaud's syndrome/phenomenon

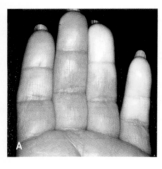 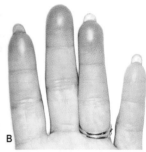

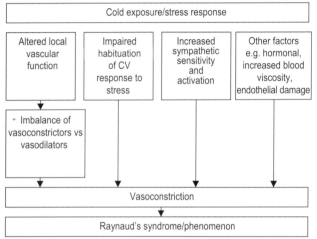

FIGURE 1.35

Raynaud's phenomenon

A Sharply demarcated pallor of the distal fingers resulting from the closure of the digital arteries; **B** cyanosis of the fingertips.

Reproduced, with permission, from Kumar V, Abbas AK, Fausto N, Aster J, Robbins and Cotran Pathologic Basis of Disease, Professional Edition, 8th edn, Philadelphia: Saunders, 2009: Fig 11-28.

Description

Raynaud's syndrome/phenomenon occurs in the digits from various stimuli, resulting in peripheral hypoperfusion followed by hyperaemia. It has three 'colour' phases:

1 white – blanching associated with vasoconstriction of the blood vessels
2 blue – cyanosis
3 red – when blood flow is restored and hyperaemia results.

Condition/s associated with

Common

- Raynaud's phenomenon

Less common

- Vasculitis
  - » Buerger's disease
- Autoimmune/connective tissue disorders
  - » Scleroderma (systemis sclerosis)
  - » Systemic lupus erythematosus
  - » CREST syndrome
  - » Sjögren's syndrome
  - » Dermatomyositis
  - » Polymyositis
  - » Rheumatoid arthritis
- Drugs
  - » Beta blockers

Mechanism/s

Raynaud's syndrome occurs due to an exaggerated vasoconstrictive response causing transient cessation of blood flow to the digits.[72-75]

The cause of this abnormal vasoconstrictive response is multifactorial:

1 *Increased sympathetic nerve activation (centrally and peripherally mediated)* – in response to cold temperatures or stressful situations, enhanced sympathetic nerve activation leads to vasoconstriction of the arterioles in the digits. Larger numbers of alpha-2-adrenoreceptors may result in more pronounced vasoconstriction.[72-75]

2 *Impaired habituation of the cardiovascular response to stress* is also thought to contribute. Habituation is the gradual extinction of a response to a stimulus over time. In normal individuals, ongoing exposure to a stress results in habituation, and decreasing incidence and duration of the response.[72,73]

3 *Local vascular factors* – an imbalance between local vasoconstrictive factors (endothelin, 5-HT, thromboxane [TXA] and other cyclo-oxygenase [COX] pathway products) and vasodilatory factors (nitric oxide [NO])[72,73] may also exist in Raynaud's syndrome.

- » Local endothelin may not produce enough NO for vasodilatation.[73]
- » Repeated vasospasm causes oxidative stress and reduced NO production, thus decreasing vasodilatation.[72]
- » Inappropriately greater production of endothelin and thromboxane (TXA_2) in response to cold also occurs, leading to marked vasoconstriction.[72,73]
- » In some studies, a higher than normal endothelin-1, a potent vasoconstrictor, was seen in patients with primary Raynaud's syndrome.[73]

4 *Other factors.* Some of these include:

- » oestrogen – causing sensitisation of vessels to vasoconstriction[72,73]
- » increased blood viscosity[73]
- » decreased amounts of calcitonin gene-related peptide (CGRP) neurons – impairing normal nerve sensitivity, activation and vasodilatation[73]
- » endothelial damage.

Secondary Raynaud's syndrome

Structural vascular abnormalities (in addition to the factors outlined above) are thought to play a role in Raynaud's phenomenon occurring secondary to an underlying disease process.

In scleroderma (systemic sclerosis), abnormal proliferation of intimal cells results in endothelial cell damage. Abnormal endothelial cells then exacerbate vasospasm by:[73,75]

- perturbing smooth muscle cells, causing them to proliferate and contract
- enhancing pro-coagulant activity and inhibitors of fibrinolysis, thus promoting microthrombi
- promoting inflammation through release of adhesion factors.

Other factors thought to contribute in systemic sclerosis include:[73]

- raised levels of angiotensin II – a vasoconstrictor
- lack of compensatory angiogenesis to meet the demands of proliferated intima – leading to ischaemia.

Saddle nose deformity

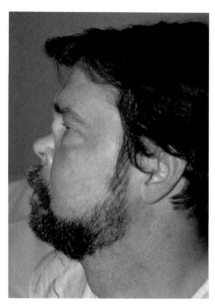

FIGURE 1.36
Saddle nose deformity

Reproduced, with permission, from Firestein GS, Budd RC, Harris ED et al., Kelley's Textbook of Rheumatology, 8th edn, Philadelphia: WB Saunders, 2008: Fig 82-5.

Description
Collapse of the middle section of the nose relative to the tip and dorsum, like a saddle.

Condition/s associated with

More common
- Trauma
- Iatrogenic – nasal surgery

Less common
- Wegener's granulomatosis
- Relapsing polychondritis
- Cocaine use, complication
- Congenital syphilis – rare

Mechanism/s
Destruction of the nasal septum or support cartilage results in the deformity. Direct trauma or prior surgery is the most common aetiology.

Wegener's granulomatosis
Wegener's granulomatosis is an autoimmune vasculitic disorder characterised by necrotising granulomas affecting the small blood vessels of the upper and lower airways. It is thought that immune complex deposition or an autoimmune response results in inflammation and damage/destruction of the vessels and their surrounding structures.

Relapsing polychondritis
Relapsing polychondritis is an autoimmune chronic inflammatory disorder resulting in the destruction of cartilage – in particular auricular and nasal cartilage.[23]

Sign value
Saddle nose deformity occurs in up to 65% of relapsing polychondritis, and 9–29% of patients with Wegener's granulomatosis.[23]

Sausage-shaped digits (dactylitis)

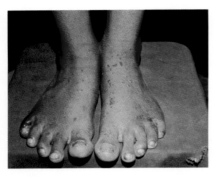

FIGURE 1.37
Sausage-shaped digits (dactylitis) in a patient with psoriatic arthritis

Reproduced, with permission, from Tyring SK, Lupi O, Hengge UR, Tropical Dermatology, 1st edn, London: Churchill Livingstone, 2005: Fig 11-16.

Description
Fusiform swelling of multiple digits such that it is difficult to visualise the individual joints (e.g. PIP, DIP).[76] Or, more simply, fingers or toes that are so swollen they look like sausages. Dactylitis typically affects multiple digits, whereas flexor tenosynovitis is a distinct entity usually only present in one digit.

Condition/s associated with

More common
- HLA-B27 spondyloarthropathy
  - » Psoriatic arthritis
  - » Ankylosing spondylitis
  - » Reactive arthritis
  - » Enteropathic arthritis (associated with inflammatory bowel disease)
- Sickle cell anaemia – paediatric

Uncommon
- Tuberculosis
- Gout
- Sarcoidosis
- Disseminated gonorrhoea

Mechanism/s

Spondyloarthropathies
Irritation of the flexor tendons, flexor tendon sheath and surrounding soft tissues due to pro-inflammatory cytokines results in pronounced diffuse inflammation of the digits.[77,78]

Tuberculosis dactylitis
A variant of tuberculous osteomyelitis whereby TB granulomas invade the short tubular bones of the hands and feet and then the surrounding tissues, causing inflammation and swelling.[77]

Syphilitic dactylitis
A manifestation of congenital syphilis where the syphilitic spirochetes invade perichondrium, bone, periosteum and marrow and thus inhibit osteogenesis. Inflammation from the invasion is another contributing factor to pain and swelling of the digits.[77]

Sarcoid dactylitis
Sarcoid non-caseating granulomas invade bone and soft tissue, causing swelling and inflammation.[77]

Sickle cell dactylitis
In sickle cell anaemia, a haemoglobin S-gene mutation results in rigid and 'sickle'-shaped red blood cells under hypoxic conditions. Acute sickling in the peripheral circulation results in digital ischaemia and painful fusiform digital swelling. It typically occurs in the paediatric population.

Sign value

In regards to patients with seronegative spondyloarthropathy, sausage-shaped digits have a sensitivity of 17.9% and a specificity of 96.4%.[79] The development of dactylitis may be a marker for progression of psoriatic arthritis,[80] being present in 16–24%[80] of reported cases, with lifetime incidence and prevalence of 48% and 33%, respectively.[81] It is seen in only 4% of tuberculosis[77] cases.

Identification of sausage-shaped digits or dactylitis in an adult should prompt an evaluation for a seronegative spondyloarthropathy. Development of dactylitis in a child of African or Mediterranean descent should prompt evaluation for sickle cell disease.

Sclerodactyly

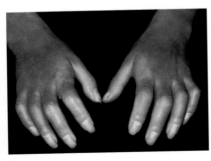

FIGURE 1.38
Sclerodactyly with flexion contractures

Reproduced, with permission, from Firestein GS, Budd RC, Harris ED et al., Kelley's Textbook of Rheumatology, *8th edn, Philadelphia: WB Saunders, 2008: Fig 47-12.*

Condition/s associated with

- Scleroderma (systemic sclerosis)
- CREST syndrome (i.e. **C**alcinosis, **R**aynaud's phenomenon, **O**esophageal dysmotility, **S**clerodactyly, **T**elangiectasia)

Mechanism/s

In scleroderma, T cells infiltrate the skin and set in motion a cascade of events including *abnormal fibroblast and growth factor stimulation*. This in turn leads to increased production of *extracellular matrix, fibrillin and type 1 collagen* and other factors. Ultimately this results in fibrosis and thickening of the skin.

Sign value

Skin thickening is seen more often in diffuse scleroderma (27%) than in limited disease (5%).[82]

Description

Thickening and tightening of the skin covering the digits.

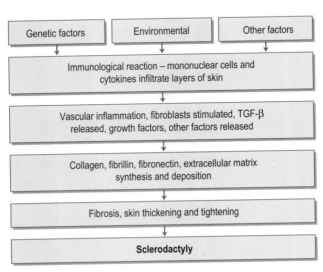

FIGURE 1.39
Proposed mechanism of sclerodactyly

Shawl sign

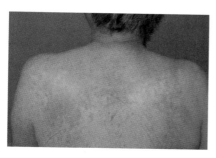

FIGURE 1.40
Shawl sign
Note discolouration over the posterior shoulder and neck.

Reproduced, with permission, from Hochberg MC et al., Rheumatology, 5th edn, Philadelphia: Mosby, 2010: Fig 144-7.

Description

A confluent, violaceous, macular rash over the posterior shoulders and neck.

Condition/s associated with

- Dermatomyositis

Mechanism/s

Complement and antibody mediated microvascular injury likely results in the development of the rash.[83] Dermatomyositis is a systemic inflammatory disorder primarily of muscle and skin characterised by microvascular damage due to antibody complex and complement deposition. Genetic predisposition, viruses and UV light are all thought to play a role.[83]

Sign value

Although not pathognomonic, the shawl sign is strongly associated with dermatomyositis. In up to 30% of cases of dermatomyositis, skin manifestations occur.

Simmonds–Thompson test

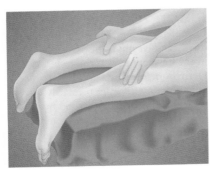

FIGURE 1.41
Simmonds–Thompson test
The calf muscles are squeezed, and the test
is positive if there is no ankle plantarflexion.

Description

With the patient lying prone on the
exam table with their ankles hanging
over the end, the examiner squeezes
the calf muscle. The test is considered
positive if no movement in the ankle
(absence of plantarflexion) can be
elicited.

Condition/s associated with

• Achilles tendon rupture

Mechanism/s

Normally, squeezing the gastrocnemius
and soleus muscles results in shortening
of the distance between the Achilles
tendon insertion site and distal femur,
causing plantarflexion.[84] If the Achilles
tendon is ruptured, no movement
occurs.

Sign value

A positive test is generally thought to
be pathognomonic for a complete
rupture of the Achilles tendon.

Speed's test

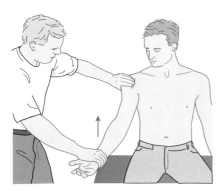

FIGURE 1.42
Speed's test
The examiner actively resists the patient lifting the extended arm.

Description

The patient sits or stands with the shoulder in 90° flexion, elbow extended and the palm facing up (supinated). The patient attempts to lift the arm up against resistance from the examiner. The test is positive if tenderness is elicited.

Condition/s associated with

- Biceps tendonitis
- SLAP lesion (**S**uperior **L**abral tear from **A**nterior to **P**osterior) – an injury of the glenoid labrum

Mechanism/s

Traction on an inflamed biceps tendon or pressure on a labral tear will result in tenderness.

Sign value

Holtby et al., in predicting biceps pathology and SLAP lesions, reported a sensitivity of 32%, a specificity of 75%, a positive likelihood ratio of 1.28 and a negative likelihood ratio of 0.91.[85] This test has limited value.

Subcutaneous nodules (rheumatoid nodules)

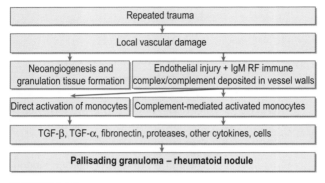

FIGURE 1.43
Mechanism of rheumatoid nodule formation

Description
Visible and palpable subcutaneous nodules typically occur over bony prominences and/or extensor surfaces.

Condition/s associated with
- Rheumatoid arthritis

Mechanism/s
Thought to be mediated via Th-1 inflammatory response.[86] Trauma over bony prominences causes local vessel damage that leads to new blood vessel growth and granulomatous tissue formation. Endothelial injury results in accumulation of immune complexes and stimulates monocytes to secrete IL-1, TNF, TGF-β, prostaglandins and other factors, including proteases, collagenases and fibronectin. This ultimately leads to angiogenesis, fibrin deposition and formation of the characteristic rheumatoid nodule.[86,87]

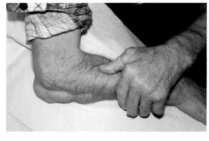

FIGURE 1.44
Large rheumatoid nodules are seen in a classic location along the extensor surface of the forearm and in the olecranon bursa

Reproduced, with permission, from Goldman L, Ausiello D, Cecil Medicine, 23rd edn, Philadelphia: Saunders, 2007: Fig 285-9.

Sign value
Seen in 20–25% of seropositive rheumatoid arthritis. They are the most common extra-articular manifestation of the disease. Frequency of development of nodules is associated with elevated rheumatoid factor titres.[87]

Sulcus sign

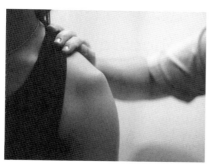

FIGURE 1.45
Sulcus sign
Note the slight dimple under the acromion.

Reproduced, with permission, from DeLee JC, Drez D, Miller MD, DeLee and Drez's Orthopaedic Sports Medicine, 3rd edn, Philadelphia: Saunders, 2009: Fig 17H2-16.

Description

With the patient's arm relaxed and hanging by the side, the examiner looks at the shoulder area. If chronic subluxation is suspected, the examiner may apply traction to the arm to elicit the sign. Dimpling of the skin between the acromion and humeral head is a positive test.

Condition/s associated with

- Anterior shoulder dislocation
- Anterior shoulder subluxation

Mechanism/s

In the setting of anterior shoulder dislocation, the head of the humerus moves inferiorly relative to the glenohumeral joint. This causes traction of the skin overlying the glenohumeral joint, and a dimple over the space between the acromion and the humeral head may be seen.

Sign value

Anterior shoulder dislocation is often apparent on inspection with the arm held anteriorly and internally rotated. Radiographs should be obtained to confirm the diagnosis.

Supraspinatus test (empty-can test)

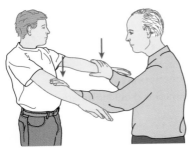

FIGURE 1.46
Supraspinatus or empty-can test

Description

The patient sits or stands with the shoulder in 90° flexion, 30° abduction, with the elbow extended and the thumbs pointing towards the ground, as if emptying two cans. The examiner applies downward pressure as the patient attempts to lift the arms up. The test is positive if the patient experiences tenderness or is unable to hold up their arm.

Condition/s associated with

- Supraspinatus tear
- Supraspinatus tendonitis
- Supraspinatus impingement

Mechanism/s

The supraspinatus muscle works in concert with the deltoid muscle during shoulder abduction and stabilises the humeral head in the glenoid fossa. Mechanical strain upon an injured supraspinatus muscle or tendon will result in tenderness and/or weakness during this manoeuvre.

Sign value

McGee et al., in a review of two studies in patients with rotator cuff muscle tears with painful supraspinatus tests, reported a sensitivity of 63–85%, a specificity of 52–55% and a positive likelihood ratio of 1.5.[2] A review of five studies of patients with rotator cuff muscle tears with weakness during testing, reported a sensitivity of 41–84%, a specificity of 58–70%, a positive likelihood ratio of 2.0 and a negative likelihood ratio of 0.5.[2]

The supraspinatus test has limited utility and may be positive in several other shoulder conditions. Detection of weakness has more diagnostic utility than tenderness alone.

Swan-neck deformity

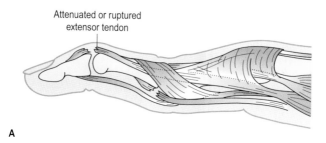

Attenuated or ruptured
extensor tendon

A

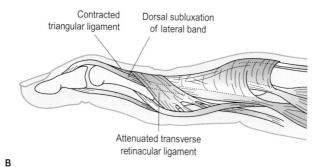

Contracted
triangular ligament

Dorsal subluxation
of lateral band

Attenuated transverse
retinacular ligament

B

FIGURE 1.47

Swan-neck deformity pathoanatomy
A Terminal tendon rupture may be associated with synovitis of DIP joint, leading to
DIP joint flexion and subsequent PIP joint hyperextension. Rupture of flexor digitorum
superficialis tendon can be caused by infiltrative synovitis, which can lead to decreased volar
support of PIP joint and subsequent hyperextension deformity; **B** lateral-band subluxation
dorsal to axis of rotation of PIP joint. Contraction of triangular ligament and attenuation of
transverse retinacular ligament are depicted.

*Based on Jupiter JB, Chapter 70: Arthritic hand. In: Canale TS, Beaty JH, Campbell's Operative
Orthopaedics, 11th edn, Philadelphia: Elsevier, 2007: Fig 70-13.*

Description

A deformity characterised by distal
interphalangeal (DIP) joint flexion and
proximal interphalangeal (PIP) joint
hyperextension in the resting digit, to
some extent resembling a swan's neck.

Condition/s associated with

Common

• Rheumatoid arthritis

Mechanism/s

A relative imbalance of flexor and
extensor tendons of the digit due to
chronic synovial inflammation.[88] A
variety of changes may result in this
deformity, whose basis is inflammatory
disruption of the collateral ligaments,
volar plates, joint capsule or invasion of
the flexor tendons.[89] The resulting
changes may be:

- attenuation or disruption of the extensor tendon on the distal phalanx, leading to unopposed flexion – and thus the flexed DIP joint
- disruption of the retinacular ligament (which helps hold the finger in flexion), leading to unopposed extensor forces at the PIP joint and PIP joint hyperextension.

Sign value

Swan-neck deformity is classically associated with rheumatoid arthritis. In patients with acute trauma with forced DIP flexion during active extension, mallet finger (i.e. extensor tendon avulsion distal to DIP joint) should be considered.

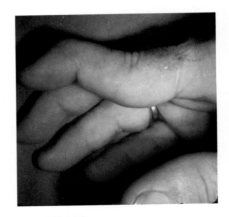

FIGURE 1.48
Swan-neck deformity

Reproduced, with permission, from Jupiter JB, Chapter 70: Arthritic hand. In: Canale TS, Beaty JH, Campbell's Operative Orthopaedics, 11th edn, Philadelphia: Elsevier, 2007: Fig 70-14.

Telangiectasia

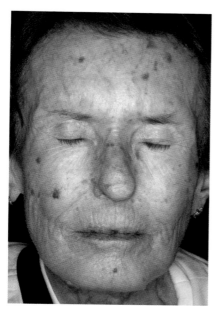

FIGURE 1.49
Telangiectasia associated with systemic sclerosis (scleroderma)
Note the skin tightening around the lips.

Reproduced, with permission, from Habif TP, Clinical Dermatology, 5th edn, Philadelphia: Mosby, 2009: Fig 17-30.

Description

Permanent dilatation of superficial peripheral vessels resulting in blanching red lesions on the skin. Telangiectasia may present as a fine red line or a punctum (dot) with radiating lines.[41]

Condition/s associated with

There are numerous conditions associated with telangiectasia, including but not limited to those listed in Table 1.2.

TABLE 1.2
Telangiectasia-associated conditions

Systemic diseases
Carcinoid syndrome
Ataxia–telangiectasia
Mastocytosis
Dermatomyositis
Scleroderma – especially periungual telangiectasia
Systemic lupus erythematosus
Hereditary haemorrhagic telangiectasia
Liver cirrhosis

General mechanism/s

Telangiectasias are predominantly *persistently dilated small capillaries and venules.* The exception to this is hereditary haemorrhagic telangiectasia, as these lesions are *arteriovenous (AV) malformations.*

Hereditary haemorrhagic telangiectasia (HHT)

HHT is an autosomal dominant disorder causing development of AV malformations, due to a genetic abnormality of the TGF-β receptor. The TGF-β pathway is known to modulate vascular architecture, matrix formation and basement membrane development.[90]

Scleroderma

The underlying mechanism for telangiectasia in scleroderma is unknown. It is presumed that there is endothelial injury, leading to aberrant angiogenesis and the development of new vessels. It has been suggested that the TGF-β pathway may be involved.[90]

Spider naevus

See 'Spider naevus' in Chapter 6, 'Gastroenterological signs'.

Sign value

Location and characteristics of telangiectasia can assist in diagnosis.

- Periungual telangiectasia (telangiectasia next to the nails) is said to be highly suggestive of SLE, scleroderma or dermatomyositis.[91]

- Broad macules with a polygonal or oval shape, known as *mat telangiectasias*, are associated with CREST syndrome.[91]

- Telangiectasias in adulthood that are located around the mucous membranes, extremities and under the nails are associated with hereditary haemorrhagic telangiectasia.

Thomas' test

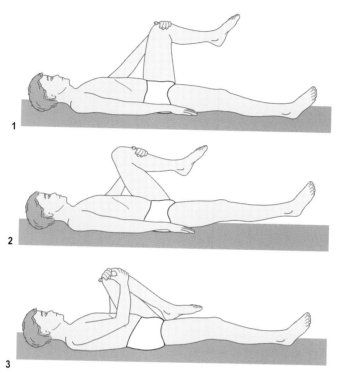

FIGURE 1.50
Performance of Thomas' test

Description

With the patient lying supine, the knee and hip on the 'normal' side are flexed, with the knee held against the chest. A positive test occurs if the opposite leg rises off the table.

Condition/s associated with

- Hip flexion contracture – fixed flexion deformity
- Iliotibial band syndrome
- Normal ageing/stiffness

Mechanism/s

Drawing up the knee and flexing one side of the hip rotates the pelvis. In order to keep the alternate leg flat on the bed, the hip flexors and rectus femoris must stretch enough to allow the leg to lie flat. In other words, if the hip flexors are contracted, the affected leg will rise as the pelvis rotates.

Sign value

There is limited value in this sign.

Tinel's sign

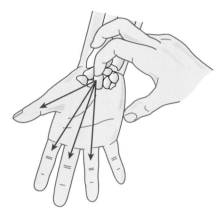

FIGURE 1.51
Completing Tinel's test
Tapping over the wrist causes pins and needles in the fingers.

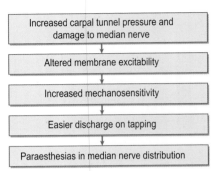

FIGURE 1.52
Mechanism of Tinel's test

Description

Paraesthesias in a median nerve distribution occur when the examiner taps with a finger at the distal wrist over the median nerve. It should be noted that Tinel's original description was not specific for the median nerve but rather for the sensation of 'pins and needles' arising from any injured nerve tested in this way.

Condition/s associated with

• Carpal tunnel syndrome

Mechanism/s

In carpal tunnel syndrome, there is increased pressure in the carpal tunnel and resulting damage to the median nerve. It is thought that this damage results in altered mechanosensitivity[92] of the median nerve, possibly due to an abnormally excitable membrane. So, when lightly struck through the skin, the inflamed nerve functions abnormally.

Sign value

D'Arcy et al. reported Tinel's sign had limited or no value in distinguishing people with carpal tunnel syndrome from those without.[62] A review of several studies reported a sensitivity of 25–60%, a specificity of 64–80%, a positive likelihood ratio of 0.7–2.7 and a negative likelihood ratio of 0.5–1.1. Neither Tinel's sign nor Phalen's sign reliably rule in or rule out carpal tunnel syndrome.[92]

Trendelenburg's sign

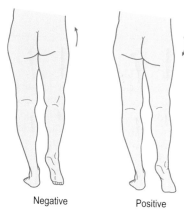

Negative   Positive

FIGURE 1.53
Trendelenburg test
Note that the positive test on the right
indicates a problem with the left hip
abductors – remember 'the sound side sags'.
*Based on Goldstein B, Chavez F, Phys Med
Rehabil State Art Rev 1996; 10: 601–630.*

Description

The patient is asked to stand on one
leg while bending the other knee so
the foot is held off the ground. For the
sign to be present, the pelvis must be
seen to 'drop' on the unsupported side.
Confusingly, the pathology is *not*
located on the 'dropped' side, but in
the opposite leg, hence the saying 'the
sound side sags'.

Condition/s associated with

- Gluteus medius muscle weakness
  - » Superior gluteal nerve palsy
    – iatrogenic
  - » Lumbar radiculopathy
  - » Sequelae of hip joint pathology
    - Osteoarthritis
    - Slipped femoral capital
      epiphysis (SCFE) – paediatrics
    - Legg–Calve–Perthes disease
      – paediatrics

Mechanism/s

The gluteus medius muscle originates
from the iliac crest and inserts into
the greater trochanter of the femur.
Normally when we stand on one leg,
the gluteus medius muscle abducts the
hip joint to maintain normal alignment
of the pelvis. With gluteal medius
weakness, the sound side (the side
opposite to the stance leg) sags, or tilts
downwards.

Sign value

Given the number of potential causes, a
positive Trendelenburg sign is fairly
non-specific; however, it is never
normal and should be investigated.

True leg length inequality (anatomic leg length inequality)

Description

The leg length is measured from the anterior iliac spine to the medial malleolus. There is no clear definition as to what constitutes a significant discrepancy. Some authors suggest that it is not clinically relevant until there is more than 20 mm difference between legs.[93]

Condition/s associated with

- Fracture – hip, femur, tibia
- Dislocation – hip, knee
- Post-surgical shortening
- Congenital disorders

Mechanism/s

True, or anatomic, leg length equality relates to the actual length of the bones and anatomical structures making up the hip and the lower limb. Therefore, any problem in the anatomy that constitutes the leg length (from the head of the femur down to the ankle) may cause a discrepancy. For example, abnormalities in growth plates during development may lead to one leg being longer than the other. Aberrant healed fractures can also lead to a shortened leg.

Sign value

A leg length discrepancy is a non-specific sign. It should be interpreted in the context of the patient's history.

Ulnar deviation

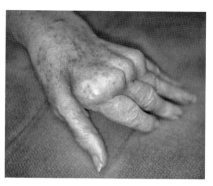

FIGURE 1.54
Ulnar deviation and subluxation
The hand shows typical manifestations of
end-stage erosive changes around the
metacarpophalangeal joints, with volar and
ulnar drift of the fingers.

*Reproduced, with permission, from Firestein GS,
Budd RC, Harris ED et al., Kelley's
Textbook of Rheumatology, 8th edn,
Philadelphia: WB Saunders, 2008: Fig 66-5.*

Description

Displacement of the metacarpophalangeal and/or radiocarpal joint
towards the ulnar aspect of the wrist.

Condition/s associated with

- Rheumatoid arthritis

Mechanism/s

Metacarpophalangeal (MCP) joint

MCP joints are condylar and are able
to move in two planes. They are less
stable than interphalangeal joints.
Progressive inflammatory changes from
rheumatoid arthritis result in stretching
of the joint capsule and ligaments,
causing instability. Extrinsic forces on
the joints tend to pull in a direction of
ulnar deviation. Possible factors
include:[87,88]

- the normal tendency of fingers to
  move towards the ulnar side on
  flexion

- inflammation of the
  carpometacarpal (CMC) joints in
  the 4th and 5th fingers causes
  further spread of the metacarpals in
  flexion, producing an 'ulnarly'
  directed force on the extensor
  tendons

- stretching of the collateral ligaments
  of the MCP joints, accessory
  collateral ligaments or flexor
  tunnels that permits volar
  displacement of the proximal
  phalanges.

Radiocarpal ulnar deviation

Progressive inflammatory changes lead
to progressive synovitis of the wrist
joint and carpal bones, including the
scaphoid. Abnormal wrist mechanics
develop due to translocation of the
carpal bones relative to the radius, and
imbalance of mechanical forces.[87]

Sign value

Ulnar deviation of the MCP joints is
classically associated with rheumatoid
arthritis.

V-sign

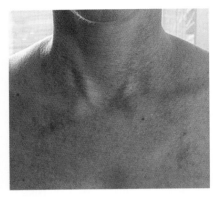

FIGURE 1.55
Irregular patchy erythema with associated prominent telangiectasias in a woman with dermatomyositis

Reproduced, with permission, from Shields HM et al., Clin Gastroenterol Hepatol *2007; 5(9): 1010–1017.*

Description

A confluent, macular, violet/red rash seen over the anterior neck and upper chest. Often found in a V-shape similar to the neck of a shirt.

Condition/s associated with

• Dermatomyositis

Mechanism/s

Complement- and antibody-mediated microvascular injury likely results in the development of the rash.[94] Dermatomyositis is an inflammatory myopathy characterised by microvascular damage and destruction of muscle by antibody complex and complement deposition. Genetic predisposition, viruses and UV light are all thought to play a role.[83]

Sign value

Although not pathognomonic, the V-sign is highly suggestive of dermatomyositis. In up to 30% of cases, skin manifestations including the V-sign may occur before development of the characteristic muscle weakness.

Valgus deformity

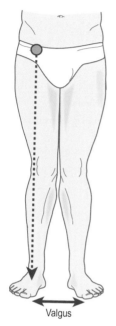
Valgus

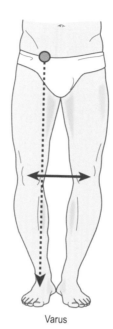
Varus

FIGURE 1.56
Examples of valgus and varus deformities of the knees

Description
Angulation of the distal bone of a joint away from the midline of the body.

Condition/s associated with
Associated conditions are given in Table 1.3.

Mechanism/s

Hallux valgus
Anatomical, biomechanical and pathological factors contribute to the formation of hallux valgus. Some of those identified include:[95]

- Limited soft tissue stabilising the 1st MTP joint results in forces pushing the toe laterally being relatively unrestrained.

- Owing to the anatomy of the metatarsocuneiform joint, increased pressure under the first metatarsal (e.g. from excessive pronation) will tend to displace the first metatarsal.

- Inflammatory joint disease may precipitate the formation of hallux valgus by damaging ligaments and altering normal joint alignment.

TABLE 1.3
Valgus deformity-associated conditions

Hip	Knee	Ankle	Toe
Osteochrondrosis	Cerebral palsy	Paralytic	Biomechanical
	Idiopathic	Osteochrondrosis	Congenital
	Blount's disease		Osteochrondrosis
	Rickets		Psoriatic arthritis
	Paralytic		Multiple sclerosis
	Osteochrondrosis		Cerebral palsy
	Rheumatoid arthritis		Rheumatoid arthritis
	Osteoarthritis		Intra-articular damage
			Connective tissue disorders

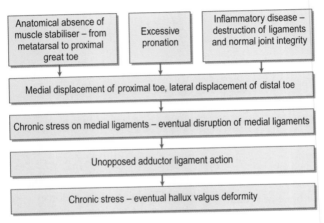

FIGURE 1.57
Factors involved in the mechanism of hallux valgus

Knee valgus (genu valgum)

Genu valgum may be caused by a number of disorders. Basic mechanisms for a number of these conditions are shown in Table 1.4.

Sign value

Valgus deformity has limited utility. Aetiologies differ largely depending upon the site of the deformity.

TABLE 1.4

Genu valgum mechanism/s

Condition	Basic mechanism
Vitamin D deficiency	A lack of vitamin D leads to abnormal bone mineralisation, softer-than-normal bones, abnormal bone regrowth and bowing of the legs. Mechanical forces play a role in bone regrowth
Paget's disease	Invasion with paramyxovirus leads to abnormal activation of osteoclasts and aberrant osteoblast activity. Deformation of the bone and knee can lead to anatomical changes and valgus deformity
Osteochrondrosis	Interrupted blood supply, especially to the epiphysis, leads to necrosis and then later bone regrowth – resulting in abnormal formation of femur and knee joint – and eventually a valgus deformity
Neuromuscular disorders	Weak quadriceps, gastrocnemius and hip abductors may cause knees to enter valgus position[49]

Varus deformity

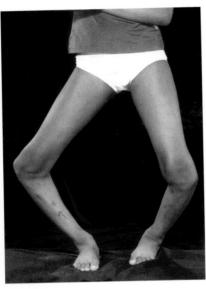

FIGURE 1.58
Bowing of both legs in infantile Blount's disease

Reproduced, with permission, from Harish HS, Purushottam GA, Wells L, Chapter 674: Torsional and angular deformities. In: Kliegman RM et al., Nelson Textbook of Pediatrics, 18th edn, Philadelphia: Saunders, 2007: Fig 674-8.

Description
Angulation of the distal bone of a joint towards the midline.

Condition/s associated with
Associated conditions are given in Table 1.5.

Mechanism/s

Coxa vara
Present if the angle between the femoral neck and shaft is less than 120°.

Congenital
Congenital coxa vara may present in infancy or later in childhood. It is often bilateral and characterised by progressive bowing of the femur and a defect in the *medial* part of the neck of the femur.[49]

Rickets
Pressure placed on the femoral neck of abnormally mineralised bone distorts its normal architecture.

Perthes' disease

Although the underlying cause of Perthes' disease is unknown, there is a loss of blood supply to the femoral head. Avascular necrosis of the femoral head results in distortion of the normal bony alignment of the femur.

Genu varum

Genu varum or 'bow-leggedness' is normal in many children up to 2 years.[96,97] It should be differentiated from Blount's disease.

Blount's disease

The underlying mechanism of genu varum in Blount's disease is unknown. Abnormal growth of the medial tibial epiphyseal growth plate causes progressive varus deformity at the knee joint.[97]

Hallux varus

Hallux varus is comprised of medial deviation of the first metatarsophalangeal (MTP) joint, supination of phalanx and interphalangeal flexion or claw toe. It results from an imbalance between osseous, tendon and capsuloligamentous structures at the first MTP joint.[98]

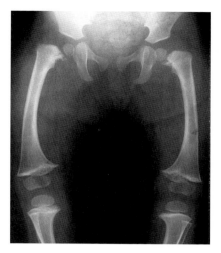

FIGURE 1.59
Metaphyseal chondrodysplasia, type Schmid
There is bilateral coxa vara, the metaphyses are splayed and irregular, and there is lateral bowing of the femora.

Reproduced, with permission, from Adam A, Dixon AK (eds), Grainger & Allison's Diagnostic Radiology, *5th edn, New York: Churchill Livingstone, 2008: Fig 67.13.*

Sign value

Aetiologies differ largely depending upon the site of the deformity.

TABLE 1.5
Varus deformity-associated conditions

Hip	Knee	Ankle	Toe
Congenital disorders (e.g. cleidocranial dysplasia, Gaucher's disease)	Physiological – common	Trauma	Complication from bunion surgery
Perthes' disease	Blount's disease	Iatrogenic	Trauma
Development dysplasia of hip	Rickets	Congenital	Burn injury with contracture
Slipped capital femoral epiphysis (SCFE)	Trauma		Rheumatoid arthritis
Rickets	Infection		Psoriatic arthritis
Osteomyelitis	Tumour		Charcot–Marie–Tooth (CMT) disease
Paget's disease	Skeletal dysplasia		Avascular necrosis
Trauma			

Yergason's sign

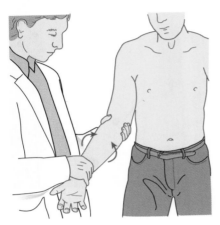

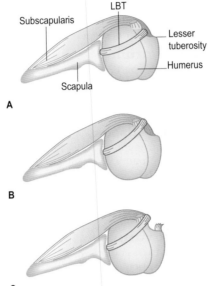

LBT
Subscapularis
Lesser tuberosity
Humerus
Scapula

A

B

C

FIGURE 1.60
Yergason's sign

FIGURE 1.61
Yergason's sign pathoanatomy
Overhead view of the subscapularis muscle, long head of the biceps tendon (LBT) and bicipital groove. **A** Intact structure depicting normal anatomy; **B** partial tear of the subscapularis tendon from the attachment on the lesser tubercle, with the LBT subluxed over the lesser tubercle into the subscapularis muscle; **C** complete tear of the subscapularis tendon from the attachment on the lesser tubercle, with the LBT subluxed over the lesser tuberosity and the subscapularis tendon.
Based on Pettit RW et al., Athletic Training Edu J *2008; 3(4): 143–147.*

Description

The examiner stands in front of the patient, who has their arms flexed to 90° at the elbow and the palms facing downwards (pronated). The patient then tries to supinate the forearm against resistance from the examiner.

Condition/s associated with

- Biceps tendonitis
- SLAP lesion (**S**uperior **L**abral tear from **A**nterior to **P**osterior) – an injury of the glenoid labrum

Mechanism/s

The long head of biceps is the main supinator of the arm. With resistance against supination, the muscle and tendon are stressed and any inflammation or damage is exacerbated, resulting in tenderness.

The long head of biceps travels in the bicipital groove of the humerus and originates on the lip of the glenoid labrum. The fibrous extension of the subscapularis muscle covers the long head of the biceps tendon and holds it in place.[99] If this fibrous extension is ruptured, the biceps tendon is susceptible to subluxation.

Sign value

Holtby et al., in predicting biceps tendon pathology and SLAP lesions, reported a sensitivity of 43%, a specificity of 79%, a positive likelihood ratio of 2.05 and a negative likelihood ratio of 0.72.[85]

Yergason's test has limited utility, although performs better than Speed's test.

1

References

1. Solomon DH, Simel DL, Bates DW, Katz JN, Schaffer JL. Does this patient have a torn meniscus of ligament of the knee? Value of physical examination. *JAMA* 2001;**286**(13): 1610–19.
2. McGee S. Chapter 53: Examination of the musculoskeletal system. In: *Evidence Based Physical Diagnosis*. 2nd ed. St Louis: Saunders; 2007.
3. Hegedus EJ, Cook C, Hasselblad V, Goode A, McCrory DC. Physical examination tests for assessing a torn meniscus in the knee: a systematic review with meta-analysis. *J Orthop Sports Phys Ther* 2007;**37**(9):541–50.
4. Scholten R, Deville W, Opstelten W, Bijl D, van der Plas CG, Bouter L. The accuracy of physical diagnostic tests for assessing meniscal lesions of the knee: a meta-analysis. *J Fam Pract* 2001;**50**(11):938–44.
5. Woodward TW, Best TM. The painful shoulder: Part 1. Clinical evaluation. *Am Fam Physician* 2000;**61**(10):3079–88.
6. Brady RJ, Dean JB, Skinner TM, Gross MT. Limb length inequality: clinical implications for assessment and intervention. *J Orthop Sports Phys Ther* 2003; **33**(5):221–34.
7. Tennant TD, Beach WR, Meyers JF. A review of special tests associated with shoulder examination. Part II: Laxity, instability and superior labral anterior and posterior (SLAP) lesions. *Am J Sports Med* 2003;**31**:301–7.
8. T'Jonck L, Staes F, Smet L, Lysens R. The relationship between clinical shoulder tests and the findings in arthroscopy examination. *Geneeskunde Sport* 2001;**34**:15–24.
9. Lo IKY, Nonweiler B, Woolfrey M, Litchfield R, Kirkley A. An evaluation of the apprehension, relocation and surprise tests for anterior shoulder instability. *Am J Sports Med* 2004;**32**:301.
10. Speer KP, Hannafin JA, Altchek DW, Warren RF. An evaluation of the shoulder relocation test. *Am J Sports Med* 1994;**22**:177–83.
11. Alexander CJ. Heberden's and Bouchard's nodes. *Ann Rheum Dis* 1999;**58**:675–8.
12. Fassbender HG. *Pathology of Rheumatic Diseases*. New York: Springer; 1975.
13. Collins DH. *The Pathology of Articular and Spinal Diseases*. London: Edward Arnold; 1949. pp. 109–13.
14. Sokoloff L. The pathology of osteoarthritis and the role of ageing. In: Nuki G, editor. *The Aetiopathogenesis of Osteoarthrosis*. Tunbridge Wells: Pitman Medical; 1980. pp. 1–15.
15. Kellegran JH, Lawrence JS, Bier F. Genetic factors in generalized osteoarthritis. *Ann Rheum Dis* 1963;**22**:237–55.
16. Stecher RM, Hersch AH. Heberden's nodes: the mechanism of inheritance in hypertrophic arthritis of the fingers. *J Clin Invest* 1944;**23**:699–704.
17. Thaper A, Zhang W, Wright G, Doherty M. Relationship between Heberden's nodes and underlying radiographic changes of osteoarthritis. *Ann Rheum Dis* 2005;**64**:1214–16.
18. Coons MS, Green SM. Boutonnière deformity. *Hand Clin* 1995;**11**(3):387–402.
19. Likes RL, Ghidella SD. Boutonnière deformity. *eMedicine*. Available: http://emedicine.medscape.com/article/1238095-overview [11 Aug 2010].
20. Nalebuff EA, Millender LH. Surgical treatment of the boutonnière deformity in rheumatoid arthritis. *Orthop Clin North Am* 1975;**6**(3):753–63.
21. Rosen A, Weiland AJ. Rheumatoid arthritis of the wrist and hand. *Rheum Dis Clin North Am* 1998;**24**(1):101–28.
22. Fox A, Kang N. Reinserting the central slip – a novel method for treating boutonnière deformity in rheumatoid arthritis. *J Plast Reconstr Aesthet Surg* 2009;**62**(5):e91–2.
23. Firestein GS, Budd RC, Harris ED, et al. *Kelley's Textbook of Rheumatology*. 8th ed. Philadelphia: WB Saunders Company; 2008.
24. Cibere J, et al. Reliability of the knee examination in osteoarthritis. *Arthritis Rheum* 2004;**50**(2):458–68.

1

25. Gogus F, Kitchen J, Collins R, Kane D. *Reliability of physical knee examination for effusion: verification by musculoskeletal ultrasound.* Presentation: 2008 Annual Scientific Meeting of American College of Rheumatology, San Francisco, 2008. Available: http://acr.comfex.com/acr/2008/webprogram/paper2759.htm [22 Nov 2010].

26. Patel P, Werth V. Cutaneous lupus erythematosus: a review. *Dermatol Clin* 2002;**20**: 373–85.

27. Orgretmen A, Akay A, Bicakci C, Bicakci HC. Calcinosis cutis universalis. *JEADV* 2002;**16**:621–4.

28. Neuman WF, DiStefano V, Mubryan BJ. The surface chemistry of bone. III. Observations of the role of phosphate. *J Biol Chem* 1951;**193**:227–36.

29. Cousins MAM, Jones DB, Whyte MP, Monafo WW. Surgical management of calcinosis cutis universalis in systemic lupus erythematosus. *Arthritis Rheum* 1997; **40**:570–2.

30. Frykberg RG, Armstrong DG, Giurnli J, et al. Diabetic foot disorders: a clinical practice guideline. American College of Foot and Ankle Surgeons. *J Foot Ankle Surg* 2000; **39**(Suppl. 5):s1–60.

31. Jeffcoate WJ, Game F, Cavanagh PR. The role of proinflammatory cytokines in the cause of neuropathic osteoarthropathy (acute Charcot foot) in diabetes. *Lancet* 2005; **366**:2058–61.

32. Jeffcoate WJ. Theories concerning the pathogenesis of acute Charcot foot suggest future therapy. *Curr Diab Rep* 2005;**5**:430–5.

33. Nabarro JD. Diabetes in the United Kingdom: a personal series. *Diabet Med* 1991;**8**:59–68.

34. Fabrin J, Larsen K, Holstein PE. Long term follow up in diabetic Charcot feet with spontaneous onset. *Diabetes Care* 2000;**23**:796–800.

35. Altman R, Asch E, Block D, et al. Development of criteria for the classification and reporting of osteoarthritis: classification of osteoarthritis of the knee. *Arthritis Rheum* 1986;**29**:1039–49.

36. Drake EL, Vogl W, Mitchell AW. *Gray's Anatomy for Students.* Philadelphia: Elsevier; 2005.

37. Murrell GAC, Walton JR. Diagnosis of rotator cuff tears. *Lancet* 2001;**357**:769–70.

38. Dinnes J, Loveman E, McIntyre L, Waugh N. The effectiveness of diagnostic tests for the assessment of shoulder pain due to soft tissue disorders: a systematic review. *Health Technol Assess* 2003;**7**(29):1–166.

39. Park HB, et al. Diagnostic accuracy of clinical tests for different degrees of subacromial impingement syndrome. *J Bone Joint Surg Am* 2005;**87**:1446–55.

40. Kutsumi K, Amadio PC, Zhao C, Zobitz ME, Tanaka T, An KN. Finkelstein's test: a biomechanical analysis. *J Hand Surg [Am]* 2005;**30**(1):130–5.

41. Anderson DM. *Dorlands Illustrated Medical Dictionary.* 30th ed. Philadelphia: Saunders; 2003.

42. Mendese G, Mahalingam M. Histopathology of Gottron's papules – utility in diagnosing dermatomyositis. *J Cutan Pathol* 2007;**34**:793–6.

43. Stone JH, Sack KE, McCalmont TH, Connolly KM. Gottron papules? *Arthritis Rheum* 1995;**38**(6):862–5.

44. McFarland EG, Muvdi-Garzon J, Xiaofeng J, et al. Clinical and diagnostic tests for shoulder disorders: a critical review. *Br J Sports Med* 2010;**44**:328–33.

45. Calis M, Akgun K, Birtane M, et al. Diagnostic values for clinical diagnostic tests in subacromial impingement syndrome. *Ann Rheum Dis* 2000;**59**:44–7.

46. Macdonald PB, Clark P, Sutherland K. An analysis of the diagnostic accuracy of the Hawkins and Neer subacromial impingement signs. *J Shoulder Elbow Surg* 2000;**9**: 299–301.

47. Iaccarino L, et al. The clinical features, diagnosis and classification of dermatomyositis. *J Autoimmun* 2014;**48–49**:122–7.

48. Wheeless CR III. *Wheeless orthopedics online.* Available: http://www.wheelessonline.com/ [October 2010].

49. Canale TS, Beaty JH. *Campbell's Operative Orthopaedics.* 11th ed. Philadelphia: Elsevier; 2007.

50. Lee JK, Yao L, Phelps CT, et al. Anterior cruciate ligament tears: MR imaging compared with arthroscopy and clinical test. *Radiology* 1988;**166**(3):861–4.

51. Gibbs MR, English JC, Zirwas J. Livedo reticularis: an update. *J Am Acad Dermatol* 2005;**52**(6):1009–18.

52. Freeman R, Dover JS. Autonomic neurodermatology (part 1): erythromelalgia, reflex sympathetic dystrophy and livedo reticularis. *Semin Neurol* 1992;**12**:385–93.

53. Kester S, McCarty DL, McCarty GA. The antiphospholipid antibody syndrome in the emergency department setting – livedo reticularis and recurrent venous thrombosis. *Ann Emerg Med* 1992;**21**:207–11.

54. Scholten RJ, Devillé WL, Opstelten W, Bijl D, van der Plas CG, Bouter LM. The accuracy of physical diagnostic tests for assessing meniscal lesions of the knee. A meta-analysis. *J Fam Pract* 2001;**50**(11):938–44.

55. Sallay PI, Poggi J, Speer FP, Garrett WE. Acute dislocation of the patella. A correlative pathoanatomic study. *Am J Sports Med* 1996;**24**(1):52–60.

56. Kastelein M, Luijsterburg PA, Wagemakers HP, et al. Diagnostic value of history taking and physical examination to assess effusion of the knee in traumatic knee patients in general practice. *Arch Phys Med Rehabil* 2009;**90**:82–6.

57. Bernard TN. *The role of the sacroiliac joints in low back pain: basic aspects of pathophysiology, and management.* Available: http://www.kalindra.com/bernard.pdf [28 Feb 2011].

58. Stuber KJ. Specificity, sensitivity and predictive values of clinical tests of the sacroiliac joint: a systematic review of the literature. *J Can Chiropr Assoc* 2007;**51**(1):30–41.

59. Broadhurst NA, Bond MJ. Pain provocation tests for the assessment of sacroiliac joint dysfunction. *J Spinal Disord* 1998;**11**(4):341–5.

60. Dreyfuss P, Michaelsen M, Pauza K, McLarty J, Bogduk N. The value of medical history and physical examination in diagnosing sacroiliac joint pain. *Spine* 1996; **21**(22):2594–602.

61. Seror P. Phalen's test in the diagnosis of carpal tunnel syndrome. *J Hand Surg* 1988; **13-B**(4):383–5.

62. D'Arcy CA, McGee S. Does this patient have carpal tunnel syndrome? *JAMA* 2000; **283**(23):3110–17.

63. Szepietowski JC, Salomon J. Do fungi play a role in psoriatic nails? *Mycoses* 2007;**50**: 437–42.

64. Szepietowski JC, Salomon J. The nail changes in psoriasis. In: Liponzencic J, Pasic A, editors. *Suvremene Sponznaje o Psorijazi Zagreb.* Medicinska Naklada; 2004. pp. 55–9.

65. Jiaravuthisan MM, Sasseville D, Vender RB, Murphy F, Muhn CY. Psoriasis of the nail: anatomy, pathology, clinical presentation, and a review of the literature on therapy. *J Am Acad Dermatol* 2007;**57**(1):1–27.

66. Crawford GM. Psoriasis of the nails. *Arch Derm Syphilol* 1938;**38**:583–94.

67. Samman PD, Fenton DA. *The Nails in Disease.* 5th ed. London: Butterworth-Heineman Ltd; 1994.

68. Kaur I, Saraswat A, Kumar B. Nail changes in psoriasis: a study of 167 patients. *Int J Dermatol* 2001;**40**:597–604.

69. Faber EM, Nall L. Nail psoriasis. *Cutis* 1992;**50**:174–8.

70. Lavaroni G, Kokelj F, Pauluzzi P, Trevisan G. The nails in psoriatic arthritis. *Acta Derm Venereol Suppl (Stockh)* 1994;**186**:113.

71. Saloman J, Szeptietowski JC, Proniewicz A. Psoriatic nails: a prospective clinical study. *J Cutan Med Surg* 2003;**7**:317–21.

72. Herrick AL. Pathogenesis of Raynaud's phenomenon. *Rheumatology (Oxford)* 2005;**44**: 587–96.

73. Cooke JP, Marshall JM. Mechanisms of Raynaud's disease. *Vasc Med* 2005;**10**:293–307.

74. Bakst R, Merola JF, Franks AG Jr, Sanchez M. Raynaud's phenomenon: pathogenesis and management. *J Am Acad Dermatol* 2008;**59**(4):633–53.

75. Wigley FM. *Pathogenesis of Raynaud phenomenon.* Uptodate. Last updated 3 October 2010. Available: http://www.uptodate.com [1 Mar 2011].

76. Rothschild BM, Pingitore C, Eaton M. Dactylitis: implications for clinical practice. *Semin Arthritis Rheum* 1998;**28**:41–7.

77. Oliveri I, Scarano E, Padula A, Giassi V, Priolo F. Dactylitis, a term for different digit diseases. *Scand J Rheumatol* 2006;**35**:333–40.

78. McGonagle D, Pease C, Marzo-Ortega H, O'Connor P, Emery P. The case of classification of polymyalgia rheumatica and remitting seronegative symmetrical synovitis with pitting edema as primarily capsular/entheseal based pathologies. *J Rheumatol* 2000; **27**:837–40.

79. Oliveri A, et al. Editorial: Dactylitis or 'sausage-shaped' digit. *J Rheumatol* 2007;**34**(6): 1217–20.

80. Oliveri I, Barozzi L, Pierro A, De Matteis M, Padula A, Pavlica P. Toe dactylitis in patients with spondyloarthropathy: assessment by magnetic resonance imaging. *J Rheumatol* 1997;**24**:926–30.

81. Brockbank JE, Stein M, Schentag CT, Gladman DD. Dactylitis in psoriatic arthritis: a marker for disease severity? *Ann Rheum Dis* 2005;**64**:188–90.

82. Silver RM, Medsger TA Jr, Bolster MB. Chapter 77: Systemic sclerosis and scleroderma variants: clinical aspects. In: Koopman WJ, Moreland LW, editors. *Arthritis and Allied Conditions.* Philadelphia: Lippincott Williams & Wilkins; 2005.

83. Sontheimer RD, Costner MI. Chapter 157: Dermatomyositis. In: Wolff K, Goldsmith LA, Katz SI, Gilchrest B, Paller AS, Leffell DJ, editors. *Fitzpatrick's Dermatology in General Medicine.* 7th ed. Available: http://proxy14.use.hcn.com.au/content.aspx?aID =2992330 [3 Oct 2010].

84. Scott BW, Al Chalabi A. How the Simmonds–Thompson test works. *J Bone Joint Surg* 1992;**74-B**(2):314–15.

85. Holtby R, Razmjou H. Accuracy of the Speed's and Yergaon's tests in detecting biceps pathology and SLAP lesions: comparison with arthroscopic findings. *Arthroscopy* 2004; **20**(3):231–6.

86. Hessian P, Highton J, Kean A, et al. Cytokine profile of the rheumatoid nodule suggests that it is a Th1 granuloma. *Arthritis Rheum* 2003;**24**:334–8.

87. Garcia-Patos V. Rheumatoid nodule. *Semin Cutan Med Surg* 2007;**26**:100–7.

88. Rosen A, Weiland AJ. Rheumatoid arthritis of the wrist and hand. *Rheum Dis Clin North Am* 1998;**24**(1):101–28.

89. Beaty JH, Canale TS, et al. Finger deformities caused by rheumatoid arthritis. In: Canale TS, Beaty JH, editors. *Campell's Operative Orthopedics.* 11th ed. Philadelphia: Elsevier; 2007.

90. Mould TL, Roberts-Thomson PJ. Pathogenesis of telangiectasia in scleroderma. *Asian Pac J Allergy Immunol* 2000;**18**:195–200.

91. Bolognia JL, Braverman IM. Chapter 54: Skin manifestations of internal disease. In: Fauci AS, Braunwald E, Kasper DL, et al., editors. *Harrison's Principles of Internal Medicine.* 17th ed. Available: http://proxy14.use.hcn.com.au/content.aspx?aID =2864525 [28 Nov 2010].

92. Urbano FL. Tinel's sign and Phalen's maneuver: physical signs in carpal tunnel syndrome. *Hosp Phys* 2000; July:39–44.

93. Friberg O. Clinical symptoms and biomechanics of lumbar spine and hip joint in leg length inequality. *Spine* 1983;**8**(6):643–51.

94. Crowson N, Magro C. The role of microvascular injury in the pathogenesis of cutaneous lesions in dermatomyositis. *Hum Pathol* 1996;**27**(1):15–19.

95. Ferrari J. *Hallux valgus deformity (bunion).* In: Eiff P, editor. http://www.uptodate.com [22 Feb 2010].

96. Holsalka HS, Gholve PA, Wells L. Chapter 674: Torsional and angular deformities. In: Kliegman RM, et al., editors. *Nelson Textbook of Pediatrics*. 18th ed. Philadelphia: Saunders; 2007.

97. Rab GT. Chapter 11: Pediatric orthopedic surgery. In: Skinner HB, editor. *Current Diagnosis & Treatment in Orthopedics*. 4th ed. Available: http://proxy14.use.hcn.com.au/content.aspx?aID=2315794 [14 Oct 2010].

98. Bevernage BD, Leemrijse T. Hallux varus: classification and treatment. *Foot Ankle Clin N Am* 2009;**14**:51–65.

99. Karlsson J. Physical examination tests are not valid for diagnosing SLAP tears: a review. *Clin J Sport Med* 2010;**20**(2):134–5.

CHAPTER 2

RESPIRATORY SIGNS

Accessory muscle breathing

Respiratory system revisited

Apart from the lungs, the respiratory system is made up of three main components: the central control centre, sensors and effectors.

The brainstem contains several centres in the pons and medulla, which (in addition to other parts of the brain) regulate inspiration and expiration. It receives information from a variety of receptors that monitor the partial pressure of oxygen and carbon dioxide as well as the stretch and compliance of the lung and irritants in the lung and upper airways. The central control system sends messages via nerve fibres such as the phrenic nerve to control respiratory rate and depth of breathing, in response to the data it receives.

Damage, disruption or alterations to any of these three – brainstem, nerves, receptors – can cause specific signs.

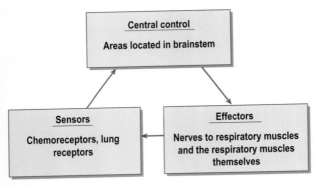

FIGURE 2.1
Simplified respiratory control
Based on West JB, West's Respiratory Physiology, 7th edn, Philadelphia: Lippincott Williams & Wilkins, 2005: Fig 8-1.

CLINICAL PEARL

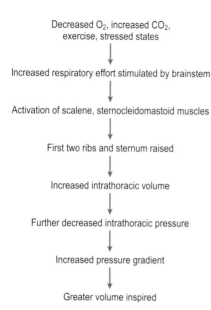

Decreased O$_2$, increased CO$_2$, exercise, stressed states

↓

Increased respiratory effort stimulated by brainstem

↓

Activation of scalene, sternocleidomastoid muscles

↓

First two ribs and sternum raised

↓

Increased intrathoracic volume

↓

Further decreased intrathoracic pressure

↓

Increased pressure gradient

↓

Greater volume inspired

FIGURE 2.2
Physiology behind accessory muscle respiration

VIDEO 2.1 ▶

Video 2.1 Access through Student Consult.

Description

Normal inspiration involves only the diaphragm. Expiration occurs passively due to elastic recoil of the lungs. When inspiratory effort requires the use of the sternocleidomastoid, scalene, trapezius, internal intercostal and abdominal muscles, the 'accessory muscles' of breathing are said to be in use.

Condition/s associated with

Any state resulting in an increased effort of breathing:

- Chronic obstructive pulmonary disease (COPD)
- Asthma
- Pneumonia
- Pneumothorax
- Pulmonary embolism
- Congestive heart failure (CHF)

Mechanism/s

In times of increased respiratory effort, the accessory muscles of breathing are invoked to exaggerate the normal respiratory process. Use of the accessory muscles can create more negative intrathoracic pressure on inspiration (pulling more air in and possibly causing *tracheal tug*) and more positive pressure on expiration (pushing air out).

On inspiration, the scalene and sternocleidomastoid muscles help lift and expand the chest wall, allowing for a decrease in intrathoracic pressure and increased air entry.

On expiration, the abdominal muscles help push air out of the lungs.

Sign value

The use of accessory muscles is a non-specific finding but is valuable in assessing the severity of respiratory difficulty (i.e. the 'work' of breathing). More than 90% of acute exacerbations of COPD present with accessory muscle use.[1] One study showed a sensitivity of 39% and specificity of 89% with a PLR of 4.75.[2] In children, accessory muscle use is a clear sign of increased respiratory effort.

Agonal respiration

VIDEO 2.2 ▷

Video 2.2 Access through Student Consult.

Description
Slow inspirations with irregular pauses. Patients are often described as gasping for air. Agonal breathing is usually closely followed by death unless intervention is provided.

Condition/s associated with
Any aetiology leading to imminent death.

Mechanism/s
Agonal respiration is thought to be a brainstem reflex, providing a last-ditch respiratory effort for the body to try to save itself. It is thought of as the last respiratory effort before terminal apnoea.[3]

Sign value
Without intervention, agonal respiration heralds impending death. Studies have shown that recognition of agonal breathing may improve recognition of cardiac arrest,[4] and implementation of protocols designed to identify agonal breathing over the phone can significantly increase the diagnosis of cardiac arrest by emergency dispatchers.[5] It is absolutely a sign that must be managed without delay.

CLINICAL PEARL

Apneustic breathing (also apneusis)

2

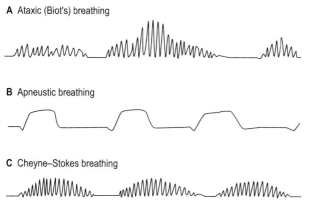

A Ataxic (Biot's) breathing

B Apneustic breathing

C Cheyne–Stokes breathing

FIGURE 2.3
Graphical representation of different respiratory patterns
http://what-when-how.com/acp-medicine/ventilatory-control-during-wakefulness-and-sleep-part-2/

Description

Apneusis (Greek *a pneusis*, 'not breathing') is characterised by prolonged periods of deep, gasping inspirations interrupted by occasional and insufficient expiration brought on by elastic recoil of the lung. Apneustic breathing involves repetitive gasps, with pauses at full inspiration lasting a few seconds.

The breathing pattern is represented in Figure 2.3.

Condition/s associated with

• Brainstem injury

Mechanism/s

The mechanism of apneusis is unclear but is most likely related to brainstem and, in particular, pontine dysfunction.

Apneustic breathing was believed to be caused by unopposed activity of the neurons in the lower pons (which facilitate inspiration). It is seen in patients with upper pontine lesions with bilateral vagotomy. However, more recent reports have shown that apneusis can be reproduced with midpontine lesions, ablation of the dorsal group of respiratory neurons and achondroplasia affecting the distal medulla and upper cervical spinal cord,[6] as well as in patients with normal vagal efferents.

Sign value

Given the variety of situations in which apneustic breathing may occur and its unclear mechanism, it cannot reliably be used to localise a lesion, apart from suggesting possible brainstem dysfunction. Given that it is a rare sign, there is little evidence to support its value.

Apnoea

Description
A pause in breathing.

Condition/s associated with

Central sleep apnoea (CSA)

- Brainstem injuries – stroke, encephalitis, cervical trauma
- Congestive heart failure (CHF)
- Opiates
- Obesity-related hypoventilation syndrome (Pickwickian syndrome)

Obstructive sleep apnoea (OSA)

- Obesity
- Micrognathia
- Alcohol
- Adenotonsillar hypertrophy

Mechanism/s
Apnoeas can be classified into central or obstructive, depending on the location of the causal pathology.

Central sleep apnoea
In central apnoeas, a lack of *respiratory drive* from the respiratory centre causes a break in breathing. There is a complex array of factors contributing to this form of apnoea.

- Injury to the brainstem ventilatory/respiratory centres (see Figure 2.1) – which normally regulate breathing – can cause diminished, inconsistent or absent respiratory drive.
- Opiate drugs, working via the *mu* receptors in the brainstem, decrease the central drive to breathe, even though the required networks remain intact.

- In obesity hypoventilation syndrome, it is thought that the body cannot compensate for the obstructed respiratory mechanics. This, combined with blunted chemoreceptor sensitivity, causes apnoea – although the mechanism is not clear.[7]
- Patients with motor neuron disease, myasthenia gravis, polio and other neurodegenerative diseases have a central respiratory drive but this drive does *not get transmitted* to the respiratory muscles to enable effective ventilation.
- *Cheyne–Stokes breathing* is a form of central sleep apnoea and is discussed in Chapter 3, 'Cardiovascular signs'.

Obstructive sleep apnoea

> **VIDEO 2.3** ▶
>
> Video 2.3 Access through Student Consult.

The negative pressure of inspiration leads to collapse of the airway, causing a temporary obstruction or occlusion of the nasopharynx and oropharynx. Most commonly, the tongue and palate move into opposition with the posterior pharyngeal wall, causing obstruction of the airway.[8]

Anything that crowds or destabilises the airway (e.g. micrognathia, adenotonsillar hypertrophy, obesity or acromegaly) may contribute to collapse and obstruction.

Alcohol can relax the normal stabilising muscles of the pharynx.

Obstructive apnoeas can be witnessed but can also be detected on polysomnography.

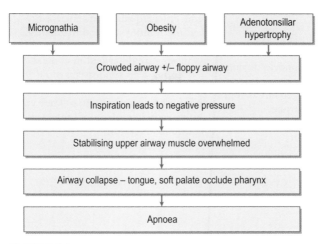

FIGURE 2.4
OSA mechanism

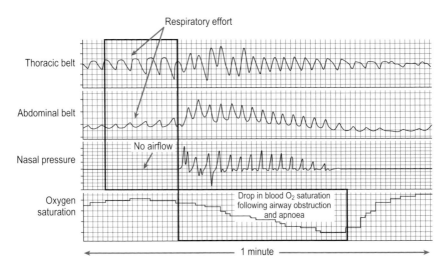

FIGURE 2.5
Polysomnogram of obstructive sleep apnoea in a patient with heart failure

Khayat R et al. Sleep-disordered breathing in heart failure: identifying and treating an important but often unrecognized comorbidity in heart failure patients. Journal of Cardiac Failure 2013; 19(6): Fig 4.

Sign value

Obstructive apnoea is an important clinical sign. There is substantial evidence that persistent apnoeas during sleep adversely affect glucose control and blood pressure management as well as increasing the risk of stroke, coronary artery disease and heart failure, among many other complications. Obstructive apnoeas reduce sleep quality, and increase daytime somnolence and irritability. They should be suspected if these symptoms are described in context.

Central sleep apnoeas are often manifestations of underlying diseases and must be monitored for. They are always pathological and if present may require intervention.

Asterixis

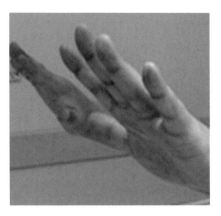

FIGURE 2.6
Asterixis

Goodman CC, Snyder TE. Differential Diagnosis for Physical Therapists: Screening for Referral, *4th edn, Philadelphia, PA: WB Saunders/Elsevier, 2007. In: Goodman CC, Screening for Gastrointestinal, Hepatic/Biliary, and Renal/Urologic Disease.* Journal of Hand Therapy *2010; 23(2): 140–157.* © *2010.*

Description

When the patient is asked to hold their arms extended with wrists dorsiflexed, the hands move in a 'flap' that is brief, rhythmless and of low frequency (3–5 Hz). Asterixis may be bilateral or unilateral. It is more simply described as a failure to hold a set pose owing to an interruption of muscle tone or posture. It is more easily understood when observed rather than described.

Condition/s associated with

More common

- Hypercapnia (e.g. CO_2 retention in COPD)
- Liver disease – see also Chapter 6, 'Gastroenterological signs'
- Renal failure
- Alcoholism

Less common

- Central nervous system (CNS) ischaemia or haemorrhage
- Drug-induced (e.g. clozapine)
- Electrolyte abnormalities (e.g. hypokalaemia and hypomagnesemia)
- Unilateral asterixis – thalamic stroke

Mechanism/s

The mechanism for asterixis in any of the aforementioned situations is unclear. The final common pathway is equally nebulous; however, several pathological mechanism/s have been postulated:[9]

- diffuse, widespread dysfunction of CNS function
- dysfunction of sensorimotor integration between the parietal lobe and midbrain
- episodic dysfunction of neuronal circuits involved in sustained muscle contraction due to focal or generalised neurochemical imbalance
- abnormality of the motor field in the cerebral cortex
- motor cortex pathologically slowed.

Sign value

Although not specific for a disorder, asterixis in a patient requires investigation and correlation with other clinical signs and history.

Asymmetrical chest expansion

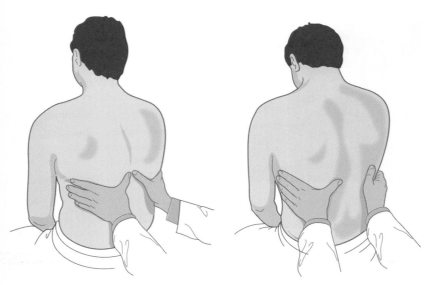

FIGURE 2.7
Palpation to detect asymmetry of chest expansion, a sign of pleural effusion
Accuracy of the physical examination in evaluating pleural effusion. Cleveland Clinic Journal of Medicine *2008; 75(4).*

Description

The clinician is positioned behind the patient, usually looking down at the clavicles (upper lobe movement) or palpating the chest wall (lower lobes). As the patient breathes, uneven extension of the chest wall in inspiration or retraction on expiration may be observed. This may manifest itself as an absolute difference or a slight lag in expansion.

Condition/s associated with

More common

- Pneumonia
- Pleural effusion

- Flail chest
- Foreign body
- Pneumothorax

Less common

- Unilateral diaphragm paralysis
- Haemothorax
- Musculoskeletal abnormality (e.g. kyphoscoliosis)
- Neuropathy
- Pulmonary fibrosis – localised

Mechanism/s

Symmetrical bilateral expansion of the chest wall is reliant on normal musculature, nerve function and lung compliance. Therefore, any abnormality unilaterally affecting a

Pleural effusion

↓

Decreased lung compliance on affected side

↓

Decreased expansion on inspiration relative to normal side

FIGURE 2.8
Mechanism of pneumonia

nerve, muscle or the compliance of the lungs may produce an asymmetrical expansion.

Pneumonia, pleural effusions

If pneumonia (consolidation of the airways) and/or pleural effusions (fluid in the pleural space) are present, the normal compliance of the lung is reduced. When inspiration occurs, the affected lung will have decreased expansion compared to normal.

Foreign body

In the lung blocked by a foreign body, air cannot get past the larger airways to the small airways to allow normal expansion.

Flail segment

A flail chest or flail segment is usually caused by trauma. Sections of ribs become detached from the chest wall. As the segment is no longer attached to the expanding chest on inspiration, it is susceptible to negative intrathoracic pressure. This pressure sucks the flail segment inwards on inspiration and pushes it out on expiration (opposite to the intact remaining chest wall).

Kyphoscoliosis

Progressive forward and/or lateral curvature of the spine (kyphoscoliosis) may become so severe that it mechanically depresses one lung over the other and causes decreased chest expansion on one side.

Unilateral diaphragm paralysis

If unilateral diaphragmatic paralysis occurs for any reason, the side of the affected diaphragm will not contract, affecting lung expansion.

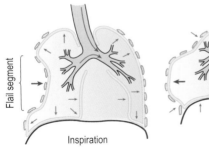 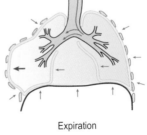

Flail segment

Inspiration   Expiration

FIGURE 2.9
Flail segment mechanism
Based on Aggarwal R, Hunter A. BMJ. http://archive.student.bmj.com/issues/07/02/education/52.php [28 Feb 2011].

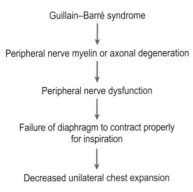

Guillain–Barré syndrome

↓

Peripheral nerve myelin or axonal degeneration

↓

Peripheral nerve dysfunction

↓

Failure of diaphragm to contract properly
for inspiration

↓

Decreased unilateral chest expansion

FIGURE 2.10
Mechanism of unilateral chest expansion

Sign value

Asymmetrical chest expansion is always pathological. While there have been very few studies, asymmetrical chest expansion was shown to be one of the most effective signs in predicting the presence of a pleural effusion, ahead of vocal resonance and vocal fremitus. It was an independent predictor of pleural effusion[10] with an odds ratio of 5.22, sensitivity of 74% and specificity of 91%.

Asynchronous respiration

Description

Abnormal breathing consisting of an abrupt inward motion near, or at the end of, inspiration, shortly followed by an outward movement continuing for a variable period of time while the chest is still moving inwards. The pattern is represented in Figure 2.11. The double movement is visibly irregular, but it is very difficult to identify the different elements with the naked eye.

Condition/s associated with

- COPD
- Respiratory distress

Mechanism/s

Asynchronous breathing is related to the strong movements of chest wall accessory muscles during forced expiration, which push the diaphragm down and the abdomen out.[11,12]

Sign value

Associated with poorer prognosis, poorer ventilatory mechanics in patients with COPD[12,13] and increased need for mechanical ventilation.

2

Chest wall movements:

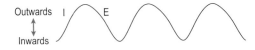

Abdominal wall movements:

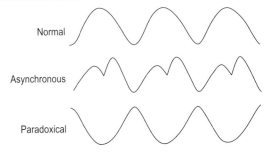

FIGURE 2.11

Respiratory abdominal movements

Chest movements are depicted in the first row. 'I' denotes inspiration and 'E' denotes expiration. Upward-sloping lines on the drawing indicate outward body wall movements; downward-sloping lines indicate inward movements. In normal persons, the abdominal and chest wall movements are completely in sync. In asynchronous breathing, only expiratory abdominal movements are abnormal. In paradoxical abdominal movements, both inspiratory and expiratory abdominal movements are abnormal.

McGee S, Evidence Based Physical Diagnosis, *3rd edn, St Louis: Elsevier, 2012: p. 151, Fig 18-2.*

Ataxic (Biot's) breathing

A Ataxic (Biot's) breathing

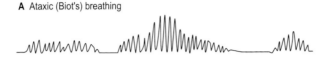

B Apneustic breathing

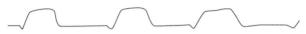

C Cheyne–Stokes breathing

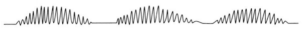

FIGURE 2.12
Graphical representation of different respiratory patterns
http://what-when-how.com/acp-medicine/ventilatory-control-during-wakefulness-and-sleep-part-2/

Description

A breathing pattern characterised by its erratic rate and depth, alternating with interspersed episodes of apnoea.[14] See Figure 2.12(a). It can be also seen on polysomnogram in Figure 2.13.

Condition/s associated with

More common

- Stroke

Less common

- Some neurodegenerative disorders (e.g. Shy–Drager syndrome)
- Meningitis
- Chronic opioid abuse
- Fatal familial insomnia – rare

Mechanism/s

The specific mechanism is not clear.

As in many breathing abnormalities, it is thought to be caused by disruption of the normal respiratory systems of the brainstem, in particular medullary impairment.[15]

Sign value

There is some evidence to support this breathing pattern localising pathology to the medulla. In a case series of 227 patients with medullary strokes, all but 12 experienced ataxic breathing.[16]

2

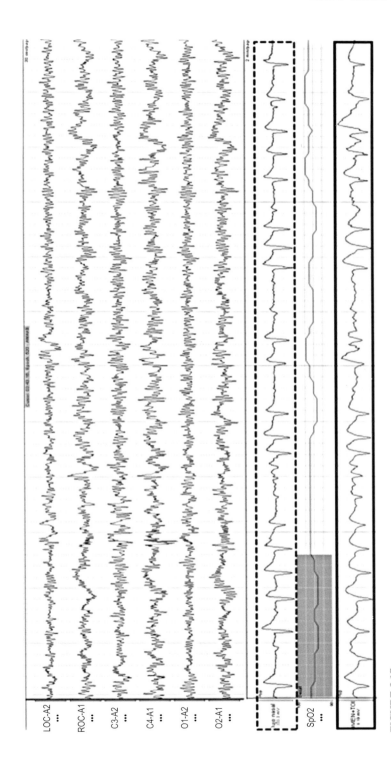

FIGURE 2.13

Biot's breathing in a patient with hypercapnic respiratory failure and homozygous methionine mutation of the PrP gene in fatal familial insomnia

A pattern of periodic shallow breathing (nasal pressure, into the dot line square) with equal irregularities in the respiratory effort channels (into the continuous line square) alternating with apnoea periods was observed while the patient was awake.

Casas-Mendez LF et al. Biot's breathing in a woman with fatal familial insomnia: is there a role for noninvasive ventilation? J Clin Sleep Med 2011; 7(1): 89–91.

Barrel chest

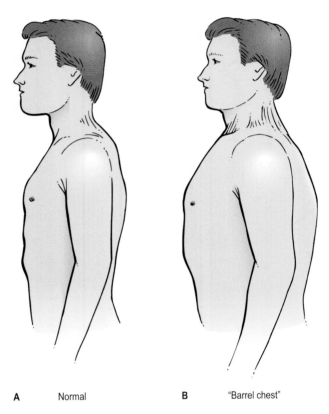

A   Normal   B   "Barrel chest"

FIGURE 2.14
Barrel chest
Swartz MH, Textbook of Physical Diagnosis: History and Examination, *6th edn, St Louis: Mosby, 2004.*

Description

A ratio of anteroposterior (AP) to lateral chest diameter of greater than 0.9. The normal AP diameter should be less than the lateral diameter and the ratio of AP to lateral should lie between 0.70 and 0.75.

Condition/s associated with

- Chronic bronchitis
- Emphysema
  Also occurs in elderly people without disease.

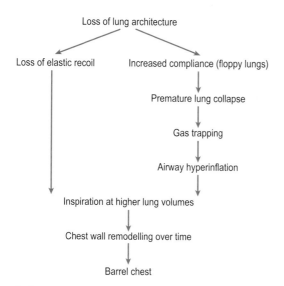

FIGURE 2.15
Mechanism of barrel chest in emphysema

Mechanism/s

Considered to be due to over-activity of the scalene and sternocleidomastoid muscles, which lift the upper ribs and sternum.[11] With time, this overuse causes remodelling of the chest.

In chronic obstructive pulmonary disease, there is a chronic airflow limitation that results in increased end-expiratory volumes and chronic hyperinflation.

Chronic hyperinflation reduces airway resistance and improves elastic recoil at the expense of higher lung volumes. Over time this leads to chest wall remodelling and barrel chest abnormality.[17]

Bradypnoea

Description

An unusually slow rate of breathing, usually defined in an adult as less than 8–12 breaths per minute.

Condition/s associated with

Bradypnoea may occur in any condition or state that affects the respiratory/ventilatory centres of the brain or brainstem.

More common

- Drugs – opiates, benzodiazepines, barbiturates, anaesthetic agents
- Respiratory failure
- Brain injury and raised intracranial pressure
- Hypothyroidism
- Excess alcohol consumption

Less common

- Hypothermia
- Uraemia
- Metabolic alkalosis

Mechanism/s

Bradypnoea can be caused by:

- decreased central nervous system output – i.e. a defect or reduction in central respiratory drive that diminishes messages 'telling' the body to breathe (e.g. brain injury, raised ICP, opiate overdose)
- disorders in the nerves connecting to the respiratory muscles (e.g. motor neuron disease)
- disorders of the muscles associated with breathing (e.g. muscle tiredness in respiratory failure)
- respiratory compensation in response to a metabolic process (e.g. in response to metabolic alkalosis, the body will reduce respiration in an attempt to retain carbon dioxide and acids).

Sign value

Although not specific, bradypnoea in an unwell patient is often a sign of serious dysfunction and requires immediate attention. In asthma and respiratory failure, bradypnoea often precedes respiratory arrest.

Breath sounds

Description

Breath sounds refer to noises auscultated over the lung fields on respiration. The sounds may be normal or have pathological associations. Their characteristics and differences are summarised in Table 2.1.

Mechanism/s

The general mechanism of breath sounds relates to flow of air through different airways *and* the filtering properties of the surrounding tissue, air, fluid or matter in between the airways and the clinician's stethoscope.

Airflow

Three types of airflow have been described, two of which contribute to the development of sounds heard on auscultation:[18]

1 *Laminar airflow* is present in small peripheral airways. It is very slow and generally inaudible.

2 *Vorticose airflow* is faster than laminar flow and present in the medium-sized branching airways. Branching creates airflow with different layers, velocities and eddies of flow, all of which can produce sound.

3 *Turbulent airflow* is very rapid, complex and typical of large central airways (trachea and major bronchi). Air is colliding against itself and the walls of the large airways, producing a loud noise.

Sound filtering

Each of the three flows produce sounds of different pitch (measured in hertz [Hz]). The differing characteristics of the lung (e.g. normal tissue versus abnormal, fluid versus solid matter) alter transmission of these sounds to the clinician's ears.

Healthy lung tissue and alveolar air usually surround the bronchi and bronchioles, acting as a low-frequency filter or muffler. This allows transmission of low-frequency sounds (e.g. 100–200 Hz) but filters out higher frequencies (30–500 Hz). Consolidation, oedema and pleural fluid are better at transmitting higher frequencies. This altered transmission is the cause of the different pathological breath sounds and other respiratory signs such as vocal resonance. The relative differences in frequency are shown in Figure 2.16.

Breath sounds: vesicular or normal

AUDIO 2.1 ◀

Audio 2.1 Access through Student Consult.

Description

Vesicular or normal breath sounds can be heard over the lung fields and are low pitched and soft. The inspiratory portion of the sound is longer than the expiratory and there is no pause between these phases. An example of vesicular breath sounds can be heard on Audio 2.1.

Vesicular breath sounds can be conceptualised and contrasted with bronchial breath sounds. Figure 2.17 shows that vesicular breath sounds have a longer inspiratory limb and bronchial breath sounds a more prominent expiratory phase.

CLINICAL PEARL

TABLE 2.1
Characteristics of breath sounds

	Duration of sounds	Intensity of expiratory sound	Pitch of expiratory sound	Locations where heard normally
Vesicular*	Inspiratory sounds last longer than expiratory sounds.	Soft	Relatively low	Over most of both lungs
Bronchovesicular	Inspiratory and expiratory sounds are about equal.	Intermediate	Intermediate	Often in the 1st and 2nd interspaces anteriorly and between the scapulae
Bronchial	Expiratory sounds last longer than inspiratory ones.	Loud	Relatively high	Over the manubrium, (larger proximal airways)
Tracheal	Inspiratory and expiratory sounds are about equal.	Very loud	Relatively high	Over the trachea in the neck

*The thickness of the bars indicates intensity; the steeper their incline, the higher the pitch.
http://o.quizlet.com/vgB7cqi80QSCQbzNk1fDwQ_m.png

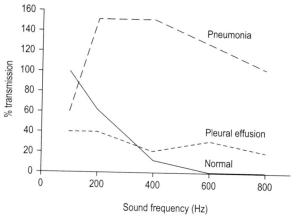

FIGURE 2.16
Transmission of sound to the chest wall
In this experiment, a speaker emitting pure musical tones of different frequencies was placed in the mouth of patients with normal lungs (solid line), pneumonia (long dashes) or pleural effusion (short dashes). Microphones on the chest wall recorded the transmission of each frequency. (For purposes of comparison, 100% transmission is the transmission of 100 Hz in normal persons.)

McGee S, Evidence Based Physical Diagnosis, *3rd edn, St Louis: Elsevier, 2012: Fig 28-2.*

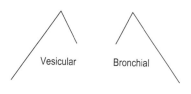

(c) 2006, Kanchan Ganda, M.D.

FIGURE 2.17
Differences between vesicular and bronchial breath sounds
http://ocw.tufts.edu/Content/24/lecturenotes/ 311144/312054_medium.jpg

Condition/s associated with

• Normal lung fields

Mechanisms

Lung sounds are produced by vertical and turbulent flow.[19]

Several studies[20,21] have suggested that the inspiratory portion of the vesicular breath sound is *regionally* produced by turbulence in the lobar, segmental and smaller peripheral airways, while expiratory elements of vesicular breath sounds are attributed to flow through the larger airways. Contrary to popular belief, vesicular breath sounds are NOT produced by air entering the vesicles or alveoli.[22]

Vesicular breath sounds are transmitted sounds from the airways which are *muffled or filtered* by air-filled alveoli, so only lower frequencies are transmitted. Low frequencies are not well heard by the human ear and therefore seem softer than bronchial breath sounds.

Sign value

Vesicular breath sounds provide the baseline with which to compare other sounds and their recognition is therefore essential in identifying and understanding abnormalities.

Breath sounds: bronchial

Description

Loud, harsh, high-pitched breath sounds that are normal if heard over the tracheobronchial tree but abnormal if heard over lung tissue on auscultation. As opposed to vesicular breath sounds, the expiratory portion of the cycle is longer and there is often a pause between inspiration and expiration.

Condition/s associated with

- Normal over trachea
- Pneumonia
- Pleural effusion – heard above the actual effusion
- Adjacent to large pericardial effusion
- Atelectasis
- Tension pneumothorax

Mechanism/s

As previously explained under 'Breath Sounds', bronchial breath sounds are not normally heard over the lung fields,

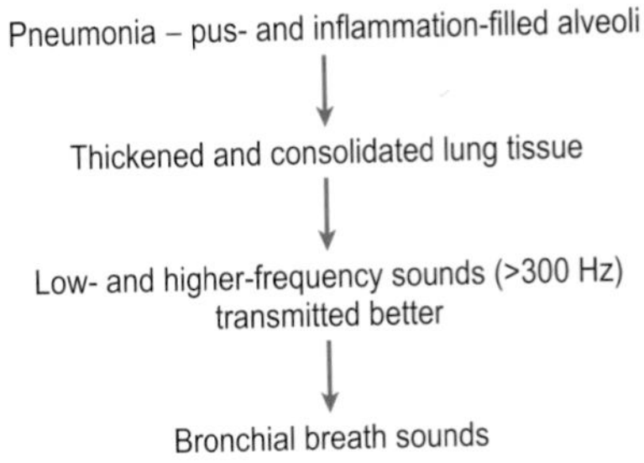

Pneumonia – pus- and inflammation-filled alveoli

↓

Thickened and consolidated lung tissue

↓

Low- and higher-frequency sounds (>300 Hz) transmitted better

↓

Bronchial breath sounds

FIGURE 2.18
Mechanism of bronchial breath sounds

as the chest wall and alveoli muffle higher-frequency sounds. In the presence of consolidation, however, the alveolar 'filter' is replaced by a medium (such as pus) that transmits sound (and higher frequencies), better[23] allowing bronchial breath sounds to be heard.

Atelectasis/collapse mechanism/s

Bronchial breath sounds can also be heard in the presence of alveolar collapse or atelectasis. In these conditions the alveoli are compressed by fluid (e.g. pleural fluid) or have collapsed owing to poor inspiration (e.g. being bed bound or pain restricting breathing). Collapsed alveoli also act as an effective transmitter of sound and higher frequencies.

Sign value

In patients with cough and fever, bronchial breath sounds suggest pneumonia (sensitivity 14, specificity 96%, LR 3.3)[11] and are a valuable sign.

CLINICAL PEARL

Breath sounds: reduced or diminished

Audio 2.3 Access through Student Consult.

Description

Low-intensity, soft breath sounds (compared to vesicular).

Condition/s associated with:

- Emphysema/chronic obstructive pulmonary disease
- Pleural effusion
- Low flow states – elderly patients, poor inspiration

- Low transmission states – muscular or obese body habitus

2

Mechanism/s

Breath sounds are related to the intensity of *flow (sound energy)* as well as the *transmission* of the sounds through the lungs and chest wall. Abnormalities of either element will diminish breath sounds.

Emphysema/chronic obstructive pulmonary disease mechanism/s

Decreased transmission of breath sounds due to airway destruction and increased gas trapping creating muffling

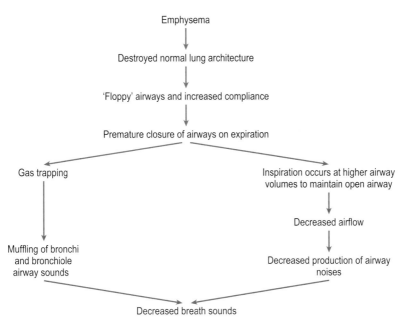

FIGURE 2.19
Mechanisms of decreased breath sounds in emphysema

Pneumonia/consolidation – bronchial breath sounds or diminished breath sounds?

Consolidation with pus, as happens with pneumonia, has been described as producing diminished and bronchial breath sounds.

How is this possible?

If the consolidation *blocks off* airways that are also surrounded by consolidation, then there will be no flow and no sound (i.e. decreased breath sounds).

If the underlying airways are *patent* and surrounded by consolidated material, then bronchial breathing is heard.

Thus it is the patency of the airways which determines what is heard.

---

of noise is thought to contribute to the diminished breath sounds present in COPD.[18] However, some research has suggested decreased production of airway noises due to decreased airflow may be the predominant cause.[24]

Low flow states

The production of vesicular breath sounds is dependent on flow. This is influenced by respiratory effort. In patients with poor respiratory effort due to any cause (e.g. drug-induced respiratory depression, age and frailty, neuromuscular disease), flow rates will be lower and therefore breath sounds softer. In cases of foreign body obstruction, there is no flow past the blockage and therefore no sound is generated.

Low transmission states

Even if airflow is normal, the transmission of lung sounds can be impeded by pulmonary or extra-pulmonary factors.[22]

Obesity is one example of an extrapulmonary impedance. Excess adipose tissue prevents the normal transmission of lung sounds during auscultation. Within the chest, the presence of gas (pneumothorax) or fluid (pleural fluid) between the airways and stethoscope may also reduce transmission.[22]

Sign value

Breath sounds have been extensively researched and have variable value depending on clinical context. Table 2.2 summarises a selection of studies reviewing altered breath sounds. Like all signs, they need to be interpreted in the light of presentation and augmented with appropriate additional tests.

More recent studies are now looking at the use of computerised lung sound analysis to improve specificities of the sounds traditionally heard via stethoscope. Initial reviews suggest this technology may be of value.[25]

TABLE 2.2
Breath sounds and vocal resonance*

Finding (reference)[+]	Sensitivity (%)	Specificity (%)	Likelihood ratio[+] if finding is	
			Present	Absent
Breath sound score				
Detecting chronic airflow obstruction[13,23]				
≤9	23–46	96–97	**10.2**	–
10–12	34–63	–	**3.6**	–
13–15	11–16	–	NS	–
≥16	3–10	33–34	**0.1**	–
Diminished breath sounds				
Detecting pleural effusion in hospitalised patients	88	83	**5.2**	**0.1**
Detecting chronic airflow obstruction[37,39,51,52]	29–82	63–96	**3.2**	0.5
Detecting underlying pleural effusion in mechanically ventilated patient[53]	42	90	**4.3**	0.6
Detecting asthma during methacholine challenge testing[54]	78	81	**4.2**	**0.3**
Detecting pneumonia in patients with cough and fever[55-57,60]	15–49	73–95	2.3	0.8
Asymmetrical breath sounds after intubation				
Detecting right main-stem bronchus intubation[62,63]	28–41	98–99	**24.4**	0.7

2

TABLE 2.2

Breath sounds and vocal resonance—cont'd

Finding (reference)[†]	Sensitivity (%)	Specificity (%)	Likelihood ratio[‡] if finding is	
			Present	Absent
Bronchial breath sounds				
Detecting pneumonia in patients with cough and fever[55]	14	96	**3.3**	NS
Egophony				
Detecting pneumonia in patients with cough and fever[55,57,64]	4–16	96–99	**4.1**	NS
Diminished vocal resonance				
Detecting pleural effusion in hospitalised patients	78	88	**6.5**	**0.3**

Diagnostic standard: For chronic airflow obstruction, FEV_1 <40% predicted (breath sound score) or FEV_1/FVC (%) ratio <0.6 to 0.7 (diminished breath sounds); for underlying pleural effusion, chest radiography or (if mechanically ventilated) computed tomography; for asthma, FEV_1 decreases ≥20% during methacholine challenge; for pneumonia, infiltrate on chest radiograph; for right main–stem intubation, chest radiograph[62] or direct endoscopic visualisation.[63]

[†]*Definition of findings: For breath sound score, see text; for diminished vocal resonance intensity, the transmitted sounds from the patient's voice when reciting numbers, as detected by a stethoscope on the patient's posterior chest, are reduced or absent.*

[‡]*Likelihood ratio (LR) if finding present = positive LR; LR if finding absent = negative LR.*

NS, not significant.

McGee S, Evidence Based Physical Diagnosis, 3rd edn, St Louis: Elsevier, 2012: EBM Box 28-1.

Breath sound score/intensity – a more objective assessment

The breath sound score developed by Pardee[26] is a more systematic approach to identifying and scoring breath sounds. The clinician assesses by:

1. Listening to the chest in six locations
   » bilateral upper anterior chest
   » bilateral midaxillae
   » bilateral posterior bases
2. Scoring each site for inspiratory sounds

   0 – absent
   1 – barely audible
   2 – faint but definitely heard
   3 – normal
   4 – loud

3. Adding up the points

A very low score is specific but not sensitive for chronic obstructive lung disease, and a very high score significantly decreases the likelihood of chronic obstructive lung disease being present.

2

Cough reflex

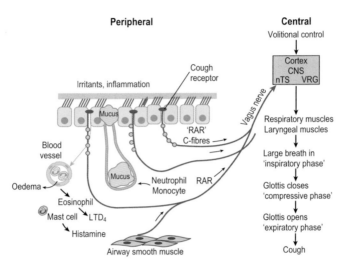

FIGURE 2.20
Cough reflex
LTD_4 = anti-leucotriene D_4

*Based on Chung KF, Management of cough. In: Chung KF, Widdicombe JG, Boushey HA (eds),
Cough: Causes, Mechanisms and Therapy, Oxford: Blackwell, 2003: pp. 283–97.*

Description
A short, explosive expulsion of air.

Condition/s associated with
- Acute cough (<3–4 weeks duration)

More common
- Upper respiratory tract infection
- Common cold
- Asthma
- Inhaled particles
- Inhaled foreign body
- Bronchitis
- Aspiration
- Pneumonia
- Exacerbation of congestive heart failure
- Exacerbation of COPD
- Bronchiolitis – in children
- Croup – in children
- Pulmonary embolism

Less common
- Pertussis
- Tracheomalacia
- Vasculitis

Chronic cough (>8 weeks duration)
- Postnasal drip
- Bronchiectasis
- Bronchitis
- COPD
- Asthma
- Gastro-oesophageal reflux disease (GORD)

- Angiotensin-converting enzyme (ACE) inhibitor side effect
- Interstitial lung disease

Mechanism/s

The cough reflex may be broken down into sensory, inspiratory, compressive and expiratory phases.

To initiate cough, vagal pulmonary receptors (made up of rapidly adapting receptors, slowly adapting receptors, C-fibres and other receptors[27,28]) sense mechanical and/or chemical stimulus in the airways and transmit signals back to the brainstem and cortex, initiating the cough reflex – this is the *sensory phase*. Any irritation, from inflammation of infection or chronic inflammation in COPD to direct stimulation from a foreign body or particles, is sensed and initiates the cough sequence.

During the *inspiratory phase*, a large breath in is stimulated to 'stretch' the expiratory muscles and allow them to produce greater positive intrathoracic pressure on expiration. This allows the body to push out more air faster with force.[29]

In the *compressive phase*, the glottis is closed after inspiration to maintain lung volume, while intrathoracic pressure is building.

Finally, during the *expiratory phase*, the glottis opens and air is pushed out because of the high positive intrathoracic pressure.

Sign value

As cough is such a common presentation or associated sign, it is essential that it be put into clinical context in order to be valuable. If this is done, it can be of assistance in diagnosis of a condition:

- A productive cough with coloured sputum (see 'Sputum' in this chapter) is much more likely to be from an infective cause with/ without underlying lung disease.

- A dry or minimally productive cough developing and lingering over months, on a background history of extensive cigarette smoking, may lead a clinician to consider lung cancer or COPD as a potential cause.
- Cough in the setting of exercise or night-induced wheeze may suggest underlying airway hyper-responsiveness and asthma.

In the setting of specific diseases, the development of cough may also suggest disease type:

- Cough as a presenting symptom in lung cancer is more often associated with central lesions within the airways where the cough receptors are located (e.g. squamous cell and small cell lung cancers).[30] It should be noted that, although cough is present in more than 65% of patients with lung cancer at diagnosis, cancer represents less than 2% of causes of chronic cough.[30]
- In an immunocompromised patient, the development of cough should raise the suspicion that opportunistic or atypical infections are present.

Character of cough

Classic characteristics of cough, particularly in children, have long been described by clinicians and caregivers (as seen in Table 2.3) and can assist diagnosis.[31]

While these descriptions may help narrow the field, data on the sensitivity and specificity of these characteristics are limited.[31]

TABLE 2.3
Classically recognised cough

Cough type	Suggested underlying process
Barking or brassy cough	Croup, tracheomalacia, habit cough
Honking	Psychogenic
Paroxysmal (with or without inspiratory 'whoop')	Pertussis and parapertussis
Staccato	Chlamydia in infants
Cough productive of casts	Plastic bronchitis/asthma
Chronic wet cough in mornings only	Suppurative lung disease

Based on Chang AB, Landau LI, Van Asperen PP et al., Med J Aust *2006; 184(8): 398–403; with permission.*

Crackles (rales)

AUDIO 2.4A 🔊

Audio 2.4A Access through Student Consult.

AUDIO 2.4B 🔊

Audio 2.4B Access through Student Consult.

AUDIO 2.4C 🔊

Audio 2.4C Access through Student Consult.

Description

Non-continuous, explosive popping sounds heard more often on inspiration but which can also be present on expiration. Crackles may be described as fine or coarse. Coarse crackles are associated with the larger airways and fine crackles with smaller branches.

Inspiratory crackles[22]

- Normally present in dependent lung areas
- Not transmitted to mouth
- Not influenced by cough

- May be influenced by gravity, posture
- Shorter duration – 5 msec, higher frequency

Expiratory crackles

- Late inspiration/expiration
- Heard throughout lung, transmitted to mouth
- Can change or disappear on coughing
- Longer duration – 15 msec, lower frequency

Condition/s associated with

There are many causes of crackles, the common ones being:

- asthma
- COPD
- bronchiectasis
- pulmonary oedema/congestive heart failure
- pneumonia
- lung cancer
- interstitial lung disease (pulmonary fibrosis).

Common causes of crackles and their features are summarised in Table 2.4.

TABLE 2.4
Characteristics of common crackles

Pulmonary fibrosis	Short duration crackles, mid to late inspiratory fine crackles[32]
Bronchiectasis	Coarse, early to mid inspiratory[33]
COPD	Scanty, early, low pitched, ending before mid-point of inspiration.[33] End-point is later than crackles in bronchiectasis
Heart failure	Late inspiratory crackles,[34] quickly resolve with appropriate treatment
Pneumonia	Mid inspiratory, coarse, similar to bronchiectasis in acute period.[33] During recovery, end inspiratory and short, similar to pulmonary fibrosis[35]
Sarcoidosis	Fine, mid to late inspiratory – fewer in nature than pulmonary fibrosis and differing locations

Mechanism/s

In all types of crackles, either altered architecture of the lung parenchyma (e.g. from pulmonary fibrosis) and/or the accumulation of secretions with accompanying inflammation or oedema causes the airways to narrow, obstruct or collapse.

Inspiratory crackles (more common) occur when the negative pressure of inspiration causes airways that have previously collapsed to 'pop' open.[36] Once open, there is a sudden equalisation of pressure on either side of the obstruction, resulting in vibrations of the airway wall, creating the sound.

Expiratory crackles are more controversial in terms of their mechanism. Two theories have been proposed:

1 The 'trapped gas hypothesis' suggests that there are areas of airway collapse and that the positive pressure of expiration forces these open, causing crackles as they burst apart.

2 Recent studies have shown that expiratory crackles are more likely to be due to sudden collapse or closure of some areas on expiration[36] (i.e. the pressures needed to keep small airways open are not maintained when breathing out and so these smaller areas collapse).

Bronchiectactic crackle mechanism/s

The destruction of elastic and muscular components of the bronchi walls that occurs in bronchiectasis can cause the bronchi to collapse on end expiration. The sudden opening at inspiration is thought to generate the crackle.[33]

COPD crackle mechanism/s

The most common cause of crackles in COPD are probably airway secretions.[33] Continuous crackles throughout inspiration and expiration have been described and are attributed to the opening and closing of bronchi, due to destruction of normal lung parenchyma and support structures.[33]

Pneumonia crackle mechanism/s

Pneumonia may present with crackles in two ways:

1 Acutely – owing to infiltration of inflammatory cells, pus and oedema which fill or narrow the airways. Inspiration may abruptly open these blocked airways and generate sound.

2 Later – in the resolving stage of illness it is thought that oedema decreases but inflammatory cells are still present. The lung becomes drier, leading to reduced compliance in some parts, causing segmental airway collapse.[33]

Sign value

A very valuable sign.

Even if heard with normal breathing, crackles are most likely pathological. Various types of crackles have been shown to be associated with different pathologies:

- Fine, late inspiratory crackles and pulmonary fibrosis: sensitivity 81%, specificity 86%, positive likelihood ratio (PLR) 5.9.[37] These fine crackles can be heard BEFORE the development of radiological abnormalities in pulmonary fibrosis patients,[38] making them very valuable in identifying early disease and monitoring for drug toxicity (e.g. amiodarone lung fibrosis).

- Coarse or fine, late or pan-inspiratory crackles and elevated left atrial pressure in patients with a cardiomyopathy and congestive heart failure: PLR 3.4.[39]

- Early inspiratory crackles and chronic airflow obstruction: specificity 97–98%, PLR 14.6[39] and in detecting severe disease in patients with chronic airflow obstruction: sensitivity 90%, specificity 96% and, if present, PLR 20.8.[40]

- Auscultation has been found to be as accurate as CT in identifying areas of asbestosis lung disease and may have a role in non-invasive screening.[22,39,41]

Expiratory crackles are a lot less common, especially in COPD, are not specific and are present in many other lung complaints.

The reduction of crackle duration may have potential as an outcome measure for respiratory therapy intervention.[42] Similarly, advanced computerised techniques to assess respiratory sounds have shown promise in objective diagnosis[43,44] and outcome following intervention.[45]

2

Dahl's sign and tripod position

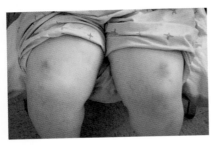

FIGURE 2.21
Dahl's sign

Rebick G, Morin S, The thinker's sign. Canadian Medical Association Journal 2008; 179(6): 611, Fig 1A. © 2008.

Description
Bilateral, symmetric, slanting regions of hyperpigmentation on anterior thighs. It is often associated with the tripod position.

Condition/s associated with
- COPD

Mechanism/s
This sign is seen in long-term, chronic respiratory illness. It is caused by patients spending long periods of time in the tripod position (i.e. with elbows resting on the epidermis of the thighs), resulting in hyperpigmented, hyperkeratotic plaques.[46]

Tripod mechanism/s
Patients in respiratory distress will either deliberately or unconsciously take this posture but the mechanisms behind the effect of positioning are not clear.

Studies have found there to be *reduced work of breathing and activity of the scalene and sternocleidomastoid muscles* if one leans forward, as well as an improvement in thoraco-abdominal movements.[1,47,48]

It is thought that the tripod pose leads to a reduction in diaphragmatic tension (caused by abdominal muscles) and a decrease in pressure from the viscera attached to the diaphragm – thereby allowing a better position of the diaphragm on the length–tension curve and improved mechanics.[49]

More recent studies have shown arm support in the tripod position allows for increased muscle activity of the inspiratory accessory muscles during inspiration when compared with a 'neutral' position, possibly allowing greater ventilation.[50]

Despite these changes, studies into the effect of change in posture did not demonstrate any improvement in airway obstruction, minute ventilation or oxygenation.[1,48–50] Therefore, the relief of dyspnoea obtained from assuming this pose may be attributable to other as yet unknown effects.

Sign value
Dahl's sign, while a sign of chronicity, is rarely recognised. The tripod posture that leads to Dahl's sign is an important sign of respiratory distress and should be recognised and acted on.

Dyspnoea

Description

Strictly a symptom and not a sign, dyspnoea is the subjective awareness that an increased amount of effort is required for breathing.

Condition/s associated with

- Anxiety
- Respiratory disorders – COPD, pulmonary fibrosis, pneumonia
- Cardiac disorders – heart failure
- Anaemia
- Bronchoconstriction
- Deconditioning

General mechanism/s

The mechanism of dyspnoea is complex, involving many parts of the respiratory control system (summarised in Figure 2.22). Causes can be broadly grouped by:

1 conditions in which central respiratory drive is increased ('air hunger')
2 conditions where there is an increased respiratory load ('increased work of breathing') or
3 conditions where there is lung irritation ('chest tightness', 'constriction').[51,52]

Keeping these three groups in mind will help make the common pathways easier to understand.

Common pathways

Mechanical loading, respiratory effort and 'corollary discharge'

At times of increased respiratory load or effort, there is a conscious awareness of the activation of the muscles needed to breathe. This sense of effort arises from the brainstem and increases whenever the brainstem signals to increase muscle effort, when the breathing load increases or when muscles are weakened, fatigued or paralysed.[51,52]

In other words, when the CNS voluntarily sends a signal to the respiratory muscles to increase the work of breathing, it also sends a copy to the sensory cortex telling it there is an increased work of breathing. This phenomenon is called 'corollary discharge'.[51]

Chemoreceptors

It has been shown that hypercapnia makes an independent contribution to the experience of breathlessness.[53,54] It is thought that hypercapnia may directly be sensed as 'air hunger', regardless of ventilatory drive.

Hypercapnia also leads to increased brainstem ventilatory output or drive (to blow off the excess carbon dioxide) and this leads to a corollary discharge (as explained above).

Hypoxaemia also contributes to increased ventilation and respiratory discomfort, although it plays a lesser role than hypercapnia. It is unclear whether hypoxaemia causes dyspnoea directly or via increasing ventilation that is then sensed as dyspnoea.

Mechanoreceptors

- *Upper airway receptors*. The face and upper airway have receptors (many of which are innervated by the trigeminal nerve) that can modulate dyspnoea. Mechanoreceptors in the upper airway have been shown to excite or inhibit expiratory and

2

Efferent signals   **Afferent signals**

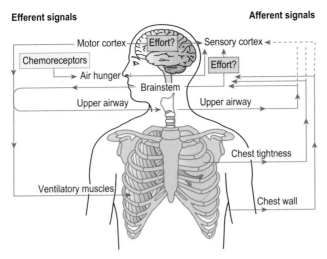

FIGURE 2.22
Mechanisms involved in the sensation of dyspnoea
Based on Manning HL, Schwartzstein RM, N Engl J Med 1995; 333(23): 1547–1553.

Chemoreceptors: which, what and where?

Peripheral chemoreceptors
- Located in carotid and aortic bodies
- Respond to pO_2, increased pCO_2 and H^+ ions

Central chemoreceptors
- Located in medulla
- Sensitive to pCO_2 **not** pO_2
- Respond to changes in pH of cerebrospinal fluid (CSF)

inspiratory muscles and modulate the intensity of dyspnoea.[51]

- *Pulmonary receptors.* The lung has three types of receptors (slowly adapting receptors, rapidly adapting receptors (RARs) and C-fibres) that transmit information back to the brainstem and brain about airway tension, lung volume and the state of the lung. These receptors can be stimulated by mechanical or chemical influences. Information detected is transmitted by the vagus nerve (CNX) back to the CNS, where, depending on the stimulus, it can be perceived as irritation, chest tightness, air hunger or increased work of breathing.

- *Chest wall receptors.* Muscle spindles and Golgi apparatus in the muscles of the chest wall function as stretch receptors, monitor 'force generation' and can detect reduced chest wall expansion, thereby contributing to dyspnoea.

Neuroventilatory dissociation

This refers to a situation where there is a mismatch between the information to the central nervous system and afferent muscle activity. For example, in neuromuscular weakness the neural effort is disproportionate to the small amount of muscle movement occurring. Alternatively, in restrictive and obstructive lung disease the neuromuscular effort may be disproportionate to the tidal volume actually achieved. If this happens it has been shown to increase dyspnoea.[51]

Deconditioning

Deconditioning lowers the threshold at which the muscles used in respiration produce lactic acidosis, causing increased respiratory neural output to reduce carbon dioxide levels.

COPD

Many factors contribute to dyspnoea in COPD:

- Hypoxaemia can stimulate peripheral chemoreceptors, increasing ventilatory drive from the brainstem.
- Hypercapnia can directly cause 'air hunger' but also increased central ventilatory drive (to blow off carbon dioxide) and corollary discharge, as discussed above.
- Increased airways resistance and hyperinflation increase the load the respiratory muscles must work against, thereby stimulating muscle receptors.
- Deconditioning via increased lactic acidosis can further contribute to dyspnoea.

Anaemia

It is still unclear what causes dyspnoea in anaemia. It is suspected that, in response to reduced blood oxygen levels, the body 'produces' tachycardia, leading to increased left ventricular end–diastolic pressure. This raised pressure then backs up into the lungs, producing an interstitial oedema that reduces lung compliance and stimulates pulmonary receptors.[55]

Alternatively, it has been suggested that a lack of oxygen produces localised metabolic acidosis and stimulation of 'ergoreceptors' (afferent receptors sensitive to the metabolic effects of muscular work).[56,57]

Heart failure

Heart failure may cause dyspnoea via two mechanisms: interstitial oedema stimulating pulmonary receptors (C–fibres), or hypoxaemia. The first cause (interstitial oedema) is the main mechanism. Interstitial fluid decreases lung compliance (which is picked up by pulmonary C–fibres) and increases the work of breathing.

Asthma

The mechanism of dyspnoea in asthma is thought to be related to an increased *sense of effort and stimulation of irritant airway receptors in the lungs.*[52]

- Bronchoconstriction and airway oedema increase the work of breathing and thus the sensation of effort.
- If hyperinflation occurs, this can change the shape of the diaphragm, affecting stretch of inspiratory muscles, making contraction less efficient and increasing mechanical load. This may lead to increased respiratory motor output and an increased sense of effort.[51]
- Irritation of airway receptors is transmitted by the vagus nerve to the CNS and perceived as chest tightness or constriction.[52]

Neuromuscular disorders

In neuromuscular disorders, central output stimulating respiration is normal; however, muscular strength is often diminished and/or the nerves stimulating the muscles may be weak or damaged. Additional central neural drive is required to activate the weakened muscles[51] and is sensed as increased respiratory effort and dyspnoea.

Pulmonary hypertension

Dyspnoea, particularly on exertion, is very common in primary pulmonary hypertension. The mechanism is dependent on the underlying aetiology.

In chronic pulmonary thrombo-embolism disease (see Figure 2.23), it is thought that pressure receptors or C-fibres in the pulmonary vasculature or right atrium are activated and interact with central systems, contributing to dyspnoea.[58]

Primary pulmonary hypertension mechanism/s

Studies of primary pulmonary hypertension[58,59] have found several physiological changes that contribute to dyspnoea. These are depicted in Figure 2.24:[59]

- relative hypoperfusion of ventilated alveoli leading to increased V/Q mismatch and increased alveolar dead space
- lactic academia occurring at a lower-than-normal rate
- hypoxaemia
- inability to increase pulmonary blood flow (and therefore systemic blood flow) to meet exercise oxygen demand.

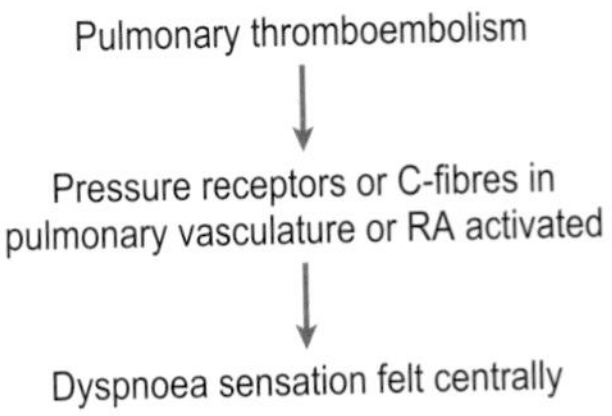

Pulmonary thromboembolism

↓

Pressure receptors or C-fibres in pulmonary vasculature or RA activated

↓

Dyspnoea sensation felt centrally

FIGURE 2.23
Mechanism of dyspnoea in pulmonary embolism

Sign value

Although a non-specific finding in isolation, dyspnoea at rest does require attention. It is often the most common feature found in patients with chronic cardiac and lung conditions.

Recent studies[60] showed the sensitivity, specificity and positive predictive value of dyspnoea at rest to be 92% (95% CI = 90–94%), 19% (95% CI = 14–24%) and 79% (95% CI = 77–82%), respectively, in patients with heart failure. Patients with dyspnoea at rest were 13% (LR = 1.13; 95% CI = 1.06–1.20) more likely to have heart failure than those without.

Given the low specificity of dyspnoea and its subjectivity, its value lies in combining it with other clinical features.[52]

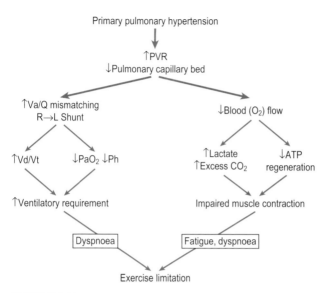

FIGURE 2.24

Pathophysiology of exercise limitation of PPH patients

Longer arrows show pathways leading to dyspnoea and fatigue with exercise. Shorter arrows indicate how each response differs from normal. PVR = pulmonary vascular resistance; Va/Q = alveolar ventilation/perfusion ratio; R = right; L = left; Vd/Vt = dead space volume/tidal volume ratio; PaO_2 = arterial O_2 pressure.

Sun X-G et al. Exercise physiology in patients with primary pulmonary hypertension. Circulation *2001; 104: p. 434, Fig 4.*

Funnel chest (pectus excavatum)

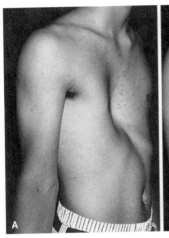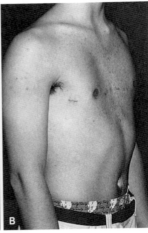

FIGURE 2.25
Funnel chest
A Prior to corrective surgery; **B** post surgery.

Reproduced, with permission, from Shamberger RC, Hendren WH III, Congenital deformities of the chest wall and sternum. In: Pearson FG, Cooper JD, et al. (eds), Thoracic Surgery, 2nd edn, Philadelphia: Churchill Livingstone, 2002: p. 1352.

Description

A congenital chest wall deformity where several ribs and the sternum grow abnormally to produce a 'sunken' or concave appearance.

Condition/s associated with

- Congenital disorder – the most common congenital chest wall abnormality
- Congenital diaphragmatic hernia

Mechanism/s

The mechanism behind the abnormal bone and cartilage growth is not known. A vast majority of cases are idiopathic.[61]

It was initially thought to be due primarily to an overgrowth of cartilage, but recent studies have disputed this.[62] A specific genetic defect has not been identified. 37% of cases have a first-degree relative with the deformity[63] and there is an association with Marfan's syndrome.[64]

Funnel chest was once believed to be caused in part by the increased work of breathing during recurrent chest infections in childhood. However, there is not a strong body of evidence to support this theory.

Sign value

Pectus excavatum can be associated with cardiac malformations and abnormal lung function.

Grunting

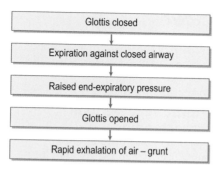

FIGURE 2.26
Mechanism of grunting

VIDEO 2.5 ▶

Video 2.5 Access through Student
Consult.

Description
A short, explosive, moaning or crying
sound heard on expiration, usually in
children or neonates.[65]

Condition/s associated with
Any cause of respiratory distress
including, but not limited to:

More common
- Paediatric
- Respiratory distress syndrome
  (hyaline membrane disease) – most
  common cause
- Meconium aspiration
- Pneumonia
- Congestive heart failure

Less common
- Sepsis
- Heart failure

Mechanism/s
In patients presenting with
intrathoracic disease, lower respiratory
tract involvement, obstruction or
collapse, grunting actually represents an
attempt to increase the functional
residual capacity.

The patient forcibly expires against a
closed glottis and, in doing so, raises
end-expiratory pressure. This helps
keep narrowed or collapsing airways
open, creating a longer time period for
the exchange of oxygen and carbon
dioxide at the alveoli.[66] The sound of
the grunt is caused by the explosive
flow of air that occurs when the glottis
opens.

Sign value
Grunting is a very valuable sign
associated with severe respiratory
distress and requires immediate
attention.

2

CLINICAL PEARL

Haemoptysis

Description
Coughing or spitting up of blood originating from the lungs or bronchial tubes.[67]

Condition/s associated with
There are many potential reasons for haemoptysis. Causes include, but are not limited to:

More common
- Infection – bronchitis, pneumonia, tuberculosis
- Cancer
- Pulmonary embolism
- Foreign body
- Airway trauma
- Idiopathic
- Pulmonary venous hypertension

Less common
- Hereditary haemorrhagic telangiectasia
- Coagulopathy
- Wegener's granulomatosis
- Goodpasture's syndrome

Mechanism/s
The common pathway to haemoptysis is disruption of and damage to vascular systems.

Cancer
Neoplasms produce haemoptysis via invasion of superficial mucosa and erosion into blood vessels. It can also be caused by a highly vascular tumour with fragile vessel walls.[67]

Pulmonary venous hypertension
Any condition that results in pulmonary venous hypertension may cause haemoptysis. For example, left ventricular failure can lead to increasingly high pulmonary venous pressures. These high pressures damage venous walls, causing blood excursion into the lung and eventually haemoptysis.

Infection
Inflammation of lung tissue can disrupt arterial and venous structures. Repetitive cough may damage the pulmonary vasculature, leading to haemoptysis.

Sign value
Although not specific to any one disorder, and bearing in mind that it must be clinically distinguished from haematemesis and other nasal or oral sources of bleeding, haemoptysis always requires investigation.

Harrison's sulcus (also Harrison's groove)

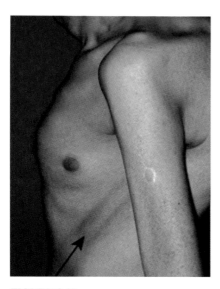

FIGURE 2.27
Pectus carinatum with prominent
Harrison's sulcus (arrow)

Douglas G, Nicol F, Robertson C, Macleod's
Clinical Examination, *13th edn, Edinburgh:
Elsevier, 2013: Fig 7.14C.*

Description
The sign present in Figure 2.27 is a
visible depression of the lower ribs
above the costal margin, at the area of
attachment of the diaphragm.

Condition/s associated with
- Rickets
- Severe asthma in childhood
- Cystic fibrosis
- Pulmonary fibrosis

Mechanism/s
Rickets is a disease specific to children
and adolescents in which growing
bones lack the mineralised calcium
required to strengthen and harden
properly (i.e. the osteoid is not
appropriately calcified). Because of this,
when the diaphragm exerts downward
tension on the weakened ribs, it pulls

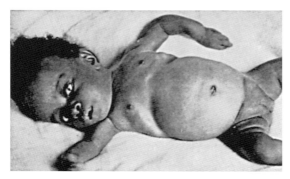

FIGURE 2.28
Deformities in rickets showing curvature of the limbs, potbelly and Harrison's groove
Kliegman RM, Behrman RE, Jenson HB, Stanton BF, Nelson Textbook of Pediatrics, *18th edn,
Philadelphia: Elsevier, 2004: Fig 195-1.*

the bones inwards, creating a flared appearance.

Similarly, if a child experiences chronic severe respiratory disease such as asthma before the bones mineralise and harden, the downward tension from the diaphragm and other accessory muscles used during increased respiratory effort can bend the ribs inwards over time.

Hoover's sign

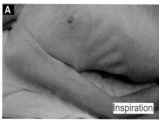
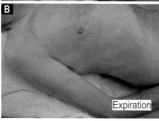

FIGURE 2.29
Hoover's sign
Note the paradoxical inspiratory retraction of the rib cage and lower intercostal interspaces on inspiration.

Based on Johnston C, Krishnaswamy N, Krishnaswamy G, The Hoover's sign of pulmonary disease: molecular basis and clinical relevance, Clin Mol Allergy *2008; 6: 8.*

Description
The paradoxical inward movement of the lower lateral costal margins on inspiration.

Condition/s associated with
• Emphysema
• Chest hyperinflation

Mechanism/s
When the chest becomes severely hyperinflated, the diaphragm often becomes stretched. As a consequence, contraction of the diaphragm at inspiration results in an inward movement,[68] bringing the costal margins with it, as opposed to normal downward movement.

Sign value
An almost forgotten sign, Hoover's sign was once reported in 77% of patients with obstructive airways disease.[69] A small, more recent study[70] found sensitivity of 58%, specificity of 86% and a PLR of 4.16 – higher than for other signs used in the detection of obstructive airways disease. Hoover's sign is also correlated with more severe disease.

Hypertrophic pulmonary osteoarthropathy (HPOA)

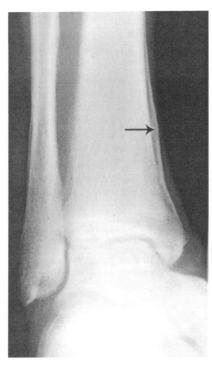

FIGURE 2.30
Hypertrophic pulmonary osteoarthropathy (HPOA)

Reproduced, with permission, from eMedicine; Goldman L, Ausiello D, Cecil Medicine, *23rd edn, Philadelphia: Saunders, 2007: Fig 189-2.*

Description

A syndrome characterised by excessive proliferation of the skin and bone at distal parts of the extremities, which can include clubbing.[71] In advanced stages of HPOA, periosteal proliferation of tubular bones and synovial effusions may be present.

Condition/s associated with

There are numerous potential causes of HPOA.

More common

- Cyanotic heart disease
- Lung cancer – most often bronchogenic or pleural (metastatic lung cancer is a rare cause)

Less common

- Inflammatory bowel disease
- Infective endocarditis

Mechanism/s

Clubbing and HPOA are thought to share a common pathogenesis. For a full description of the clubbing mechanism see 'Clubbing' in Chapter 3, 'Cardiovascular signs'.

It has been observed that patients with cyanotic heart disease commonly get clubbing and/or HPOA. It is thought that one or more factors, normally inactive in the lung, are shunted around the pulmonary vasculature via a congenital abnormality (e.g. ventricular septal defect) and are deposited in the periphery.

For example, it has been demonstrated in this setting that large platelets or megakaryocytes can gain access to the peripheral systemic circulation, rather than being broken down within the lung. Once in the extremities, they react with endothelial cells to release a variety of factors including bradykinin, platelet-derived growth factor (PDGF) and vascular endothelial growth factor (VEGF). This results in vascular hyperplasia and proliferation of periosteal layers.[71,72] This does not necessarily explain all occurrences of HPOA/clubbing and, ultimately, many mechanisms probably contribute, depending on underlying aetiology.

Other theories or observations include:

- increased exposure of peripheral tissues to VEGF,[73,74] either by ectopic or systemic production
- increased exposure of peripheral tissues to COX2-derived PGE2 generated by tumour or resulting inflammation[75]
- vagally mediated alterations in limb perfusion – vagotomy and sympatholytic drugs have been shown to reverse or improve HPOA.[74]

Lung cancer

In lung cancer, studies have shown more circulating VEGF[73,76] as well as VEGF deposition in clubbed digits. VEGF is known to produce angiogenesis and proliferation.

Sign value

HPOA is pathological and investigation as to cause is imperative, remembering it is not specific to one condition. It has been found to be a significant presenting feature in up to 20% of patients found to have lung cancer.[75]

For the value of clubbing as a sign refer to 'Clubbing' in Chapter 3, 'Cardiovascular signs'.

2

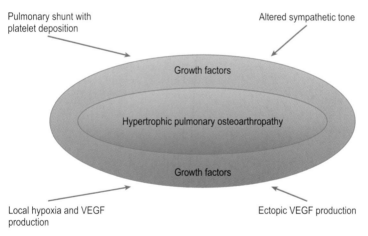

FIGURE 2.31
Factors involved in the mechanism of hypertrophic pulmonary osteoarthropathy

Hyperventilation

Description

Breathing that occurs in excess of metabolic requirements,[77] usually with an associated tachypnoea.

Condition/s associated with

There are many causes of hyperventilation. They can be broken down into three main categories:

- Psychogenic
  - » Anxiety
  - » Panic attacks
- Organic
  - » Asthma
  - » Pneumonia
  - » Bronchiectasis
  - » COPD
  - » Fibrosing alveolitis
  - » Pulmonary embolus
  - » Pain
  - » CNS disorders
  - » Hepatic disease

- Physiological
  - » Metabolic acidosis
  - » Pregnancy

Mechanism/s

There are many psychological and physical factors that can induce hyperventilation. Figure 2.32 (courtesy of Gardner)[77] demonstrates the different elements at play. A complete understanding of mechanisms for all aetiologies of hyperventilation is not generally necessary; however, there are some key components worth knowing.

Psychogenic

Hyperventilation may induce (as well as be induced by) feelings of anxiety. In patients with anxiety disorders, there is a predisposition to 'over-breathe' based on biological vulnerability, personality and cognitive variables.[78] For example, anxious patients may interpret non-specific chest pain as a heart attack, causing them to attach increased importance to the pain,

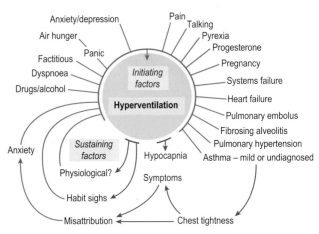

FIGURE 2.32
Factors involved in hyperventilation
Based on Gardner WN, Chest 1996; 109: 516–34.

stimulating the sympathetic nervous system and inducing tachypnoeas and hyperventilation. There is also evidence that these patients may have increased chemoreceptor sensitivity to carbon dioxide and, therefore, are more likely to over-breathe in response to a minor increase in carbon dioxide levels.

In panic disorders, the mechanism is unclear. As for anxiety, hyperventilation may induce a panic attack and vice versa. It is possible that there is a misinterpretation of physiological variables, leading to the brain believing suffocation is taking place, therefore inducing inappropriate hyperventilation as a response.[79]

Organic causes

Respiratory disease
The most researched example is asthma and, even so, the mechanism is inexact. Suggested contributing mechanism/s include:

- hypoxia stimulating hyperventilation via chemoreceptors
- hyperinflation causing stimulation of pulmonary receptors
- misinterpretation of symptoms – chest pain = heart attack, leading to a sympathetic response, tachypnoeas and hyperventilation (similar to anxiety).

Pulmonary embolism
In pulmonary embolism, the primary mechanism of hyperventilation is thought to be hypoxic drive via chemoreceptors.

CNS disorders
Brainstem injuries may cause altered breathing patterns (see 'Ataxic breathing' and 'Apneustic breathing' in this chapter and 'Cheyne–Stokes

breathing' in Chapter 3), most likely due to damage to the ventilatory centres. Hyperventilation has been associated with lesions in the pons, medulla and midbrain.

Hepatic disease
Idiopathic hyperventilation in patients with liver cirrhosis is well described and different from the arterial hypoxia and shortness of breath seen in hepatopulmonary syndrome.

Increased progesterone and oestradiol is well described in cirrhotic patients, owing to impaired breakdown. Progesterone is known to stimulate ventilation receptors in the central nervous system and hyperventilation.[80] Studies have shown a possible relationship between the increased progesterone and ventilation seen in cirrhotic patients, which may represent a possible mechanism for some degree of hyperventilation seen in cirrhotic patients.[81] Progesterone may also increase carbon dioxide sensitivity in cirrhotic patients, making them more prone to hyperventilation.

Physiological causes

Metabolic acidosis
Metabolic acidosis is a well-known cause of tachypnoea as the body attempts to 'blow off' carbon dioxide to reduce acidosis. It is an appropriate response to metabolic requirements and could be thought of in this way as opposed to grouping it with hyperventilation.

Pregnancy
During pregnancy, raised circulating progesterone combines with oestrogen to increase sensitivity to hypoxia, inducing increased ventilation by acting centrally and via the carotid body.[82]

Intercostal recession

VIDEO 2.6 ▶

Video 2.6 Access through Student Consult.

Description

This refers to the indrawn skin and soft tissue that can be seen in the intercostal spaces on inspiration during times of respiratory distress.

Condition/s associated with

Any form of respiratory distress including, but not limited to:

Common

- Hyaline membrane disease
- Pneumonia
- Bronchiolitis
- Anaphylaxis
- Croup
- Epiglottitis
- Foreign body inhalation

Mechanism/s

In times of increased respiratory effort or respiratory distress, there is increasingly negative intrathoracic pressure, pulling in the skin and soft tissues.

At these times, the accessory muscles are in use and there is a decrease in intrathoracic pressure above that present in normal inspiration. This decreased pressure 'sucks' skin and soft tissue inwards on inspiration, causing intercostal recession.

Sign value

Like accessory muscle usage, it is a non-specific sign of increased work of breathing, but nonetheless very important to notice and useful in monitoring in terms of whether treatment is improving the respiratory status of the patient.

CLINICAL PEARL

Kussmaul's breathing

VIDEO 2.7 ▶

Video 2.7 Access through Student Consult.

Description

Also described as 'air hunger', Kussmaul's breathing is typified by deep, rapid inspirations.

Condition/s associated with

Potentially any cause of metabolic acidosis.

More common

- Diabetic ketoacidosis
- Sepsis
- Lactic acidosis

Less common

- Severe haemorrhage
- Uraemia/renal failure
- Renal tubule acidosis (RTA)
- Salicylate poisoning
- Ethylene glycol poisoning
- Biliary/pancreatic fistulas
- Diarrhoea

Mechanism/s

Kussmaul's breathing is an adaptive response to metabolic acidosis. By producing deep, rapid inspirations, anatomical dead space is minimised, allowing for more efficient 'blowing off' of carbon dioxide, thus decreasing acidosis and increasing pH.

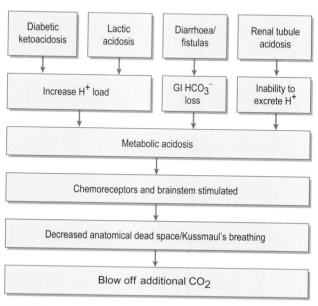

FIGURE 2.33
Kussmaul's respiration mechanism

Sign value

Although only a few studies have assessed the evidence base for Kussmaul's respiration, it is generally accepted that it is a useful sign. In children, an abnormal respiratory pattern like Kussmaul's respiration has been shown to be a very good sign of 5% or greater dehydration with a likelihood ratio of 2.0.[83]

Orthopnoea

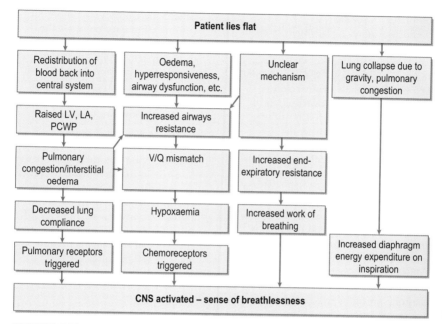

FIGURE 2.34
Mechanism of orthopnoea
LV = left ventricular; LA = left atrial; PCWP = pulmonary capillary wedge pressure.

Description

Dyspnoea that is made worse by lying in a supine position.

Although more often described as a symptom, as sleep studies become more common orthopnoea is increasingly being clinically observed. In either case, it is a useful discovery as the mechanism behind orthopnoea can assist understanding of underlying conditions.

Condition/s associated with

- Congestive heart failure (CHF)
- Bilateral diaphragm paralysis
- COPD
- Asthma

Congestive heart failure mechanism/s

Despite the fact that orthopnoea has been described in medicine for many years, its origin is still not absolutely clear. Figure 2.34 summarises the theories put forward to date.

The current accepted hypothesis for the triggering of orthopnoea is the redistribution of fluid from the splanchnic circulation and lower extremities into the central circulation which occurs while lying flat.[84]

In patients with impaired left ventricular function, the additional blood volume that is returned to the heart cannot be pumped out efficiently. Left ventricular, left atrial and, eventually, pulmonary capillary wedge

2

CLINICAL PEARL

pressure rises, resulting in pulmonary oedema, increased airways resistance, reduced lung compliance, stimulation of pulmonary receptors and, ultimately, dyspnoea.

Furthermore, replacement of air in the lungs with blood or interstitial fluid can cause a reduction of vital capacity, restrictive physiology and air trapping as a result of small airways closure.[84]

Alterations in the distribution of ventilation and perfusion result in relative V/Q mismatch, with consequent widening of the alveolar–arterial oxygen gradient, hypoxaemia and increased dead space.

Oedema of the bronchial walls can lead to small airways obstruction and produce wheezing ('cardiac asthma').[84]

When lying flat venous return is increased to the heart, increasing end–diastolic volume and pressure. The failing heart is unable to accommodate the increased venous return. End-diastolic pressures rise and are transmitted to the lungs, exacerbating a number of the above factors, and therefore producing orthopnoea.

Recent studies have found other factors that may contribute to orthopnoea in CHF patients:

- *Increased airflow resistance.* Studies have shown that airflow resistance is increased in patients with CHF when lying supine.[85] The reason for this is unclear. It may be due to increased airway hyper-responsiveness and/or airway dysfunction, bronchial mucosal swelling, thickening of the bronchial wall, peribronchial swelling and increased bronchial vein volume,[86] and loss of lung expansion forces due to loss of lung volume.

- *Increased expiratory flow limitation.* There is an increase in expiratory flow limitation in patients with CHF and this is aggravated when they lie flat,[86] making it more difficult for them to expel air from their lungs. Again, the cause of this is not clear. It is possible that when patients lie flat they lose more lung volume (as gravity collapses the lung), further impeding the ability to inspire and expire effectively. Another explanation is that blood redistributing in the lungs affects lung mechanics and increases the expiratory flow limitation.

- *Increased diaphragmatic energy expenditure.*[87] In patients with CHF who are lying flat, there appears to be a rise in diaphragmatic energy expenditure to help deal with the rise in resistive loads to the lung (which the inspiratory muscles must overcome). This increase in the work of the diaphragm also leads to orthopnoea.

Bilateral diaphragm paralysis mechanism/s

Bilateral diaphragm paralysis is a relatively rare cause of orthopnoea, but its presence can lead to prominent, immediate orthopnoea. Pathological states such as amyotrophic lateral sclerosis, trauma, spinal cord disease and multiple sclerosis lead to interruption or destruction of the phrenic nerve or its impulses, which stimulate the diaphragm to contract. When supine, the patient's abdominal contents move towards the head (due to gravity), resulting in decreased residual volume and severe dyspnoea. The diaphragm is unable to contract so cannot push the abdominal contents down.[88–90]

Orthopnoea due to bilateral diaphragm paralysis can be differentiated from that of congestive heart failure by its speed of onset (faster than congestive failure) and the presence of paradoxical abdominal movements.

COPD mechanism/s

Increased inspiratory effort owing to intrinsic PEEP and *increased airways resistance* in the supine position is proposed to contribute to orthopnoea in COPD.[91]

The destruction of lung architecture and premature airway closure on expiration, increased airway resistance and airway collapsibility present in COPD patients result in expiratory flow limitation at rest; that is, expiratory flow is at its maximum during tidal breathing and the only way it can be increased is by breathing at higher lung volumes (i.e. breathing at levels towards total lung capacity).[92]

One of the results of decreased expiratory flow is promotion of dynamic hyperinflation. This is a process where the COPD patient (who is already operating at higher lung volumes than normal), traps more gas as they breathe. This happens due to either increased respiratory rate and therefore decreased time to expire the gas, or increased flow limitation (mentioned above). This generates intrinsic PEEP or increased alveolar pressure at end expiration. As a result of higher end-expiratory pressures, more work is required to take in air on inspiration.

Dynamic flow limitation is exacerbated by lying flat, as is tidal breathing. It thus may contribute to hyperinflation, intrinsic PEEP, inspiratory work[92] and the development of orthopnoea. See Figure 2.35.

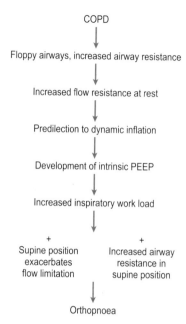

FIGURE 2.35
Mechanism of orthopnoea in COPD

Sign value

Orthopnoea is a valuable sign and relatively specific for congestive heart failure. Studies have shown a sensitivity of 42.8% and specificity of 87.51%, with a positive predictive value (PPV) of 14.5% and negative predictive value (NPV) of 96.9%.[93] As in paroxysmal nocturnal dyspnoea (PND), if the sign is absent, it can help exclude heart failure as a cause of breathlessness.

Paradoxical abdominal movements (also abdominal paradox)

Description

During normal inspiration, the diaphragm descends and the anterior abdominal wall moves outwards. For paradoxical abdominal movements to be present, the anterior abdominal wall must move outwards with expiration and inwards on inspiration.[94,95]

Condition/s associated with

- Neuromuscular disease – bilateral diaphragm weakness
- Diaphragmatic paralysis
- Diaphragmatic fatigue

Mechanism/s

When the diaphragm is paralysed or functionally impaired, breathing is dependent on the chest wall and intercostal muscles. The outward movement of the chest wall on inspiration draws the diaphragm and abdominal contents upwards, making the abdominal cavity pressure more negative, which pulls the abdominal wall inwards.[10] The weight of the abdominal contents contributes by pushing the diaphragm upwards.

Sign value

Paradoxical abdominal movements are nearly always pathological and should be investigated immediately.

Paradoxical respiration/ breathing

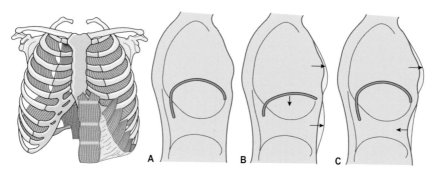

FIGURE 2.36
Normal mechanism of breathing and paradoxical breathing in neuromuscular respiratory failure
A Normal position of diaphragm; **B** normal mechanism: during inspiration, a downward movement of the diaphragm pushes the abdominal contents down and out as the rib margins are lifted and moved out, causing both the chest and abdomen to rise; **C** paradoxical breathing: with diaphragmatic weakness or paralysis, the diaphragm moves up rather than down during inspiration, and the abdomen moves in, contracting during chest rise.

Parrillo JE, Dellinger RP, Critical Care Medicine: Principles of Diagnosis and Management in the Adult, *4th edn, St Louis: Elsevier 2014: Fig 64.1.*

Description

Paradoxical breathing means the deflation of a lung, or a portion of a lung, during the phase of inspiration and the inflation of the lung during the phase of expiration. It may appear simply as inward movement of the chest on inspiration, instead of the normal outward expansion.

Condition/s associated with

Any cause of respiratory distress:

- COPD
- Pneumonia
- Airway obstruction
- Diaphragm paralysis
- Flail chest

Mechanism/s

As the diaphragm tires, the accessory muscles assume a larger role in breathing. In an effort to overcome airway obstruction, the accessory muscles produce greater negative intrathoracic pressure on inspiration. This negative pressure sucks the chest inwards on inspiration (particularly in children with compliant chest walls).

This negative pressure may also pull the diaphragm upwards, causing the abdomen to move inwards instead of out on inspiration (see 'Paradoxical abdominal movements' in this chapter).

Sign value

Paradoxical respiration is a sign of severe respiratory distress which requires immediate attention.

Paroxysmal nocturnal dyspnoea (PND)

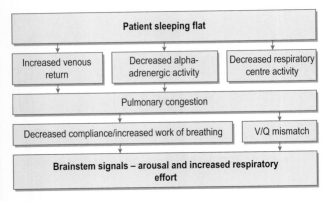

FIGURE 2.37
Mechanism of paroxysmal nocturnal dyspnoea

Description

PND is described as the sudden onset of breathlessness/respiratory distress occurring during sleep (and therefore usually at night). It may also manifest itself as coughing and wheezing fits. Classically described as a symptom, the phenomenon can be observed in the hospital setting.

Condition/s associated with

- Congestive heart failure (CHF)

Mechanism/s

Similar to orthopnoea, the mechanism has not been definitively proven. It is thought that PND occurs due to a combination of:

- increased venous return from the peripheries
- reduced adrenergic support of ventricular function that occurs during sleep – leading to the inability of the left ventricle to cope with the increased venous return.

This leads to pulmonary congestion, oedema and increased airways resistance

- normal nocturnal depression of the respiratory centre[84]
- increased pressure in the bronchial arteries, leading to airway compression.[96]

These factors cause decreased lung compliance, increased work of breathing and prompting of the pulmonary or chest wall receptors, which activate brainstem stimulation and arousal from sleep.

Alternatively, V/Q mismatch occurs causing a transient hypoxaemia that stimulates the brain to waken to correct the imbalance.

Sign value

PND is a valuable symptom/sign in assessing a patient for heart failure. With sensitivity of 37%, specificity of 89.8%, PPV of 15.3% and NPV of 96.7%, it is useful in ruling out heart failure if it is absent.[93]

Percussion

VIDEO 2.8 ▷

Video 2.8 Access through Student Consult.

The *act* of percussion is obviously not a sign; however, understanding its basis will aid interpretation of particular percussion notes, which *are* signs.

Percussion is traditionally said to produce three distinctive sounds:

1 tympany
2 resonance/hyper-resonance
3 dullness.

Different pathologies underlie the sounds that result from percussion of relevant organs. There are two theoretical mechanisms put forward to explain these sounds – the topographic percussion theory and the cage resonance theory. Anyone other than a respiratory physician would not be expected to know either, but they may assist the diligent percussor to better understand what they are doing and why.

Topographic percussion theory

The central idea in this theory is that only the physical characteristics of *tissues directly underneath* the percussive 'strike' determine the resulting sound. The body wall between the organ and percussor is not acknowledged as contributory, and the sound itself represents structures only to a depth of 4–6 cm underneath the location percussed.[97]

Cage resonance theory

Cage resonance theory states that the percussive note represents the *ease with which the body wall vibrates*. This is affected by the strength of the percussion strike, the state of the body wall and the *underlying organs*. Disease sites *distant* from the percussion strike *can* influence the note heard.[97]

Despite enthusiasm for the topographic percussion theory, the available evidence strongly supports cage resonance as the most likely mechanism.

Percussion: dullness

Description
On percussion of the chest wall and
lung fields, a shorter, dull sound of
high frequency is heard.

Condition/s associated with
• Pleural effusions
• Pneumonia

Mechanism/s
Pleural fluid dampens the normal
resonance of the lung fields, creating
the characteristic 'stony' dullness.

Sign value
Only a few variable quality studies exist
for dullness of percussion as a sign.
One review of three studies[98] found
dullness to conventional percussion one
of the best signs for predicting the
presence of a significant pleural
effusion, albeit with a wide confidence
interval (positive LR, 8.7; 95% CI,
2.2–33.8). Diacon[99] et al. compared
clinical examination to chest ultrasound
in locating pleural puncture sites with a
resulting sensitivity of 76%, specificity
of 60%, positive predictive value of
85% and negative predictive value of
45%. When compared to standard
chest radiography, the accuracy with
regard to pleural effusion is said to be
similar.[100]

Percussion: resonance/ hyper-resonance

Description

Low-pitched hollow sounds traditionally elicited over the lungs. Hyper-resonant sounds are louder and lower pitched than resonant sounds.

Condition/s associated with

- Normal lung fields – resonant
- Pneumothorax – hyper-resonant
- COPD – hyper-resonant

Mechanism/s

In hyper-resonance, over-inflated lungs allow better transmission of the low-frequency sound produced by the percussive tap.

Sign value

Hyper-resonance has been shown to have a PLR of 3.0 to 5.1 in detecting patients with chronic airflow obstruction.[101,102] It has a sensitivity and specificity of 42% and 86% respectively.[102]

In a study of 375 patients, hyper-resonance to percussion was the strongest predictor of COPD, with a sensitivity of only 20.8, but a specificity of 97.8, and likelihood ratio of 9.5.[103] After multivariate logistic regression, where pack-years, shortness of breath, and chest findings were among the explanatory variables, three physical chest findings were independent predictors of COPD, of which hyper-resonance to percussion yielded the highest odds ratio (OR = 6.7).

On a more practical level, hyper-resonance is extremely useful if a post-procedural patient develops shortness of breath or in any acute respiratory distress scenario prior to chest x-ray. Hyper-resonance in these settings requires assessment and management without delay (e.g. pneumothorax).

2

CLINICAL PEARL

Periodic breathing

Description

Believed to be a variant of Cheyne–Stokes respiration, it is characterised by regular, recurrent cycles of changing tidal volumes (TV) in which the lowest TV is less than half of the maximal TV.[104] It is also part of the spectrum of central sleep apnoea.

Condition/s associated with

- Stroke
- Subarachnoid haemorrhage
- Congestive heart failure

Mechanism/s

Thought to result from transient fluctuations or instabilities of an otherwise intact respiratory control system.[105]

Several models have been put forward to account for the described fluctuations, but central to all of them is that the pCO_2 transiently falls below the threshold to stimulate respiratory drive. Full details of the mechanisms underpinning Cheyne–Stokes breathing can be found in Chapter 3, 'Cardiovascular signs'.

In strokes and other neurological disorders, *transient disruptions of the ventilatory centres of the brainstem combined with a depressed level of consciousness* are key in the development of this breathing pattern.

Sign value

Frequently seen in patients with left ventricular heart disease, periodic breathing has been shown to be associated with lower left ventricular ejection fractions, lower cardiac indices,[106] higher capillary wedge pressures[107] and, if present at rest, this form of breathing powerfully predicts mortality.[108]

Periodic breathing may occur in up to 25% of patients following stroke.[104] It has been shown to occur if autonomic (insula) and volitional (cingulate cortex, thalamus) respiratory networks have been involved.[109]

Pigeon chest (pectus carinatum)

Description

Skeletal prominence of the chest caused by outward bowing of the sternum and costal cartilages.

Condition/s associated with

More common

- Familial
- Childhood chronic respiratory illness

Less common

- Rickets
- Marfan's syndrome

Mechanism/s

One theory has suggested that repeated contractions of the diaphragm (e.g. infections causing prolonged coughing) while the chest wall is still malleable push pliable bones outwards. Over time this causes an irreversible deformation.

Alternative theories include abnormal costal cartilage growth and sternal ossification abnormalities. The primary abnormality may vary on the subtype of carinatum.[110]

Sign value

Seen in approximately 1 in 1500 births,[111] pectus carinatum has limited value as a sign in identifying pathology. However, if seen in the context of respiratory illness or symptoms, there is value in identifying whether the abnormal structure is contributory.

2

Platypnoea/orthodeoxia

Description

Platypnoea or 'flat breathing' refers to shortness of breath while sitting or standing that is relieved by lying supine. It is the opposite of orthopnoea. Orthodeoxia refers to arterial desaturation noted when sitting up as opposed to lying down. These are not common signs but are quite striking when present.

Condition/s associated with

- Cardiac (intracardiac shunt)
  - » Atrial septal defect (ASD)
  - » Patent foramen ovale (PFO)
  - » Pneumonectomy

Usually associated with pulmonary hypertension or raised right atrial (RA) pressure (e.g. constrictive pericarditis, cardiac tamponade).

- Pulmonary (intrapulmonary right-to-left shunts)
  - » Hepatopulmonary syndrome
  - » Pulmonary diseases
  - » COPD
  - » Pulmonary embolism
- Upper airway tumour
  - » Acute respiratory distress syndrome
- Miscellaneous causes
  - » Autonomic neuropathy
  - » Acute respiratory distress syndrome (ARDS)

General mechanism/s

In general, *shunting of blood from the venous to the arterial system* can result in platypnoea/orthodeoxia. There are multiple ways in which this shunting may transpire and they are complex.[112]

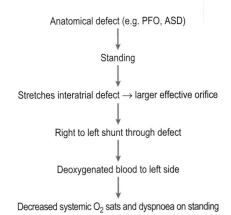

Anatomical defect (e.g. PFO, ASD)

↓

Standing

↓

Stretches interatrial defect → larger effective orifice

↓

Right to left shunt through defect

↓

Deoxygenated blood to left side

↓

Decreased systemic O_2 sats and dyspnoea on standing

FIGURE 2.38
Simplified mechanism of platypnoea/orthodeoxia

Cheng TO. Platypnea-orthodeoxia syndrome: etiology, differential diagnosis and management. Catheterization and Cardiovascular Interventions; *1999: 47: 64–66.*

For simplicity they may be divided into three categories: intracardiac shunts, pulmonary arteriovenous shunts or ventilation/perfusion mismatching.[113]

Intracardiac shunts (e.g. patent foramen ovale)

Under normal circumstances, the presence of a communication between the left and right sides of the heart would lead to left to right shunting, given that systemic pressures are higher than right-sided and pulmonary pressures. Bearing this in mind, it is proposed that a *second* functional and/or positional abnormality in/directly contributes to 'pushing' blood across the defect in a *right to left* shunt – resulting in platypnoea/orthodeoxia.[114]

Platypnoea may occur in patients with an isolated PFO or in patients with a PFO *and* secondary raised right atrial pressure. This is demonstrated in Figure 2.39. Some patients who

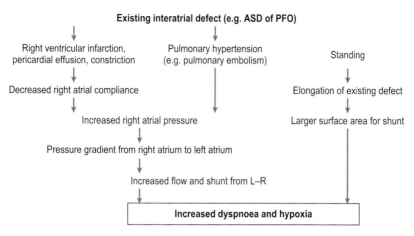

FIGURE 2.39
Mechanism of platypnoea/orthodeoxia

Cheng TO. Platypnea-orthodeoxia syndrome: etiology, differential diagnosis and management.
Catheterization and Cardiovascular Interventions; *1999: 47: 64–66.*

demonstrate platypnoea in the presence of a PFO may undergo a postural redirection of inferior vena cava (IVC) blood flow towards the atrial septum and left atrium.[112] Standing upright may stretch the interatrial communication (PFO) and allow for more streaming of venous blood from the IVC through the defect.

Changes in right atrial compliance and pressure may also facilitate increased right to left shunting and the development of platypnoea/orthodeoxia. For example, right ventricular infarction, pulmonary embolism, constrictive pericarditis or pericardial effusion can decrease right atrial compliance and increase pressure, which will contribute to further propulsion of blood across the existing defect.

Pneumonectomy

Pneumonectomy may cause increased right-sided pressures of the heart. The rise is due to the smaller pulmonary vascular bed present with a single lung. In time, the right ventricle may become less compliant than the left, elevating RV and RA pressures and producing a pressure gradient across

the atrial septal defect (ASD) or PFO, resulting in a right-to-left shunt and platypnoea.

Pulmonary arteriovenous shunts

Pulmonary arteriovenous malformations have been associated with platypnoea/orthodeoxia and are usually located in the lung bases. It is thought that when the patient sits or stands upright, increased blood flow through the basal malformations or shunts occurs due to gravity, leading to increased deoxygenated blood going to the left side of the heart, causing dyspnoea and hypoxaemia.

Hepatic

Platypnoea in liver disease is predominantly due to intrapulmonary shunting of deoxygenated blood and V/Q mismatch. The mechanism for this is multifaceted as hepatopulmonary syndrome has been shown to cause numerous pulmonary system changes which can result in altered oxygenation:[112]

- Diffuse intrapulmonary shunts are formed, mainly by pre-capillary and capillary vascular dilatations (some arteriovenous anastamoses are seen as well).[115]

- Impaired hypoxic vasoconstriction leads to deoxygenated blood passing through areas of poor gas exchange rather than being redistributed to areas of better ventilation.
- Development or worsening of V/Q mismatch.
- Pleural effusions and diaphragmatic dysfunction.

In addition to these factors, it is thought that while sitting up allows gravity to redistribute blood to the lung bases, where there are dilated pre-capillary beds, this also means that less oxygenation of blood occurs, producing hypoxaemia and dyspnoea.

It has also been shown that patients with hepatopulmonary syndrome have a hyperdynamic circulation and low pulmonary resistance, meaning there is less time for deoxygenated blood to become oxygenated in the lungs.

Pulmonary ventilation/ perfusion (V/Q) mismatching

Like the cardiac causes, pulmonary origins of platypnoea involve deoxygenated blood being shunted to the arterial system.

It is suggested that lung disease causes changes in lung mechanics, raised alveolar pressures, decreased pulmonary artery pressures leading to pulmonary artery compression and increased respiratory dead space[116] – all of which worsen V/Q mismatch and/or intrapulmonary shunts, resulting in platypnoea. When the patient is standing upright, right ventricular preload is reduced, resulting in lower output to the pulmonary arteries to the extent that alveolar pressure exceeds arterial and venous pressures. The upshot of this is that minimal blood flow is oxygenated and ventilated. Adding to this, standing and gravity cause more blood to flow to the basal segments of the lung, worsening the V/Q mismatch and causing increased dyspnoea.[113]

Sign value

Platypnoea is a rare but valuable sign; if seen it almost certainly indicates a pathology causing a shunt of blood from the venous to the arterial system.

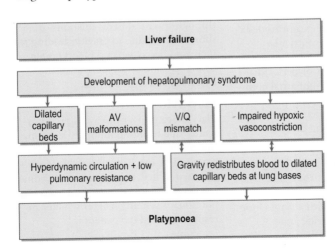

FIGURE 2.40
Mechanism of platypnoea in hepatopulmonary syndrome

Pleural friction rub

Description
A loud scratching, crackling sound heard over the lung tissue on auscultation that predominantly occurs in the expiratory phase.

Condition/s associated with

More common
- Pleurisy
- Lung cancer
- Pneumonia
- Pulmonary embolism

Less common
- Rheumatoid arthritis (RA)
- Systemic lupus erythematosus (SLE)
- Tuberculosis

Mechanism/s
The common pathway is inflammation of the pleura and loss of normal pleural lubrication.

A local process, such as one caused by infection, embolism or a systemic inflammatory state (as in RA or SLE) may result in inflammation of the pleural lining and the characteristic rubbing sound.

Pericardial or pleural rub?

Sometimes it may be difficult to determine whether a rub is pleural or pericardial, especially when some conditions may cause both and they are equally high pitched.
- *Pericardial rub*: Often has three distinct sounds – one in systole and two in diastole, which are *independent of respiration*. This rub is more 'distant' in nature and is best heard over the left lower sternal edge.
- *Pleural rub*: Generally composed of two sounds (during inspiration and expiration), this rub is *dependent on respiration* – so the sound will disappear if the patient holds his/her breath. A pleural rub sounds more superficial (i.e. closer to the chest wall).

Pursed-lip breathing (PLB)

Description

A breathing practice, often taught, which includes a long, slow expiration against pursed lips.

Condition/s associated with

- COPD

Mechanism/s

To understand the reason for pursed-lip breathing the pathophysiology behind chronic obstructive pulmonary disease must be appreciated. Inflammation of the airways ultimately leads to destruction of lung parenchyma and emphysema. The resultant reduction in elastic recoil, along with fibrosis and muscle hypertrophy, causes increased airways resistance and premature airway closing on expiration or *expiratory airflow limitation*. This results in air trapping at end expiration and, with time, hyperinflation. When coupled with periods of increased respiratory rate (during which the relative expiratory phase of respiration is short), dynamic hyperinflation occurs.

Pursing the lips allows the patient to *breathe against resistance*, thus maintaining a slow exhalation pressure within the lungs. This helps keep bronchioles and small airways open for much-needed oxygen exchange.[117,118] As such, it allows deeper breathing and improved V/Q matching.

PLB has been shown to have other physiological benefits:

- reduction in breathing frequency, a longer relative expiratory time and a reduction in intrinsic PEEP (i.e. gas trapping), and therefore less dynamic hyperinflation
- increased tidal volume
- increased expiratory airway pressure and therefore a reduction in expiratory airways collapse, expiratory flow limitation and airways resistance.[119]

Sign value

Pursed-lip breathing has become a therapeutic modality in patients with COPD to help alleviate dyspnoea. It has been shown to reduce respiratory rate and increase efficacy of ventilation, tidal volume and oxygen saturation.[120,121]

Sputum

Description

Matter/mucus ejected from the lungs, bronchi and trachea through the mouth.

Condition/s associated with

- COPD
- Pneumonia
- Tuberculosis (TB)
- Bronchiectasis
- Malignancy
- Cystic fibrosis
- Asthma

Mechanism/s

Mucus is produced by glands within the tracheobronchial tree. Irritants such as cigarette smoke or inflammation increase mucus production. Inflammation and irritation from a variety of causes can stimulate the cough reflex (see entry in this chapter) to bring up sputum.

Sign value

A very non-specific sign if produced in isolation from other signs, symptoms or history. However, a recent change in colour or quantity of sputum is worth investigating. Studies have shown:

- Sputum culture samples are of limited value in COPD unless the patient is not responding to antibiotics.[122]

- In patients with COPD, the presence of green (purulent) sputum was 94.4% sensitive and 77.0% specific for the yield of a high bacterial load, allowing timely identification of those who require antibiotics.[105]

- For patients producing white, cream or clear-coloured sputum, bacterial count was low and further testing was not warranted.[123]

- In the Australian COPDX guidelines, an increased volume and/or change of colour of sputum is used as a marker for an infective exacerbation of COPD.

- There is debate over the value of sputum and sputum Gram stain and cultures in community-acquired pneumonia.[124] One recent study[125] found sputum Gram stain to be a dependable test for early diagnosis of bacterial community-acquired pneumonia. This can assist with rational and appropriate initial antimicrobial therapy. However, there is a financial cost to the test and given that most community-acquired pneumonias are caused by streptococcus pneumonia, it may be argued that it is better to treat empirically and only test high-risk or difficult-to-treat cases.

- In tuberculosis endemic areas, sputum collection is a key tool in diagnosis and management. The diagnostic value of 'rust-coloured' sputum in TB is not clear. Microscopic examination of sputum is required.

Stertor

Description

A form of noisy breathing whose name derives from the Latin *stertere* ('to snore'), it is a sign easily appreciated with the naked ear. Unlike stridor, stertor does not have a musical quality, is low pitched and is heard only on inspiration. It is the type of breathing usually associated with nasal congestion and usually originates at the level of naso/oropharynx. It is most often heard in (and associated with) paediatric patients, especially infants, in part due to the smaller proportions of the associated anatomy.

Condition/s associated with

- Nasopharyngeal and/or oropharyngeal obstruction
- Nasal obstruction and deformity
- Adenoid hypertrophy
- Epiglottitis
- Glioma (if blocking nasal passage)

Mechanism/s

Stertor is caused by airway narrowing, causing airflow turbulence. It is usually due to oropharyngeal obstruction (i.e. above the level of the larynx). On inspiration, air flows through the extrathoracic airways into the lungs. When there is a narrowing or constriction (e.g. via inflammation), the velocity of flow through the obstruction increases and there is a pressure drop across the narrowing. This pressure drop causes the airway to narrow and/or collapse, then spring back open. The movement of the obstructed or inflamed airways, in conjunction with the pressure changes, produces the sounds of stertor.

Stridor

AUDIO 2.6 🔊

Audio 2.6 Access through Student Consult.

Description

Stridor (from the Latin *stridere*, 'to creak') is a loud, intense, monophasic sound with constant pitch. It is best heard over the extrathoracic airways and is most commonly inspiratory, but may be expiratory or biphasic in timing if a lesion below the level of the larynx is present.

Condition/s associated with

Any form of upper airway obstruction.

More common

- Foreign body
- Croup
- Peritonsillar abscess
- Aspiration

Less common

- Laryngomalacia – chronic, low-pitched stridor, most common form of inspiratory stridor in neonates
- Subglottic stenosis – chronic, common form of biphasic stridor
- Vocal cord dysfunction – chronic, common form of biphasic stridor
- Laryngeal haemangiomas
- Tracheomalacia and bronchiomalacia – expiratory stridor
- Epiglottitis

Mechanism/s

Any obstruction in the extrathoracic airways (supraglottis, glottis, subglottis

TABLE 2.5
Type of stridor and location of obstruction

Stridor type	Obstruction location
Inspiratory	Laryngeal/supraglottic lesion
Expiratory	Tracheobronchial lesion – below thoracic inlet
Biphasic	Subglottic/glottic to tracheal ring

and/or trachea) causes *narrowing and flow turbulence*. In addition, as with stertor, narrowing causes an increase in flow velocity and a pressure drop across the narrowing, causing further narrowing or temporary closure of the airway, contributing to the production of the sound (see Table 2.5).

Characteristics of stridor

The volume, pitch and phase of stridor can be helpful if attempting to localise the obstruction:[126]

- *Volume:* stridor is believed to represent a significant narrowing of the airway,[126] but a sudden drop in volume may indicate impending airway collapse.[127]

- *Pitch:*
  » High-pitched stridor is usually caused by obstruction at the level of the glottis.[128]
  » Lower-pitched stridor is often caused by higher lesions in the nose, nasopharynx and supraglottic larynx.[129]
  » Intermediate pitch usually signifies obstruction at the subglottis or below.[129]

CLINICAL PEARL

- *Phase:*
  - » Inspiratory – the obstruction is usually above the glottis.[130]
  - » Biphasic – fixed obstruction at the glottis or subglottis down to tracheal ring.[126]
  - » Expiratory – suggests collapse of the lower airways below the thoracic inlet.[126]

Sign value

Stridor is a valuable sign that can quickly identify upper airways obstruction. Once heard it is never forgotten. It must be investigated and managed quickly.

Subcutaneous emphysema/ surgical emphysema

2

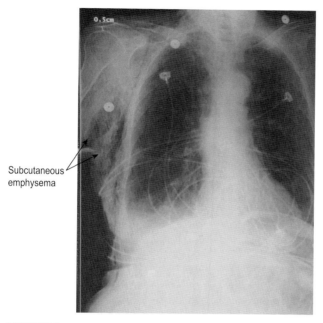

FIGURE 2.41
X-ray of subcutaneous emphysema

Reproduced, with permission, from Roberts JR, Hedges JR, Clinical Procedures in Emergency Medicine, *5th edn, Philadelphia: Saunders, 2009: Fig 10-12.*

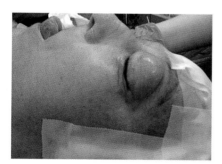

FIGURE 2.42
Subcutaneous emphysema of the eyelid

Girnius AK, Ortega R, Chin LS. Subcutaneous emphysema of the eyelid on emergence from general anesthesia after a craniotomy. Journal of Clinical Anesthesia *2010; 22(5): Fig 1, Elsevier.*

Description

Air or gas present within the subcutaneous layer of the skin. On palpation there will be a crackling feeling (much like pressing bubble wrap) along with obvious changes to the skin texture.

Condition/s associated with

Blunt or sharp trauma causing puncture of gastrointestinal organs or lungs.

- Pneumothorax
- Pneumomediastinum
- Barotrauma
- Oesophageal rupture

Mechanism/s

Subcutaneous emphysema is caused by air or gas reaching the subcutaneous layer of the skin.

Skin from the neck, mediastinum and retroperitoneal space is *connected by fascial planes* and it is these planes that allow air to track from one space to another.[131]

Typically, subcutaneous emphysema is caused by sharp or blunt trauma to the lungs. If the lung is punctured (whether at the parietal or visceral pleura), air is able to track up the peri-vascular sheaths, into the mediastinum and from there enter subcutaneous tissues.

Similarly, in barotrauma, excess pressure in the lungs may cause the alveoli to burst, allowing air to travel below the visceral pleura, up to the hilum of the lung, along the trachea and into the neck.

Sign value

A valuable sign; subcutaneous emphysema in the presence of chest wall trauma usually indicates a more serious thoracic injury involving an air-containing structure of the thorax.[132]

Tachypnoea

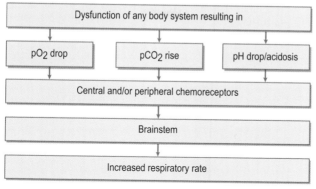

FIGURE 2.43
Simplified mechanism of tachypnoea

Description

A respiratory rate measured above 20 breaths per minute.

Condition/s associated with

Tachypnoea may be produced by many different system pathologies including:

- Cardiac
- Respiratory
- CNS
- Infectious
- Psychogenic
- Pain

Mechanism/s

Any state causing a derangement in oxygen (hypoxia), pCO_2 (hypercapnia) or acid/base status (acidosis) will stimulate respiratory drive and increase respiratory rate.

Tachypnoea occurs *in most situations as a compensatory response to either a drop in pO_2 (hypoxaemia) or a rise in pCO_2 (hypercapnia)*. Central chemoreceptors in the medulla and peripheral chemoreceptors in the aortic arch and carotid body measure a combination of these variables and send messages to the central ventilatory systems to increase respiratory rate and tidal volume to compensate for any fluctuations.[133]

Sign value

Tachypnoea is a very valuable vital sign and is unfortunately often neglected when routine observations are performed. Studies reviewing tachypnoea have shown:

- Predicting cardiopulmonary arrest – sensitivity of 0.54, specificity of 0.83, odds ratio of 5.56.[134]
- In unstable patients, the change in respiratory rate is better at predicting an at-risk patient than heart rate or blood pressure.[135]
- Unwell patients with a higher respiratory rate had a higher risk of death.[136]
- Over half of all patients suffering a serious adverse event on general hospital wards had a respiratory rate greater than 24 breaths/minute.[137]

2

CLINICAL PEARL

- In predicting negative outcomes (ICU admission or death) in community-acquired pneumonia, respiratory rate of greater than 27 had sensitivity of 70%, specificity of 67%, PPV of 27% and NPV of 93%.[133]

New onset or change in rate of tachypnoea requires quick and thorough investigation. It may herald ominous decompensation.

Tracheal tug

VIDEO 2.10 ▷

Video 2.10 Access through Student Consult.

Description

Downward displacement of the thyroid cartilage during inspiration.

Condition/s associated with

Most common

- Respiratory distress/COPD (Campbell's sign)

Less common

- Arch of aorta aneurysm (Oliver's sign)

Mechanism/s

Tracheal tug – Campbell's sign

Patients in respiratory distress have increased work of breathing and the *movements of the chest wall, muscles and diaphragm* are transmitted along the trachea, pulling it rhythmically downwards.

An alternative cause of tracheal tug occurs in patients who have *intercostal weakness but preserved diaphragmatic*

strength. This can be caused by muscle relaxants and deep sedation from anaesthetic agents and is due to the unopposed action of the crura pulling on the diaphragm, which also pulls the pericardium and lung structures during inspiration.

Tracheal tug – Oliver's sign

Tracheal tug in this situation refers to downward displacement of the cricoid cartilage in time with ventricular contraction, in the presence of an aortic arch aneurysm. With the patient's chin lifted, the clinician can grasp the cricoid cartilage and push it upwards. This movement brings the aortic arch and the aortic aneurysm (if present) closer to the left main bronchus (which it overrides). The pulsation of the aorta and the aneurysm is then transmitted up the bronchus to the trachea, creating Oliver's sign.

Sign value

There is limited evidence as to value; however, tracheal tug is generally accepted as a sign of increased work of breathing.

Oliver's sign is much rarer than the tracheal tug seen with COPD and/or respiratory distress.

Trepopnoea

Description

Dyspnoea which is worse when the patient is lying on one side (in lateral decubitus position), which is relieved by lying on the opposite side.

Condition/s associated with

- Unilateral lung disease
- Congestive heart failure – dilated cardiomyopathy
- Lung tumour

Mechanism/s

Unilateral lung disease

When the patient lies on the side of the 'good' lung, gravity increases blood flow to the lower lung and improves oxygenation.

Congestive heart failure

These patients prefer to lie on their right side. The cause of this preference is as yet unclear.

Recent studies[138] suggest that lying on the right side enhances *venous return and sympathetic activity*. It is also thought that the right lateral position allows changes to the *hydrostatic forces* on the right and left ventricles, which can reduce lung congestion.

Other potential contributing factors include:[139]

- positional improvements in lung mechanics – the enlarged heart is not causing atelectasis by pushing on the lung
- less airway compression
- in patients with decreased compliance of the left ventricle, its compression has a greater impact on filling pressures. This occurs when lying in the left lateral position.

Lung tumour

Gravity causes tumours to compress the lungs and/or vasculature, depending on location. Therefore, a tumour of sufficient size in a significant site can cause a transient V/Q mismatch, hypoxia/hypercarbia and breathlessness.

Sign value

There is limited evidence on the sensitivity and specificity values; however, trepopnoea is pathological and requires investigation. A recent small study has suggested that trepopnoea in heart failure may be more common than initially thought and is present in up to 51% of patients.

Vocal fremitus/tactile fremitus

Description

The vibration felt when placing the hands on the back of a patient and asking them to speak (usually the phrase 'ninety-nine'). The vibration is decreased in bigger areas of air, fat, fluid or tumour, whereas it is increased in areas of consolidation. Symmetrical fremitus may be physiological, whereas asymmetrical fremitus should always be considered abnormal.

Condition/s associated with

- Pneumonia – increased vocal fremitus
- Pneumothorax – decreased fremitus
- Pleural effusion – decreased fremitus
- COPD – decreased fremitus
- Tumour

Mechanism/s

As discussed in 'Vocal resonance' in this chapter, variation in vocal fremitus can be explained by the manner in which various *voice frequencies are transmitted through tissue or fluid*.

In pneumonia, consolidation *augments lower frequencies* (such as the human voice) and thus is more likely to be felt as a stronger vibration. Large pleural effusions decrease the *transmission of low frequencies* and thus diminish vocal fremitus.

Sign value

See box under 'Vocal resonance'.

2

Vocal resonance

Description

Vocal resonance refers to the character of the patient's voice heard with the stethoscope over the posterior lung fields. Normally a patient's voice is muffled and difficult to understand in this situation but in consolidated areas it will be heard clearly.

Classically, the changes in vocal resonance seen with disease are:

- bronchophony – voice is louder than normal
- pectoriloquy – whispered words are clearly heard, also called 'whispering pectoriloquy'
- aegophony – the voice has a nasal, bleating quality (like a goat); implies high resonance.

Condition/s associated with

Changes in vocal resonance are classically associated with:

- Consolidation: tumour, pneumonia
- Pleural effusion

Mechanism/s

The differences in vocal resonance are determined by the *transmission frequency (Hz)* and the physical properties of

Inflammation, consolidation and pus
↓
Transmission of low and high frequencies
↓
Increased vocal resonance

FIGURE 2.44
Mechanism of increased vocal resonance

normal lungs, fluid and consolidation. These elements are common to the mechanism/s of '*breath sounds*'.

Normal lung tissue filters out lower-frequency sounds and transmits high-frequency sounds.[10] Human voices are *generally lower in frequency* and, therefore, are not well transmitted.

Consolidated lungs transmit *low and higher frequencies effectively* and so a patient's voice is heard clearly and easily over a consolidated area.

Large effusions (due to the physical properties of fluid) *reduce the transmission of lower frequencies*[11,140,141] and therefore voices are muffled or less audible.

Sign value

In patients with cough and fever, aegophony has very good specificity for detecting pneumonia – sensitivity of 4–16%, specificity of 96–99%.[11]

Vocal fremitus versus vocal resonance

Vocal fremitus and resonance are always taught but probably under-utilised as clinical signs. One study[10] looking at pleural effusions showed the following diagnostic utility:
- *Reduced vocal fremitus*: sensitivity 82%, specificity 86%, PPV 0.59, NPV 0.95, PLR 5.67, NLR 0.21
- *Reduced vocal resonance*: sensitivity 76%, specificity 88%, PPV 0.62, NPV 0.94, PLR 6.49, NLR 0.27.

CLINICAL PEARL

Wheeze

Description

Continual high-pitched 'musical' sounds heard at the end of inspiration or at the start of expiration.

Condition/s associated with

- Asthma
- Respiratory tract infections
- COPD
- Foreign body aspiration: bronchial foreign bodies in children may present with a 'triad' of unilateral wheeze + cough + decreased breath sounds.

Mechanism/s

Airway narrowing allows airflow-induced oscillation of airway walls, producing acoustic waves.[142] As the airway lumen becomes smaller, the airflow velocity increases, resulting in vibration of the airway wall and the tonal quality.

Sign value

A wheeze on normal quiet expiration or inspiration is most likely pathological. The longer and more high pitched the wheeze, the more severe the obstruction is.[143] Changes of extent and pitch[144] should be monitored when assessing response to treatment in chronic obstructive pulmonary disease. Wheeze monitoring has also been used to good effect in assessing asthma severity and response to treatment.[145]

Remember that having a wheeze implies that the patient has enough air movement to produce one. Beware the wheezing patient who suddenly becomes silent, as this may mean air movement is so *low* that a wheeze cannot be produced. If this happens, respiratory arrest may be imminent.

Monophonic versus polyphonic wheeze

Monophonic wheeze

A wheeze with a single note that starts and ends at different points in time. The classic example is caused by a tumour in the bronchi. The pitch and timing is fixed as the tumour itself is static.

A child with a fixed foreign body may have a monophonic wheeze.

Polyphonic wheeze

A wheeze with several different tones starting and finishing at the same time. It is heard when a fixed compression occurs in multiple bronchi at the same time. Can be present in COPD and in healthy people at end expiration. It is caused by second- or third-order bronchi closing at the same time at end expiration, as the pressures within the airway keeping them patent are reduced.

References

1. O'Neill S, McCarthy DS. Postural relief of dyspnoea in severe chronic airflow limitation: relationship to respiratory muscle strength. *Thorax* 1983;**38**:595–600.

2. Mattos WL, et al. Accuracy of clinical examination findings in the diagnosis of COPD, but the interrelator reliability was poor. *J Bras Pneumol* 2009;**35**(5):404–8.

3. Perkin RM, Resnik DB. The agony of agonal respirations: is the last gasp necessary? *J Med Ethics* 2002;**28**:164–9.

4. Perkins GD, Walker G, Christensen K, Hulme J, Monsieurs KG. Teaching recognition of agonal breathing improves accuracy of diagnosing cardiac arrest. *Resuscitation* 2006;**70**:432–7.

5. Roppolo LP, Westfall A, Pepe PE, et al. Dispatcher assessments for agonal breathing improve detection of cardiac arrest. *Resuscitation* 2009;**80**(7):769–72.

6. Mador JM, Tobin MJ. Apneustic breathing: a characteristic feature of brainstem compression in achrondroplasia? *Chest* 1990;**97**(4):877–83.

7. Eckert DJ, Jordan AS, Merchia P, Malhotra A. Central sleep apnoea: pathophysiology and treatment. *Chest* 2007;**131**:595–607.

8. Douglas BT, Phillipson EA. Chapter 74: Sleep disorders. In: Mason RJ, Murray JF, Broaddus VC, Nadal JA, editors. *Murray and Nadal's Respiratory Medicine*. 4th ed. 2010. Available: http://www.mdconsult.com.ezproxy1.library.usyd.edu.au/das/book/body/185300500-5/957919650/1288/689.html#4-u1.0-B0-7216-0327-0..50077-X-cesec7_4145 [28 Feb 2011].

9. Gokula RM, Khasnis A. Asterixis. *J Postgrad Med* 2003;**49**:272–5.

10. Kalantri S, Joshi R, Lokhande T, et al. Accuracy and reliability of physical signs in the diagnosis of pleural effusion. *Respir Med* 2007;**101**:431–8.

11. McGee S. *Evidence Based Physical Diagnosis*. 2nd ed. St Louis: Saunders; 2007.

12. Ashutosh K, Gilbert R, Auchincloss JH, Peppi D. Asynchronous breathing movements in patients with chronic obstructive pulmonary disease. *Chest* 1975;**67**:553–7.

13. Gilbert R, Ashutosh K, Auchincloss JH, et al. Prospective study of controlled oxygen therapy: poor prognosis of patients with asynchronous breathing. *Chest* 1977;**71**:456–62.

14. Frank JI. Abnormal breathing patterns. In: Hanley DF, Einhaupl KM, Bleck TP, Diringer MN, editors. *Neurocritical care*. Heidelberg: Springer-Verlag; 1994. p. 366.

15. Howard RS, Rudd AG, Wolfe CD, et al. Pathophysiological and clinical aspects of breathing after stroke. *Postgrad Med J* 2001;**77**:700–2.

16. North JB, Jennett S. Abnormal breathing patterns associated with acute brain damage. *Arch Neurol* 1974;**31**:338.

17. Silbernagl S, Lang F. *Color Atlas of Pathophysiology*. New York: Thieme; 2010. p. 82.

18. Mangione S. *Physical Diagnosis Secrets*. 2nd ed. St Louis: Elsevier; 2007.

19. Gnitecki J, Moussavi Z. Separating heart sounds from lung sounds. *IEEE Eng Med Biol Mag* 2007;**26**(1):20–9.

20. Loudon R, Murphy RLH. State of the art: lung sounds. *Am Rev Respir Dis* 1984;**130**:663–73.

21. Stahlheber C, et al. Breath sound assessment. Available: http://emedicine.medscape.com/article/1894146-overview#showall [17 Sept 2014].

22. Bohadana A, Izbicki G, Kraman S. Fundamentals of lung auscultation. *NEJM* 2014;**370**(21):744–51.

23. Ceresa CC, Johnston I. Auscultation in the diagnosis of the respiratory disease in the 21st century. *Postgrad Med J* 2008;**84**:393–4.

24. Schreur HJ, Sterk PJ, Vanderschoot J, et al. Lung sound intensity in patients with emphysema and in normal subjects at standardised airflows. *Thorax* 1992;**47**:674–9.

25. Gurugn A, et al. Computerized lung sound analysis as diagnostic aid for the detection of abnormal lung sounds: A systematic review and meta-analysis. *Respir Med* 2011;**105**(9):1396–403.

26. Pardee NE, Martin CJ, Morgan EH. A test of the practical value of estimating breath sound intensity. Breath sounds are related to measured ventilatory function. *Chest* 1976;**70**(3):341–4.

27. Canning BJ. Anatomy and neurophysiology of the cough flex. *Chest* 2006;**129**:33S–47S.

28. Polverino M, et al. Anatomy and neuro-pathophysiology of the cough reflex arc. *Multidiscip Respir Med* 2012;**7**:5.

29. McCool D. Global physiology and pathophysiology of cough. *Chest* 2006;**129**:48S–53S.

30. Kvale PA. Chronic cough due to lung tumours; ACCP evidence based clinical practice guidelines. *Chest* 2006;**129**:147S–153S.

31. Chang AB, Landau LI, Van Asperen PP, et al. Cough in children: definitions and clinical evaluation. *Med J Aust* 2006;**184**(8):398–403.

32. Dalmasso F, et al. A computer system for timing and acoustical analysis of crackles: a study in cryptogenic fibrosing alveolitis. *Bull Eur Physiopathol Respir* 1984;**20**:139–3.

33. Piirila P, Sovijarvi ARA. Crackles: recording, analysis and clinical significance. *Eur Respir J* 1995;**8**:2139–48.

34. Nath AR, Capel LH. Inspiratory crackles – early and late. *Thorax* 1974;**29**:223.

35. Piirila P. *Acoustic properties of cough and crackling lung sounds in patients with pulmonary diseases. Doctoral thesis.* Helsinki: Helsinki University; 1992 ISBN 951-801-900-2.

36. Vyshedskiy A, Alhashem RM, Paciej R, et al. Mechanism of inspiratory and expiratory crackles. *Chest* 2009;**135**(1):156–64.

37. Badgett RG, Tanaka DJ, Hunt DK, et al. Can moderate chronic obstructive pulmonary disease be diagnosed by historical and physical findings alone? *Am J Med* 1993;**94**:188–96.

38. Cottin V, Cordier J-F. Velcro crackles: The key for early diagnosis of idiopathic pulmonary fibrosis? *Eur Respir J* 2012;**40**(3):519–21.

39. Al Jarad N, Strickland B, Bothamley G, et al. Diagnosis of asbestosis by a time expanded wave form analysis, auscultation and high resolution computed tomography: a comparative study. *Thorax* 1993;**48**:347–53.

40. McGee S. *Evidence Based Physical Diagnosis.* 3rd ed. St Louis: Elsevier; 2012.

41. Murphy RL Jr, et al. Crackles in the early diagnosis of asbestosis. *Am Rev Respir Dis* 1984;**129**:375–9.

42. Marques A. Are crackles an appropriate outcome measure for airway clearance techniques. *Respir Care* 2012;**57**(9):1468–75.

43. Ponte D, et al. Characterisation of crackles from patients with fibrosis, heart failure and pneumonia. *Med Eng Phys* 2013;**35**:448–56.

44. Flietstra B, et al. Automated analysis of crackles in patients with interstitial pulmonary fibrosis. *Pulm Med* 2011;**2011** doi: 10.1155/2011/590506.

45. Marques A, et al. Computerised adventitious respiratory sounds as outcome measures for respiratory therapy: a systematic review. *Respir Care* 2014;**59**(5):765–76.

46. Miller PE, Houston BA. Dahl's sign. *N Engl J Med* 2014;**371**:357. doi:10.1056/NEJMicm1309904.

47. Sharp JT, Druz WS, Moisan T, Foster J, Machnach W. Postural relief of dyspnea in severe chronic obstructive pulmonary disease. *Am Rev Respir Dis* 1980;**122**:201–11.

48. Meysman M, Vincken W. Effect of body posture on spirometric values and upper airway obstruction indices derived from the flow-volume loop in young nonobese subjects. *Chest* 1998;**114**:1042–7.

2

49. Bhatt SP, et al. Effect of tripod position on objective parameters of respiratory function in stable chronic obstructive pulmonary disease. *Indian J Chest Dis Allied Sci* 2009;**51**(2):83–5.

50. Kim K-S, et al. Effects of breathing maneuver and sitting posture on muscle activity in inspiratory accessory muscles in patients with chronic obstructive pulmonary disease. *Multidiscip Respir Med* 2012;**7**:9.

51. Scano G, Ambrosino N. Pathophysiology of dyspnoea. *Lung* 2002;**180**:131–48.

52. Manning HL, Schwartzstein RM. Pathophsyiology of dyspnoea. *N Engl J Med* 1995;**133**(23):1547–53.

53. Chanon T, Mullholland MB, Leitner J, Altose MD, Cherniack NS. Sensation of dyspnoea during hypercapnia, exercise and voluntary hyperventilation. *J Appl Physiol* 1990;**68**:2100–6.

54. O'Donnell DE, Sannii R, Anthonisen NR, Younes M. Expiratory resistance loading in patients with severe chronic airflow limitation: an evaluation of ventilatory mechanics and compensatory responses. *Am Rev Resp Dis* 1987;**138**:1185–91.

55. Schwartzstein R, Stoller JK, Hollingsworth H. Physiology of dyspnoea. *Uptodate* November 2009;version 19.1.

56. Clark AL, Peipoli M, Coats AJ. Skeletal muscle and the control of ventilation on exercise: evidence of metabolic receptors. *Eur J Clin Invest* 1996;**25**:299.

57. Clark A, Volterrani M, Swan JW, et al. Leg blood flow, metabolism and exercise in chronic stable heart failure. *Int J Cardiol* 1996;**55**:127.

58. Sajkov D, Latimer K, Petrovsky N. Dyspnea in pulmonary arterial hypertension, pulmonary hypertension. In: Sulica R, Preston I, editors. *Bench Research to Clinical Challenges, InTech.* 2011. pp. 191–208 http://www.intechopen.com/articles/show/title/dyspnea-in-pulmonary-arterial-hypertension.

59. Sun X-G, et al. Exercise physiology in patients with primary pulmonary hypertension. *Circulation* 2001;**104**:429–35.

60. Ahmed A, Allman RM, Aronow WS, DeLong JF. Diagnosis of heart failure in older adults: predictive value of dyspnoea at rest. *Arch Gerontol Geriatr* 2004;**38**(3): 297–307.

61. Koumbourlis AC. Pectus excavatum: pathophysiology and clinical characteristics. *Paediatr Respir Rev* 2009;**10**(1):3–6.

62. Nakaoka T, Uemura S, Yano T, Nakagawa Y, Tanimoto T, Suehiro S. Does overgrowth of costal cartilage cause pectus excavatum? A study on the lengths of ribs and costal cartilage in asymmetric patients. *J Paediatr Surg* 2009;**44**(7):1333–6.

63. Shamberger RC. Congenital chest wall deformities. *Curr Probl Surg* 1996;**33**(6):469–542.

64. Kelly RE. Pectus excavatum: historical background, clinical picture, preoperative evaluation and criteria for operation. *Semin Pediatr Surg* 2008;**17**(3):181.

65. Mathers LH, Frankel LR. Stabilization of the critically ill child. In: Behrman RE, Kliegman RM, Jenson HB, editors. *Nelson Textbook of Pediatrics.* 17th ed. Philadelphia: WB Saunders; 2003. pp. 279–96.

66. Ely E. Grunting respirations: sure distress. *Nursing* 1989;**19**(3):72–3.

67. Bidwell JL, Pachner RW. Haemoptysis: diagnosis and management. *Am Fam Physician* 2005;**77**(7):1253–60.

68. Gilmartin JJ, Gibson GJ. Mechanisms of paradoxical rib motion in patients with chronic obstructive pulmonary disease. *Am Rev Respir Dis* 1986;**134**:683–7.

69. Gilmartin JJ, Gibson GJ. Abnormalities of chest wall motion in patients with chronic airflow obstruction. *Thorax* 1984;**39**:264–71.

70. Garcia-Pachon E. Paradoxical movement of the lateral rib margin (Hoover's sign) for detecting obstructive airway disease. *Chest* 2002;**122**:651–5.

71. Martinez-Lavin M, Vargas AL, Rivera-Viñas M. Hypertrophic osteoarthropathy: a palindrome with a pathogenic condition. *Curr Opin Rheumatol* 2008;**20**:88–91.

72. Martinez-Lavin M. Exploring the cause of the oldest clinical sign of medicine: finger clubbing. *Semin Arthritis Rheum* 2007;**36**:380–5.

73. Olan F, Portela M, Navarro C, et al. Circulating vascular endothelial growth factor concentrations in a case of pulmonary hypertrophic osteoarthropathy. Correlation with disease activity. *J Rheumatol* 2004;**31**:614–16.

74. Dhawan R, Mehwish AK. Hypertrophic osteoarthropathy. *Medscape* 2014; http://emedicine.medscape.com/article333735 [29 Sept 2014].

75. Kozak KR, et al. Hypertrophic osteoarthropathy pathogenesis: a case highlighting the potential role for cyclooxygenase-2-derived prostaglandin E2. *J Thorac Oncol* 2012;**7**(12):1877–8.

76. Silveira L, Martínez-Lavín M, Pineda C, et al. Vascular endothelial growth factor in hypertrophic osteoarthropathy. *Clin Exp Rheumatol* 2000;**18**:57–62.

77. Gardner WN. The pathophysiology of hyperventilation disorders. *Chest* 1996;**109**:516–34.

78. Bass C, Kartsounis L, Lelliott P. Hyperventilation and its relationship to anxiety and panic. *Integr Psych* 1987;**5**:274–91.

79. Klein DF. False suffocation alarms, spontaneous panics and related conditions. *Arch Gen Psychiatry* 1993;**50**:306–17.

80. Lustik LJ. The hyperventilation of cirrhosis: progesterone and estradiol effects. *Hepatology* 1997;**25**(1):55–8.

81. Passino C, et al. Abnormal hyperventilation in patients with hepatic cirrhosis: role of enhanced chemosensitivity to carbon dioxide. *Int J Cardiol* 2012;**54**(1):22–6.

82. Hannhart B, Pickett CK, Moore LG. Effects of estrogen and progesterone on carotid body neural output responsiveness to hypoxia. *J Appl Physiol* 1990;**68**:1909–16.

83. Steiner MJ, DeWalt DA, Byerley JS. Is this child dehydrated? *JAMA* 2004;**291**:2746–54.

84. Kusumoto FM. Chapter 10: Cardiovascular disorders: heart disease. In: McPhee SJ, Hammer GD, editors. *Pathophysiology of Disease: An Introduction to Clinical Medicine.* 6th ed. 2010. Available: http://www.accesspharmacy.com/content.aspx?aID=5367630 [13 Mar 2011].

85. Yap JC, Moore DM, Cleland JG, et al. Effect of supine posture on respiratory mechanics in chronic left ventricular failure. *Am J Respir Crit Care Med* 2000; **162**(4 Pt 1):1285–91.

86. Duguet A, Tantucci C, Lozinguez O, et al. Expiratory flow limitation as a determinant of orthopnea in acute left heart failure. *J Am Coll Cardiol* 2000;**35**:690–700.

87. Nava S, Larvovere M, Fanfulla F, et al. Orthopnea and inspiratory effort in chronic heart failure patients. *Respir Med* 2003;**97**(6):647–53.

88. Yelgec NS, et al. Severe orthopnea is not always due to heart failure: a case of bilateral diaphragm paralysis. *J Emerg Med* 2013;**45**(6):922–3.

89. Kumar N, Folger WN, Bolton CF. Dyspnea as the predominant manifestation of bilateral phrenic neuropathy. *Mayo Clin Proc* 2004;**79**:1563–5.

90. Celli BR. Respiratory management of diaphragm paralysis. *Semin Respir Crit Care Med* 2002;**23**:275–81.

91. Loubna E, et al. Orthopnea and tidal expiratory flow limitation in patients with stable COPD. *Chest* 2001;**119**(1):99–104.

92. Tantucci C. Expiratory flow limitation definition, mechanisms, methods, and significance. *Pulm Med* 2013;**2013**.

93. Ekundayo OJ, Howard VJ, Safford MM, et al. Value of orthopnea, paroxysmal nocturnal dyspnoea, and medications in prospective population studies of incident heart failure. *Am J Cardiol* 2009;**104**(2):259–64.

94. Mier-Jedrzejowicz A, Brophy C, Moxham J, Green M. Assessment of diaphragm weakness. *Am Rev Respir Dis* 1988;**137**:877–83.

95. Chan CK, Loke J, Virgulto JA, et al. Bilateral diaphragmatic paralysis: clinical spectrum, prognosis and diagnostic approach. *Arch Phys Med Rehabil* 1998;**69**:976–9.

96. Mann DL. Chapter 227: Heart failure and cor pulmonale. In: Kasper DL, Braunwald E, Fauci AS, et al., editors. *Harrison's Principles of Internal Medicine*. 17th ed. 2008. Available: http://www.accesspharmacy.com/content.aspx?aID=2902061 [28 Feb 2011].

97. McGee SR. Percussion and physical diagnosis: separating myth from science. *Dis Mon* 1995;**41**(10):641–92.

98. Wong C, et al. Does this patient have a pleural effusion? *JAMA* 2009;**301**(3): 309–17.

99. Diacon AH, Brutsche MH, Soler M. Accuracy of pleural puncture sites: a prospective comparison of clinical examination with ultrasound. *Chest* 2003;**123**:436–41.

100. Diaz-Guzman E, Budev MM. Accuracy of physical examination in evaluating pleural effusion. *Cleve Clin J Med* 2008;**75**(4):297–303.

101. Badgett RG, Tanaka DJ, Hunt DK, et al. Can moderate chronic obstructive pulmonary disease be diagnosed by historical and physical findings alone? *Am J Med* 1993;**94**:188–96.

102. Badgett RG, et al. The clinical evaluation for diagnosing obstructive airways disease in high risk patients. *Chest* 1994;**106**:1427–31.

103. Oshaug K, Halvorsen PA, Melbye H. Should chest examination be reinstated in the early diagnosis of chronic obstructive pulmonary disease? *Int J Chron Obstruct Pulmon Dis* 2013;**8**:369–77.

104. North JB, Jennett S. Abnormal breathing patterns associated with acute brain damage. *Arch Neurol* 1974;**31**:338.

105. Pien GW, Pack AI. Chapter 79: Sleep disordered breathing. In: Mason RJ, et al., editors. *Murray and Nadel's Textbook of Respiratory Medicine*. 5th ed. Philadelphia: Saunders/Elsevier; 2010.

106. Lanfranchi PA, Braghiroli A, Bosimini E, et al. Prognostic value of nocturnal Cheyne–Stokes respiration in chronic heart failure. *Circulation* 1999;**99**:1435–40.

107. Mortara A, Sleight P, Pinna GD, et al. Abnormal awake respiratory patterns are common in chronic heart failure and may prevent evaluation of autonomic tone by measures of heart rate variability. *Circulation* 1997;**96**:246–52.

108. Bard RL, Gillespie BW, Patel H, Nicklas JM. Prognostic ability of resting periodic breathing and ventilatory variation in closely matched patients with heart failure. *J Cardiopulm Rehabil Prev* 2008;**28**:318–22.

109. Hermann DM, Siccoli M, Kirov P, Gugger M, Bassetti CL. Central periodic breathing during sleep in acute ischemic stroke. *Stroke* 2007;**38**:1082–4.

110. Desmarais TJ, Keller MS. Pectus carinatum. *Curr Opin Pediatr* 2013;**25**:375–81.

111. Shamberger RC. Congenital chest wall deformities. In: O'Neill J, Rowe MI, Grosfeld JL, et al., editors. *Pediatric Surgery*. 5th ed. St Louis: Mosby; 1998. p. 787.

112. Natalie AA, Nichols L, Bump GM. Platypnea-orthodeoxia, an uncommon presentation of patent foramen ovale. *Am J Med Sci* 2010;**339**(1):78–80.

113. Rodigues P, et al. Platypnea-orthodexia syndrome in review: defining a new disease? *Cardiology* 2012;**123**:15–23.

114. Cheng TO. Platypnea-orthodeoxia syndrome: etiology, differential diagnosis and management. *Catheter Cardiovasc Interv* 1999;**47**:64–6.

115. Rodriguez-Roisin R, Krowka MJ. Hepatopulmonary syndrome – a liver induced lung vascular disorder. *N Engl J Med* 2008;**358**(22):2378–87.

116. Hussain SF, Mekan SF. Platypnea-orthodeoxia: report of two cases and review of the literature. *South Med J* 2004;**97**(7):657–62.

117. Mueller R, Petty T, Filley G. Ventilation and arterial blood gas exchange produced by pursed-lips breathing. *J Appl Physiol* 1970;**28**:784–9.

118. Tiep BL, Burns M, Kao D, et al. Pursed lips breathing training using ear oximetry. *Chest* 1986;**90**:218–21.

2

119. Puente-Maetsu L, Stringer W. Hyperinflation and its management in COPD. *Int J COPD* 2006;**1**(4):381–400.

120. Breslin EH. The pattern of respiratory muscle recruitment during pursed-lip breathing. *Chest* 1992;**101**:75–8.

121. Thoman RL, Stroker GL, Ross JC. The efficacy of pursed-lips breathing in patients with chronic obstructive pulmonary disease. *Am Rev Resp Dis* 1966;**93**: 100–6.

122. Stockley RA, O'Brien C, Pye A, Hill SL. Relationship of sputum color to nature and outpatient management of acute exacerbations of COPD. *Chest* 2000;**117**(6):1638–45.

123. Johnson A. Sputum color: potential implications for clinical practice. *Respir Care* 2008;**53**(4):450.

124. Morris CG, Safranek S, Neher J. Clinical inquiries. Is sputum evaluation useful for patients with community-acquired pneumonia? *J Fam Pract* 2005;**54**(3):279–81.

125. Anevlavisa S, Petrogloub N, Tzavarasb A, et al. A prospective study of the diagnostic utility of sputum Gram stain in pneumonia. *J Infect* 2009;**59**(2):83–9.

126. Mancuso RF. Stridor in neonates. *Pediatr Clin North Am* 1996;**43**(6):1339–56.

127. Holinger LD. Etiology of stridor in the neonate, infant and child. *Ann Otol Rhinol Laryngol* 1980;**89**:397–400.

128. Grundfast KM, Harley EH. Vocal cord paralysis. *Otolaryngol Clin North Am* 1989;**22**:569–97.

129. Richardson MA, Cotton RT. Anatomic abnormalities of the pediatric airway. *Pediatr Clin North Am* 1984;**31**:821–34.

130. Ferguson CF. Congenital abnormalities of the infant larynx. *Ann Otol Rhinol Laryngol* 1967;**76**:744–52.

131. Findlay CA, Morrisey S, Paton JY. Subcutaneous emphysema secondary to foreign body aspiration. *Paediatr Pulmonol* 2003;**36**(1):81–2.

132. Rosen P, Barkin RM. Chapter 42: Pulmonary injuries. In: Marx JA, Hockberger RS, Walls RM, et al., editors. *Rosen's Emergency Medicine.* 7th ed. 2009. Available: http://www.mdconsult.com.ezproxy2.library.usyd.edu.au/book/player/book.do?method=display&type=bookPage&decorator=header&eid=4-u1.0-B978-0-323-05472-0..00042-6-s0185&displayedEid=4-u1.0-B978-0-323-05472-0..00042-6-s0190&uniq=187207748&isbn=978-0-323-05472-0&sid=962896223#lpState=open&lpTab=content sTab&content=4-u1.0-B978-0-323-05472-0..00042-6-s0185%3Bfrom%3Dtoc%3 Btype%3DbookPage%3Bisbn%3D978-0-323-05472-0 [28 Feb 2011].

133. Cheng AC, Black JF, Buising KL. Respiratory rate the neglected sign: letter to editor. *Med J Aust* 2008;**189**(9):531.

134. Fieselmann JF, Hendry MS, Helms CM, Wakefield DS. Respiratory rate predicts cardiopulmonary arrest for internal medicine inpatients. *J Gen Intern Med* 1993;**8**(7):354–60.

135. Subbe CP, Davies RG, Williams E, et al. Effect of introducing the Modified Early Warning score on clinical outcomes, cardio-pulmonary arrests and intensive care utilisation in acute medical admissions. *Anaesthesia* 2003;**58**:797–802.

136. Goldhill DR, McNarry AF, Mandersloot G, et al. A physiologically-based early warning score for ward patients: the association between score and outcome. *Anaesthesia* 2005;**60**:547–53.

137. Cretikos M, Chen J, Hillman K, et al. The Objective Medical Emergency Team Activation Criteria: a case–control study. *Resuscitation* 2007;**73**:62–72.

138. Fujita MS, Tambara K, Budgell MS, Miyamoto S, Tambara K, Budgell B. Trepopnea in patients with chronic heart failure. *Int J Cardiol* 2002;**84**:115–18.

139. Schneider de Araujo B. Trepopnea may explain right-sided pleural effusion in patients with decompensated heart failure. *Am J Emerg Med* 2012;**30**(6):925–31.

140. Buller AJ, Dornhorst AC. The physics of some pulmonary sounds. *Lancet* 1956;**2**:649–52.

141. Baughman RP, Loudon RG. Sound spectral analysis of voice transmitted sound. *Am Rev Respir Dis* 1986;**134**:167–9.

142. Earis J. Lung sounds. *Thorax* 1992;**47**:671–2.

143. Marini JJ, Pierson DJ, Hudson LD, Lakshminarayan S. The significance of wheeze in chronic airflow obstruction. *Am Rev Respir Dis* 1979;**120**:1069–72.

144. Baughman RP, Loudon RG. Quantitation of wheezing in acute asthma. *Chest* 1984;**86**(5):718–22.

145. Bentur L. Wheeze monitoring in children for assessment of nocturnal asthma and response to therapy. *Eur Respir J* 2003;**21**(4):621–6.

CHAPTER 3

CARDIOVASCULAR SIGNS

Apex beat (also cardiac impulse)

Description

The normal cardiac impulse or 'apex beat' should be felt in the left fifth intercostal space in the midclavicular line over an area 2–3 cm^2 in diameter.[1]

The normal impulse is described as a brief outward thrust occurring in early systole and will disappear before S2 is heard. It coincides with isovolumetric contraction.

Apex beat: displaced

Description

Normally the apex beat of the heart is palpated in the left fifth intercostal space in the midclavicular line. A 'displaced' apex beat usually implies that the impulse is felt lateral to the midclavicular line or more distally.

Condition/s associated with

Similar conditions to the pressure- and volume-loaded beats described below.

More common

- Skeletal abnormality – scoliosis or pectus excavatum
- Left ventricular enlargement of any cause – apex is usually displaced downwards and laterally
- Right ventricular enlargement of any cause – apex is displaced laterally
- Cardiomyopathies and dilatation of the heart
- Congestive heart failure
- Valvular heart disease

Less common

- Situs inversus dextrocardia/isolated dextrocardia
- Intra-thoracic disorders e.g. tension pneumothorax, large right pleural effusion

Mechanism/s

The displacement of the apex beat is related to changes in the heart size, whether via hypertrophy of the muscle (e.g. aortic stenosis and left ventricular hypertrophy), dilatation of the heart (e.g. dilated cardiomyopathy) or displacement of the heart (tension pneumothorax). With enlargement and/or dilatation of the heart, the apex moves laterally/downwards.

3

Sign value

If detected, a valuable sign.

Kelder et al. found after a review of over 700 patients that in suspected heart failure, a displaced apex had the strongest predictive value out of clinical signs assessed.[2]

One systematic review of 10 000 patients looked at history, examination findings, chest radiography and natriuretic peptides. A displaced apex beat had a pooled PLR (Positive Likelihood Ratio) of 16 (8.2–30.9) for left ventricular systolic dysfunction, which was higher than the other elements analysed in the systematic review.[3]

The displaced apex beat may not be frequently detected; thus its absence does not rule out systolic dysfunction.

Apex beat: double or triple impulse

Description

The sensation on palpation of the apex beat that there are two or three impulses felt during a cardiac cycle.

Condition/s associated with

- Hypertrophic obstructive cardiomyopathy
- Aortic stenosis

Mechanism/s

In hypertrophic cardiomyopathy, a combination of a stiff, thickened myocardium with or without left ventricular outflow tract obstruction leads to higher left ventricular and left atrial end diastolic pressures. A forceful atrial contraction can be felt (one ripple), a sensation of outward systolic thrust with rapid ejection early in systole is then palpated (second ripple), then a sustained late slow ejection of blood from the ventricle can be sensed (third ripple).

The mechanism in aortic stenosis is similar with hypertrophy of the myocardium secondary to the stenosed aortic valve. A left ventricular outflow tract obstruction, however, is not present.

Sign value

Although minimal research on it as a sign, if present it may have some value in increasing the likelihood of the presence of left ventricular hypertrophy.

Apex beat: hyperdynamic apical impulse/volume-loaded

Description

On palpation of the praecordium, the apex beat will be diffuse (i.e. over an area greater than 3 cm^2), with a large amplitude, but quickly disappearing.

Condition/s associated with

Classically associated with situations of volume overload and hypermetabolic states.[1,4,5]

More common

- Aortic and mitral regurgitation
- Thyrotoxicosis
- Sympathetic nervous system activation
- Anaemia

Less common

- Patent ductus arteriosus
- Ventricular septal defect

Mechanism/s

In hyperdynamic states, the impulse felt is simply an exaggeration of the normal cardiac beat.

In *volume-overloaded* states, the Frank–Starling mechanism produces a more forceful ventricular contraction.

Sign value

The hyperdynamic impulse is related to increased left ventricular volume.[6] It is unlikely to be found in mitral stenosis, as in this condition left ventricular filling is impaired. If mitral stenosis is suspected in the presence of a hyperdynamic impulse, other valvular pathology should be looked for.

In assessing left ventricular size, one study demonstrated that an apical impulse over an area greater than 3 cm^2 had a sensitivity of 92% with 91% specificity for an enlarged ventricle (PPV 86% and NPV 95%).[7]

3

Apex beat: left ventricular heave/sustained apical impulse/pressure-loaded apex

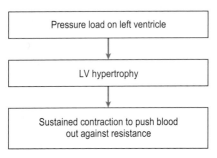

FIGURE 3.1
Sustained apical impulse or left ventricular heave mechanism

Description
Used to define an apex beat that is holosystolic in nature (that lasts through systole to S2).

Condition/s associated with

More common
Classically seen in *pressure-loaded* states:

- Hypertension
- Aortic stenosis
- Hypertrophic obstructive cardiomyopathy

Less common
- Dilated heart
- After myocardial infarction

Mechanism/s
In order to compensate for the increased *pressure load* on the left ventricle, the ventricle enlarges in size, making it more likely to be palpable. In conditions of increased afterload, ejection of blood out of the left ventricle is prolonged throughout systole, giving the impression of a sustained impulse through to S2.

Sign value
Although not extensively researched, a left ventricular heave has been shown in one study to be superior to electrocardiography in predicting left ventricular hypertrophy[8] (sensitivity 88%, specificity 78%). The presence of a sustained apical impulse does increase the probability of left ventricular hypertrophy being present.

Apex beat: tapping

Description

A tapping apex beat is a short, sharp systolic 'tap' felt where the apex beat would normally be. It is the palpable equivalent to a loud S1.

Conditions associated with

• Mitral stenosis

Mechanism/s

One suggested mechanism is that reduced ventricular filling caused by stenosis over the mitral valve results in a shortened outward movement of the apex, which creates the short, sharp tapping quality.

An alternative theory is that the stenosed valve provides an obstruction to blood flow into the left ventricle, resulting in elevated left atrial pressures which delay mitral valve closure. Instead of slowly gliding shut, the thickened leaflets are 'slammed' closed under higher pressure at the start of systole,[9] resulting in a palpable S1.

Sign value

Limited studies on this sign but if present it does suggest severe mitral stenosis.

3

Arterial pulse

The arterial pulse waveform can be difficult to classify and is an often-neglected clinical sign. The differences between pulse patterns may be subtle and therefore difficult (or impossible) for the expert as well as the novice to detect clinically without intra-arterial monitoring. They are discussed as a group for ease of comparison, and the important clinical pulse forms are highlighted. In order to understand the mechanism/s that create alternative pulse waveforms and the differences between them, a basic revision of the normal arterial waveform and some important definitions are first explained.

Key concept explained
The normal arterial waveform

Like the jugular venous pulse, the arterial pulse has a waveform, as shown in Figure 3.2. The waveform and arterial pressure are made up of two main components: the *pulse wave* (or pressure wave) and the *wave reflection*.

Pulse wave
The pulse wave is the pressure felt against the finger when palpating a pulse and represents the wave produced by left ventricular contraction.

Wave reflection
The waveform felt when taking a pulse, which is visible on monitoring, is created by more than just the pulse wave or forward flow of systole. Narrowing and bifurcation of blood vessels cause impedance, which forces the pressure wave to be reflected back on itself, and the systolic blood pressure and waveform to be amplified. The easiest analogy to use is that of waves in the ocean: if one wave travelling in one direction hits another wave heading in the opposite direction, the resulting collision is larger than the two independent waves.[10]

Anacrotic limb or upstroke
The anacrotic or ascending limb of the arterial waveform mainly reflects the pressure pulse produced by left ventricular contraction.[11]

Dicrotic limb and dicrotic notch
The dicrotic or descending limb of the waveform represents the decreasing pressure after left ventricular contraction. The dicrotic notch represents the closure of the aortic valve and retrograde or regurgitant flow across the valve.

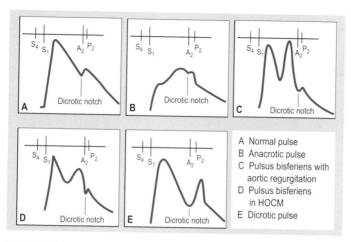

FIGURE 3.2
Configurational changes of the carotid pulse
A Normal pulse; **B** anacrotic pulse; **C** pulsus bisferiens; **D** pulsus bisferiens; **E** dicrotic pulse.
Based on Chatterjee K, Bedside evaluation of the heart: the physical examination. In: Chatterjee K et al. (eds), Cardiology. An Illustrated Text/Reference, *Philadelphia: JB Lippincott, 1991: Fig 48.5.*

TABLE 3.1
Summary of pulse types

Pulse name	Key features	Condition/s
Alternans	Alternating strong and weak beats	Advanced left ventricular failure
Anacrotic	Slow rising, late peaking, interrupted upstroke	Aortic stenosis
Bigeminal	Two pulses in rapid succession then long pause	Severe heart failure Hypovolaemia Sepsis Benign
Bisferiens	2 beats per cardiac cycle – BOTH in systole. Accentuated notch	Aortic regurgitation HOCM
Dicrotic	2 beats per cardiac cycle – one in systole, one in diastole	Myocardial dysfunction or low stroke volumes WITH intact systemic resistance
Pulsus parvus et tardus	Low amplitude and late peaking	Aortic stenosis
Pulus paradoxus		Cardiac tamponade Severe asthma

Important concept explained
The Venturi principle

The Venturi principle is central to understanding the mechanism of arterial pulse signs. It states that when fluid flows through a constricted pipe (in this case a blood vessel), the pressure of the fluid (blood) drops. This causes constriction of the vessel (see Figure 3.3).

The importance of this will be demonstrated in the clinical signs following.

Venturi principle

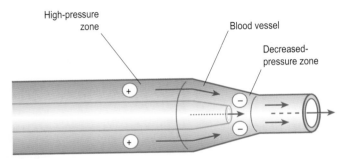

FIGURE 3.3
Schematic representation of the venturi principle

Based on Vender JS, Clemency MV, Oxygen delivery systems, inhalation therapy, and respiratory care. In: Benumof JL (ed), Clinical Procedures in Anesthesia and Intensive Care, Philadelphia: JB *Lippincott, 1992: Fig 13-3.*

Arterial pulse: anacrotic pulse

Description
A slow rising pulse that gives the impression of an interruption of the upstroke of the pulse on the ascending limb of the waveform (see Figure 3.2B). The peak of the limb is also closer to the second heart sound.

Condition/s associated with
- Aortic stenosis

Mechanism/s
Like pulsus tardus (see 'Pulsus tardus' in this section), the anacrotic pulse of aortic stenosis can be attributed to *prolonged ventricular ejection* and the *Venturi effect in the aorta*.[10] The stenosis, or narrowing of the aortic valve, means it takes longer to eject blood out of the left ventricle. This longer ejection time delays the upstroke of the pulse so the peak occurs closer to the second heart sound. Valvular narrowing creates a Venturi effect that further reduces the diameter of the arterial lumen, thus giving the feeling of an interrupted upstroke on palpation.

Sign value
If present, an anacrotic pulse is specific for severe aortic stenosis. Being able to elicit this sign can be useful in both observed clinical exam settings and in evaluating the emergent patient who presents with shortness of breath and an aortic stenotic murmur.

3

CLINICAL PEARL

Arterial pulse: bigeminal

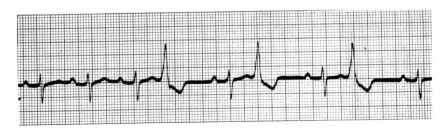

FIGURE 3.4
A short run of bigeminal rhythm is present

Surawicz B, Knilans TK, Chou's Electrocardiography in Clinical Practice, *6th edn,
Philadelphia: Elsevier, 2008: Fig 17.1.*

Definition

As the name suggests, this is a double
or twinned pulse (*bi* – 'two' and
geminus – 'twins'). Two beats of a
peripheral pulse occur in rapid
succession, followed by a long pause,
then another two beats in rapid
succession. It is an irregular pulse.

Condition/s associated with

- Severe heart failure
- Hypovolaemic shock
- Cardiac tamponade
- Sepsis
- Benign

Mechanism/s

The bigeminal pulse is created by a
normal sinus beat followed by a
premature contraction. The premature
beat has less stroke volume; therefore,
the strength of the pulse varies between
the two beats.

Arterial pulse: dicrotic

Description

In a dicrotic pulse, there are two beats per cardiac cycle, one during systole and the second in diastole. If the patient is being intra-arterially monitored, a dicrotic pulse will produce a characteristic 'M'-shaped waveform (see Figure 3.2).

Condition/s associated with

Generally seen in younger patients with low cardiac output states and elevated systemic vascular resistance:

- Cardiomyopathy/heart failure[12]
- Post valve replacement surgery[13]
- Sepsis
- Hypovolaemia
- Heart failure

Mechanism/s

In a dicrotic pulse, there is an accentuated diastolic dicrotic wave after the dicrotic notch (aortic valve closure).

Low stroke volume combined with *intact arterial vascular resistance* must be present for a dicrotic pulse to occur.[13,14]

In patients with a normal arterial pulse (see Figure 3.2), a dicrotic wave (thought to be caused by rebounding of blood against the aortic valve) is measurable on waveform analysis but is too low in amplitude to be felt on palpation and is hidden by the larger normal systolic wave.

In disease states resulting in low stroke volume, the systolic wave is smaller, making it easier to palpate the dicrotic wave. When combined with an intact arterial system (which amplifies the rebound of the pulse during diastole), the dicrotic pulse may be felt.[12-14]

Sign value

There is some evidence that a dicrotic pulse noticed after valve surgery carries a worse prognosis;[14] however, the pulse (if felt) is frequently confused with pulsus bisferiens and, therefore, may have limited value as a sign.

3

Arterial pulse: pulsus alternans

Description

A regular pulse that has alternating strong and weak beats. This can be identified at the bedside but can also be seen on arterial waveform at cardiac catheterisation as seen in Figure 3.5.

Condition/s associated with

- Advanced left ventricular failure[15-19]
- Aortic valve disease

Mechanism/s

Several mechanisms have been proposed,[14] two of which are associated with the most evidence:

1 *Frank–Starling theory* – in left ventricular dysfunction there is a decrease in cardiac output that causes a raised end-diastolic volume. This raised volume allows for greater myocardial stretch and, via the Frank–Starling mechanism, causes the next

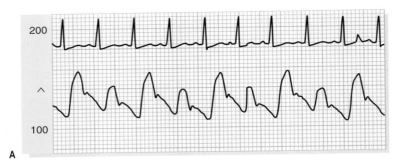

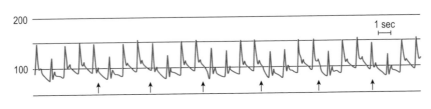

FIGURE 3.5
Beat-to-beat variability in arterial pressure waveform morphologies
A Pulsus alternans; **B** pulsus paradoxus. The marked decline in both systolic blood pressure and pulse pressure during spontaneous inspiration (arrows) is characteristic of cardiac tamponade.

Ragosta M, Cardiac Catheterization, *Philadelphia: Saunders, 2010; Ch 6, 58-74. © 2010 Saunders; Mark JB*, Atlas of Cardiovascular Monitoring, *New York: Churchill Livingstone, 1998: Figs 3-3, 18-10.*

contraction to be more forceful (the strong beat). After the strong beat, the end–diastolic volume is smaller and hence the next beat is weaker.

2 *Inherent beat-to-beat variability* – this theory is based on the concept that there is inherent beat-to-beat variability in myocardial contractility (i.e. that the myocardium can vary its inotropic state and, therefore, the force of contraction from one beat to the next).

Other suggested mechanisms include:[15]

• failure of the ventricle to completely relax after a strong beat, causing incomplete filling in diastole

• alternations of preload and afterload

• sympathetic system and baroreceptor influences

• alternations of cardiac action potentials

• variations in intracellular calcium[10,20] – in diastolic left ventricular dysfunction, ejection duration is prolonged due to slowed calcium reuptake.

Sign value

There are few well-conducted studies on the value of pulsus alternans as a sign. However, if present, studies have shown pulsus alternans to have a reasonable correlation with left ventricular dysfunction.[16-19]

3

Arterial pulse: pulsus bisferiens

Description

As seen in Figure 3.2A, the 'normal' pulse is characterised by two systolic peaks separated by a mid-systolic dip. Often only the first systolic peak is felt when taking a pulse. The first systolic peak is the percussion wave caused by rapid left ventricular ejection, and the second peak is created by the wave hitting the peripheral vessels and being reflected back.

In pulsus bisferiens, both peaks are accentuated, resulting in *two systolic peaks* of the pulse with a mid-systolic dip being palpable. These characteristics are seen in both Figure 3.2C and Figure 3.6.

Condition/s associated with

More common

- Aortic regurgitation
- Aortic regurgitation with milder aortic stenosis
- Hypertrophic cardiomyopathy

Less common

- Large patent ductus arteriosus – rare
- Arteriovenous fistula – rare

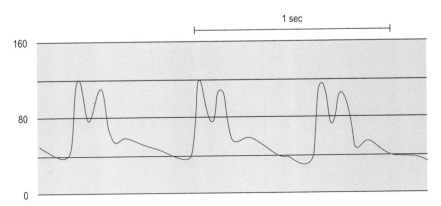

FIGURE 3.6
Pulsus bisferiens – note the two systolic peaks

General mechanism/s

In aortic regurgitation with aortic stenosis, the Venturi effect causes the abnormal pulse. Rapid blood flow through the aortic valve sucks in the walls of the aorta. This momentarily reduces the flow and produces a notch between the systolic peaks of the arterial waveform.[21-23]

This is the same principle as the mechanism underlying the anacrotic pulse. However, in aortic stenosis the Venturi effect reduces a *normal* amplitude pulse whereas, in the setting of aortic regurgitation, the initial pulse amplitude is *higher* as there is a large stroke volume from vigorous systolic contraction. Due to this higher output state and the additional regurgitant volume being ejected from the ventricle, the first systolic peak of the pulse becomes more obvious (see Figure 3.2D).[10]

Hypertrophic cardiomyopathy

In hypertrophic cardiomyopathy, there is a sharp rapid upstroke of the carotid pulse in systole, owing to a hyperdynamic contraction due to hypertrophy, followed by rapid decline due to left ventricular outflow obstruction. The Venturi effect may also draw the anterior mitral valve leaflet towards the interventricular septum, exacerbating the outflow tract obstruction and producing a more significant 'notch'. The second pulse peak is thought to be related to the reflected wave.[24]

Sign value

Although documented in patients with moderate and severe aortic regurgitation,[21-23] detailed studies on its evidence base are lacking. It is rarely discovered at the bedside and, therefore, is arguably of limited value as a clinical sign.

3

Arterial pulse: pulsus parvus et tardus

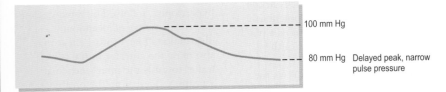

100 mm Hg

80 mm Hg   Delayed peak, narrow
pulse pressure

FIGURE 3.7
Pulsus parvus et tardus (small amplitude with a slow upstroke) associated with aortic stenosis.
Andreoli TE, Benjamin IJ, Griggs RC, Wing EJ. In: Andreoli and Carpenter's Cecil Essentials of Medicine, *8th edn, Philadelphia: Elsevier, 2011: Chapter 4, 32–45, Figure 4.2.*

Description
Pulsus parvus et tardus refers to a carotid pulse that is of small volume (parvus) on palpation and delayed (tardus) in its peak (i.e. the peak is closer to the second heart sound).

Condition/s associated with
• Aortic stenosis

Mechanism/s
Aortic stenosis causes a decrease in the rate of ejection of blood from the left ventricle, while at the same time the duration of ejection is prolonged. Consequently, amplitude is decreased resulting in a smaller pulsation.

The delayed nature of the pulse is thought to be caused by the combined effects of:

• flow stenosis causing a decrease in rate of ejection of blood out of the left ventricle
• compliance of the vessel distal to the stenosis
• Venturi effect.

The stenosed aortic valve reduces the speed at which blood is ejected out of the left ventricle into the aorta.

When blood flows through a stenosis, there is a pressure drop and a decrease in the rate of ejection of blood into the aorta. This is exacerbated by the Venturi effect, which sucks in the arterial wall, narrowing the arterial lumen and further delaying the arterial pulse.

Studies[25] have shown that decreased compliance of the post-stenotic vessel damps the arterial waveform at high frequencies, decreasing downstream pulsatility, contributing to the production of a delayed pulse.

Sign value
Unlike other arterial pulse signs, which can be difficult to palpate and recognise at the bedside, pulsus parvus et tardus can be readily felt, and is important in assessing a patient with a systolic murmur, as well as a key examination finding.

Pulsus parvus is moderately valuable in predicting moderate to severe aortic stenosis if present,[26,27] with a sensitivity of 74–80% and specificity of 65–67% for severe aortic stenosis, and a likelihood ratio for severe aortic stenosis of 2.3.

Pulsus tardus has reasonable evidence as a clinical sign in the setting of severe aortic stenosis.[28] Normally, the pulse should be felt close to S1; the closer the pulse is to S2, the more significant the stenosis. Studies[26,27,29,30] have shown a sensitivity of 31–90% and specificity of 68–93% with a PLR for severe aortic stenosis of 3.7.

Arterial pulse: sinus arrhythmia

Description

The normal physiological changes of the heart rate during inspiration and expiration can be demonstrated by feeling the peripheral pulse rate. On inspiration the heart rate quickens, on expiration it slows.

Condition/s associated with

None, it is physiological.

Mechanism/s

Heart rate is predominantly mediated by the medulla and the parasympathetic nervous system via the nucleus ambiguus and, subsequently, through the vagus nerve (CNX) to the sino-atrial node. On expiration, the vagus nerve is stimulated and acts at the sino-atrial node to slow the heart down, whereas the opposite occurs on inspiration. When we breathe in, inhibitory signals are triggered and act on the nucleus ambiguus and then the vagus nerve to inhibit the parasympathetic signal to the heart. The heart rate then quickens.

Sign value

As it is a normal physiological process, if absent a pathological neuronal process may be present. In general it has limited value as a sign.

Bradycardia

Description

A heart rate of less than 60 beats per minute.

Condition/s associated with

The individual causes of bradycardia are too numerous to list. They include, but are not limited to:

More common

- Myocardial infarction
- Sinus node disease
- Drugs (e.g. beta blockers, calcium channel blockers, amiodarone)
- Hypothyroidism
- AV nodal disease
- Heart block
- Degeneration/ageing of the heart

Less common

- Cellular hypoxia
- Myocarditis
- Electrolyte imbalances
- Inflammatory disease (e.g. SLE)
- Obstructive sleep apnoea
- Haemochromatosis
- Congenital defect

Mechanism/s

The individual mechanisms for each underlying cause of bradycardia are numerous. In terms of a final common pathway, bradycardia is caused by:

- an interruption to or blocking of the conduction of electrical impulses in the heart

or

- an increase in vagal tone to the heart.

The disturbance can be present at the SA node, AV node, bundle of His or left or right bundle branches.

Myocardial infarction

May cause heart block, particularly if the right coronary artery (which feeds the AV and SA nodes in the majority of people) is occluded. Failure to deliver blood to the nodes causes ischaemia and, thus, SA and AV node dysfunction.

Cellular hypoxia

Decrease in oxygen from any cause (although usually ischaemic) can cause depolarisation of the SA node membrane potential, causing bradycardia; severe hypoxia completely stops pacemaker activity.

Sinus node disease

Damage to or degeneration of the sinus node leads to a number of problems, such as discharging at an irregular rate or pauses or discharges with subsequent blockage. All of these irregularities may cause bradycardia.

Heart block

Damage or disruption at the atria, AV node, bundle of His or in the bundle branches may slow conduction around the heart and cause heart block.

Electrolyte imbalances

Potassium, in particular, influences the membrane activity of cardiac myocytes as well as the SA and AV nodes. Significant variations in potassium concentration will affect membrane polarisation and heart rate. Bradycardia is more associated with hyperkalaemia than hypokalaemia, although it may be present with either.

3

Haemochromatosis

Iron infiltration that damages both the myocytes and conduction system of the heart has been shown to cause bradycardia.

Drugs

Drugs act by a variety of mechanisms to precipitate bradycardia:

- Calcium channel blockers inhibit the slow inward Ca^{+2} currents during SA node action potentials.

- Beta blockers and muscarinics act directly at the autonomic receptors, blocking sympathetic activity or enhancing parasympathetic activity.

- Digoxin enhances vagal tone to the AV node, slowing the heart rate.

Sign value

With so many potential causes of bradycardia, the specificity of the sign for a given disease is low. However, if noted in a patient who should otherwise have a normal heart rate, it warrants immediate attention.

Buerger's sign

Description

In patients with suspected vascular disease, when the patient lies on their back with a leg elevated for at least a few minutes, the foot becomes white; the patient is then quickly sat upright with legs hanging down and the limb turns dark red.

Condition/s associated with

• Peripheral vascular disease

Mechanism/s

Partial or total occlusion of the arteries of the leg by emboli or thrombosis leads to limited vascular flow to the distal leg and foot. Raising the leg further worsens arterial blood flow to the limb, causing the foot to become white. When the foot is then placed close to the ground, gravity assists flow to the distal limb and, along with compensatory peripheral vasodilatation (in response to poor perfusion), the leg quickly turns red.

Sign value

A positive Buerger's sign indicates severe limb-threatening ischaemia and should be treated immediately.

3

Capillary return decreased/delayed

Description

The time taken for a distal capillary bed to regain normal colour after sufficient pressure has been applied to cause blanching.[31] Delayed capillary return is usually described as a return to normal colour which takes longer than 2–3 seconds.

Condition/s associated with

- Dehydration
- Hypovolaemia
- Peripheral vascular disease
- Decreased peripheral perfusion (e.g. heart failure)

Mechanism/s

The normal components of peripheral perfusion are complex. Normal capillary perfusion is based on the driving pressure, arteriolar tone, capillary patency and density.[31] These, in turn, are influenced by a number of factors such as noradrenaline, angiotensin II, vasopression, endothelin 1 and thromboxane A2, all of which cause arteriolar vasoconstriction and may decrease capillary return, whereas prostacyclin, nitric oxide and local metabolites all may produce vasodilatation and increase capillary return. The interplay between these elements is thought to alter the ability of the blood to refill post blanching. There is limited scientific evidence to support this theory.[31]

Dehydration mechanism/s

In dehydration, the body's compensatory system tries to redistribute available fluid from the periphery to the central vasculature to maintain preload and, ultimately, cardiac output. The sympathetic nervous system is also invoked, resulting in peripheral vasoconstriction via local and neurohormonal mechanisms. This leads to decreased peripheral perfusion of the distal capillary beds and decreased or delayed capillary return.

Decreased peripheral perfusion mechanism/s

In heart failure, there is a lack of forward flow or 'driving pressure' to perfuse the distal capillary beds effectively. The body also compensates for poor forward flow by activating the sympathetic nervous system, the renin–angiotensin system, vasopressin and other factors that increase arteriolar tone, cause vasoconstriction and alter the time for distal capillary beds to refill.

Shocked state mechanism/s

In 'shocked' states (particularly sepsis), it is thought that an imbalance between vasoconstrictor and vasodilator substances and endothelial dysfunction occurs with the result that normal regulation of microvascular blood flow is impaired.[31]

Other factors, including arteriovenous shunting, 'no flow' capillaries, intermittent flow capillaries, increased capillary permeability and interstitial oedema, as well as leukocyte- and red-blood-cell-derived thrombi, may decrease functional capillary density and capillary refill.[31]

Sign value

As a sign, capillary refill or return suffers from significant inter-rater variability. Additionally, factors such as temperature and age can vary the time for refilling without pathology being present. Evidence is more robust in children (where it is used frequently) and is still very useful in adults if obviously deranged.

• One study found a capillary refill time (CRT) of >3 seconds suggests a fluid deficit greater than 100ml/kg in paediatric patients.[32]

• One systematic review found CRT was one of the strongest warning signs for serious paediatric infections in developed countries.[33]

• A review of studies including 478 patients found capillary refill time as the most useful individual sign for predicting 5% dehydration in children with a PLR of 4.1 with sensitivity 60% and specificity 85%.[34]

3

Cardiac cachexia

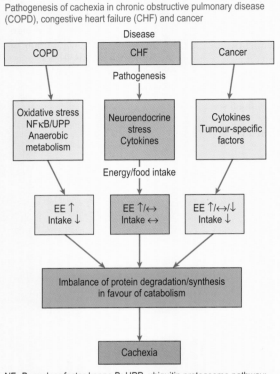

Pathogenesis of cachexia in chronic obstructive pulmonary disease (COPD), congestive heart failure (CHF) and cancer

NFκB, nuclear factor-kappa B; UPP, ubiquitin proteasome pathway; EE, energy expenditure.

FIGURE 3.8
Pathogenesis of cachexia in chronic obstructive pulmonary disease (COPD), congestive heart failure (CHF) and cancer

Stephens NA, Fearon KCH. Anorexia, cachexia and nutrition, Medicine *2007; 36(2): Fig 3.*

Description

A state seen in heart failure, where the patient has significant body wasting that affects all types of tissue but especially lean tissue. A current definition proposed is an unintentional non–oedematous weight loss of >6% of previous weight over a period of 6 months, regardless of BMI and in the absence of other cachetic states[35] (such as cancer or hyperthyroidism).

Condition/s associated with

- Congestive heart failure (CHF)

Mechanism/s

The pathway to cardiac cachexia is multi-factorial and complex. Key elements thought to be involved include:

- *Neuroendocrine abnormalities* – counter-regulatory responses to heart failure cause increased levels of angiotensin II, aldosterone, renin and catecholamine activity. These, in turn, increase basal energy expenditure and cause a catabolic shift in energy.[35]

- *Immune system activation* – myocardial injury, increased gut wall oedema and bacteria can induce an immune response, which causes an over-expression of TNF-α and other cytokines. This brings about an increased metabolic rate, decreased protein synthesis, increased proteolysis and other catabolic processes.[35,36]

- *Neuroendocrine, immunological and other factors* affect the orexigenic (increased energy intake) and the anorexigenic (decreased energy intake) pathways to favour decreased energy intake and appetite.

- *Malabsorption* – gut wall oedema in CHF reduces absorption of nutrients and may alter permeability, allowing endotoxins to enter the circulation and further stimulate the immune system.[35]

- *Cellular hypoxia* – chronic low cardiac output deprives cells of normal required amounts of oxygen, producing less efficient metabolism and a shift towards catabolism rather than anabolism.[37]

Sign value

Although only seen in 13–36% of CHF patients,[35] the onset of cardiac cachexia heralds a poor prognosis.

3

Carotid bruit

Description

A high-pitched, blowing systolic murmur heard on auscultation of the carotid arteries.

Condition/s associated with

More common

- Carotid artery stenosis

Less common

- AV malformations

High flow states:

- Anaemia
- Thyrotoxicosis

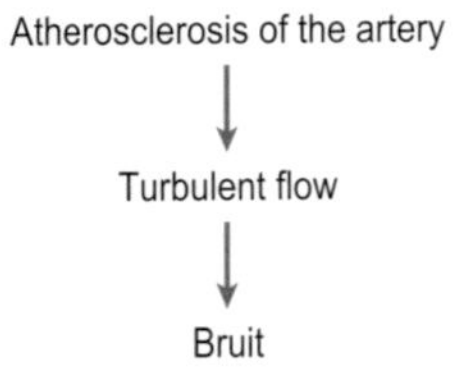

Atherosclerosis of the artery

↓

Turbulent flow

↓

Bruit

FIGURE 3.9
Mechanism of a bruit

Mechanism/s

Atherosclerosis of the common, internal or external carotid artery leads to turbulent flow, causing the bruit.

Sign value

A well studied sign of mixed value. It is present in approximately 1% of the normal adult population.[38]

In a completely asymptomatic patient, there is evidence that carotid bruits are associated with an increased risk of cerebrovascular and cardiac events.[39]

In the setting of an identified carotid stenosis, the presence of a bruit triples stroke risk.[39] However, use of bruit as a diagnostic tool has shown that it has only a variable ability to pick up high-grade stenosis with sensitivity ranging from 29% to 76% and specificity ranging from 61% to 94% (PLR from 1.6 to 5.7).[40-44]

In summary, in an asymptomatic patient who has a carotid bruit, further investigation is probably necessary. However, the characteristics of the bruit are not predictive of the level of underlying stenosis.

Cheyne–Stokes breathing

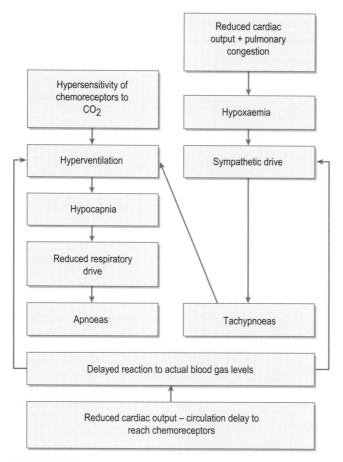

FIGURE 3.10
Flow diagram of Cheyne–Stokes respiration

VIDEO 3.1 ▶

Video 3.1 Access through Student Consult.

Description

Cheyne–Stokes respiration is technically described as a breathing pattern characterised by alternating apnoeas and tachypnoeas with a crescendo–decrescendo pattern of tidal volume. In practice, what will be seen is a rhythmic waxing and waning of the depth of respiration. The patient breathes deeply for a short time and then breathes very shallowly or stops breathing altogether.[45] The clinical sign can also be depicted on a polysomnogram seen in Figure 3.11. When looking at the flow, in the chest and abdomen leads there is rhythmic movement, followed by an apnoea.

3

CLINICAL PEARL

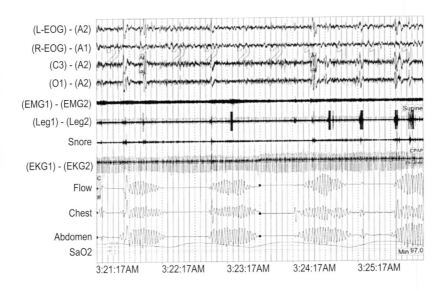

(L-EOG) - (A2)
(R-EOG) - (A1)
(C3) - (A2)
(O1) - (A2)
(EMG1) - (EMG2)
(Leg1) - (Leg2)
Snore
(EKG1) - (EKG2)
Flow
Chest
Abdomen
SaO2

3:21:17AM   3:22:17AM   3:23:17AM   3:24:17AM   3:25:17AM

FIGURE 3.11
Polysomnogram of a patient with Cheyne-Stokes respiration. Note the periods of airflow
and chest movement and then periods of apnoea

Condition/s associated with

More common

- Congestive heart failure[45]
- Stroke

Less common

- Traumatic brain injury
- Brain tumours
- Carbon monoxide poisoning
- Morphine administration

Mechanism/s

Underlying damage or changes to the brainstem respiratory centre (which is responsible for involuntary respiration).

Mechanism/s in congestive heart failure

Several metabolic changes that affect chemoreceptors, the autonomic nervous system and the brainstem have been identified:

- Hypersensitivity of central chemoreceptors in the brainstem to changes in arterial blood carbon dioxide levels can lead to hyperventilation. This 'blowing off' causes a significant drop in carbon dioxide levels resulting in a central apnoea[46,47] (i.e. a drop in respiratory drive). The apnoea allows carbon dioxide to accumulate, stimulate respiratory drive and start the cycle again.

- Hypoxaemia due to lowered cardiac output and pulmonary congestion induces hyperventilation, leading to hypocapnia and an apnoea.[48]

- Hypoxaemia and hypercapnia combine to increase the sensitivity of the central breathing centre and cause an imbalance in respiration.[49]

- Heart enlargement and pulmonary congestion reduce pulmonary reservoirs of oxygen and carbon

194

dioxide, especially during sleep, making the respiratory cycle more variable and less stable.

- With circulation delay, decreased cardiac output means it takes longer for oxygenated blood to reach peripheral chemoreceptors and help regulate ventilation. In contrast, the respiratory centre in the medulla can sense changes in pH and stimulate respiration to lower carbon dioxide immediately via the nervous system. The relatively slow feedback system of circulation means that changes to blood gas concentrations are often delayed and not truly representative,[48] causing an under- or over-activation of respiration and an ineffective feedback system to ventilatory regulation in the medulla.

- Increased levels of adrenaline have been seen in patients with CHF[49] due to over-activation of the sympathetic nervous system. Adrenaline increases minute ventilation, thus potentially increasing the 'blowing off' of carbon dioxide, causing hypocapnia and apnoea.

Sign value

A valuable sign, Cheyne–Stokes breathing is common in patients with an ejection fraction of less than 40%[49] and is seen in 50% of patients with CHF.[48] Studies have shown that patients with heart failure who experience Cheyne–Stokes breathing have a worse prognosis than those who do not.

3

Clubbing

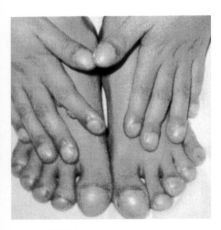

FIGURE 3.12
Clubbing of fingers and toes

Reproduced, with permission, from Marx JA, Hockberger RS, Walls RM et al. (eds), Rosen's Emergency Medicine, *7th edn, Philadelphia: Mosby, 2009: Fig 29.2.*

Description

A characteristic bulging of the distal finger and nail bed, often described in stages:

1 Softening of the nail bed, causing a spongy feeling when the nail is pressed
2 Loss of the normal <165° angle between nail bed and fold
3 Convex nail growth
4 Thickening of the distal part of the finger
5 Shine and striation of the nail and skin

Condition/s associated with

Clubbing has a large number of differential diagnoses. The vast majority of clubbing is bilateral. Unilateral clubbing is very rare and has been seen in patients with hemiplegia, dialysis fistulas and ulnar artery AV malformations.

Pulmonary and neoplastic causes are by far the most common causes (see Table 3.2).

Mechanism/s

Many theories have been developed that attempt to explain clubbing; however, the mechanism for each aetiology is still unclear. Vasodilatation and proliferation of the distal nail beds is thought to be key and has been demonstrated in small MRI studies;[50] however, why vasodilatation occurs and what other contributing elements are present is not known. The lungs are thought to play a role in stopping factors that may precipitate clubbing from reaching the distal circulation. This theory is supported by observation that patients with untreated patent ductus arteriosus (PDA) demonstrate clubbing that is confined to the feet. The PDA is thought to provide an avenue for blood from the pulmonary artery which bypasses the lungs and is shunted into the descending aorta.

The most currently accepted explanation involves *platelets and platelet-derived growth factor (PDGF)*.[51] This theory does not explain unilateral clubbing and is not applicable to all cases where clubbing is present.

It is hypothesised that in healthy individuals, megakaryocytes are broken down into fragments in the lungs and these fragments become platelets. If this fragmentation does not occur, whole megakaryocytes can become wedged in the small vessels of distal extremities. Once trapped, they release PDGFs, which recruit cells and promote proliferation of muscle cells and fibroblasts. This cell proliferation

TABLE 3.2
Causes of bilateral clubbing

Neoplastic	Pulmonary
Bronchogenic carcinoma Lymphoma Pleural tumours	Cystic fibrosis Asbestosis Pulmonary fibrosis Sarcoidosis Hypertrophic pulmonary osteoarthropathy (HPOA)
Cardiac	**Gastrointestinal**
Cyanotic heart disease Endocarditis	Inflammatory bowel disease Liver disease Coeliac disease
Infectious	**Endocrinological**
Tuberculosis Infective endocarditis HIV	Thyroid disease

causes the characteristic appearance of clubbing.

Therefore, any pathology that affects normal pulmonary circulation (such as cardiac shunts or lung disease) may allow whole megakaryocytes to enter the peripheral circulation unfragmented.

In bowel disease, it is suggested that the polycythaemia and arteriovenous malformations of the lung seen in some instances contribute to this process. In addition, vascular endothelial growth factor (VEGF) has been isolated in some patients with lung cancer and hypertrophic pulmonary osteoarthropathy (HPOA) and is likely to contribute to hyperplasia of the distal digits.

Sign value

Clubbing is almost always pathological and should be investigated; however, its absence does not exclude underlying disease.

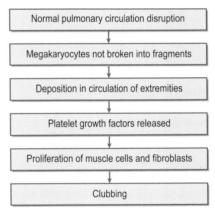

FIGURE 3.13
Proposed mechanism of clubbing

Crackles (also rales)

Description

Popping, crackling, rattling or clicking sounds heard on lung auscultation that may be inspiratory or expiratory in timing.

Condition/s associated with

More common

- Left heart failure/pulmonary oedema – classically mid- to end-inspiratory
- Pneumonia
- Atelectasis
- Bronchiectasis
- Bronchitis
- Interstitial lung disease

Mechanism/s

Heart failure

In left heart failure, raised left ventricular and atrial pressures back up into the lung vasculature. When pulmonary vasculature pressure increases above 19mm Hg, a transudate of fluid enters the lung interstitium and alveoli. The alveoli are filled with fluid and collapse. When the patient breathes in, the alveoli are filled with air and 'pop' open, causing inspiratory crackles.

Other

Accumulation of phlegm, debris, mucus, blood or pus in the alveoli or

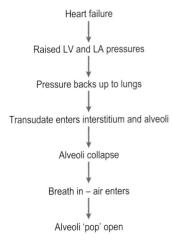

Heart failure

↓

Raised LV and LA pressures

↓

Pressure backs up to lungs

↓

Transudate enters interstitium and alveoli

↓

Alveoli collapse

↓

Breath in – air enters

↓

Alveoli 'pop' open

FIGURE 3.14
Mechanism of crackles in heart failure

small airways as a result of pneumonia, haemoptysis, inflammatory disorder or any other aetiology will cause the alveoli to collapse and then potentially be 'popped' open, creating crackles.

Sign value

Crackles or rales are the most common sign in acute heart failure – seen in up to 66–87% of patients.[52,53] In the setting of acute heart failure without concomitant lung pathology, crackles are highly specific for heart failure. They are less valuable in chronic heart failure as the compensatory increased lymphatic drainage will shift fluid away more effectively.

Cyanosis

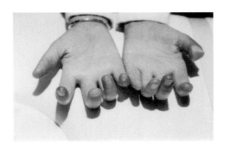

FIGURE 3.15
Photograph of hands of a 22-year-old female patient with SLE of 2 years duration Extreme peripheral vasospasm and cyanosis was associated with early terminal gangrene in the right thumb (bandaged) and later several other digits.

Williams RC, Autoimmune disease etiology – a perplexing paradox or a turning leaf? Autoimmun Rev 2007-03-01Z, 6(4): 204–208, Fig. 2. Copyright © 2006.

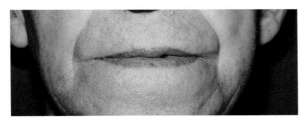

FIGURE 3.16
Central cyanosis of the lips
Douglas G, Nicol F, Robertson C, Macleod's Clinical Examination, *13th edn, Fig 3.6.*

Cyanosis: central

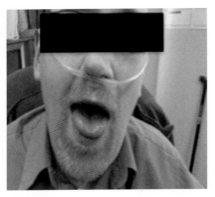

FIGURE 3.17
Central cyanosis

McMullen SM, Ward P. Cyanosis. The American Journal of Medicine *2013; 126(3): Fig B.*

Description
A blue/purple discolouration of the tongue, lips and mucous membranes.

Condition/s associated with

More common
- Cardiac
  - » Congenital heart disease – The five Ts and two Es
  - » **T**ransposition of the great arteries
  - » **T**etralogy of Fallot
  - » **T**ricuspid Atresia
  - » **T**runcus arteriosus
  - » **T**otal anomalous pulmonary venous return
  - » **E**bstein's anomaly
  - » **E**isenmenger physiology
  - » Heart failure
- Respiratory
  - » V/Q mismatches (e.g. due to pneumonia)
  - » Hypoventilation

Less common
- Cardiac
  - » Transposition of the great arteries
  - » Eisenmenger's syndrome
- Haematological
  - » Methaemoglobinaemia
  - » Sulfhaemoglobinaemia
- Respiratory
  - » Pulmonary venous fistulas
  - » Intrapulmonary shunts

Mechanism/s
In central cyanosis, the key point is that *deoxygenated blood is leaving the heart.* That is, deoxygenated blood is present in the arterial circulation even before it reaches the periphery. This is due to *low oxygen saturation and/or abnormal haemoglobin.*

Cardiac
In cardiac causes of central cyanosis, the main issue is the mixing or shunting of venous blood into arterial blood, leading to decreased oxygen saturation. In many of the congenital heart defects there is a physical deformity or connection allowing mixing of the venous and arterial blood. For example, in Tetralogy of Fallot, the ventricular septal defect results in mixing across the ventricles. This means the blood leaving the left side of the heart already has a lower-than-normal oxygen saturation.

Respiratory
A V/Q mismatch or shunting of blood through the lungs, without adequate oxygenation, will increase the quantity of deoxygenated haemoglobin that passes out of the lungs, leading to reduced oxygen saturation.

Haematological

Methaemoglobinemia is a disorder whereby the normal ferrous haemoglobin ($Fe2+$) is replaced by methaemoglobin ($Fe3+$).

Methaemoglobin is formed by the oxidation of ferrous to ferric haemoglobin and is incapable of oxygen transport. The oxygen dissociation curve is shifted leftward, reducing oxygen delivery and leading to tissue hypoxia. This can be a primary hereditary cause or, more commonly, an acquired condition.

Several chemicals or drugs (dapsone, amyl nitrate, sulfonamides among many others) may precipitate the oxidation.

Once methaemoglobin is present in sufficient quantities, oxygen cannot be released at the peripheries. Tissue hypoxia may occur along with increased levels of deoxygenated haemoglobin and thus cyanosis may be present. A methaemoglobin level of 1.5 g/dL or 15% of total haemoglobin can produce cyanosis.[54]

3

Central cyanosis

A blue/purple discolouration of the skin and mucous membranes caused by an *absolute* increase in the quantity of deoxygenated haemoglobin in the *capillary or venule blood*.

The two final common pathways that can result in enough deoxygenated haemoglobin to cause cyanosis are:
1. an increase in venous blood in the area of cyanosis
2. a reduction in oxygen saturation (SaO_2).

The amount of deoxygenated haemoglobin needed to cause cyanosis is 50 g/L (5 g/dL). It is important to note that the total amount of haemoglobin influences the level of oxygen desaturation that needs to occur before cyanosis.

For example, in a severely anaemic patient with a haemoglobin level of 60 g/L (6 g/dL), the proportion of haemoglobin that is deoxygenated (reduced) may be 60% (36 g/L or 3.6 g/dL) and the patient would still not be cyanotic. Conversely, in a patient who is polycythaemic with a haemoglobin level of 180 g/L (18 g/dL), the deoxygenated haemoglobin may be only approximately 28% (50 g/L or 5 g/dL) and the patient may be cyanotic.

In other words, it is the *absolute* amount of deoxygenated haemoglobin that causes cyanosis, *not* the relative amount.[55]

CLINICAL PEARL

Cyanosis: peripheral

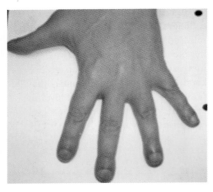

FIGURE 3.18
Peripheral cyanosis

McMullen SM, Ward P. Cyanosis. The American Journal of Medicine *2013; 126(3): Fig A.*

Description

Blue/purple discolouration of the extremities, often in the fingers.

Condition/s associated with

Common

- Cold exposure
- Decreased cardiac output (e.g. CHF)
- Raynaud's phenomenon (see Chapter 1, 'Musculoskeletal signs')

Less common

- Arterial and venous obstruction

Mechanism/s

Peripheral cyanosis is caused by the *slowing of blood flow and increased oxygen extraction* in the extremities.

When human bodies are exposed to cold, peripheral vasoconstriction occurs to maintain warmth. This leads to reduced blood flow to the periphery and effectively more time for oxygen to be taken out of the blood – hence more deoxygenated blood is present.

Similarly, in CHF, decreased cardiac output leads to vasoconstriction (to maintain blood pressure and venous return), which decreases blood flow to peripheral areas.

Ewart's sign

Description

A combination of the following signs:

- Dullness to percussion over the left scapula
- Aegophony (increased vocal resonance)
- Bronchial breath sounds over the left lung

Condition/s associated with

- Pericardial effusion

Mechanism/s

A large pericardial effusion can compress the left lung, causing consolidation and/or atelectasis, which alters percussive resonance. If the effusion enlarges sufficiently to collapse and/or consolidate the lung, increased vocal resonance and bronchial breath sounds will be heard. (For a discussion of the mechanism of increased vocal resonance and bronchial breath sounds, see Chapter 2, 'Respiratory signs'.)

3

Hepatojugular reflux (also abdominojugular reflux)

VIDEO 3.2 ▶

Video 3.2 Access through Student Consult.

Description

Pressing firmly over the right upper quadrant (liver area) causes the jugular venous pressure (JVP) to become more obvious and sometimes visibly higher. A positive hepatojugular reflux is present if there is an increase in JVP of more than 3 cmH$_2$O for longer than 15 seconds.

Condition/s associated with

- Any cause of right ventricular dysfunction – systolic or diastolic dysfunction
- Heart failure and volume overload
- Elevated right ventricular afterload
- Cor pulmonale

  Note: This sign is NOT seen in cardiac tamponade.

Mechanism/s

Putting pressure on the right upper quadrant assists in venous return to the right side of the heart via the inferior vena cava. In patients in a stressed or a pathological state, venoconstriction also leads to peripheral veins being less compliant or 'flexible' than normal[56] and therefore any additional venous return is likely to lead to increased pressure, such as central venous pressure, exemplified by a raised JVP.

In addition, the increased volume of blood returning to the right side of the heart is met with raised end-systolic and -diastolic pressures in the right atrium and ventricle (due to right-sided dysfunction e.g. dilated right ventricle restricted by pericardium in constrictive pericarditis or pre-existing high filling pressures in the setting of heart failure) and venous blood and pressure is 'backed up' into the jugular veins. *The right ventricle cannot accommodate additional venous return.*

Sign value

This is a useful and commonly used test to help assess venous pressures at the bedside. It is sensitive but not specific to any particular disorder and must be taken in clinical context.

- In the presence of dyspnoea, can predict heart failure: PLR 6.0, NLR −0.7834.[57]
- In the presence of dyspnoea, can predict elevated pulmonary capillary wedge pressure >15 mmHg: PLR 6.7, NLR 0.08.[57]
- Detecting elevated left heart diastolic pressures, with sensitivity of 55–84%, specificity of 83–98%, PLR 8.0, NLR 0.3.[58]

If dyspnoea is not present, search for alternative causes of the reflex.

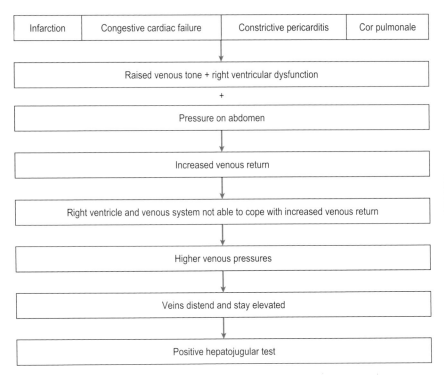

| Infarction | Congestive cardiac failure | Constrictive pericarditis | Cor pulmonale |

Raised venous tone + right ventricular dysfunction

+

Pressure on abdomen

Increased venous return

Right ventricle and venous system not able to cope with increased venous return

Higher venous pressures

Veins distend and stay elevated

Positive hepatojugular test

FIGURE 3.19
Mechanism of hepatojugular reflux

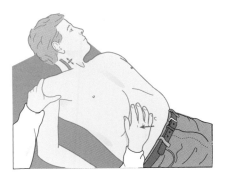

FIGURE 3.20
Hepatojugular reflux

Hypertensive retinopathy

Refers to pathological changes seen in retinal vessels owing to (or as a marker of) hypertension. Some of these changes have also been used as markers for severity of underlying hypertension.

Sign value

There has recently been renewed interest in hypertensive retinopathy as a marker, prognostic indicator and risk factor for disease.[59-61]

- Mild and moderate hypertensive retinopathy is associated with a 1–2-fold increase in the risk of hypertension.

- Mild and moderate hypertensive retinopathy is associated with a 1–8-fold increase in the risk of stroke.

- Mild hypertensive retinopathy is associated with a 2–3-fold increase in the risk of coronary artery disease.

- Moderate hypertensive retinopathy is associated with increased risk of cognitive decline.

A recent study[62] with a mean of 13-years follow-up re-enforced the above finding and found that people with moderate hypertensive retinopathy were more likely to have stroke (moderate versus no retinopathy: multivariable hazard ratios, 2.37 [95% confidence interval, 1.39–4.02]).

Furthermore, even in patients with treated hypertension, hypertensive retinopathy was related to an increased risk of cerebral infarction (mild retinopathy: hazard ratio, 1.96 [95% confidence interval, 1.09–3.55]; and moderate retinopathy: hazard ratio, 2.98 [95% confidence interval, 1.01–8.83]).

Hypertensive retinopathy may predict the long-term risk of stroke, independent of blood pressure, even in treated patients with good hypertension control.

Hypertensive retinopathy: arteriovenous (AV) nipping (or AV nicking)

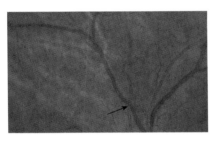

FIGURE 3.21
AV nipping/nicking

Based on Yanoff M, Duker JS (eds),
Ophthalmology, *3rd edn, St Louis: Mosby,*
2008: Fig 6-15-2.

Description

An enlarged retinal arteriole that crosses a vein can press down and cause swelling distal to the crossing. The vein will have an hourglass appearance on either side of the intersection.

Condition/s associated with

• Hypertension

Mechanism/s

Persistently elevated blood pressure causes hyperplasia of the arteriolar media and intimal thickening.[59] The enlarged vessel impinges on the underlying vein, giving it a 'nipped in' appearance.

3

Hypertensive retinopathy: copper and silver wiring

Description

Refers to the abnormal colouring of the arterioles seen through an ophthalmoscope. In copper wiring, the arterioles appear reddish-brown; in silver wiring, the vessels look grey.

Condition/s associated with

- Hypertension

Mechanism/s

The *distortion of the normal light reflex* of the retinal vessels is the cause of both discolourations.

In copper wiring, the sclerosis and hyalinisation spreads throughout the arterioles, continually thickening them. As this thickening continues, the light reflex *becomes more diffuse* and the retinal arterioles become red-brown in appearance.

In silver wiring, worsening sclerosis increases the optical density of the vessel wall, making it look 'sheathed'. If the entire vessel becomes sheathed, it will look like a silver wire.

Hypertensive retinopathy: cotton wool spots

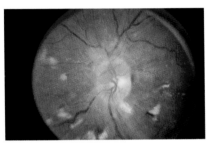

FIGURE 3.22
Cotton wool spots
White lesions with fuzzy margins, seen here approximately one-fifth to one-quarter disk diameter in size. Orientation of cotton wool spots generally follows the curvilinear arrangement of the nerve fibre layer.

Reproduced, with permission, from Effron D, Forcier BC, Wyszynski RE, Chapter 3: Funduscopic findings. In: Knoop KJ, Stack LB, Storrow AB, Thurman RJ, The Atlas of Emergency Medicine, 3rd edn, McGraw-Hill. Available: http://proxy14.use.hcn.com.au/content.aspx?aID=6000554 [2 Apr 2010].

Description

Small areas of yellow-white discolouration on the retina, often described as puffy white patches.

Condition/s associated with

More common

- Diabetes – most common
- Hypertension – common

Less common

- Central retinal vein occlusion
- Branch retinal vein occlusion
- HIV – rare
- Pancreatitis – rare

Mechanism/s

Principally due to damage and swelling of the nerve fibres.

Prolonged hypertension results in distortion and blocking of retinal arterioles, blockage of axoplasmic flow (of proteins, lipids etc along the axon of the neuron) and a build-up of intracellular nerve debris in the nerve fibre layer. These insults result in swelling of the layer.

3

Hypertensive retinopathy: microaneurysms

Description

Small, round, dark red dots on the retinal surface that are smaller than the diameter of major optic veins (see Figure 3.23). They often herald a progression to the exudative phase of hypertensive retinopathy.

Condition/s associated with

- Diabetes
- Hypertension

Mechanism/s

As progression of hypertensive retinopathy occurs, there is capillary occlusion ischaemia and degeneration of the vascular smooth muscle, endothelial cell necrosis and formation of tiny aneurysms.

Hypertensive retinopathy: retinal haemorrhage

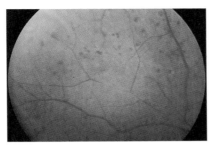

FIGURE 3.23
Dot and blot haemorrhages and microaneurysms

Reproduced, with permission, from Yanoff M, Duker JS (eds), Ophthalmology, 3rd edn, St Louis: Mosby, 2008: Fig 6-20-2.

Description
Bleeding that occurs in or spills onto the retina. Can be 'dot and blot' or 'streaking' in appearance.

Condition/s associated with
More common
- Hypertension
- Diabetes
- Trauma

Less common
- Retinal vein occlusions
- Retinal artery occlusions

Mechanism/s
Prolonged hypertension leads to intimal thickening and ischaemia. This causes degeneration of retinal blood vessels to the point where they leak plasma and bleed onto the retina.[60]

3

Hypertrophic obstructive cardiomyopathy murmur

Description

A systolic ejection murmur heard loudest at the lower left sternal border that does not radiate to the carotids.

Condition/s associated with

- Hypertrophic *obstructive* cardiomyopathy (often said to be with a gradient >30mmHg)

Mechanism/s

Hypertrophic cardiomyopathy is an autosomal dominant condition that is associated with a number of gene mutations encoding for a variety of proteins in the cardiac sarcomere. The net result of the mutation is inappropriate hypertrophy of the myocardium. This hypertrophy may include the septum and result in obstruction of the left ventricular outflow tract. The obstruction and murmur is significantly contributed to by *systolic anterior motion* of the anterior leaflet of the mitral valve. That is, in systole the anterior leaflet of mitral valve is dragged into the left ventricular outflow tract towards the septum, causing the obstruction of flow out of the left ventricle and turbulent flow.

Systolic anterior motion of the anterior leaflet was once thought to be due to the already narrowed outflow tract (as a result of septal hypertrophy) causing a pressure drop and sucking the leaflet towards the septum and into the left ventricular outflow tract.

Recent evidence indicates that this is not the predominant mechanism but drag (the pushing force of flow) directly 'pushes' slightly abnormally sized and placed (as a result of hypertrophy of the myocardium) leaflets forwards into the outflow tract. Further abnormalities in the septum may direct abnormal flows towards the leaflets which catch and push them towards the septum.

Mechanism/s of dynamic manoeuvres on outflow tract murmurs.

Outflow tract gradients which are seen in hypertrophic obstructive cardiomopathies are:

- decreased by anything that decreases myocardial contractility (beta blockers)

- decreased by anything that increases ventricular volume arterial pressure (squatting, handgrip exercises)

- increased by a decrease in arterial pressure or ventricular volume (Valsalva, nitrates, dehydration)

- increased by an increase in contractility.

Examples of the mechanisms of these principles are shown in Figures 3.24, 3.25 and 3.26.

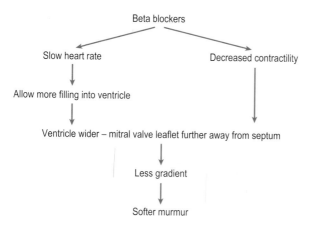

FIGURE 3.24
Mechanism of HOCM murmur change with beta blockers

3

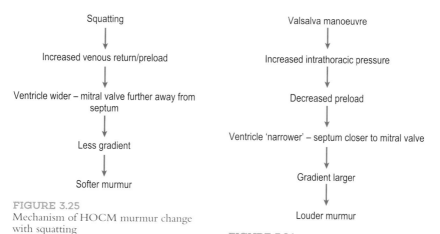

FIGURE 3.25
Mechanism of HOCM murmur change
with squatting

FIGURE 3.26
Effect of standing on Valsalva on HOCM
murmur

Janeway lesions

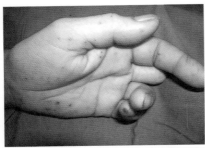

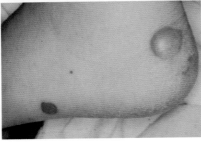

FIGURE 3.27
Janeway lesions

Based on Mandell GL, Bennett JA, Dolin R, Mandell, Douglas, and Bennett's Principles and Practice of Infectious Diseases, 7th edn, Philadelphia: Churchill Livingston, 2009: Fig 195-15.

Definition

Non-tender, haemorrhagic macules or papules often found on the palms or soles – especially on thenar or hypothenar eminences.[63]

Condition/s associated with

- Bacterial endocarditis – traditionally reported with the acute form of the disease

Mechanism/s

The underlying mechanism is still under debate. Janeway lesions are thought to be caused by septic micro-emboli deposited in peripheral sites.[64] However, histological research[63] still suggests that an immunological vasculitic process may play a role in some lesions.

Sign value

Janeway lesions have limited value as a sign, appearing in only 4–10% of patients with bacterial endocarditis.[65] If present, investigations for other signs of bacterial endocarditis should be performed.

For other signs of bacterial endocarditis, see also 'Osler's nodes', 'Roth spots' and 'Splinter haemorrhages' in this chapter.

Jugular venous pressure (JVP)

The signs associated with jugular venous pressure (JVP) are some of the first and most useful to be introduced to students studying cardiology. Jugular venous pressure is still the cornerstone of bedside assessment of volume/left ventricular filling pressure. It is integral to diagnostic and management decisions even while other more sophisticated tests are undertaken.

Key concept explained
JVP what does it actually measure?

When casting a knowing look at the internal jugular vein (and sometimes the external jugular vein), both of which drain via the superior vena cava into the right atrium, the clinician is using its features to estimate central venous pressure (CVP). CVP refers to right atrial pressure and, providing there is no tricuspid stenosis, right ventricular diastolic pressure.

This in turn is influenced by parts of the circuit seen in Figure 3.28.

These include the blood volume itself, the right ventricle, the pulmonary artery, the lungs, the pulmonary veins and the left side of the heart. Changes or dysfunction along this circuit at any point may cause changes to the JVP. For example, a decrease in circulating blood volume such as occurs in dehydration, may cause the JVP to be low, whereas a decrease in compliance due to infarction of the right ventricle will lead to decreased relaxation of the right ventricle and increased pressure for the given volume, and therefore a higher jugular venous pressure. Understanding the flow and circuit in Figure 3.28 is crucial in understanding the different causes of change to the JVP.

3

CLINICAL PEARL

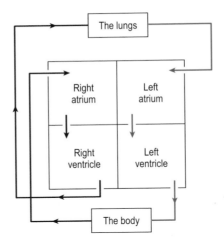

FIGURE 3.28
Stylised diagram of the pulmonary and systemic circuits
Interruptions or changes in pressures along the circuits cause changes in pressure upstream of the underlying pathology.

JVP: Kussmaul's sign

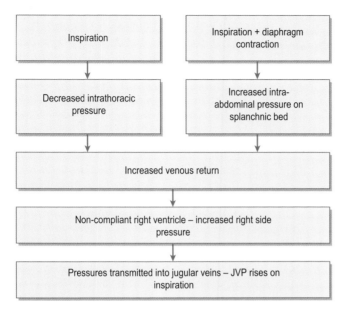

FIGURE 3.29
Mechanism of Kussmaul's sign

VIDEO 3.3 ▶

Video 3.3 Access through Student Consult.

Description

Rather than the expected decline in the level of jugular venous pressure on inspiration as venous blood is returned to the heart, a paradoxical rise in the JVP is seen when the patient breathes in.

Condition/s associated with

More common

- Severe heart failure
- Right ventricular infarction
- Pulmonary embolus

Less common

- Tricuspid stenosis
- Constrictive pericarditis

Mechanism/s

Kussmaul's sign is thought to be caused by a combination of *increased venous return* to the heart in conjunction with a *constricted or non-compliant right ventricle*.

The process occurs as follows:

- Normal inspiration requires a decrease in intrathoracic pressure. This helps draw venous blood back towards the thorax.
- Contraction of the diaphragm on inspiration increases abdominal pressure and further increases venous return from an engorged splanchnic bed.[66]

- A non-compliant right ventricle, owing to constrictive pericarditis, failure of the right ventricle or increased right ventricular afterload (pulmonary embolus), cannot accommodate the venous return, and right atrial pressure exceeds the fall in pleural pressure.[67]
- The blood then backs up into distended neck veins.

Sign value

Kussmaul's sign may be present in less than 40% of constrictive pericarditis cases; however, its specificity for an underlying pathology is very high. If present it needs to be investigated.

JVP: raised

Description

This refers to the level of venous pulsation in the jugular veins relative to the sternal angle. The JVP is elevated if visible higher than 3 cm from the sternal angle with the patient reclining at 45°.

The JVP is an indirect measure of right ventricular filling pressure. If filling pressure is raised, JVP is raised. It also has a predictable relationship with pulmonary wedge pressure and is useful in assessing volume status and left ventricular function.

Identifying and measuring the JVP can be challenging. Some authors have suggested a simplified test – noting a lack of collapse of the JVP on inspiration – as one way to identify patients with raised central venous pressures.[68]

Condition/s associated with

- Heart failure
- Volume overload
- Cardiac tamponade
- Pericardial effusion
- Pulmonary hypertension

Mechanism/s

Contributing factors include:

- In patients with heart failure, the peripheral veins are abnormally constricted due to increased tissue oedema and sympathetic stimulation. This has the effect of increasing the blood volume in the central venous system – i.e. the thoracic vena caval system that enters the right side of the heart.

- *Volume overload* – like any pump system, ventricular function cannot manage excess intravascular volume indefinitely. Eventually, overload will lead to increased ventricular end-systolic and end-diastolic volume and pressure, which in turn backs up through the atrium and is transmitted into the jugular veins – either directly from the right-sided dysfunction or via the lungs in left heart failure.

- *Right ventricular systolic failure* – decreased right ventricular output leads to increased end-systolic pressure, which is transmitted back to cause increased right atrial pressure. The pressure is then transmitted back into the venous system, raising venous pressure and the JVP.

- *Right ventricular diastolic failure* (e.g. constrictive pericarditis, cardiac tamponade) – increased stiffness or decreased compliance of the right ventricle means end-diastolic pressure is higher for a given volume during filling. The pressure is then 'backed-up' into the venous and jugular venous system.

- *Compression or infiltration* (e.g. thoracic outlet syndrome, tumour invasion) – compression of the superior vena cave or internal jugular vein by any mass or anatomical abnormality will impede venous drainage and cause a raised jugular venous pressure.

Sign value

Correctly identifying the JVP can be difficult. Correct identification of the jugular veins occurs in 72–94% of patients.[69] The accuracy of the assessment of CVP by visualising the JVP was called into question by four studies[70-73] which found a poor correlation between JVP and invasive monitoring of venous pressure. These studies were based on a very difficult population group of critically ill patients, a majority of which were on mechanical ventilators.

Several studies have confirmed the value of a raised JVP.

TABLE 3.3
Value of jugular venous pressure

Predicting raised central pressure	Prognostic value	Pericardial disease
Predicting CVP >8 cmH$_2$O: sensitivity 47–92%, specificity 93–96%, LR if present 9.0[60,73]	Predicting heart failure admissions: RR 1.32[74]	Cardinal finding of cardiac tamponade in 100% of cases
Detecting CVP >12 cmH2O: sensitivity 78–95%, specificity 89–93%, LR if present 10.4 and if absent 0.1.52	Predicting death from heart failure: RR 1.37.[74]	Seen in 98% of patients with constrictive pericarditis
Predicting PCWP >18 mmHg: sensitivity 57%, PPV 95%, NPV 47%.[75] However, if the raised JVP was absent, the specificity was 93% for PCWP <18 mmHg	A study of over 7000 patients with heart failure and a raised JVP found that it may be a marker of higher burden of sickness and poor outcomes[76]	

JVP: the normal waveform

In well people, the JVP has a predictable waveform that is visible during cardiac catheterisation (as depicted in Figure 3.30). Each section represents a change in right atrial and jugular venous pressure:

a – represents the contraction of the right atrium and the end of diastole

c – marks the start of right ventricular contraction and blood flow, causing the tricuspid valve to bulge into the right atrium

x – or '*x-descent*' occurs when the atrium relaxes and the tricuspid valve is pulled down to the apex of the heart. In normal patients it is the predominant waveform

v – represents atrial filling pressure after ventricular contraction and follows just after S2

y – or '*y-descent*' marks the filling of the ventricle after the tricuspid valve opens

In short, *a*, *c* and *v* all represent relative increases in atrial pressure, while *x* and *y* represent decreasing atrial pressure. Often the *a* and *c* components are too close in timing to see except in certain clinical situations. With this in mind, abnormalities of the different parts of the waveforms can be identified.

3

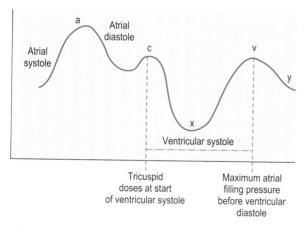

Graph of level of JVP with time

FIGURE 3.30
The normal JVP waveform

JVP waveform variations: *a*-waves – cannon

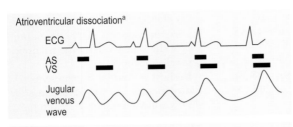

Atrioventricular dissociation[a]

ECG

AS
VS

Jugular
venous
wave

[a]Produces occasional giant a waves.
AS = atrial systole; ECG = electrocardiography; VS = ventricular systol

FIGURE 3.31
Atrioventricular dissociation
Chiaco C. The jugular venous pressure revisited. Cleveland Clinic Journal of Medicine 2013; 80(10): 641, Fig 2.

Description

A large, abrupt flicker/flicker of the *a*-wave that occurs after S1 and *on* the carotid pulse upstroke. Cannon *a*-waves usually do not have the prominent descent that occurs with large *v*-waves (see 'JVP waveform variations: *v*-waves – large' in this chapter).

Condition/s associated with

More common

- AV dissociation and complete heart block

Less common

- Atrial flutter
- Ventricular tachycardia
- Ventricular ectopics
- Atrial premature beats
- Junctional premature beats
- Severe tricuspid stenosis
- 1st degree heart block with markedly prolonged PR interval

Mechanism/s

The underlying mechanism for almost all causes of cannon *a*-waves is a disparity in timing between atrial and ventricular contraction, resulting in atrial contraction against a closed tricuspid valve.

The *a*-wave represents the onset of atrial contraction during which there is an expected minor increase in atrial pressure, as the atrial size is momentarily reduced. Normally, the tricuspid valve opens and atrial pressure drops as blood flows into the ventricle, then ventricular systole occurs and the tricuspid valve closes again.

When a disparity between atrial contraction and ventricular relaxation occurs (regardless of the cause), the atrium contracts vigorously against a closed tricuspid valve, causing a wave of increased pressure from the atrium into the jugular veins – the cannon *a*-wave.

In all of the causes of cannon *a*-waves listed here, there is some degree of atrial/ventricular dyssynchrony, when the atrium is beating at various points in time against a closed tricuspid valve.

For example, in atrial flutter the atria are beating 2–4 times as fast as the ventricle, depending on the AV block. This means that at regular intervals the atrium will be contracting against a valve recently shut after the previous ventricular contraction.

In complete heart block, the atria and ventricles are operating with different pacemakers that are stimulating contractions at different times.

3

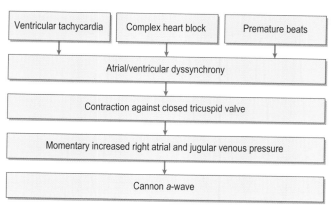

FIGURE 3.32
Mechanism underlying cannon *a*-waves

JVP waveform variations: *a*-waves – prominent or giant

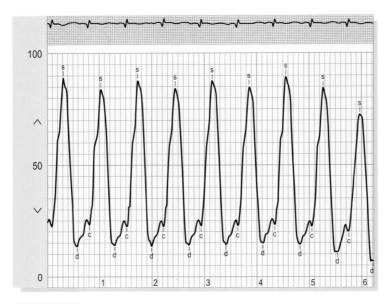

FIGURE 3.33

Patients with right ventricular hypertrophy caused by pulmonary hypertension often have prominent '*a*' waves on the right ventricular pressure waveform

Ragosta M, Cardiac Catheterisation an Atlas and DVD, *Elsevier: p. 71, Fig 6-30.*

Description

An abnormally large and abrupt outward movement of the jugular vein that occurs before the first heart sound. The 'prominent' *a*-wave *precedes* ventricular systole and the carotid pulse upstroke. They can be difficult to witness on clinical examination other than noting a prominent pulsation that is timed *before ventricular systole* but can be easily recognised on cardiac catheterisation as shown in Figure 3.33.

Condition/s associated with

- Right ventricular hypertrophy
  - » Pulmonary stenosis
  - » Pulmonary hypertension
- Tricuspid stenosis
- Mitral stenosis resulting in pulmonary hypertension

Mechanism/s

Raised right atrial pressure from resistance to ventricular filling is the common final pathway. In pulmonary stenosis and pulmonary hypertension, a higher effective afterload on the right ventricle reduces right ventricular stroke volume and raises end-systolic ventricular pressure, which backs up to cause raised right atrial pressure. This may cause (or be exacerbated by) right ventricular hypertrophy, further increasing resistance to filling and end–diastolic pressure.

In tricuspid stenosis, less blood flows into the ventricle in diastole, leaving a higher volume and pressure in the right atrium at the end of diastole. The atrium then contracts against an already raised pressure, further increasing the prominence of the *a*-wave.

Potential areas of confusion explained
Prominent versus cannon a-waves

Prominent *a*-waves and cannon *a*-waves are hard to see and difficult to differentiate.

Two helpful tips to remember when looking at the JVP:
1. Prominent *a*-waves occur before ventricular systole (i.e. **not in time** with the carotid pulse and before S1).
2. Cannon *a*-waves occur with ventricular systole (i.e. **in time** with the carotid pulse and after S1).

3

JVP waveform variations: v-waves – large

VIDEO 3.4 ▌▶

Video 3.4 Access through Student Consult.

Description

Usually found in patients with an elevated JVP, v-waves will appear as a large systolic outward distension and rise of the JVP with carotid pulsation. There is usually prominent venous collapse visible after the v-wave and S2 then occurs. This can be visualised on venous waveform and is depicted in Figure 3.34.

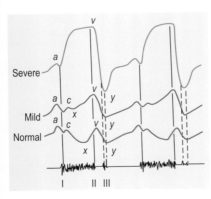

FIGURE 3.34

Normal jugular venous waveform (bottom), mild TR (middle) and severe TR (top), with corresponding phonocardiogram With severe TR, 'ventricularisation' of the jugular venous waveform is seen, with a prominent v-wave and rapid y-descent. The x-descent is absent.

Abrams J, Synopsis of Cardiac Physical Diagnosis, 2nd edn, Elsevier, 2001: 25–35. In: Braunwald's Heart Disease: A Textbook of Cardiovascular Medicine, 10th edn, Philadelphia: Elsevier, 2015.

Condition/s associated with

- Tricuspid regurgitation
- Pulmonary hypertension
- Severe mitral regurgitation

Mechanism/s

The height of the v-wave is determined by right atrial compliance and by the volume of blood returning to the right atrium. The volume may return from the superior vena cava or as a result of tricuspid regurgitation via an incompetent tricuspid valve. Increased right atrial blood volume, due to regurgitant flow from the right ventricle during systole, leads to increased right atrial pressure that is then transmitted up into the jugular vein, leading to the characteristic v-wave distention.

In pulmonary hypertension, pressure from the pulmonary artery backs up through to the right ventricle and then the right atrium.

Sign value

The presence of large v- or cv-waves on clinical examination significantly supports the diagnosis of tricuspid regurgitation in one study with sensitivity 37%, specificity 97% and PLR 10.9 to 31.4.[77]

Alternatively, on cardiac catheterisation a slightly different conclusion was drawn. The absence of large v-waves and raised JVP was specific for the absence of moderate or severe tricuspid regurgitation (a good negative predictive value).[78] If one suspects the presence of tricuspid regurgitation, observation for large v-waves and palpation for a pulsatile liver is essential.

CLINICAL PEARL

JVP waveform variations: x-descent – absent

Description

The loss of the characteristic descent in JVP waveform that normally coincides with systole.

Condition/s associated with

- Tricuspid regurgitation
- Atrial fibrillation

Mechanism/s

Normally, the x-descent is caused by the floor of the atrium drawing downwards during systole (see discussion under 'JVP waveform variations: x-descent – prominent'). In tricuspid regurgitation, the regurgitant volume offsets the normal drop in pressure caused by ventricular systole.

In atrial fibrillation, an x-descent is thought to be absent due to poor right ventricular contraction combined with a degree of tricuspid regurgitation.[79]

3

JVP waveform variations: x-descent – prominent

Description

The x-descent occurs in the jugular venous waveform after atrial contraction, during ventricular systole, and is timed with the carotid pulse.

The x-descent represents the decrease in JVP, which occurs due to:

- atrial relaxation
- the tricuspid valve being pulled downwards during ventricular systole
- ejection of blood volume from the ventricles.

All of these aspects enlarge or relax the atrium, decreasing the atrial pressure.

A prominent x-descent is faster and larger than normal. It is a sign that shows that forward venous flow only occurs during systole.

It is a challenging sign to identify on clinical exam but has been proven on cardiac catheterisation.

Condition/s associated with

- Cardiac tamponade/pericardial effusion

Mechanism/s

A prominent x-descent is an exaggeration of the normal waveform descent. In cardiac tamponade, compression of the chambers of the heart leads to elevated right atrial pressure. This raised pressure eventually blocks the forward flow of venous blood (i.e. filling) from the jugular vein into the atrium during diastole.

When the atrium relaxes and the ventricles contract in systole, the tricuspid valve is pulled down towards the apex of the heart, and there is a momentary increase in atrial volume and decrease in atrial pressure, allowing a *rapid descent* in atrial pressure and the JVP.

Sign value

Often a difficult sign to see, and there is limited evidence on the prevalence of a prominent x-descent; nonetheless, if suspected, cardiac tamponade must be excluded.

JVP waveform variations: y-descent – absent

Description

The y-descent represents the drop in right atrial pressure that occurs when the tricuspid valve opens and blood flows into the right ventricle during diastole. This can be seen clinically and is represented on pressure waveforms in Figure 3.35.

Condition/s associated with

Most common

• Cardiac tamponade

Less common

• Tricuspid stenosis

3

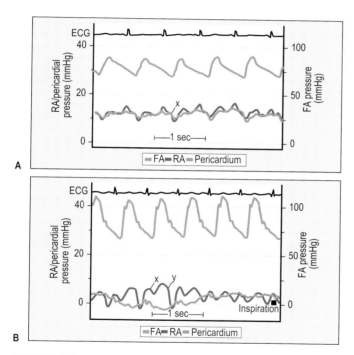

A

B

FIGURE 3.35

Absent y-descent in cardiac tamponade

Femoral, right atrial and pericardial pressure before (**A**) and after (**B**) pericardiocentesis in a patient with cardiac tamponade. Note that before pericardiocentesis, there is an x-descent but no y-descent. Post pericardiocentesis there is an increase in femoral artery pressure and a decrease in right atrial pressure and the y-descent is now visible.

Modified from Lorell BH, Grossman W, Profiles in constrictive pericarditis, restrictive cardiomyopathy and cardiac tamponade. In: Baim DS, Grossman W (eds), Grossman's Cardiac Catheterization, Angiography, and Intervention, 6th edn, Philadelphia: Lippincott Williams & Wilkins, 2000: p. 832.

Mechanism/s

Any pathology that may limit or prevent ventricular filling in diastole will cause an absent y-descent.

In cardiac tamponade, pressure from pericardial fluid surrounding the heart leads to a higher left ventricular diastolic pressure, which impedes filling of the ventricle during diastole and thus blunts the y-descent.[80]

Rarely, in tricuspid stenosis the filling of the right ventricle is impaired by the stenotic tricuspid valve. Therefore, right atrial pressure remains higher than normal and an impaired pressure descent occurs.

JVP waveform variations: y-descent – prominent (Friedrich's sign)

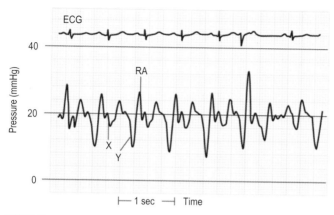

FIGURE 3.36
Prominent y-descent in constrictive pericarditis
Right atrial (RA) pressure recording from a patient with constrictive pericarditis. Note the elevation in pressure and prominent y-descent corresponding to rapid early diastolic right atrial emptying.

Reproduced, with permission, from Goldman L, Ausiello D, Cecil Medicine, 23rd edn, Philadelphia: Saunders, 2007: Fig 77-11.

Description

A faster and more prominent descent of the JVP during diastole, coinciding with the drop in right atrial pressure that occurs after opening of the tricuspid valve.

Seen on physical examination as an abrupt collapse of the neck veins during diastole.

Condition/s associated with

More common

• Constrictive pericarditis

Less common

• Right ventricular infarction
• ASD
• Atrial fibrillation

Mechanism/s

In constrictive pericarditis, early diastolic filling is not inhibited but filling becomes impaired in the last two-thirds of diastole when the expanding ventricle hits the rigid pericardium. Once this occurs, the pressure rises again to a higher-than-normal level.

The y-descent appears accentuated as it descends from a higher-than-normal right atrial pressure.

Sign value

A prominent y-descent has been found to occur in about one-third of patients with constrictive pericarditis and two-thirds of patients with right ventricular infarction, although studies are limited and it is often difficult to see in a clinical setting. Presence of the y-descent is valuable when interpreting waveforms on cardiac catheterisation to diagnose constrictive pericarditis.

The presence of a rapid y-descent excludes the diagnosis of pericardial tamponade (see 'JVP waveform variations: y-descent – absent').

Descents *x* vs *y*

There can be some confusion over x-descents prominent or absent and y-descents prominent or absent, especially when discussing constrictive pericarditis and cardiac tamponade.

Put simply:
- x-descent prominent with y-descent absent – think cardiac tamponade
- x-descent variable with y-descent prominent – think constrictive pericarditis.

Mid-systolic click

Description

A non-ejection systolic click, heard shortly after S1, with radiation to the axilla. It is best heard with the diaphragm of the stethoscope over the apex with the patient in the left lateral position.

The mid-systolic click may occur in isolation or in conjunction with a late systolic mitral regurgitation murmur.

Condition/s associated with

- Mitral valve prolapse

Mechanism/s

In mitral valve prolapse, the leaflets, especially the anterior leaflet, protrude into the atrium in systole. The mid-systolic click occurs when the *anterior leaflet prolapses into the atrium, putting tension on the chordae tendinae. The click corresponds to the sudden tensing of the chordae tendinae.*[81]

Mechanisms of dynamic manoeuvres

In mitral valve prolapse, as the left ventricle chamber decreases in size in systole, the papillary muscles and/or the chordae fail to maintain tension on the mitral valve, and it prolapses with a brief regurgitant period into the left atrium.

To help elicit the sign and diagnosis, additional manoeuvres are performed. Manoeuvres or conditions which decrease venous return (Valsalva, tachycardia or an increase in contractility) allow for less tension on the valve and chordae tendinae, so prolapse will occur earlier and closer to S1, as depicted in Figure 3.37.

Conversely, manoeuvres (e.g. squatting, bradycardia or decreased contractility) that increase venous return and diastolic filling, and increase ventricular volume, help to maintain tension along the chordae and to keep the valve shut and not prolapse, or prolapse later in the cycle towards S2.

Sign value

A staple in physician clinical examinations when present, this sign is very specific for mitral valve prolapse; however, prolapse may be present without a mid-systolic click occurring.

3

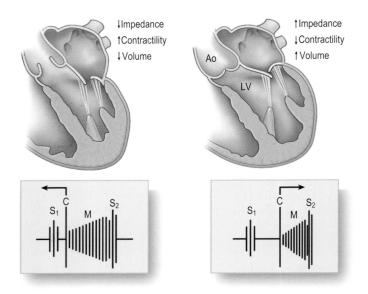

FIGURE 3.37

Dynamic auscultation in mitral valve prolapse

Any manoeuvre that decreases LV volume (e.g. decreased venous return, tachycardia, decreased outflow impedance, increased contractility) worsens the mismatch in size between the enlarged mitral valve and LV chamber, resulting in prolapse earlier in systole and movement of the click (C) and murmur (M) towards the first heart sound (S1). Conversely, manoeuvres that increase LV volume (e.g. increased venous return, bradycardia, increased outflow impedance, decreased contractility) delay the occurrence of prolapse, resulting in movement of the click and murmur towards the second heart sound (S2).[82]

Ao = aorta.

Mann DL et al., Braunwald's Heart Disease: A Textbook of Cardiovascular Medicine, *10th edn, Philadelphia: Elsevier, 2015: Fig 63.40. (Modified from O'Rourke RA, Crawford MH. The systolic click-murmur syndrome: clinical recognition and management. Curr Probl Cardiol 1976; 1: 9.)*

Mitral facies

Description

A purple or plum-coloured malar flush.

Condition/s associated with

• Mitral stenosis

It should be noted that many causes of low cardiac output can cause mitral facies.

Mechanism/s

Low cardiac output with severe pulmonary hypertension leads to chronic hypoxaemia and skin vasodilatation.

3

Mottling

Description

Patchy skin discolouration often starting around the knees.[83]

Condition/s associated with

- Sepsis
- Shocked states

Mechanism/s

Skin mottling is likely due to *heterogenic small vessel vasoconstriction* and has been shown to reflect abnormal skin microperfusion.[83]

A recent study in patients with septic shock showed skin perfusion was inversely related to the degree of mottling (i.e. as skin perfusion decreases the mottling increases).[83]

It is likely poor skin perfusion causing mottling in septic shock is related to the known complex interplay of cytokines, endothelial dysfunction and abnormal microcirculation.

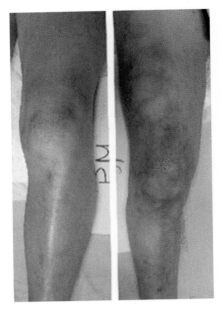

FIGURE 3.38
Skin mottling

Ait-Oufell H. Mottling score predicts survival in septic shock. Intensive Care Medicine *2011; 37: 803.*

Sign value

Skin mottling has long been associated with severe illness and a poor prognosis. There is recent evidence to support this,[83] demonstrating mottling's relationship to other parameters that reflect organ perfusion, such as arterial lactate level or diuresis.

A high mottling score (more mottling = higher score, [score 0–1 OR 1; score 2–3 OR 16, 95% CI (4–81); score 4–5 OR 74!, 95% CI (11–1568), p = 0.0001]) has been strongly associated with 14-day mortality. The higher the mottling score, the earlier death occurred (p = 0.0001) and patients whose mottling score decreased during the resuscitation period had a better prognosis (14-day mortality 77 vs 12%, p = 0.0005).[83]

Murmurs

The appreciation and classification of murmurs is an important clinical skill. Even with increased availability of echocardiography, being able to recognise a murmur impacts on diagnostic formulation, as well as decisions about further testing.

Although the six components of timing, intensity, pitch, shape, location and radiation are all required for a complete description of a murmur as a clinical sign, murmurs in this chapter will be listed, in the first instance, according to their timing and in the following order: systolic, diastolic or continuous. Table 3.4 matches the characteristics of the murmur with a likely cardiac pathology or vice versa. The underlying mechanism is then explained under the heading for that pathology.

TABLE 3.4
Summary of murmurs

Timing	Shape	Best heard	Common cause
Systolic			
'Ejection' systolic	Mid- to late-peaking	Aortic area radiating to carotid	Aortic stenosis
	Crescendo–decrescendo	Pulmonic area with inspiration	Pulmonary stenosis
Pansystolic/holosystolic	Flat	Apex radiating to left axilla	Mitral regurgitation
		4th intercostal space at left sternal edge to right sternal edge increasing with inspiration	Tricuspid regurgitation (Carvello's sign)
		4th–6th intercostal spaces	VSD
Late systolic	As for mitral regurgitation but with an associated mid-systolic click	Apex radiating to left axilla	Mitral regurgitation associated with MV prolapse
Diastolic			
Early	Decrescendo	Left sternal edge (aortic area)	Aortic regurgitation
	Decrescendo	Pulmonic area on full inspiration	Pulmonary regurgitation
Mid-to-late	Decrescendo	Mitral area with the bell and patient in left lateral decubitus position	Mitral stenosis
	Crescendo–decrescendo	4th intercostal space at lower left sternal edge	Tricuspid stenosis
Continuous			
	'Machinery'	Left upper chest	PDA

Murmurs – systolic: aortic stenotic murmur

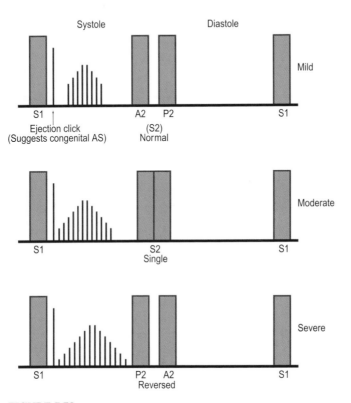

FIGURE 3.39

Timing and shape of an aortic stenotic murmur

Based on Talley N, O'Connor S, Clinical Examination, *6th edn, Sydney: Elsevier Australia, 2009: Fig 4.48A.*

Description

A mid-to-late-peaking ejection systolic murmur best heard over the aortic area of the praecordium that radiates to the carotid arteries. It is late-peaking and ceases before A2. Manoeuvres that increase stroke volume (e.g. squatting) will increase the volume of the murmur, while manoeuvres increasing afterload (e.g. standing and Valsalva) will reduce volume.

Condition/s associated with

- Age-related degeneration/ calcification – most common cause
- Rheumatic heart disease – common cause

- Congenital bicuspid valve and calcification
- Congenital aortic stenosis

Mechanism/s

Most causes of aortic stenosis eventually result in progressive damage to and calcification of the valvular apparatus, leading to narrowing or obstruction of the area of the valve and/or stiffening of the leaflets. Blood flowing over the stenotic valve in systole causes the murmur. The mechanisms leading to this common pathway vary depending on the underlying pathology.

Age-related degeneration ('senile calcification')

This was initially thought to be due to normal, continuous mechanical stress over many years. The current proposed mechanism involves inflammatory changes, lipid accumulation, up-regulation of immunological mediators and ACE activity leading to *calcification and bone formation.*[28]

Rheumatic heart disease

In all instances of rheumatic heart disease, a type 2 hypersensitivity reaction to group A streptococcus (GAS) causes damage to the heart valve.

Antibodies directed against the M protein of the GAS cross-react and act against normal myocardium, joints and other tissues by virtue of molecular mimicry. The M protein antigen of the GAS 'looks like' normal self-antigens, which are attacked by the body's immune system.

The resulting reaction leads to the characteristic changes of rheumatic heart disease:

- fusion of the commissures and cusps
- adhesion formation and stiffening of the leaflets

- thickening of leaflet edges
- shortened, thickened chordae tendinae.

Consequently, valve area is diminished and the valve cannot open widely or efficiently.

Dynamic manoeuvres mechanisms

Manoeuvres such as squatting increase venous return, stroke volume, flow across the valve and thus the murmur. The strain of Valsalva, which decreases venous return, has the opposite effect on the intensity of the murmur. See Figure 3.40.

Sign value

This sign is best used in conjunction with other clinical findings. If present, it is of reasonable value in determining the presence of aortic stenosis (sensitivity of 96%, specificity of 71%, PLR 3.3[84,85]). The likelihood of the aortic stenosis is further increased in the presence of a delayed carotid upstroke, absent S2 (due to the late peaking murmur) and a humming quality to the murmur.

The radiation of the murmur is very helpful in identifying aortic stenosis. Should a systolic murmur radiate from the aortic area across the praecordium to the apex in a 'broad apical-to-base pattern', the LR is 9.7.[77]

The absence of certain findings also aids in the *exclusion* of aortic stenosis as the cause of the murmur. Studies have shown that the absence of the characteristic aortic stenotic murmur is very helpful in excluding aortic stenosis with an LR of 0.10,[84,85] as is the absence of radiation of the murmur to the carotids, LR 0.2 (0.1–0.3).[77]

The intensity of the murmur does not indicate severity. Body size and cardiac output are more important determinants.[85] In fact, a softer aortic stenotic murmur may indicate more severe disease.

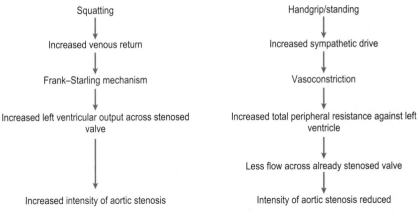

FIGURE 3.40
Dynamic manoeuvres and aortic stenosis

Murmurs – systolic: mitral regurgitation murmur

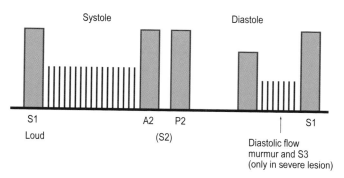

FIGURE 3.41
Timing and shape of mitral regurgitation murmur

Reproduced, with permission, from Talley N, O'Connor S, Clinical Examination, *6th edn, Sydney: Elsevier Australia, 2009: Fig 4.46A.*

AUDIO 3.3

Audio 3.3 Access through Student Consult.

See also 'Mid-systolic click' in this chapter.

Description

A high-pitched, pan-systolic, blowing murmur heard loudest at the apex and radiating to the left axilla. It varies little with beat-to-beat changes in stroke volume.

Condition/s associated with

Any damage or disruption to the mitral apparatus (mitral leaflets, chordae tendinae, papillary muscles, mitral annulus) can cause mitral regurgitation so there are numerous potential causes.

More common causes

- Mitral valve prolapse
- Rheumatic heart disease
- Infective endocarditis
- Myxomatous degeneration
- Cardiomyopathy
- Ischaemic heart disease

General mechanism/s

To cause a mitral regurgitation murmur, the underlying disease or pathology must disrupt the mitral apparatus so that the valve does not close effectively. Thus, during systole a jet of blood moves back across into the left atrium. This turbulent regurgitant jet moving across an incompletely closed valve causes the murmur.

Rheumatic heart disease

Thickening of the valve leaflets and stiffening of the commissures prevents normal closure of the mitral valve.

Infective endocarditis

In infective endocarditis, infection of the valve and the resulting inflammatory process can destroy any part of the valvular apparatus, rendering the valve unable to close or remain closed effectively during systole.

Cardiomyopathy

In dilated cardiomyopathy of any cause, the left ventricle enlarges, as does the mitral annulus. Consequently, the mitral leaflets are unable to effectively cover the valvular orifice, allowing a regurgitant jet of blood back into the left atrium.

Ischaemic heart disease

In ischaemic heart disease, a myocardial infarction may cause mitral regurgitation through a variety of mechanisms:

- papillary muscle rupture or elongation causing leaflet prolapse
- dysfunction of the papillary muscles preventing tightening of the chordae tendinae and effective closure of the mitral valve
- regional remodelling and changes in ventricular size and function that cause annular dilatation and affect papillary muscle function and mitral leaflet coaptation.

Myxomatous degeneration

A genetic defect in the composition of the collagen in the valvular apparatus allows *stretching and elongation of the leaflets and chordae tendinae*. This increases the risk of the chordae rupturing and leaflets prolapsing into the left atrium on systole.

Dynamic manoeuvres mechanism

As with aortic regurgitation, any manoeuvre that increases systemic vascular resistance will increase pressure against forward flow, increase backward flow and augment the mitral regurgitative murmur. A failure of the

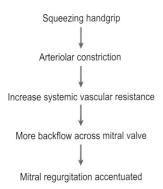

Squeezing handgrip

↓

Arteriolar constriction

↓

Increase systemic vascular resistance

↓

More backflow across mitral valve

↓

Mitral regurgitation accentuated

FIGURE 3.42
Dynamic manoeuvres mechanism

murmur to accentuate on this manoeuvring may suggest the presence of an alternate diagnosis.

Sign value

The characteristic mitral regurgitation murmur has moderate value in detecting the presence of mitral regurgitation with a sensitivity of 56–75%, specificity of 89–93% and an LR of 5.4.[86,87] It does not, however, indicate the severity of the regurgitation.

Specifically, the radiation of the systolic murmur is also helpful in predicting mitral regurgitation. A 'broad apical pattern', with the murmur extending from the fourth or fifth intercostal space to the midclavicular or anterior axillary line, has a PLR of 6.8 for significant mitral regurgitation.[77]

The absence of a mitral regurgitation murmur is very good at predicting absence of significant mitral regurgitation, with an LR of only 0.2 if absent.[86,87] The presence of an S3 is variably associated with severe mitral regurgitation.

Murmurs – systolic: pulmonary stenotic murmur

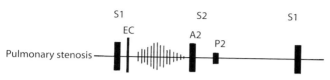

FIGURE 3.43
Timing and shape of a pulmonary stenotic murmur
Reproduced, with permission, from Keane JF et al. (eds), Nadas' Pediatric Cardiology, *2nd edn, Philadelphia: Saunders, 2006: Fig 31-6.*

3

AUDIO 3.4 🔊

Audio 3.4 Access through Student Consult.

Description

Classically, the pulmonary stenotic murmur is described as a systolic crescendo–decrescendo ejection murmur. It is heard best in the pulmonary area of the praecordium and increases with inspiration.

Condition/s associated with

- Congenital heart disease – most common cause
- Carcinoid syndrome – uncommon
- Rheumatic heart disease – rare

Mechanism/s

As in other forms of stenotic lesions, turbulent blood flow across either abnormally functioning leaflets or a constricted valve orifice causes the pulmonary stenotic murmur.

Congenital

Abnormalities in development of the valvular, subvalvular or peripheral pulmonary arteries can cause a pulmonary stenotic murmur. Abnormalities include, but are not limited to, dysplastic irregularly thickened valve leaflets, a smaller-than-normal annulus and bicuspid valves.

Carcinoid syndrome

Carcinoid syndrome produces pulmonary stenosis via the deposition of plaques on or around the pulmonary valve, obstructing the orifice and/or affecting the valve opening. The cause of the plaques is thought to be associated with high serotonin levels that stimulate fibroblast proliferation[88] and activation; however, the exact mechanism is still unclear.

Murmurs – systolic: tricuspid regurgitation murmur (also Carvello's sign)

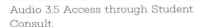

FIGURE 3.44
Tricuspid regurgitation is a pan-systolic murmur, heard over the left sternal edge, that is louder on inspiration

Reproduced, with permission, from Libby P et al., Braunwald's Heart Disease: A Textbook of Cardiovascular Medicine, *8th edn, Philadelphia: Saunders, 2007: Fig 11.9B.*

AUDIO 3.5 🔊

Audio 3.5 Access through Student Consult.

Description

A high-pitched, pan-systolic murmur that gets louder on inspiration, heard best over the left sternal edge in the fourth intercostal space.

Condition/s associated with

A variety of diseases may cause tricuspid regurgitation. Most commonly, it is secondary to dilatation of the right ventricle and not to disease of the valve itself. Causes of tricuspid regurgitation include:

More common

- Any cause of right ventricular dilatation – most common cause
- Rheumatic heart disease
- Infective endocarditis

Less common

- Ebstein's anomaly and other congenital abnormalities

- Prolapse
- Carcinoid syndrome
- Papillary muscle dysfunction
- Connective tissue disease
- Trauma

General mechanism/s

An incompetent tricuspid valve allows blood to flow back from the right ventricle to the right atrium during systole. *The flow across the incompetent valve causes the murmur.*

The augmentation of the murmur with inspiration is likely due to inspiration causing a large increase in effective regurgitance and tricuspid annular enlargement, which despite a decline in regurgitant gradient, causes a notable increase in volume.[89]

As in other valvular disorders, a malfunction or anomaly in the valve itself, the annulus[90] or any other part of the valvular apparatus that does not allow *normal coaptation of valve leaflets* can cause tricuspid regurgitation.

Right ventricular dilatation

This is the *most common* cause of tricuspid regurgitation. In itself, the valve is normal. Right ventricular failure and dilatation of any cause (e.g. myocardial infarction, pulmonary hypertension, mitral valve disease leading to secondary right ventricular dilatation including the tricuspid annulus) does not allow proper coaptation of the leaflets, leading to regurgitation during systole.

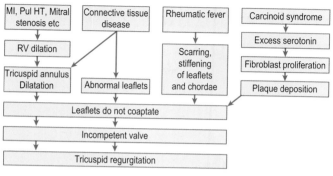

FIGURE 3.45
Mechanisms of tricuspid regurgitation

Based on Pennathur A, Anyanwu AC (eds). Seminars in Thoracic and Cardiovascular Surgery *2010; 22(1): 79–83.*

Carcinoid syndrome

Excessive serotonin stimulates fibroblast proliferation and plaque development, and deposition on the endocardium and valvular apparatus causes the tricuspid valve to adhere to the ventricular wall.[91]

Connective tissue disease

Abnormalities in the connective tissue and collagen produce a floppy valve and may also produce dilatation of the annulus, both of which contribute to poor coaptation of leaflets.

Rheumatic fever

As in mitral and aortic rheumatic heart disease (see 'Aortic stenotic murmur', 'Mitral regurgitation murmur'), scarring and stiffening of the valve and the chordae tendinae reduces mobility and the ability of the valve to close properly.

Sign value

If present, it has a strong PLR (14.6)[86] for mild-to-severe tricuspid regurgitation being present. Additional signs may aid the identification of triscuspid regurgitation. Early systolic outward movement of the neck veins (*v*- or *cv*-waves, LR of 10.9) and hepatic pulsation (LR 12.1) significantly increase the likelihood that tricuspid regurgitation is present.[77]

If not present, this does not rule out mild-to-severe tricuspid regurgitation – NLR of 0.8.[86]

3

Murmurs – systolic: ventricular septal defect murmur

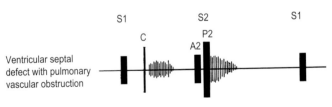

S1 S2   S1

C P2

A2

Ventricular septal defect with pulmonary vascular obstruction

FIGURE 3.46
Timing and shape of ventricular septal defect murmur
Based on Avery ME, First LP (eds), Pediatric Medicine, *Baltimore: Williams & Wilkins, 1989.*

AUDIO 3.6 🔊

Audio 3.6 Access through Student Consult.

Description
A pan-systolic, high-pitched murmur heard best in the fourth to sixth intercostal spaces that does *not* radiate to the axilla and does not increase with inspiration.

Condition/s associated with
- Ventricular septal defect

Mechanism/s
A pressure gradient across the defect and turbulent flow are the principal factors involved in the mechanism.

 The left ventricle experiences much higher pressure than the right ventricle. The septal defect allows blood to go from a region of high pressure to the low pressure of the right ventricle. Turbulent flow across the orifice creates the murmur.

Dynamic manoeuvres mechanism
Manoeuvres such as squatting and isometric handgrip exercises increase systemic vascular resistance. This in turn increases afterload on the left ventricle, raising left ventricular pressures, which leads to more blood being pushed across the ventricular septal defect, producing a louder murmur. This is depicted in Figure 3.47.

Sign value
The intensity of the murmur may be a guide to the size of the defect – the smaller the defect, often the louder the murmur.[92]

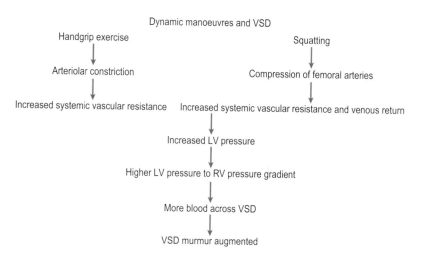

FIGURE 3.47
Murmurs – diastolic: aortic regurgitation murmur

3

Murmurs – diastolic: aortic regurgitation

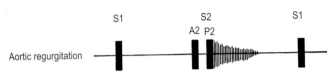

FIGURE 3.48
Timing and shape of an aortic regurgitation (AR) murmur
Reproduced, with permission, from Keane JF et al. (eds), Nadas' Pediatric Cardiology, *2nd edn, Philadelphia: Saunders, 2006: Fig 33-20.*

AUDIO 3.7 🔊

Audio 3.7 Access through Student Consult.

Description
A high-pitched, decrescendo, blowing diastolic murmur that is best heard over the aortic area of the praecordium.

Condition/s associated with
Any process that can lead to damage to or destruction of the aortic valve, including but not limited to:

More common
- Rheumatic valve disease
- Bacterial endocarditis
- Connective tissue disorders (e.g. Marfan's syndrome)
- Bicuspid aortic valve

Less common
- Age-related degenerative change
- Aortic dissection
- Syphilis
- Takayasu disease
- Ankylosing spondylitis
- Other inflammatory diseases (e.g. SLE, Reiter's syndrome)

Mechanism/s
The final common pathway for aortic regurgitation (AR) is damage to and/or incompetence of the valvular apparatus – this causes blood to flow back into the left ventricle in diastole. The characteristic murmur is the sound of blood moving back across the damaged aortic valve.

The different diseases causing AR can affect either the valve cusps and leaflets or the aortic root and are mediated by a number of immunological, degenerative and/or inflammatory mechanisms, or else via a traumatic process.

Dynamic manoeuvres mechanisms
The aortic regurgitant murmur is dependent on flow back across an incompetent valve. Therefore, in theory, any manoeuvre, such as handgrip or standing, which increases systemic vascular resistance will push more blood back across the valve and accentuate the murmur.

Sign value
Hearing an AR murmur warrants further investigation. Aortic regurgitation can be differentiated from pulmonary regurgitation by the fact

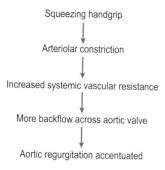

Squeezing handgrip

↓

Arteriolar constriction

↓

Increased systemic vascular resistance

↓

More backflow across aortic valve

↓

Aortic regurgitation accentuated

FIGURE 3.49
Dynamic manoeuvres mechanism

that it occurs later in the cardiac cycle (i.e. after A2, rather than after P2 as occurs in pulmonary regurgitation). It is a valuable sign whose absence is a good indication that moderate to severe AR is absent (LR 0.1).[93] Its sensitivity and specificity in predicting moderate to severe regurgitation are 88–98% and 52–88%, respectively.[86,94-96]

Similarly, the presence of an AR murmur significantly increases the chance of the presence of mild or more serious AR (LR 8.8–32.0).[93] Contrary to popular belief there is some evidence that the loudness of the murmur does correlate with severity;[97] however, it is still taught that the length of the murmur is associated with severity more than the loudness. The presence of a widened pulse pressure and collapsing pulse pressure with the characteristic murmur greatly increases the chance of significant aortic regurgitation being present.

3

Murmurs – diastolic: eponymous signs of aortic regurgitation

AR has classically been associated with a large number of eponymous signs (see Table 3.5). Although these are interesting to elicit and impressive to recite, the mechanisms underlying them and their true value are often unclear.

TABLE 3.5
Eponymous signs of aortic regurgitation (AR)

Sign	Description	Mechanism	Sign value
Austin Flint murmur	A low-pitched rumbling murmur, starting in mid-diastole and finishing at end of diastole. It is best heard over the cardiac apex with the patient leaning forward and breathing out. Mitral stenosis must be absent.	Postulated mechanisms include: • Regurgitant aortic blood flow traps leaflets of the mitral valve, leading to a form of mitral stenosis • Fluttering of mitral valves due to the AR jet flow • Endocardial vibrations caused by AR jets	Opinions vary as to the value of the sign. An Austin Flint murmur is most likely to be heard in the setting of severe aortic regurgitation and has wide variations in sensitivity from 25% to 100%, depending on the study.[98] Another review has suggested that the presence of the murmur indicates moderate to severe AR with LR of 25[99]
Becker's sign	Pulsation of the retinal arteries		Limited evidence
Corrigan's sign (water hammer or collapsing pulse)	Rapid visible arterial pulsations with a noticeable increase in amplitude of peripheral pulses	Increased arterial wall compliance	Corrigan's sign is of limited usefulness with sensitivity of 38–95% and specificity of 16% for presence of AR[98]
De Musset's sign	Rhythmic head bobbing in synchrony with the heart beat	Unclear	Limited evidence
Duroziez's sign	To-and-fro murmur or 'machinery' murmur heard over the femoral artery in diastole and systole, when compressed with a stethoscope	Systolic murmur caused by forward flow into distal artery; diastolic murmur caused by AR back towards heart	Sensitivity of 35–100%, specificity of 33–81% for presence of significant AR; studies lack consistent quality and power[98]

TABLE 3.5

Eponymous signs of aortic regurgitation (AR)—cont'd

Sign	Description	Mechanism	Sign value
Gerhardt's sign	Pulsatile spleen		Limited evidence
Hill's sign	Higher systolic blood pressure in the legs than the arms. If the foot/arm blood pressure difference is greater than 60 mmHg or if there is an increase in the popliteal/brachial gradient of more than 20 mmHg, this is a positive Hill's sign	No clear understanding of the underlying mechanism	Conflicting evidence from limited studies: • A recent study showed no true increase in intra-arterial lower extremity blood pressures compared to upper limb blood pressures in patients with AR[100] • Another study showed the popliteal/brachial gradient predicted severity of AR with an increase in gradient >20 mmHg with a sensitivity of 89%, but the sign does not distinguish between mild and absent AR[99] • In predicting presence of AR, specificity of 71–100% and sensitivity ranging from 0% to 100%[99]
Mayne's sign	A fall in diastolic blood pressure of >15 mmHg with arm elevation		Limited evidence
Müller's sign	Pulsatile uvula		Limited evidence
Quincke's sign	Exaggerated pulsations of the capillary nail bed. May be accentuated by depressing and releasing the distal end of the nail		Limited evidence
Traube's sign	A sharp or 'pistol shot'-like sound heard over the femoral artery	Sudden expansion and tensing of vessel walls in systole[58]	Limited evidence

3

Murmurs – diastolic: Graham Steell murmur

Audio 3.8 Access through Student Consult.

Description

A high-pitched, early diastolic, blowing decrescendo murmur best heard in the pulmonary area of the praecordium on full inspiration. It is a pulmonary regurgitative murmur in the setting of pulmonary hypertension.

Condition/s associated with

- Pulmonary regurgitation (PR) with pulmonary hypertension – often secondary to lung disease. (Note: PR does *not* cause pulmonary hypertension!)

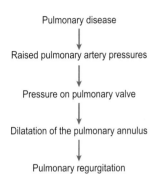

Pulmonary disease

↓

Raised pulmonary artery pressures

↓

Pressure on pulmonary valve

↓

Dilatation of the pulmonary annulus

↓

Pulmonary regurgitation

FIGURE 3.50
Mechanism of diastolic murmur

Mechanism/s

Pulmonary hypertension (usually above 55–60 mmHg) leads to increased pressure on the pulmonary valve and annulus. *Dilatation of the annulus occurs* and the valve becomes incompetent. The high-flow jet of blood across the incompetent valve creates the murmur.

Murmurs – diastolic: mitral stenotic murmur

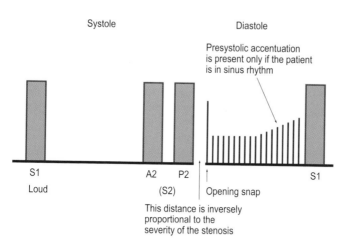

Systole   Diastole

Presysystolic accentuation is present only if the patient is in sinus rhythm

S1   Loud

A2   P2 (S2)

Opening snap

This distance is inversely proportional to the severity of the stenosis

S1

FIGURE 3.51

Timing and shape of a mitral stenotic murmur

Based on Talley N, O'Connor S, Clinical Examination, *6th edn, Sydney: Elsevier Australia, 2009: Fig 4.45A.*

AUDIO 3.9

Audio 3.9 Access through Student Consult.

Description

A diastolic low-pitched, rumbling murmur best heard with the bell of the stethoscope over the mitral area of the praecordium with the patient in the left lateral decubitus position.

Condition/s associated with

- Rheumatic heart disease – almost exclusively
- Congenital mitral stenosis – rare

Mechanism/s

Diastolic blood flow across a damaged, narrow valve.

The immunological mechanism in rheumatic heart disease is discussed under 'Aortic stenotic murmur' under 'Murmurs – systolic' in this chapter. It is thought that repeated acute subclinical rheumatic attacks, continued chronic rheumatic activity or haemodynamic trauma leads to progressive fibrosis, calcification and thickening of the valvular apparatus[28] and causes poor leaflet opening during diastole and narrowing of the valvular orifice.

With the valve narrowed, the blood flow across it in diastole is turbulent and produces the characteristic murmur.

Sign value

The mitral stenotic murmur can be difficult to auscultate and is becoming less common in developed countries with the decline in rheumatic heart disease. The murmur is very specific for mitral stenosis and should be investigated if heard.

Murmurs – diastolic: opening snap (OS)

Audio 3.10 Access through Student Consult.

Source: Robert J. Hall Heart Sounds Lab, Texas Heart Institute CHI St. Luke's Medical.

Description

Brief, sharp, high-pitched sound heard in early diastole.

Condition/s associated with

• Mitral stenosis

Mechanism/s

It is most likely caused by the sudden stop in movement of the mitral dome into the left ventricle, combined with a sudden increase in the velocity of blood moving from the atrium into the ventricle.[101]

Put more simply, the stenotic calcified valve tends to form a 'dome' shape during diastole, as the left ventricle attempts to suck blood into its cavity. Although initially mobile, the calcification of the valve will abruptly stop further movement, causing an opening snap.[102]

Sign value

There is limited evidence on the value of this sign. However, there are some characteristics that assist in assessing the degree of mitral stenosis:

• The A2-to-opening snap interval is inversely proportional to the degree of left atrial to left ventricle diastolic pressure gradient. In other words, the shorter the interval between A2 and the opening snap, the larger the gradient and the worse the stenosis.[28]

• The length of the murmur is a guide to the severity – NOT the loudness. The murmur will persist for as long as the left atrioventricular pressure gradient exceeds 3mmHg.[103]

• The louder the S1 or opening snap, the less the mitral valve is actually calcified.[101]

• Very severe mitral stenosis may not be associated with an opening snap – the valve may be too stiff to open fast enough for a snap to occur.

Murmurs – diastolic: pulmonary regurgitation murmur

Description

In the absence of significant pulmonary hypertension, described as an early decrescendo murmur heard best over the third and fourth intercostal spaces on the left sternal edge. As with other right-sided murmurs, it will become louder on inspiration.

Condition/s associated with

More common

- Pulmonary hypertension – most common cause, especially in association with Eisenmenger's syndrome
- Post-surgical repair of Tetralogy of Fallot in which the pulmonary valve has been cut across
- Dilated pulmonary artery – idiopathic or secondary to a connective tissue disorder (e.g. Marfan's syndrome)
- Infective endocarditis

Less common

- Congenital malformations of the structure of the valvular apparatus
- Rheumatic heart disease – rare
- Carcinoid syndrome – rare

Mechanism/s

A pulmonary regurgitation (PR) murmur is caused by an incompetent pulmonary valve allowing blood to flow back across from the pulmonary artery to the right ventricle in diastole. Regardless of the underlying cause, this can be due to:

- dilatation of the valve ring
- dilatation of the pulmonary artery
- abnormal valve leaflet morphology
- congenital abnormalities pertaining to the valve.

Dilatation of the valve ring as a result of prolonged pulmonary hypertension is the most common cause and mechanism (see 'Graham Steell murmur' in this section).

Dilatation of the pulmonary artery, thereby effectively 'outgrowing' the pulmonary valve, may occur idiopathically or in connective tissue disorders.[28]

Sign value

Mild degrees of pulmonary regurgitation are common within the community. However, the presence of a significant murmur increases the likelihood of pulmonary regurgitation, LR 17.0.[86]

The absence of a murmur does not rule out the presence of pulmonary regurgitation, NLR 0.9.[86]

3

Murmurs – diastolic: tricuspid stenotic murmur

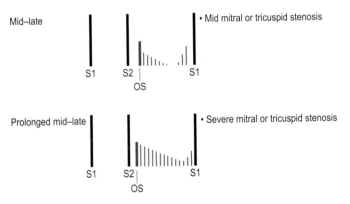

FIGURE 3.52
Timing and shape of tricuspid stenotic murmur
Reproduced, with permission, from Blaustein AS, Ramanathan A. Tricuspid valve disease. Cardiology Clinics 1998; 16(3): 551–572.

AUDIO 3.11

Audio 3.11 Access through Student Consult.

Description
A soft, diastolic, crescendo–decrescendo murmur heard loudest over the tricuspid area of the praecordium (lower left sternal edge in the fourth intercostal space).

It is often seen and confused with mitral stenosis, and it is also seen with tricuspid regurgitation.

Condition/s associated with

More common
- Rheumatic heart disease – most common[104]

Less common
- Congenital tricuspid atresia and other congenital abnormalities
- Carcinoid syndrome
- Tumours – rare

Mechanism/s
Turbulent diastolic flow across a narrowed, damaged or abnormal tricuspid valve causes the murmur.

As with other valves affected by rheumatic heart disease, thickened valve leaflets, stiffened commissures and shortened and stiff chordae tendinae restrict valve opening and cause blood flow across the valve to be turbulent.

Only 5% of tricuspid stenosis is clinically significant;[104] however, a tricuspid stenotic murmur is always abnormal and warrants investigation.

Murmurs – continuous: patent ductus arteriosus murmur

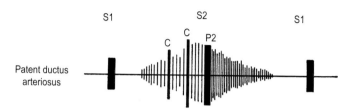

FIGURE 3.53

Timing and shape of a patent ductus arteriosus murmur

Reproduced, with permission, from Keane JF et al. (eds), Nadas' Pediatric Cardiology, *2nd edn, Philadelphia: Saunders, 2006: Fig 35-3.*

AUDIO 3.12

Audio 3.12 Access through Student Consult.

Description

A persistent, 'machinery' murmur that exists throughout systole and diastole, which is best heard over the left upper chest.

Condition/s associated with

- Patent ductus arteriosus

Mechanism/s

For a continuous murmur to exist, there must be a persistent gradient over structures in diastole and systole.

In patent ductus arteriosus, where there is persistent connection between the aorta and pulmonary artery (as seen in Figure 3.54), blood flows from the high-pressure system of the aorta into the lower-pressure pulmonary artery, producing the 'first half' of the murmur. In diastole there is still a higher pressure in the aorta than in the pulmonary artery, so blood continues to go across the patent ductus – producing the 'second half' of the murmur.

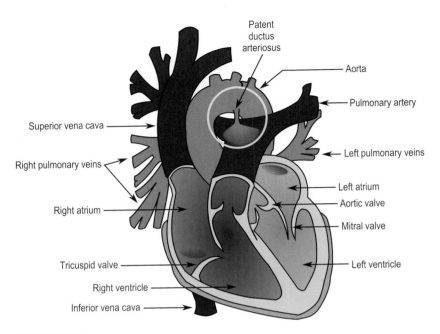

FIGURE 3.54

Patent ductus arteriosus

Adsllc_commonswiki, https://en.wikipedia.org/wiki/Patent_ductus_arteriosus#/media/File:Patent_ductus _arteriosus.svg.

Osler's nodes

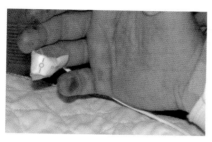

FIGURE 3.55
Osler's nodes in infective endocarditis

Reproduced, with permission, from Goldman L, Ausiello D, Cecil Medicine, *23rd edn, Philadelphia: Saunders, 2007: Fig 76-2.*

Definition

Tender, red–purple, slightly raised, cutaneous nodules often with a pale surface. Most frequently found over the tips of the fingers and toes, but can be present on the thenar eminences[63] and are often painful.

Condition/s associated with

More common

• Bacterial endocarditis

Less common

• SLE
• Disseminated gonococcus
• Distal to infected arterial catheter

Mechanism/s

As in the case of Janeway lesions, the mechanism behind this sign is still unclear. Osler's nodes are thought to differ from Janeway lesions by having an underlying immunological or vasculitic process; however, some histological studies have shown evidence to also support an embolic process.

Sign value

Estimated to be seen in only 10–25% of bacterial endocarditis.[105] The low sensitivity makes the absence of Osler's nodes of limited value.

For other signs of bacterial endocarditis, see 'Janeway lesions', 'Roth spots' and 'Splinter haemorrhages' in this chapter.

3

Passive leg raise with blood pressure or pulse pressure change

Description

With the patient lying supine and blood pressure monitored, the legs are raised to 45°. Changes in blood pressures and pulse pressures are noted over the next few minutes. An elevation in blood pressure or an increase in pulse pressure >12% suggests a positive test. This is a test to measure volume responsiveness in critically ill patients.

The best way to perform a passive leg raise (PLR) manoeuvre is to elevate the lower limbs to 45° (using automatic bed elevation or a wedge pillow) while at the same time placing the patient in the supine from a 45° semirecumbent position.

Conditions/s associated with

- Any critically ill patient

Mechanism/s

This test is used to assess fluid responsiveness (i.e. whether the patient is fluid depleted, or would benefit from any further fluid or a fluid challenge – saline infusion or otherwise). Passive leg raising is a manoeuvre that mimics rapid fluid loading. It transiently and reversibly increases venous return by shifting venous blood from the legs to the intrathoracic compartment. It has been shown to increase right and left ventricular preload, which in turn may lead to an increase in stroke volume and cardiac output.[106]

Sign value

A number of studies have found PLR to be better at predicting fluid responsiveness in patients than other tests, including echocardiographic markers of volume status.[107-110] A recent meta analysis has confirmed the value of the test in predicting fluid responsiveness in adults.[106]

Transfer of blood from the legs and abdominal compartments

= test for fluid responsiveness

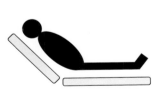

Passive leg raising

FIGURE 3.56
Passive leg raising
The passive leg test consists of measuring the haemodynamic effects of a leg elevation up to 45°. A simple way to perform the postural manoeuvre is to transfer the patient from the semirecumbent posture to the passive leg raising position by using the automatic motion of the bed.

Marik et al. Surviving sepsis: going beyond the guidelines. Annals of Intensive Care 2011; 1(1): Fig 4.

Pericardial knock

Audio 3.13 Access through Student Consult.

Description

An early-diastolic, high-pitched sound heard best between the apex of the heart and the left sternal border.

Condition/s associated with

• Constrictive pericarditis

Mechanism/s

The sudden slowing of blood flow into the ventricle in early diastole that occurs when the ventricle meets the rigid pericardial sac.[111,112]

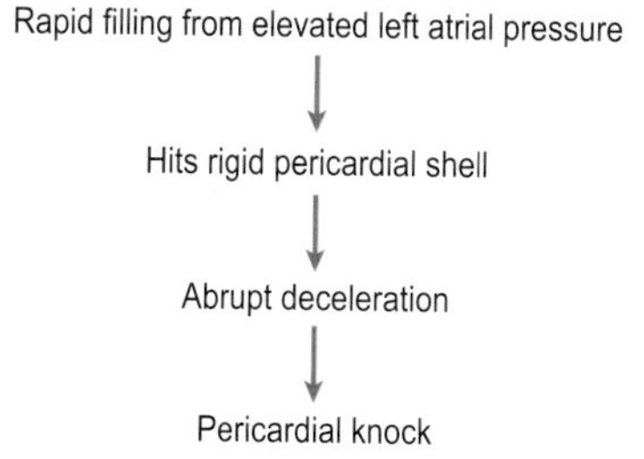

Rapid filling from elevated left atrial pressure

↓

Hits rigid pericardial shell

↓

Abrupt deceleration

↓

Pericardial knock

FIGURE 3.57
Mechanism of pericardial knock

Sign value

Classically taught as one of the cardinal signs of constrictive pericarditis, it may be seen in 24–94% of patients with this condition.[111,112]

Potential areas of confusion explained
The third heart sound versus pericardial knock

The mechanism is similar to that of the third heart sound, and differentiating the two can be difficult. However, a pericardial knock is a high-pitched sound whereas the third heart sound is classically a low-pitched sound. As always, history and other clinical signs should be used to assist in differentiation.

Pericardial rub

AUDIO 3.14 ◀

Audio 3.14 Access through Student Consult.

Description

A grating or scratching sound heard throughout the cardiac cycle. It is classically described as having three components, one during diastole and two during systole.

Condition/s associated with

• Pericarditis

Mechanism/s

Inflammation causes the pericardial and visceral surfaces of the pericardium (which are normally separated by a small amount of fluid) to rub together.

Peripheral oedema

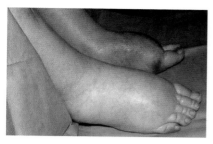

FIGURE 3.58
Peripheral oedema

Rangaprasad L et al., Itraconazole associated quadriparesis and edema: a case report. Journal of Medical Case Reports *2011; 5: 140.*

Definition

An abnormal accumulation of fluid under the skin or within body cavities, causing swelling of the area or indentations on firm palpation.

Condition/s associated with

Diseases associated with peripheral oedema are numerous. Main causes include:

More common

- Congestive cardiac failure
- Liver disease
- Nephrotic syndrome
- Renal failure
- Venous insufficiency
- Drug side effects
- Pregnancy

Less common

- Hypoalbuminaemia
- Malignancy

Mechanism/s

The mechanism underlying peripheral oedema is dependent on the underlying pathology. However, regardless of aetiology, either one or a combination of the following factors is present:

1 increased venous or hydrostatic pressure – raising capillary hydrostatic pressure (increased pressure pushing fluid out)
2 reduced interstitial hydrostatic pressure (reduced pressure pushing fluid into vessels)
3 decreased plasma oncotic pressure (decreased proteins keeping fluid in the vessel)
4 increased interstitial oncotic pressure (increased proteins trying to draw fluid out of vessels)
5 increased capillary leakiness
6 blocked lymphatic system – decreased ability to draw fluid and proteins away from interstitium and return them to the normal circulation.

Mechanism in heart failure

Increased venous hydrostatic pressure causes a transudative process in which fluid is 'pushed out' of vessels into the interstitium. It is normally seen in the context of *right* heart failure.

Factors contributing to this include:

- *Increased plasma volume* – decreased cardiac output (either via right or left heart failure) leads to renal hypoperfusion. In response to this, the RAAS is activated and salt and water are retained, leading to increased venous and capillary hydrostatic pressure.

3

CLINICAL PEARL

- *Raised venous pressure* – ventricular dysfunction leads to increased end-systolic and/or end-diastolic pressures – these pressures are transmitted back to the atrium and then to the venous system, increasing venous and capillary hydrostatic pressure.
- Increased hydrostatic pressure forces fluid out of venous vessels into surrounding tissues.
- The lymphatic system is unable to keep up with the task of reabsorbing additional interstitial fluid and oedema develops.

Liver disease

Contrary to popular belief, the main factor in the development of oedema in liver failure is *vasodilatation of the splanchnic bed*. It is not necessarily a consequence of the liver failing to produce its normal proteins (leading to hypoalbuminaemia), although this may contribute.

In liver failure, increased nitric oxide and prostaglandins are present in the splanchnic circulation. This vasodilates the splanchnic vessels, leading to more blood being 'pooled' there, with less effective circulating volume driven through the kidneys, leading to an aberrant neurohormonal response that results in increased salt and water retention through the RAAS, increasing hydrostatic pressure.[113]

Nephrotic syndrome

The mechanism of oedema in nephrotic syndrome has not been

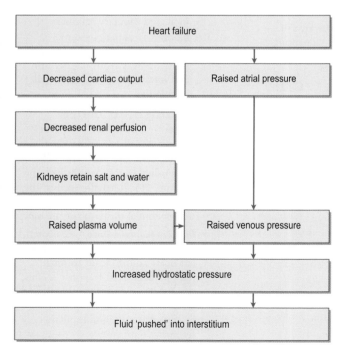

FIGURE 3.59
Peripheral oedema in heart failure

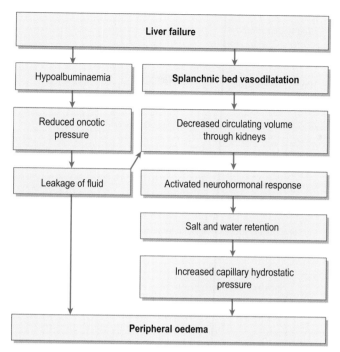

FIGURE 3.60
Peripheral oedema in liver failure

completely worked out. Factors involved include:

- Massive protein loss through the kidneys and hypoalbuminaemia, decreased plasma oncotic pressure (i.e. there are fewer proteins keeping fluid in) so fluid leaks out.

- Loss of circulating volume triggers a neurohormonal response with increased salt and water retention, increasing capillary hydrostatic pressure – pushing fluid out.

- Blunted hepatic protein synthesis contributes to the low quantity of proteins in the serum.

- Blunted atrial natriuretic response (ANR) – the normal response to volume overload is to excrete more salt and thus water out via the kidneys.

- The renal impairment seen in nephrotic and nephritic syndromes does not allow the 'normal' amount of salt to be excreted, thus fluid is retained. This is possibly the predominant mechanism in the absence of massive protein loss.[113]

Sign value

Peripheral oedema is a useful sign when present; however, its absence does not exclude heart failure (sensitivity 10%, specificity 93%[114]) with only 25% of patients with chronic heart failure under 70 years of age having oedema.

In liver failure, the development of peripheral oedema, and in particular ascites, heralds a poor prognosis.

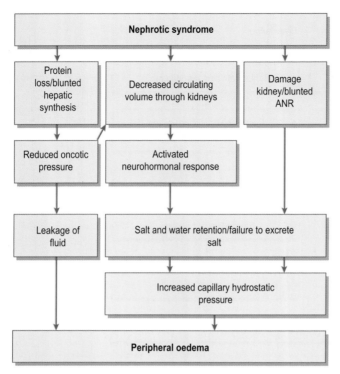

FIGURE 3.61
Peripheral oedema in nephrotic syndrome

Pulse pressure

Pulse pressure is calculated as systolic blood pressure minus diastolic blood pressure. The normal range is 40 mmHg. A variation in pulse pressure has significant clinical implications. The determinants of pulse pressure are not straightforward. The key elements are thought to be arterial resistance, arterial compliance and stroke volume/cardiac output.[115]

3

Pulse pressure: narrow

Description

A pulse pressure that is less than 20 mmHg.

Condition/s associated with

Common

- Heart failure
- Aortic stenosis
- Hypovolaemia – shock

Less common

- Hypertrophic cardiomyopathy
- Mitral stenosis

Mechanism/s

Systolic blood pressure represents the *maximum* pressure in systole, whereas diastolic pressure represents the *minimum* pressure in the arteries when the heart is in diastole. *Decreased cardiac output and increased systemic resistance* form the common pathway to a narrowed pulse pressure.

In practice, this means that any condition that results in a reduced cardiac output (systolic blood pressure) with maintained resistance of the arterial tree (diastolic pressure) can cause a narrow pulse pressure.

Cardiac failure

In heart failure, a low stroke volume (due to heart dysfunction) leads to more sympathetic outflow and higher (or maintained) systemic vascular resistance in order to preserve blood pressure and assist venous return to the heart. Therefore, systolic blood pressure is lowered (due to decreased cardiac output) and diastolic blood pressure is maintained (increased systemic vascular resistance), creating a narrow pulse pressure.

Shock

In the early stages of hypovolaemic shock, catecholamine levels are high as the body tries to raise peripheral vascular resistance and thus maintain venous return to the heart. This boost in peripheral vascular resistance increases diastolic blood pressure and, as a consequence, narrows the pulse pressure.

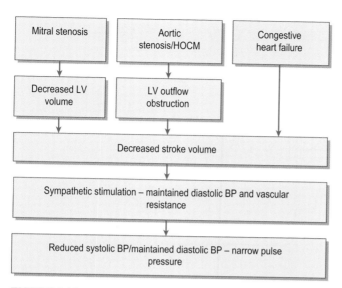

FIGURE 3.62
Narrow pulse pressure mechanism

Pulse pressure variation

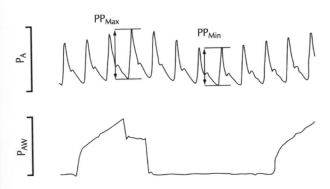

FIGURE 3.63

Schematic representation of pulse pressure variation on mechanical ventilation

P_A = arterial pressure; P_{AW} = airway pressure; PP_{Max} = maximum pulse pressure after a positive pressure breath; PP_{Min} = minimum pulse pressure after a positive pressure breath. Note the variation in PP between inspiration (the 'hump' in the bottom line) and expiration (flat line on the bottom airway pressure line).

Gunn SR, Pinsky MR. Implications of arterial pressure variation in patients in the intensive care unit, MD. Current Opinion in Critical Care *2001; 7: 212–217, Fig 4.*

Definition

Pulse pressure variation refers to the difference between the pulse pressure at inspiration versus expiration and is usually only measured on mechanically ventilated patients. A pulse pressure variation of >12% across the respiratory cycle is considered significant.[116] It is observed on an arterial line trace and is exemplified in Figure 3.66.

Condition/s associated with:

- Normal respiration variation
- Volume deplete status

Mechanism/s

Variation in the arterial waveform reflects the response by the cardiovascular system to preload changes. It is a way in which to see where a patient 'is' on the Frank–Starling curve.

Essential to understanding the mechanism and concept of pulse pressure variation is an understanding of the idea of preload dependency, the Frank–Starling curve and the physiology of mechanical respiration.

In the critically ill patient, the main reason for fluid challenge is to increase stroke volume (i.e. to ascertain whether the patient is a volume responder). According to the Frank–Starling curve, as preload increases, left ventricular volume and cardiac output will increase until the maximum overlap of the actin–myosin filaments occurs (i.e. the optimum level of preload is met).[117] *After* this point more filling with fluid will not significantly add to left ventricular volume and output. *Below* this point, additional preload (volume boluses or filling) will be of benefit and the ventricles/patient deemed to be 'preload dependent'. This is represented in Figure 3.64. If the patient is on the

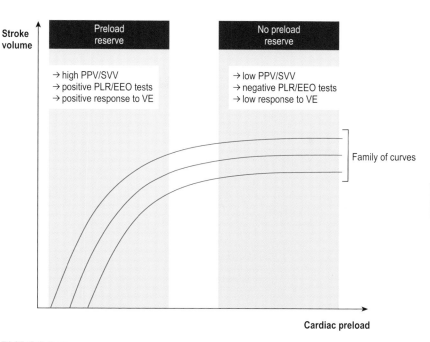

Stroke volume

Preload reserve	No preload reserve
→ high PPV/SVV	→ low PPV/SVV
→ positive PLR/EEO tests	→ negative PLR/EEO tests
→ positive response to VE	→ low response to VE

Family of curves

Cardiac preload

FIGURE 3.64

Conceptualisation of the Frank–Starling curve, response to fluid bolus and pulse pressure variation

Marik et al. Surviving sepsis: going beyond the guidelines. Annals of Intensive Care *2011; 1(1): Fig 1.*

steep part of the curve they are still preload dependent; if on the flat part of the curve, additional preload will not make much difference. Looking at pulse pressure variation is a way in which to see if patients are on the steep part of the curve and would benefit from additional preload or 'filling'.

Mechanical ventilation has relatively predictable changes in cardiovascular physiology, which contribute to pulse pressure variation and the ability to monitor variation. The ventilator delivers intermittent positive pressure, as opposed to the negative pressure generated by inspiration in normal spontaneous breathing. This positive pressure increases pleural pressure and decreases the pressure gradient in the chest, which facilitates venous return to the right atrium and ventricle. At the same time there is an increase in

transpulmonary pressure and lung volume, which increases right ventricular afterload.[117]

A reduction in venous return plus an increase in right ventricular afterload results in decreased right ventricular stroke volume (forward flow). This decreases left ventricular preload and therefore reduces left ventricular stroke volume. A summary of these changes can be seen in Figure 3.65. The degree of decrease in left ventricular stroke volume seen during the ventilator cycle is known to be proportional to the Frank–Starling curve[118] and is greatest when the ventricles of the patient are operating on the steep part of the curve[117] (i.e. when they are preload dependent and therefore benefit from filling).

An example of these concepts is displayed in Figure 3.66.

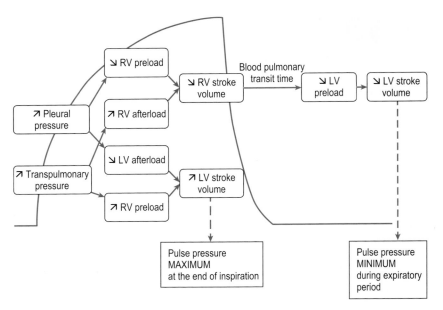

FIGURE 3.65

Heart–lung interactions: haemodynamic effects of mechanical ventilation

The cyclic changes in left ventricular (LV) stroke volume are mainly related to the expiratory decrease in LV preload due to the inspiratory decrease in right ventricular (RV) filling.

Reproduced, with permission, from Critical Care/Current Science Ltd.
Marik et al. Hemodynamic parameters to guide fluid therapy. Annals of Intensive Care *2011, 1: 2.*

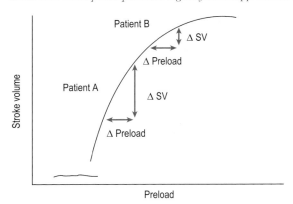

Δ Preload, change in preload after a positive pressure breath, Δ SV, change in stroke volume resulting from a positive pressure breath.

FIGURE 3.66

Stroke volume changes with differing preloads

Patient's LVSV is on the 'steep portion' of the Frank–Starling curve. Changes in preload will result in large changes in LVSV and systolic and pulse pressure (i.e. preload responsive). Patient B's curve is relatively flat and identical changes in preload will not alter LVSV as much as Patient A.

Gunn SR, Pinsky MR. Implications of arterial pressure variation in patients in the intensive care unit, MD. Current Opinion in Critical Care *2001; 7: 213.*

Pulse pressure is known to be determined by left ventricular stroke volume, heart rate and arterial tone.[118] The latter two factors remain relatively constant over the course of a breath; therefore, any alteration in arterial pressure is primarily due to changes in left ventricular stroke volume. By this logic, significant variation in pulse pressure can be used to indicate a preload dependent patient.

Sign value

In assessing whether a mechanically ventilated patient would benefit from additional preload via additional fluids, pulse pressure variation has been well validated and is highly predictive of fluid responsiveness,[117] making it a very valuable sign. A systematic review of 29 studies on mechanically ventilated patients found:

- The pooled correlation coefficients between the baseline pulse pressure variation, stroke volume variation, systolic pressure variation, and the change in stroke/cardiac index were 0.78, 0.72 and 0.72, respectively. The area under the receiver operating characteristic curves were 0.94, 0.84 and 0.86, respectively.
- The sensitivity, specificity and diagnostic odds ratio were 0.89, 0.88 and 59.86 for the pulse pressure variation.

More recently the concept has also been shown to be useful in spontaneously breathing patients.[119]

- The area under the receiver operator characteristic curve for pulse pressure variation was 0.87 (95% CI 0.74–0.99; $p < 0.0001$).
- Pulse pressure variation was correlated with increase in systolic arterial pressure ($r2 = 0.32$; $p < 0.001$) and mean arterial pressure ($r2 = 0.10$; $p = 0.037$).

Pulse pressure variation has been shown to be a reliable sign of volume responsiveness in critically ill ventilated patients. There is also some evidence for its use in spontaneously breathing patients. It is less useful in patients with concomittent arrhythmias (e.g. atrial fibrillation).

3

273

Pulse pressure: widened

Description

A pulse pressure that is greater than 55–60 mmHg.

Condition/s associated with

Most common

- Old age
- Aortic regurgitation
- Septic shock – end-stage
- High cardiac output states
- Hyperthyroidism

Mechanism/s

Old age

The factors determining pulse pressure in healthy patients are complex and cannot be explained by one model. However, *decreased arterial compliance and increasing pulse wave velocity* are thought to be central to the widened pulse pressure seen in older patients.

As humans age there is fragmentation and disruption of the lamina of the artery and alteration in the collagen-to-elastin ratio. These changes make the arteries stiffer and less compliant. When this occurs the artery loses its ability to accommodate the pressure rise that normally occurs in systole and so the pressure increases even further (see Figure 3.67).

A second model has shown that greater arterial stiffness results in faster transmission of the arterial waveform, as there is less compliance or 'give' in the arteries to damp the waveform. A consequence of this is the faster return of the wave and augmentation of the systolic pressure, further raising systolic pressure and, therefore, pulse pressure.[55]

In summary, just knowing that increased arterial stiffness/decreased compliance and increased pulse wave velocity are present would be more than enough to explain increased pulse pressure in older patients.

Septic shock

In 'warm' septic shock, the principal cause of a widened pulse pressure is vasodilatation, increased endothelial permeability and reduced peripheral vascular resistance.

Infection causes an immunological inflammatory reaction. Humoral and innate immune responses are activated, leading to recruitment of white blood cells and release of a number of cytokines, including TNF-α, IL-8, IL-6, histamine, prostaglandins and nitric oxide. These cytokines increase *vascular permeability and systemic vasodilatation*, reducing systemic vascular resistance and diastolic blood pressure and, hence, widening the pulse pressure.

It should be noted that septic shock can present (especially early on) as 'cold' shock with the peripheral vasculature shut down and peripheral vascular resistance maintained.

Aortic regurgitation

The high pulse pressure can be attributed to the high-volume flow from the left ventricle into the ascending aorta during systole. The diastolic decay of the pulse is attributed to the backflow into the ventricle and to forward flow through peripheral arterioles.[10]

Hyperthyroidism

Thyroid hormone has many effects on the cardiovascular system and sequelae include increased blood volume, increased cardiac inotropy and decreased vascular resistance, which all contribute to widened pulse pressure.

Excess thyroid hormone increases thermogenesis in the peripheral tissues, causing vasodilatation and decreased systemic vascular resistance and diastolic blood pressure. In addition, T3 also has the direct effect of decreasing vascular resistance.

At the same time, thyroid hormone is a positive inotrope and chronotrope and also increases haematopoesis and blood volume, therefore increasing cardiac output and systolic blood pressure.

Sign value

A widened or increased pulse pressure is a very valuable sign, depending on the clinical situation in which it is encountered.

Pulse pressure is an independent predictor of mortality and morbidity in normotensive and hypertensive patients.[120,121] Furthermore, some studies suggest that pulse pressure is a better indicator of risk than diastolic and systolic blood pressure,[122-124] although not all studies agree with this.

There is strong evidence that a higher pulse pressure increases the risk of atrial fibrillation[125] and the risk of

3

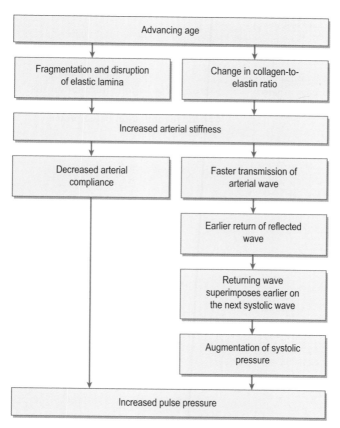

FIGURE 3.67
Mechanism of widened pulse pressure in old age

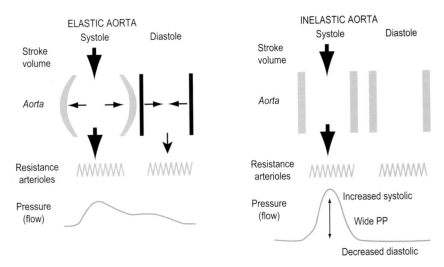

FIGURE 3.68
Widened pulse pressure and stiff vessels
Based on Lip GYH, Hall JE, Comprehensive Hypertension, *1st edn, Elsevier, 2007: Fig 11-3.*

heart failure and that treating chronic widened pulse pressure or isolated systolic hypertension reduces the risk of adverse outcomes.[126]

Widened pulse pressure in the setting of a diastolic murmur greatly increases the likelihood of significant aortic regurgitation being present.

Pulsus paradoxus

Description

Dr Adolph Kussmaul first named this sign in 1873 when he noticed that there was a discrepancy between the absence of a peripheral pulse and a corresponding heart beat on inspiration in patients with constrictive pericarditis. The paradox refers to the fact that heart sounds can be heard on auscultation but a radial pulse cannot be felt.

The definition of pulsus paradoxus is usually an inspiratory fall in systolic blood pressure exceeding 10 mmHg.[127] It is elicited by inflating the blood pressure cuff to above systolic pressure and noting the peak systolic pressure during expiration. The cuff is then deflated until the clinician can hear the Korotkoff sounds during inspiration and expiration and this pressure value is noted. When a difference between these two pressures of greater than 10 mmHg occurs, pulsus paradoxus is present.[128] It is depicted in Figure 3.69.

Condition/s associated with

More common

- Cardiac tamponade
- Asthma

Less common

- Large pulmonary embolus
- Tension pneumothorax
- Large pleural effusions
- Acute myocardial infarction
- Volvulus of the stomach
- SVC obstruction
- Diaphragmatic hernia
- Constrictive pericarditis (it is commonly argued that it does not occur in constrictive pericarditis – see the box 'Potential areas of

3

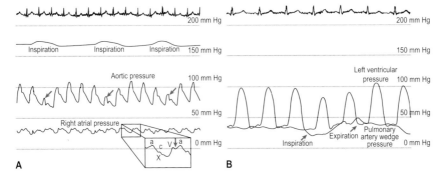

FIGURE 3.69

Pulsus paradoxus

A shows the electrocardiogram, the respirogram and the tracings of aortic pressure and right atrial pressure. There was an elevated right atrial pressure with an X descent but blunting of the Y descent (solid arrow). On inspiration, there was a 30 mmHg decrease in aortic systolic pressure as well as a decrease in pulse pressure (open arrows) – findings that constitute pulsus paradoxus. The tracings of left ventricular pressure and pulmonary-artery wedge pressure (**B**) show that the pulsus paradoxus is caused by underfilling of the left ventricle during inspiration (due to a drop in the initial pressure gradient between the pulmonary-artery wedge pressure and the left ventricular diastolic pressure).

Wu LA, Nishimura RA. Pulsus paradoxus. New England Journal of Medicine 2003; 349: 666.

CLINICAL PEARL

confusion explained – pulsus paradoxus versus Kussmaul's sign in constrictive pericarditis and cardiac tamponade' below)

General mechanism/s

In a healthy person the radial pulse decreases in amplitude on deep inspiration. This is because breathing in causes a decrease in intrathoracic pressure, drawing more venous blood into the right ventricle. The right ventricle enlarges and the interventricular septum impinges on the left ventricle, impeding blood flow into the left ventricle. In addition, during inspiration the lungs expand, allowing more blood to pool in the pulmonary vasculature. This increase of blood pooling in the lungs combines with the impingement on the left ventricle to decrease stroke volume from the left ventricle, reducing peripheral pulses.

The mechanism behind pulsus paradoxus is an exaggeration of this normal respiratory physiology and in general can be caused by the following factors:[128,129]

- a limitation in the increase of inspiratory blood flow to the right ventricle and pulmonary artery
- greater than normal pooling of blood in the pulmonary circulation (a theory that has been recently put into question)
- wide variations in intrathoracic blood pressure during inspiration and expiration – with the pulmonary pressure being more negative compared to the left atrium; as a result, blood is pulled back from the left atrium to the pulmonary veins during inspiration, thereby decreasing the amount of blood available for stroke volume[129]

- impedance of venous return to the left ventricle caused by bulging of the interventricular septum.

A recent study completed by Xing et al.[130] suggests the respiratory intra-thoracic pressure change (RIPC) (i.e. the change in pressure during respiration) affects pressures in the left and right ventricle, resulting in a pressure gradient across the inter-ventricular septum which then moves it left or right.

Cardiac tamponade

Fluid within the pericardial sac places pressure on all chambers of the heart and impairs left ventricular filling but does not impair right ventricular filling to the same extent.[128] Inspiration brings with it increased right ventricular filling compared to left ventricular filling, and the pushing across of the inter-ventricular septum into the left ventricle further impairs left ventricular filling. When impaired left ventricular filling is combined with pooling of blood in the lungs on inspiration, it exaggerates the normal decrease of left atrial and ventricular filling on inspiration. In addition to this, pulmonary venous pressure tends to be lower than the pressure in the left atrium, resulting in a decrease in left ventricular filling as more blood is pulled back towards the pulmonary veins.[128]

Massive pulmonary embolism

A massive pulmonary embolism causes right ventricular dysfunction or failure. Less blood is pumped out of the right ventricle due to high pulmonary artery pressure. This decreased right ventricular output, coupled with pooling of blood in the lungs, reduces left atrial and ventricular filling and consequently decreases stroke volume.[128]

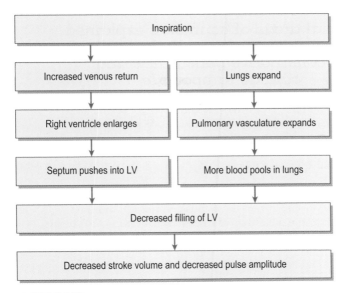

FIGURE 3.70
Normal variations in pulse with the respiratory cycle

Respiratory disorders

The main mechanism in respiratory disorders is thought to be unusually wide intrathoracic variations that are transmitted to the aorta and right side of the heart.[128,129]

In episodes of airways resistance (e.g. asthma, or loaded breathing), the negative intrathoracic pressure seen on inspiration is greater than normal (sometimes down to −30 to −20 cm of water), and on expiration the intrathoracic pressure is higher. The net result of this is an exaggeration of the normal physiological response outlined previously.[131]

During inspiration with airways resistance, the increased negative intrathoracic pressure draws more blood into the right ventricle and right pulmonary arteries, leaving less blood in the left side of the heart, resulting in a smaller stroke volume.[131] At the same time, it may have transmitted effects to

the vascular tree to increase left ventricular afterload.[132]

During expiration the opposite occurs, with more blood moving to the left side of the heart, giving a greater stroke volume. Thus, airways resistance exaggerates the normal process, resulting in pulsus paradoxus.

Sign value

If accurately demonstrated, pulsus paradoxus is an extremely useful sign. In one study[133] it had sensitivity of 98%, specificity of 83%, PLR of 5.9 and NLR of 0.03. Although an alternative pooled analysis[134] found sensitivity of 82%, given its reasonably high sensitivity and low NLR, in the setting of a pericardial effusion the absence of pulsus paradoxus suggests cardiac tamponade is not present.

In the setting of asthma, it is a foreboding sign indicating imminent respiratory failure.

Potential areas of confusion explained
Pulsus paradoxus versus Kussmaul's sign in constrictive pericarditis and cardiac tamponade

There is often confusion regarding the pathological settings in which pulsus paradoxus and Kussmaul's sign occur. Classically, pulsus paradoxus occurs in cardiac tamponade and Kussmaul's sign in constrictive pericarditis, and the two are mutually exclusive. The reasoning behind this is as follows.

In constrictive pericarditis, the normal negative intrathoracic pressure present on inspiration is not passed through the rigid pericardial shell to the atria and ventricles of the heart. As a result, on inspiration, the normal right-sided augmented *filling does not occur*, and the *septum does not impinge* on the left ventricle (as occurs in pulsus paradoxus) and *does not affect left ventricular stroke volume* in the same way as it does in cardiac tamponade.

In severe pericardial constriction, inspiration does not draw venous blood back to the heart, but it coincides with elevated right atrial and ventricular pressures and distends jugular veins instead, as the heart cannot accumulate returning blood resulting in Kussmaul's sign.
 • Constrictive pericarditis = Kussmaul's sign
 • Cardiac tamponade = pulsus paradoxus

Although this is the simple rule to follow, it should also be mentioned that pulsus paradoxus can be seen in up to one-third of cases of constrictive pericarditis.[47]

Radial–radial delay

Description

A disparity between the timing of pulses felt when simultaneously palpating the left and right radial pulse.

Condition/s associated with

- Coarctation of the aorta
- Subclavian stenosis due to aneurysm

Mechanism/s

A coarctation or narrowing of the aorta occurs before the origin of the left subclavian artery, limiting the blood flow and causing a pressure drop distal to the narrowing. The pulse wave will arrive later in the left arm and the amplitudes of the left and right pulses will be different.

Sign value

Limited evidence of the value of the sign. It should be noted that a majority of coarctations occur distal to the subclavian artery and therefore radial–radial delay is often absent.

3

Radio-femoral delay

Description

Reduced amplitude and delayed timing of the pulses in the lower body with respect to the pulses in the upper body are classic features of aortic coarctation.[10]

Condition/s associated with

- Coarctation of the aorta

Mechanism/s

Similar to aortic stenosis, coarctation will cause a decrease in the rate of ejection of blood because of vessel narrowing and the Venturi effect sucking the walls inwards, creating a reduction in the flow and amplitude of the pulse distal to the occlusion.

In addition, the following factors are essential in the mechanism of a pulse seen in any type of coarctation:[10]

- The coarctation creates a pulse wave reflection site that is much closer to the heart. This means the pulse wave is reflected earlier and faster, creating a higher blood pressure proximal to the stricture.

- There are fewer cushioning properties (i.e. less compliance of the arterial segment involved proximal to the coarctation), further increasing blood pressure at or just prior to the stricture.

- The flow and pressure pulsations are damped in the long and dilated collateral vessels that form to provide flow distal to the coarctation.[10]

Sign value

There is limited evidence as to the value of the sign and it can be difficult to elicit. The presence of the systolic murmur heard under the left clavicle or under the left scapular caused by turbulent flow across the coarctation is said to be more common.

Right ventricular heave

Description

On palpation along the left parasternal border, a sustained impulse that peaks in early- to mid-systole which 'lifts' the examiner's hand.

Condition/s associated with

Situations in which increased right ventricular pressure load and right ventricular hypertrophy are present.[1]

More common

- Pulmonary embolism
- Pulmonary hypertension

Less common

- Tetralogy of Fallot
- Severe mitral regurgitation
- Severe mitral stenosis

General mechanism/s

Increased pressure load causes right ventricular hypertrophy and displacement of the right ventricle closer to the chest wall.

Mitral regurgitation

In mitral regurgitation, the left atrium provides a cushion under the heart while increased volume in systole displaces the ventricle anteriorly,[1] causing the cardiac impulse to be felt for longer and the sensation of a right ventricular heave. This is very uncommon.

3

Roth spots

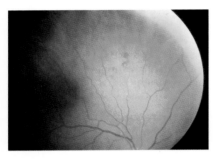

FIGURE 3.71
Roth spots

Reproduced, with permission, from Talley N, O'Connor S, Clinical Examination, *6th edn, Sydney: Elsevier Australia, 2009: Fig 4-42.*

Description
Round, white-centred retinal haemorrhages.

Condition/s associated with
While initially thought to be pathognomonic for subacute bacterial endocarditis, Roth spots are seen in many conditions including:

More common
- Infective endocarditis
- Anoxia

Less common
- Myelodysplastic syndromes
- Intracranial haemorrhage
- Diabetes
- Shaken baby syndrome

Mechanism/s
Roth spots are *not* caused by bacterial emboli. The currently accepted theory is based on capillary rupture and fibrin deposition.

By this mechanism, insult causes rupturing of the retinal capillaries, followed by extrusion of whole blood, leading to platelet activation, the coagulation cascade and a platelet fibrin thrombus. The fibrin appears as the white lesion within the haemorrhage.[135]

The initial insult varies depending on underlying pathology:

- It is suggested that in subacute bacterial endocarditis, thrombocytopenia secondary to a low-grade disseminated intravascular coagulopathy can prompt capillary bleeding in the retinal vasculature.
- Anaemia may cause further anoxic insult to retinal capillaries in patients with subacute bacterial endocarditis and leukaemia.
- Raised venous pressure may lead to capillary endothelial ischaemia and rupture of the capillary.

Sign value
Given the many possible causes of Roth spots and the fact that they are only seen in less than 5%[105] of patients with bacterial endocarditis, their value as a sign independent of other clinical signs is limited.

For other signs of bacterial endocarditis, see 'Janeway lesions', 'Osler's nodes' and 'Splinter haemorrhages' in this chapter.

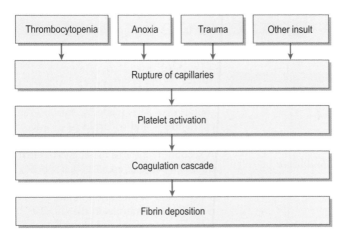

FIGURE 3.72
Roth spots mechanism

S1 (first heart sound): normal

Description

The characteristic sound heard on auscultation which corresponds with closure of the mitral and tricuspid valves.

Mechanism/s

Traditional teaching tells us that the sound of an S1 is made by the closure of the mitral and tricuspid valve and there is evidence to support this.[136-138] A second hypothesis has suggested that the main cause of an S1 is that when the valves close there is a sudden deceleration of the filling blood, resulting in vibrations in the chordae tendinae, ventricles and blood.[139]

S1 (first heart sound): accentuated

AUDIO 3.16 🔊

Audio 3.16 Access through Student Consult.

Description
The first heart sound closes with greater than normal intensity.

Condition/s associated with
- Shortened PR interval[92]
- Mild mitral stenosis
- High cardiac output states
- Atrial myxoma
- Ventricular septal defect

General mechanism/s
The intensity or loudness of the first heart sound is related to the distance the leaflets travel when they are wide open to when they shut and the velocity of their closing. If the leaflets are wide open before shutting they will cause a louder noise than if initially close together. Similarly, if there is a high force or pressure slamming the valve shut, then the S1 will be increased.

Shortened PR interval
Normally, the leaflets of both the mitral and tricuspid valves have time to drift towards each other before the onset of the ventricular contraction. With a shortened PR interval, the leaflets are further apart at the onset of ventricular contraction, thus they slam shut from a wider distance and produce an accentuated S1.

Mild mitral stenosis
In mild mitral stenosis, a longer pressure gradient is formed between atrium and ventricle,[45] keeping the mitral valve leaflets open and wider apart for longer. They are similarly slammed shut from a distance at the onset of ventricular systole.

High cardiac output states
In high cardiac output states (e.g. tachycardia due to anaemia), diastole is shortened and the tricuspid and mitral valve leaflets close from wider than normal positions. In addition, if there is vigorous contraction there is a large increase in pressure relative to time and the valves are more forcibly shut.

Sign value
There are limited studies on the value of an accentuated S1. It is classically taught that a vast majority of mitral stenotic patients have a loud S1.

3

S1 (first heart sound): diminished

Description

A softer than normal first heart sound.

Condition/s associated with

- Lengthened PR interval (e.g. first-degree heart block)
- Mitral regurgitation
- Severe mitral stenosis
- Left ventricle with reduced compliance
- Poor LV function

General mechanism/s

Restricted mobility of the valves, an inability of the valves to coapt at closure, short distance for valve closure and weak ventricular contraction are the underlying causes of a soft S1.

Lengthened PR interval

A longer PR interval allows more time between atrial and ventricular contraction for the valvular leaflets to drift back towards each other;

therefore, when the ventricle does contract, the leaflets are already closer together and less sound is produced.

Mitral regurgitation

In severe mitral regurgitation, the regurgitant jet prevents the leaflets from closing together completely, diminishing the S1 sound. In less severe cases of rheumatic mitral valve disease, fibrosis and destruction of the valve leaflet may prevent effective valve closure.[140]

Severe mitral stenosis

In severe mitral stenosis, the leaflets are too stiff and fixed to move into either an open or a closed position.

Left ventricle with reduced compliance

In a less-compliant ventricle, the end-diastolic pressure is higher, which increases the speed at which the leaflets move back together. When the ventricle contracts to slam the valve shut, the leaflets are already closer together and produce less sound.[92]

S2: loud (or loud P2 – pulmonary component of second heart sounds)

Definition

Louder than normal pulmonary component of the second heart sound. Often heard only as a loud second heart sound.

Condition/s associated with

- Pulmonary hypertension

Mechanism/s

Increased pulmonary hypertension of any cause may slam shut the pulmonary valve and cause a louder than normal pulmonary component of the second heart sound.

Sign value

The evidence for a loud P2 predicting pulmonary hypertension is quite poor, with a sensitivity varying between 58% and 96%, and specificity of only 19–46%.[141] A palpable P2 is a much better sign, with a sensitivity of pulmonary hypertension of 96%.[141]

3

S3 (third heart sound)

Audio 3.17 Access through Student Consult.

Description

A dull, low-frequency extra heart sound heard in the rapid filling phase of early diastole. The cadence of the heart sounds in a patient with an S3 is said to be similar to the word 'Ken-tuck-y'.

Condition/s associated with

More common

- Often physiological in young patients (under the age of 40)
- Any cause of ventricular dysfunction may produce a third heart sound

Less common

- Other pathological causes: anaemia, thyrotoxicosis, mitral regurgitation, HOCM, aortic and tricuspid regurgitation

Mechanism/s

An abrupt limitation of left ventricular inflow during early diastole causes vibration of the entire heart and its blood contents, resulting in the S3.[142] Typically, this is seen in patients who have increased or exaggerated filling, increased volume status and a stiff, non-compliant ventricle. The higher filling pressures mean that there is a higher flow rate and louder sound when blood hits the stiff ventricle.

Heart failure mechanism

In heart failure with systolic dysfunction there is elevated atrial pressure. When the mitral valve opens

Heart failure and systolic dysfunction

↓

Raised atrial pressures

↓

Mitral valve opens

↓

Rapid filling into dysfunctional left ventricle

↓

Third heart sound S3

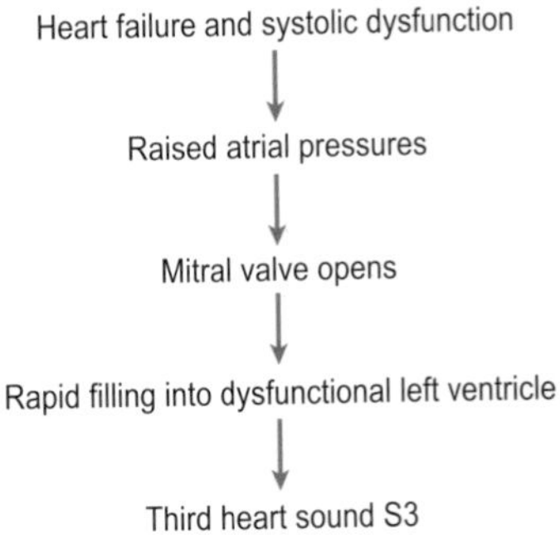

FIGURE 3.73
Mechanism of third heart sound

there is rapid filling down the pressure gradient into the stiffened dysfunctional ventricle.

Sign value

An audible third heart sound is a useful sign for left ventricular dysfunction; although its absence does not exclude heart failure. It has been shown to have negative prognostic value in patients with heart failure, with its presence proven to predict mortality and morbidity.

An S3 has been shown to predict systolic dysfunction or ejection fraction of less than 50% with 51% sensitivity and 90% specificity. There is good evidence for its value in predicting elevated left ventricular pressure (>15 mmHg) with sensitivity of 41% and specificity of 92%, with a PPV of 81 and NPV of 65.[143]

In the setting of acute chest pain, it is 95% specific in detecting myocardial infarction but only has a sensitivity of 16%.[58]

An S3 is said to be almost universally present in the setting of chronic mitral regurgitation, although the evidence for this is less clear.

S4 (fourth heart sound)

Description

The fourth heart sound is sound heard in addition to the normal S1 and S2. It is usually described as a low-pitched sound heard in late diastole with the onset of atrial contraction. This is different to the S3 or third heart sound, which is heard early in diastole.

Condition/s associated with

An S4 is typically found in conditions that cause a decrease in compliance of the left ventricle or diastolic dysfunction. Any condition causing stiffening of the left ventricle may cause an S4.

Common

- Hypertension with left ventricular hypertrophy
- Aortic stenosis
- Hypertrophic cardiomyopathy
- Ischaemic changes
- Advancing age

Less common

An S4 can also be heard in conditions where there is a rapid inflow of blood, such as anaemia (owing to a high output state) and mitral regurgitation.

Mechanism/s

Forceful contraction of the atrium pushes blood into a non-compliant left ventricle. The sudden deceleration of blood against the stiff ventricular wall produces a low-frequency vibration, recognised as the fourth heart sound.

Sign value

Evidence on the usefulness of an S4 is inconsistent. Some studies[143-145] have shown an association between a stiffened left ventricle and S4 being a pathological finding. Others did not find a valuable relationship between diastolic dysfunction and the presence of a fourth heart sound,[146] labelling it a non-specific and non-sensitive finding.

By phonographic recording, studies have shown a fourth heart sound to be present in 30–87% of heart disease patients, but also in 55–75% of people without heart disease.[147-154]

3

Skin turgor: decreased

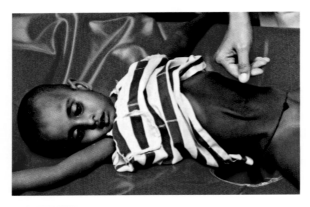

FIGURE 3.74
A child with cholera showing decreased skin turgor
From Sack DA, Sack RB, Nair GB, et al., Cholera, Lancet 2004; 363: 223–233.
Kleigman et al., Nelson Textbook of Pediatrics, Chapter 201, 1400–1403.e1. © 2016 Elsevier.

Description

A decrease in skin turgor is indicated when the skin (on the back of the hand for an adult or on the abdomen for a child) is gently pinched for a few seconds and does not return to its original state when released.

Condition/s associated with

- Age
- Dehydration
- Ehlers–Danlos syndrome

Mechanism/s

Normal skin elasticity or turgor is dependent on collagen, elastin and fluid content. In dehydrated patients, available fluid and water in the body is reabsorbed and used to supplement circulating volume. Fluid from the skin is no exception. With decreased water in the layers of the skin, turgor is decreased.

Ehlers–Danlos syndrome mechanism

In Ehlers–Danlos syndrome, there is a genetic mutation resulting in abnormal collagen synthesis. In classical Ehlers–Danlos, the mutation causes an abnormal type V collagen, whereas other forms affect different types of collagen and the extracellular matrix. Collagen is essential for skin strength and elasticity and, therefore, defects in this can produce thin and elastic skin resulting in decreased skin turgor.

Sign value

The sign of poor skin turgor suffers from high interobserver variability. As skin turgor decreases with age the most robust evidence is with regard to children. In pooled studies of 602 patients across five studies, abnormal skin turgor was associated with 5% or greater dehydration in children 2–15 years, with a sensitivity of 58% (40–75 95% CI), specificity 76% (59–93 CI) with a PLR of 2.42.[34]

Splinter haemorrhages

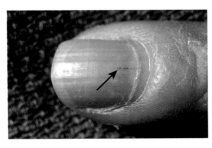

FIGURE 3.75
Splinter haemorrhages

Adams J.G., Wallace C.A, Emergency Medicine, Elsevier 2013. Courtesy Marc E. Grossman, MD, FACP.

Description

Small, red-brown lines of blood seen beneath the nails. They run in line with the nail and look like splinters caught underneath the nail.

Condition/s associated with

- Bacterial endocarditis
- Trauma
- Scleroderma
- SLE

Mechanism/s

In bacterial endocarditis, this sign is thought to be caused by emboli creating clots in capillaries under the nail, resulting in haemorrhage.

Sign value

Splinter haemorrhages are seen in only up to 15% of cases[105] of bacterial endocarditis and, therefore, have a low sensitivity. Like the other classic signs of bacterial endocarditis, they are of limited value in isolation from other signs and symptoms.

For other signs of bacterial endocarditis, see 'Janeway lesions', 'Osler's nodes' and 'Roth spots' in this chapter.

3

Splitting of the heart sounds

Splitting of the heart sounds usually refers to the ability to hear the two components of the second heart sound or S2 (closure of pulmonary and aortic valves). Different types of 'split' are caused by varying physiologies and pathologies. The splitting phenomena is conceptualised in Figure 3.76.

Splitting heart sounds: physiological splitting

Description

Hearing the aortic valve and pulmonary valve closing distinctly and separately during inspiration. They are both high-pitched sounds heard best in the pulmonary area of the praecordium.

Condition/s associated with

None, it is physiological.

Mechanism/s

The key to this sign is the pulmonary component of the second heart sound (P2) being delayed and/or closure of the aortic component of the second heart sound (A2) occurring slightly earlier than normal.

On inspiration, intrathoracic pressure becomes more negative and the lungs inflate. Lung expansion decreases resistance in the pulmonary vasculature and increases capacitance (the amount of blood in the vessels of the lungs). Because of the low resistance, blood flow through the pulmonary valve continues after systole (this is known as 'hangout'). As a consequence, there is a transient drop in the back pressure from the lungs into the pulmonary artery that is responsible for P2 closure – so the P2 occurs later.

As the lungs expand and their capacitance increases, there is a temporary drop-off in blood volume returning to the left atrium and ventricle. This reduction in filling means the next systolic contraction will have a slightly smaller stroke volume and therefore the left ventricle will empty faster and the aortic valve (A2) will close earlier. On the right side of the heart, filling of the right ventricle is accentuated on inspiration due to negative intrathoracic pressure. This leads to a greater right ventricular stroke volume which increases the time to eject blood and contributes to further delays of the closure of the pulmonary valve.

3

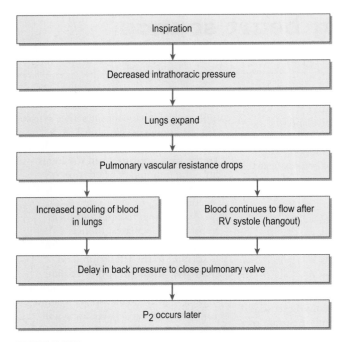

FIGURE 3.76
Mechanisms of physiological splitting

Splitting heart sounds: paradoxical (reverse) splitting

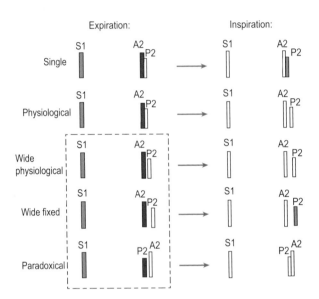

FIGURE 3.77
Paradoxical/reverse splitting of heart sounds

Based on McGee S, Evidence-Based Physical Diagnosis, *2nd edn, St Louis: Science Direct, 2007: Fig 36.1.*

AUDIO 3.19 🔊

Audio 3.19 Access through Student Consult.

Description
The opposite of physiological splitting, paradoxical splitting refers to the presentation in which the splitting of the heart sounds disappears on inspiration, while there is an audible splitting of A2 and P2 on expiration.

Condition/s associated with
- Left bundle branch block (LBBB)
- Aortic stenosis

Mechanism/s
Delaying of A2 is the final pathway for most causes of paradoxical splitting.

Aortic stenosis
In aortic stenosis, the valve becomes so stiffened and closes so slowly that it is heard after the pulmonary valve.

Left bundle branch block (LBBB)

In LBBB, the delayed depolarisation of the left ventricle causes outflow from the left ventricle to occur later and valvular closure to occur after P2.

Sign value

In the setting of aortic stenosis, it is of limited value as it only has moderate sensitivity (50%) and specificity (79%) for aortic stenosis and does not distinguish between severe aortic stenosis and minor aortic stenosis.[29] There are few studies of the value of paradoxical splitting in LBBB.

Splitting heart sounds: widened splitting

Description

Refers to a situation in which A2 and P2 are split during expiration and the timing of the split is even wider than normal during inspiration.

Condition/s associated with

- Right bundle branch block (RBBB)
- Pulmonary stenosis
- Left ventricular pacing
- Ventricular tachycardia
- Mitral regurgitation – rare

Mechanism/s

In theory, a widened split comes down to either what can make the pulmonary valve close later or what can make the aortic value close earlier.

Pulmonary stenosis

In pulmonary stenosis, the pulmonary valve is damaged and stiffened so that it is slower to close after right ventricular emptying.

Right bundle branch block (RBBB)

In RBBB the delayed depolarisation leads to delayed right ventricular contraction and delayed ejection. The closure of the pulmonary valve is therefore delayed as well.

Mitral regurgitation

A reduction in left ventricular ejection time occurs because of reduced impedance to left ventricular ejection (i.e. the blood flows out of the aortic valve but also back up to the left atrium via the incompetent mitral valve). This results in the A2 occurring earlier and therefore a splitting of the heart sounds.

Sign value

In the setting of pulmonary stenosis, the extent of S2 splitting (i.e. the time between A2–P2) is directly related to severity of pulmonary stenosis and right ventricular hypertension.[140,155]

3

Splitting heart sounds: widened splitting – fixed

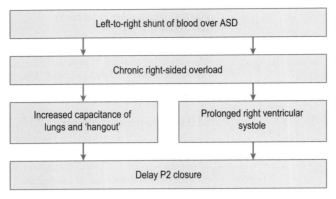

FIGURE 3.78
Mechanisms of widened fixed splitting of heart sounds

Description

Fixed splitting of S2 refers to when the time between A2 and P2 remains consistently widened throughout the inspiratory/expiratory cycle.

Condition/s associated with

• Atrial septal defect (ASD)

Mechanism/s

An ASD allows blood to flow from the left heart to the right heart circulation, causing chronic right-sided volume overload. This overload leads to a high capacitance (the lungs hold more blood), low resistance in the pulmonary system and, therefore, less pulmonary artery pressure on the pulmonary valve. Because of the volume overload, it is thought that the right ventricle takes longer to expel blood and so the pulmonary valve closes later than normal.

The reason it is 'fixed' is related to two factors. Firstly, inspiration cannot substantially increase the already raised vascular capacitance of the lungs and, secondly, the naturally occurring increased venous return to the right atrium on inspiration is offset by the blood being shunted from left to right across the ASD.[92]

Sign value

Fixed splitting has high sensitivity (92%) but lower specificity (65%) for the presence of an ASD.[156] If it is absent, it is unlikely that an ASD is present.

Tachycardia (sinus)

Description

A regular heart rate of more than 100 beats per minute.

Condition/s associated with

Sinus tachycardia is associated with a number of conditions. These may be normal physiological responses or a reaction to a pathological insult. The conditions include, but are not limited to:

More common

- Exercise
- Anxiety
- Pain
- Fever/infection
- Hypovolaemia
- Anaemia
- Decreased cardiac output (e.g. heart failure)
- Sino-atrial node dysfunction
- Pulmonary embolism
- Hyperthyroidism
- Stimulants and drugs (e.g. caffeine, beta-2 agonists, cocaine)
- Hypoxia
- Myocardial infarction

Less common

- Phaeochromocytoma

Mechanism/s

Knowing the mechanism for each cause of tachycardia is impractical. For most causes the final common pathway for the development of sinus tachycardia is activation of the sympathetic nervous system and/or catecholamine release. This can be appropriate in the case of anxiety, fear or hypovolaemia, or inappropriate in the case of a phaeochromocytoma or drugs that release (or cause the release of) catecholamines.

Mechanism in hyperthyroidism

The mechanism of tachycardia in hyperthyroidism is unique and is a result of *increased T3 levels*.

T3 has genomic (induction and expression of specific genes) and non-genomic properties that influence the production and alter the performance of myofibrillary proteins, sarcoplasmic reticula, ATPases and sodium, potassium and calcium channels. The end result is increased contractility and increased heart rate and cardiac output.[157]

Sign value

Isolated tachycardia is a very non-specific sign. Its value as a clinical sign is dependent on context. However, studies have shown the following:

- It has limited independent value in predicting hypovolaemia.[158]
- In conjunction with other variables, it has value in predicting pneumonia.[159]
- In trauma, sepsis pneumonia and myocardial infarction, tachycardia has been shown to have prognostic value in predicting increased risk of mortality.[160-164]

3

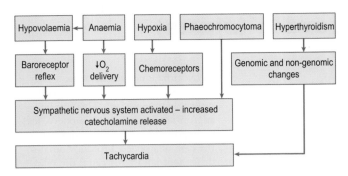

FIGURE 3.79
Mechanisms of tachycardia

Xanthelasmata

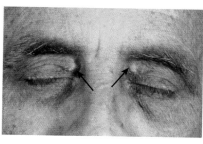

FIGURE 3.80
Xanthelasmata

Reproduced, with permission, from Rakel RE, Textbook of Family Medicine, 7th edn, Philadelphia: Saunders, 2007: Fig 44-66.

Description

Well demarcated, yellow plaques of cholesterol most often seen around eyes.

Condition/s associated with

- Hypercholesterolaemia (although only 50% of people with xanthelasmata are actually hyperlipidaemic)[165]
- Diabetes
- Fredrickson hyperlipidaemia
- Primary biliary cirrhosis

Mechanism/s

Patients with xanthelasmata have been found to have lipid abnormalities – high LDL and low HDL. However, the mechanism/s involved may vary, depending on whether the patient is normolipidaemic or hyperlipidaemic.

Hyperlipidaemic

In hyperlipidaemic patients with xanthelasmata, elevated cholesterol, mostly of the LDL type, enters through capillary walls to form the skin lesion.

Normolipidaemic

The mechanisms are less clear but those proposed include:[156,165,166]

- Local trauma and inflammation are thought to alter vascular permeability, allowing lipoproteins to enter the dermis and subsequently be taken up by dermal cells.
- Dermal macrophages, which are not regulated by the body's normal mechanisms (which limit cellular uptake of LDL cholesterol), take up cholesterol and become foam cells, which deposit themselves in the dermal layer.
- HDL, which normally removes excess cholesterol from tissues, is low in many patients with xanthelasmata; therefore, less cholesterol is being removed from the tissues and a build-up occurs.

Sign value

The value of xanthelasmata as a sign and predictor of disease is still being clarified. However, a brief summary of what is known includes:

- The prevalence of atherosclerosis in patients with xanthelasmata has varied between 15% and 69% in different studies.
- Recent studies[166-168] have shown an increased risk of ischaemic heart disease for men over 50. There was no increase in risk of heart disease shown for women, and no association with peripheral vascular disease was found in these studies.

- Patients who are hyperlipidaemic and have xanthelasmata have an increased risk of cardiovascular disease, and management should be based on cholesterol and lipoprotein abnormalities.

- In patients who are normolipidaemic, the significance of xanthelasmata is less clear, as there is a lack of sound studies and some data are conflicting.

References

1. Karnath B, Thornton W. Precordial and carotid pulse palpation. *Hosp Physician* 2002;20–4.

2. Kelder JC, Cramer MJ, Van Wijngaarden J, et al. The diagnostic value of physical examination and additional testing in primary care patients with suspected heart failure. *Circulation* 2011;**124**:2865–73.

3. Madhok V, et al. The accuracy of symptoms, signs and diagnostic tests in the diagnosis of left ventricular dysfunction in primary care: a diagnostic accuracy systematic review. *BMC Fam Pract* 2008;**9**:56.

4. Conn RD, O'Keefe JH. Cardiac physical diagnosis in the digital age: an important but increasingly neglected skill (from stethoscopes to microchips). *Am J Cardiol* 2009;**104**:590–5.

5. Basta LL, Bettinger JJ. The cardiac impulse: a new look at an old art. *Am Heart J* 1979;**97**(1):96–111.

6. Cole JS, Conn RD. Assessment of cardiac impulse using fiberoptics. *Br Heart J* 1971;**33**:463–8.

7. Eilen SD, Crawford MH, O'Rouke RA. Accuracy of precordial palpation in detecting left ventricular volume. *Ann Intern Med* 1983;**99**:628–30.

8. Conn RD, Cole JS. The cardiac apex impulse. Clinical and angiographic correlations. *Ann Intern Med* 1971;**75**:185–91.

9. Morris PD, Warriner DR, Saraf K, Morton AC. *Br J Hosp Med* 2013;**74**(2):C23–5.

10. Vlachopoulos C, O'Rourke M. Genesis of the normal and abnormal arterial pulse. *Curr Probl Cardiol* 2000;**25**(5):300–67.

11. McGhee BH, Bridges MEJ. Monitoring arterial blood pressure: what you may not know. *Crit Care Nurse* 2002;**22**:60–79.

12. Ewy G, Rios J, Marcus F. The dicrotic arterial pulse. *Circulation* 1969;**39**:655–62.

13. Smith D, Craige E. Mechanism of the dicrotic pulse. *Br Heart J* 1986;**56**:531–4.

14. Orchard RC, Craige E. Dicrotic pulse after open heart surgery. *Circulation* 1980;**62**:1107–14.

15. Euler D. Cardiac alternans: mechanisms and pathophysiological significance. *Cardiovas Res* 1999;**42**:583–90.

16. Swanton RH, Jenkins BS, Brooksby IAB, Webb-Peploe MM. An analysis of pulsus alternans in aortic stenosis. *Eur J Cardiol* 1976;**4**:39–47.

17. Noble S, Ibrahim R. Pulsus alternans in critical aortic stenosis. *Can J Cardiol* 2009; **25**(7):e268.

18. Mitchell JH, Sarnoff SJ, Sonneblick EH. The dynamics of pulsus alternans: alternating end–diastolic fiber length as a causative factor. *J Clinical Investigations* 1963;**42**:55–63.

19. Schafer S, Malloy CR, Schmitz JM, Dehmer GJ. Clinical and haemodynamic characteristics of patients with inducible pulsus alternans. *Am Heart J* 1988;**115**:1251–7.

20. Sipido K. Understanding cardiac alternans: the answer lies in the Ca^{2+} store. *Circ Res* 2004;**94**:570–2.

21. Fleming P. The mechanism of pulsus bisferiens. *Heart* 1957;**19**:519–24.

22. Ikram H, Nixon P, Fox J. The haemodynamic implications of the bisferiens pulse. *Br Heart J* 1964;**26**:452.

23. Ciesielski J, Rodbard S. Doubling of the arterial sounds in patients with pulsus bisferiens. *JAMA* 1961;**175**:475–7.

24. Chatterjee K. Examination of the arterial pulse. In: Topoj EJ, editor. *Textbook of Cardiovascular Medicine.* 1st ed. Philadelphia: Lippincott, Raven; 1997.

25. Bude RO, Rubin JM, Platt JF, Fechner KP, Adler RS. Pulsus tardus: its cause and potential limitations in detection of arterial stenosis. *Cardiovasc Radiol* 1994;**190**(3): 779184.

3

26. Forsell G, Jonasson R, Orinius E. Identifying severe aortic valvular stenosis by bedside examination. *Acta Med Scand* 1985;**218**:397–400.

27. Hoagland PM, Cook EF, Wynne J, Goldman L. Value of non-invasive testing in adults with suspected aortic stenosis. *Am J Med* 1986;**80**:1041–50.

28. Braunwald E. *Braunwald's Heart Disease: A Textbook of Cardiovascular Medicine*. 8th ed. Philadelphia: Elsevier; 2008.

29. Aronow WS, Kronzon I. Correlation of prevalence and severity of valvular aortic stenosis determined by continuous-wave Doppler echocardiography with physical signs of aortic stenosis in patients aged 62 to 100 years with aortic systolic ejection murmurs. *Am J Cardiol* 1987;**60**:399–401.

30. Aronow WS, Kronzon I. Prevalence and severity of valvular aortic stenosis determined by Doppler echocardiography and its association with echocardiographic and electrocardiographic left ventricular hypertrophy and physical signs of aortic stenosis in elderly patients. *Am J Cardiol* 1991;**67**:776–7.

31. Pickard A, et al. Capillary refill time: is it still a useful clinical sign? *Anesth Analg* 2011;**113**(1):120–3.

32. Saavedra JM, et al. Capillary refilling (skin turgor) in the assessment of dehydration. *Am J Dis Child* 1991;**145**:296–8.

33. Van den Bruel A, Haj-Hassan T, Thompson M, Butinx F, Mant D. Diagnostic value of clinical features at presentation to identify serious infection in children in developed countries: a systematic review. *Lancet* 2010;**375**:135–42.

34. Steiner MJ, et al. Is this child dehydrated? *JAMA* 2004;**291**(22):2746–854.

35. Moughrabi SM, Evangelista LS. Cardiac cachexia at a glance. *Prog Cardiovasc Nurs* 2007;**Spring**:101–3.

36. von Haehlin S, Lainscak M, Springer J, Anker SD. Cardiac cachexia: a systematic overview. *Pharmacol Ther* 2009;**121**:227–52.

37. Pittman JG, Cohen P. The pathogenesis of cardiac cachexia. *N Engl J Med* 1964;**271**:453–60.

38. Wadia NH, Monckton G. Intracranial bruits in health and disease. *Brain* 1957;**80**:492–509.

39. Sauve JS, Laupacis A, Ostbye T, et al. Does this patient have a clinically important carotid bruit? *JAMA* 1993;**270**:2843–5.

40. Ingall TJ, Homer D, Whisnat JP, Baker HL, O'Fallon WN. Predictive value of carotid bruit for carotid atherosclerosis. *Archive of Neurology* 1989;**46**(4):418–22.

41. Ziegler DR, Zileli T, Dick A, Seabaugh JL. Correlation of bruits over the carotid artery with angiographically demonstrated lesions. *Neurology* 1971;**21**(8):860–5.

42. Hankey GJ, Warlow CP. Symptomatic carotid ischaemic events: safest and most cost effective way of selecting patients for angiography, before carotid endarterectomy. *BMJ* 1990;**300**(6738):1485–91.

43. Sauve JS, Sackett DL, Taylor DW, et al. Can bruits distinguish high grade from moderate symptomatic carotid stenosis? *Clinical Res* 1992;**40**:304A.

44. Sauve JS, Thorpe KE, Sackett DL, et al. Can bruits distinguish high grade stenosis from moderate asymptomatic carotid stenosis? *Ann Intern Med* 1994;**120**(8):633–7.

45. Dorland WAN. *Dorland's Illustrated Medical Dictionary*. 30th ed. Philadelphia: Saunders; 2003.

46. Javaheri S. A mechanism of central sleep apnoea in patients in heart failure. *N Engl J Med* 1999;**341**:949–54.

47. Wilcox I, Grunstein RR, Collins FL, Berthon-Jones M, Kelly DT, Sullivan CE. The role of central chemosensitivity in central sleep apnoea of heart failure. *Sleep* 1993;**16**:S37–8.

48. Ingbir M, Freimark D, Motro M, Adler Y. The incidence, pathophysiology, treatment and prognosis of Cheyne–Stokes breathing disorder in patients with congestive heart failure. *Herz* 2002;**2**:107–12.

49. Yoshiro Y, Kryger MH. Sleep in heart failure. *Sleep* 1993;**16**:513–23.

50. Nakamura J, Halliday NA, Fukuba E, et al. The microanatomic basis of finger clubbing – a high-resolution magnetic resonance imaging study. *J Rheumatol* 2014; **41**(3):523–7.

51. Spicknall KE, Zirwas MJ, English JC. Clubbing: an update on diagnosis, differential diagnosis, pathophysiology and clinical relevance. *J Am Acad Dermatol* 2005;**52**:1020–8.

52. Tavazzi L, Maggioni AP, Lucci D, et al. Nationwide survey on acute heart failure in cardiology ward services in Italy. *Eur Heart J* 2006;**27**:1207–15.

53. ADHERE Scientific Advisory Committee: Acute Decompensated Heart Failure National Registry (ADHERE®). Core Module Q1 2006 Final Cumulative National Benchmark Report. Scios, Inc, 2006.

54. www-clinicalkey-com-au.ezproxy2.library.usyd.edu.au/#!/ContentPlayerCtrl/doPlayContent/21-s2.0-2001395/{"scope":"all","query":"Methemoglobinemia"}.

55. Braunwald E. Chapter 35: Hypoxia and cyanosis. In: Fauci AS, Braunwald E, Kasper DL, et al., editors. *Harrison's Principles of Internal Medicine*. 17th ed. 2010. Available: http://proxy14.use.hcn.com.au/content.aspx?aID=2863787.

56. Burch GE, Ray CT. Mechanism of the hepatojugular reflux test in congestive heart failure. *Am Heart J* 1954;**48**(3):373–82.

57. Wiese J. The abdominojugular reflux sign. *Am J Med* 2000;**109**(1):59–61.

58. McGee S. *Evidence Based Physical Diagnosis*. 2nd ed. St Louis: Elsevier; 2007.

59. Porta M, Grosso A, Veglio F. Hypertensive retinopathy: there's more than meets the eye. *J Hypertension* 2005;**23**(4):684–96.

60. Wong TY, Mitchell P. Hypertensive retinopathy. *N Engl J Med* 2004;**351**(22): 2310–16.

61. Grosso A, Veglio F, Porta M, Grignolo FM, Wong TY. Hypertensive retinopathy revisited: some answers, more questions. *Br J Ophalmol* 2005;**89**:1646–54.

62. Ong YT, et al. Hypertensive retinopathy and risk of stroke. *Hypertension* 2013;**62**: 706–11.

63. Gunson T, Oliver FG. Osler's nodes and Janeway lesions. *Australasian J Dermatol* 2007;**48**(4):251–5.

64. Alpert JS. Osler's nodes and Janeway lesions are not the result of small vessel vasculitis. *Am J Med* 2013;**126**(10):843–4.

65. Zetola N, Zidar DA, Ray S. Chapter 57: Infective endocarditis. In: Nilsson KR Jr, Piccini JP, editors. *The Osler Medical Handbook*. 2nd ed. Philadelphia: Johns Hopkins University; 2006.

66. Takata M, Beloucif S, Shimada M, Robotham J. Superior and inferior caval flows during respiration: pathogenesis of Kussmaul's sign. *Am J Physiol* 1992;**262**(3 Pt 2): H763–70.

67. Meyer TE, Sareli P, Marcus RH, Pocock W, Berk MR, McGregor M. Mechanism underlying Kussmaul's sign in chronic constrictive pericarditis. *Am J Cardiol* 1989;**64**: 1069–72.

68. Wood PH, Conn RD, O'Keefe JH. Simplified evaluation of the jugular venous pressure: significance of inspiratory collapse of jugular veins. *Mo Med* 2012;**109**:150–2.

69. Garg N, Garg N. Jugular venous pulse: an appraisal. *Journal of Indian Academy of Clinical Medicine* 2000;**1**(3):260–9.

70. Cook DJ. Clinical assessment of central venous pressure in the critically ill. *Am J Med Sci* 1990;**299**:175–8.

71. Connors AF, McCaffree DR, Gray BA. Evaluation of rightheart catheterization in the critically ill patients without acute myocardial infarction. *N Eng J Med* 1983;**308**:263–7.

72. Eisenberg PR, Jaffe AS. Schuste DP. Clinical valuation compared to pulmonary artery catheterization in the hemodynamic assessment of critically ill patients. *Crit Care Med* 1984;**12**:549–53.

3

73. Davison R, Cannon R. Estimation of central venous pressure by examination of jugular veins. *Am Heart J* 1974;**87**:279–82.

74. Drazner MH, Hamilton M, Fonarow G, Creaser J, Flavell C, Warner Stevenson L. Relationship between right and left sided filling pressures in 1000 patients with advanced heart failure. *J Heart Lung Transplantation* 1999;**18**(11):1126–32.

75. Butman SM, Ewy GA, Standen JR, et al. Bedside cardiovascular examination in patients with severe, chronic heart failure. *J Am Coll Cardiol* 1993;**22**:968–74.

76. Meyer P, et al. A propensity-matched study of elevated jugular venous pressure and outcomes in chronic heart failure. *Am J Cardiol* 2009;**103**:839–44.

77. McGee SR. Etiology and diagnosis of systolic murmurs in adults. *Am J Med* 2010;**123**:913–21.

78. Pitts WR, Lange RA, Cigarroa JE, Hillis D. Predictive value of prominent right atrial V waves in assessing the presence and severity of tricuspid regurgitation. *Am J Cardiol* 1999;**83**(4):617–18.

79. Constant J. Jugular wave recognition: breakthrough X' descent vs the X descent and trough. *Chest* 2000;**118**:1788–91.

80. Spodick DH. Pathophysiology of cardiac tamponade. *Chest* 1998;**113**:1372–8.

81. Terasawa Y, Tanaka M, Konno K, Niita K, Kashiwagi M. Mechanism of production of midsystolic click in a prolapsed mitral valve. *Jap Heart J* 1977;**18**(5):652–63.

82. O'Rourke RA, Crawford MH. The systolic click-murmur syndrome: clinical recognition and management. *Curr Probl Cardiol* 1976;**1**:9.

83. Ait-Oufell H. Mottling score predicts survival in septic shock. *Intensive Care Med* 2011;**37**:801–7.

84. Aronow WS, Schwartz KS, Koenigsberg M. Correlation of aortic cuspal and aortic root disease with aortic systolic ejection murmurs and with mitral annular calcium in persons older than 62 years in a long term health care facility. *Am J Cardiol* 1986;**58**:651–2.

85. Etchells E, Glenns V, Shadowitz S, et al. A bedside clinical prediction rule for detecting moderate to severe aortic stenosis. *J Gen Intern Med* 1998;**13**(10):699–704.

86. Rahko PS. Prevalence of regurgitant murmurs in patients with valvular regurgitation detected on Doppler echocardiography. *Ann Int Med* 1989;**111**(6):466–72.

87. Meyers DG, McGall D, Sears TD, et al. Duplex pulsed Doppler echocardiography in mitral regurgitation. *J Clin Ultrasound* 1986;**14**:117–21.

88. Møller JE, Connolly HM, Rubin J, Seward JB, Modesto K, Pellikka PA. Factors associated with progression of carcinoid heart disease. *N Engl J Med* 2003;**348**(11):1005–15.

89. Topilsky Y, Tribouilloy C, Michelena HI. Pathophysiology of tricuspid regurgitation circulation. *Circulation* 2010;**122**:1505–13.

90. Frater R. Tricuspid insufficiency. *J Thoracic Cardiovascular Surgery* 2001;**122**(3):427–9.

91. Simula DV, Edwards WD, Tazelaar HD, et al. Surgical pathology of carcinoid heart disease: a study of 139 valves from 75 patients spanning 20 years. *Mayo Clinical Proceedings* 2002;**77**(2):139–47.

92. Lilly LS, editor. *Pathophysiology of Heart Disease*. 3rd ed. Philadelphia: Lippincott Williams; 2003.

93. Choudhry MK, Etchells EE. Does this patient have aortic regurgitation? *JAMA* 1999;**281**(23):2231–8.

94. Aronow WS, Kronzon I. Correlation of prevalence and severity of aortic regurgitation detected by pulsed Doppler echocardiography with the murmur of aortic regurgitation in elderly patients in a long term health care facility. *Am J Cardiol* 1989;**63**:128–9.

95. Dittman H, Karsch KR, Siepel L. Diagnosis and quantification of aortic regurgitation by pulse doppler echocardiography in patients with mitral valve disease. *Eur Heart J* 1987;**8**(Suppl. C):53–7.

96. Grayburn PA, Smith MD, Handshoe R, et al. Detection of aortic insufficiency by standard echocardiography, pulse Doppler cardiography and auscultation: a comparison of accuracies. *Ann Intern Med* 1986;**104**:599–605.

97. Desjardins VA, Enriquez-Sarano M, Tajik J, et al. Intensity of murmurs correlates with severity of valvular regurgitation. *Am J Med* 1996;**100**:149–56.

98. Desjardins VA, Enriquez-Sarano M, Tajik AJ, et al. Intensity of murmurs correlates with the severity of valvular regurgitation. *Am J Med* 1996;**101**(6):664.

99. Babu AN, Kymes SM, Carpenter Fryer SM. Eponyms and the diagnosis of aortic regurgitation: what says the evidence? *Ann Intern Med* 2003;**138**:736–42.

100. Pascarelli EF, Bertrand CA. Comparison of blood pressures in the arms and legs. *N Eng J Med* 1964;**270**:693–8.

101. Muralek-Kubzdela T, Grajek S, Olasinska A, et al. First heart sound and opening snap in patients with mitral valve disease. Phonographic and pathomorphic study. *Int J Cardiol* 2008;**124**:433–5.

102. Barrington W, Boudoulas H, Bashore T, Olson S, Wooley MC. Mitral stenosis: mitral dome excursion at M1 and the mitral opening snap – the concept of reciprocal heart sounds. *Am Heart J* 1988;**115**(6):1280–90.

103. Bonow RO, et al. *Braunwald's Heart Diseases: A Textbook of Cardiovascular Medicine*. 9th ed. Philadelphia: Elsevier; 2015.

104. Ewy GA. Tricuspid valve disease. In: Alpert JS, Dalen JE, Rahimtoola SH, editors. *Valvular Heart Disease*. 3rd ed. Philadelphia: Lippincott Williams & Wilkins; 2000. pp. 377–92.

105. Goldman L, Ausiello D. *Cecil Medicine*. 23rd ed. Philadelphia: Saunders; 2007.

106. Cavallaro F, Sandroni C, Marano C, et al. Diagnostic accuracy of passive leg raising for prediction of fluid responsiveness in adults: systematic review and meta-analysis of clinical studies. *Intensive Care Med* 2010;**36**:1475–83.

107. Teboul JL, Monnet X. Prediction of volume responsiveness in critically ill patients with spontaneous breathing activity. *Curr Opin Crit Care* 2008;**14**(3):334–9. doi:10.1097/MCC.0b013e3282fd6e1e. PMID 18467896.

108. Monnet X, Rienzo M, Osman D, et al. Passive leg raising predicts fluid responsiveness in the critically ill. *Crit Care Med* 2006;**34**(5):1402–7. doi:10.1097/01. CCM.0000215453.11735.06. PMID 16540963.

109. Lamia B, Ochagavia A, Monnet X, Chemla D, Richard C, Teboul JL. Echocardiographic prediction of volume responsiveness in critically ill patients with spontaneously breathing activity. *Intensive Care Med* 2007;**33**(7):1125–32. doi:10.1007/s00134-007-0646-7. PMID 17508199.

110. Lafanechère A, Pène F, Goulenok C, et al. Changes in aortic blood flow induced by passive leg raising predict fluid responsiveness in critically ill patients. *Crit Care* 2006;**10**(5):R132. doi:10.1186/cc5044. PMC 1751046. PMID 16970817.

111. Michaels AD, et al. Computerized acoustic cardiographic insights into the pericardial knock in constrictive pericarditis. *Clin Cardiol* 2007;**30**:450–8.

112. Tyberg T, Goodyer A, Langou R. Genesis of pericardial knock in constrictive pericarditis. *Am J Cardiol* 1980;**46**:570–5.

113. Schroth BE. Evaluation and management of peripheral edema. *JAAPA* 2005;**18**(11): 29–34.

114. William D, et al. *Heart Failure: A Comprehensive Guide to Diagnosis and Treatment*. New York: Marcel Dekker; 2005.

115. Dart A, Kingwell B. Pulse pressure – a review of mechanisms and clinical relevance. *J Am Coll Cardiol* 2001;**37**:975–84.

116. Marik PE, Cavallazzi R, Vasu T, Hirani A. Dynamic changes in arterial waveform derived variables and fluid responsiveness in mechanically ventilated patients. A systematic review of the literature. *Crit Care Med* 2009;**37**:2642–7.

3

117. Marik PE, et al. Hemodynamic parameters to guide fluid therapy. *Annals of Intensive Care* 2011;**1**(1).

118. Gunn SR, Pinsky MR. Implications of arterial pressure variation in patients in the intensive care unit. *Curr Opin Crit Care* 2001;**7**:213.

119. Grassi P, et al. Pulse pressure variation as a predictor of fluid responsiveness in mechanically ventilated patients with spontaneous breathing activity: a pragmatic observational study. *HSR Proc Intensive Care Cardiovasc Anesth* 2013;**5**(2):98–109.

120. Benetos A, Rudnichi A, Safar M, Guize L. Pulse pressure and cardiovascular mortality in normotensive and hypertensive patients. *Hypertension* 1998;**32**:560–4.

121. Benetos A, Safar M, Rudnichi A, et al. Pulse pressure: a predictor of long term cardiovascular mortality in a French male population. *Hypertension* 1997;**30**:1410–15.

122. Domanski MJ, Davis BR, Pfeffer M, Kasantin M, Mitchell GF. Isolated systolic hypertension: prognostic information provided by pulse pressure. *Hypertension* 1999;**34**:375–80.

123. Fang J, Madhavan S, Cohen H, Alderman MH. Measures of blood pressure and myocardial infarction in treated hypertensive patients. *J Hypertension* 1995;**13**:413–19.

124. Chae CU, Pfeffer MA, Glynn RJ, Mitchell GF, Taylor JO, Hennekens CH. Pulse pressure and risk of heart failure in the elderly. *JAMA* 1999;**281**:634–9.

125. Mitchell GF, et al. Pulse pressure and the risk of new onset atrial fibrillation. *JAMA* 2007;**297**(7):709–15.

126. SHEP Cooperative Research Group. Prevention of stroke by antihypertensive drug treatment in older persons with isolated systolic hypertension: final results of the Systolic Hypertension in the Elderly Program (SHEP). *JAMA* 1991;**265**:3255–64.

127. Bandinelli G, Lagi A, Modesti PA. Pulsus paradoxus: an underused tool. *Internal Emergency Medicine* 2007;**2**:33–5.

128. Khasnis A, et al. Pulsus paradoxus. *J Postgrad Med* 2002;**48**:46–9.

129. Golinko RJ, Kaplan N, Rudolph AM. The mechanism of pulsus paradoxus in acute pericardial tamponade. *J Clin Invest* 1963;**42**(2):249–57.

130. Xing CY, et al. Mechanism study of pulsus paradoxus using mechanical models. *PLoS ONE* 2013;**8**(2):1–7.

131. Blaustein AS, et al. Mechanisms of pulsus paradoxus during restrictive respiratory loading and asthma. *JACC* 1986;**8**(3):529–36.

132. Hamzaoui O, Monnet X, Tebout JL. Pulsus paradoxus. Physiology in respiratory medicine. *Eur Repir J* 2013;**42**:1696–705.

133. Curtiss EL, Reddy PS, Uretsky BF, Cechetti AA. Pulsus paradoxus definition and relation to the severity of cardiac tamponade. *Am J Heart* 1988;**115**:391–8.

134. Roy CL, Minor MA, Brookhart AM, Choudhry NK. Does this patient with a pericardial effusion have cardiac tamponade? *JAMA* 2007;**297**(16):1810–18.

135. Ling R, James B. White centred retinal haemorrhages. *Postgrad Med J* 1998;**74**(876): 581–2.

136. O'Toole JD, Reddy SP, Curtiss EI, et al. The contribution of the tricuspid valve closure to the first heart sound. An intracardiac micromanometer study. *Circulation* 1976;**53**:752.

137. Waider W, Criage E. First heart sound and ejection sounds. Echocardiographic and phonocardiographic correlation with valvular events. *Am J Cardiol* 1975;**35**:346.

138. Lanaido SS, Yellin EL, Miller H, Frater RW. Temporal relation of the first heart sound to closure of the mitral valve. *Circulation* 1973;**47**:1006.

139. Luisada AA, Portaluppi F. The main heart sounds as vibrations of the cardiohemic system: old controversy and new facts. *Am J Cardiol* 1983;**52**:1133–6.

140. Chatterjee K. Auscultation of heart sounds. In: Otta CM, editor. *Uptodate*. Waltham, MA: UpToDate; 2014.

141. McGee S. *Evidence Based Physical Diagnosis*. 3rd ed. St Louis: Elsevier; 2012.

142. Shah SJ, et al. Physiology of the third heart sound: novel insights from tissue Doppler imaging. *J Am Soc Echocardiography* 2008;**21**(4):394–400.

143. Marcus GM, Gerber IL, McKeown BH, et al. Association between phonocardiographic third and fourth heart sounds and objective measures of left ventricular function. *JAMA* 2005;**293**:2238–44.

144. Homma S, Bhattacharjee D, Gopal A, et al. Relationship of auscultatory fourth heart sound to the quantitated left atrial filling fraction. *Clin Cardiol* 1991;**14**:671–4.

145. Shah SJ, et al. Association of the fourth heart sound with increased left ventricular end-diastolic stiffness. *J Cardiac Failure* 2008;**14**:431–6.

146. Meyers D, Porter I, Schneider K, Maksoud A. Correlation of an audible fourth heart sound with level of diastolic dysfunction. *Am J Med Sci* 2009;**337**(3):165–7.

147. Rectra EH, Khan AH, Piggot VM, et al. Audibility of the fourth heart sound. *JAMA* 1972;**221**:36–41.

148. Spodick DH, Quarry VM. Prevalence of the fourth sound by phonocardiography in the absence of cardiac disease. *Am Heart J* 1974;**87**:11–14.

149. Swistak M, Muschlin H, Spodick DH. Comparative prevalence of the fourth heart sound in hypertensive and matched normal persons. *Am J Cardiol* 1974;**33**:614–16.

150. Prakash R, Aytan N, Dhingra R, et al. Variability in the detection of the fourth heart sound – its clinical significance in elderly subjects. *Cardiology* 1974;**59**:49–56.

151. Benchimol A, Desser KB. The fourth heart sound in patients without demonstrable heart disease. *Am Heart J* 1977;**93**:298–301.

152. Erikssen J, Rasmussen K. Prevalence and significance of the fourth heart sound (S4) in presumably healthy middle-aged men, with particular relation to latent coronary heart disease. *Eur J Cardiol* 1979;**9**:63–75.

153. Jordan MD, Taylor CR, Nyhuis AW, et al. Audibility of the fourth heart sound: relationship to presence of disease and examiner experience. *Arch Intern Med* 1987;**147**:721–6.

154. Collins SP, Arand P, Lindsell CJ, et al. Prevalence of the third and fourth heart sounds in asymptomatic adults. *Congest Heart Fail* 2005;**11**(5):242–7.

155. Leathem A, Segal B. Auscultatory and phonocardiographic signs of pulmonary stenosis. *Br Heart J* 1957;**19**:303.

156. Perloff JK, Harvey WP. Mechanisms of fixed splitting of the second heart sound. *Circulation* 1958;**18**:998–1009.

157. Klein I, Ojama K. Thyroid hormone and the cardiovascular system. *N Engl J Med* 2001;**344**(7):501–8.

158. Brasel KJ, Guse C, Gentilello LM, Nirula R. The heart rate: is it truly a vital sign? *Journal of Trauma – Injury, Infection, and Critical Care* 2007;**62**:812–17.

159. Heckerling PS, Tape TG, Wigton RS, et al. Clinical prediction rule for pulmonary infiltrates. *Ann Intern Med* 1990;**113**(9):664–770.

160. Victorino GP, Battistella FD, Wisner DH. Does tachycardia correlate with hypotension after trauma? *J Am Coll Surg* 2003;**196**:679–84.

161. Kovar D, Cannon CP, Bentley JH, et al. Does initial and delayed heart rate predict mortality in patients with acute coronary syndromes? *Clin Cardiol* 2004;**27**:80–6.

162. Zuanetti G, Mantini L, Hernandez-Bernal F, et al. Relevance of heart rate as a prognostic indicator in patients with acute myocardial infarction: insights from the GISSI 2 study. *Eur Heart J* 1998;**19**(Suppl. F):F19–26.

163. Leibovici L, Gafter-Gvili A, Paul M, et al. TREAT Study Group. Relative tachycardia in patients with sepsis: an independent risk factor for mortality. *QJM* 2007;**100**(10):629–34.

164. Parker MM, Shelhamer JH, Natanson C, Dalling DW, Parillo JE. Serial cardiovascular variables in survivors and nonsurvivors of human septic shock: heart rate as an early predictor of prognosis. *Crit Care Med* 1987;**15**:923–9.

165. Bergman R. Xanthelasma palpebrarum and risk of atherosclerosis. *Int J Dermatol* 1998;**37**:343–9.

166. Segal P, Insull W Jr, Chambless LE, et al. The association of dyslipoproteinemia with corneal arcus and xanthelasma. *Circulation* 1986;**73**(Suppl.):1108–18.

167. Bergman R. The pathogenesis and clinical significance of xanthelasma palpebrarum. *J Am Acad Dermatol* 1994;**30**(2):235–42.

168. Menotti A, Mariotti S, Seccareccia F, et al. Determinants of all causes of death in samples of middle-aged men followed up for 25 years. *J Epidemiol Community Health* 1987;**41**:243–50.

CHAPTER 4

HAEMATOLOGICAL AND ONCOLOGICAL SIGNS

Angular stomatitis

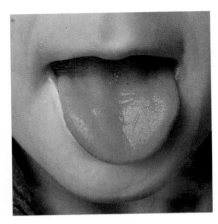

FIGURE 4.1
Angular stomatitis
Note atrophic glossitis is also present.
Reproduced, with permission, from Forbes CD, Jackson WF, Color Atlas and Text of Clinical Medicine, *3rd edn, London: Mosby, 2003.*

Description
Maculopapular and vesicular lesions grouped on the skin at the corners (or 'angles') of the mouth and mucocutaneous junction.

Condition/s associated with
More common
- Oral candidiasis
- Poorly fitting dentures
- Bacterial infection

Less common
- Nutritional deficiencies (especially riboflavin, iron and pyridoxine)
- Human immunodeficiency virus (HIV)

Nutritional deficiency mechanism/s
Iron and other nutrients are necessary to gene transcription for essential cell replication, repair and protection. Nutrient deficiency leads to impeded protection, repair and replacement of the epithelial cells on the edges of the mouth resulting in atrophic stomatitis.

Sign value
There is limited evidence on the value of angular stomatitis as a sign.

Atrophic glossitis

Description

The absence or flattening of the filiform papillae of the tongue.[1] See Figure 4.1.

Condition/s associated with

More common

Associated with micronutrient deficiency, including:

- Iron deficiency
- Vitamin B12 deficiency
- Folic acid deficiency
- Thiamine deficiency
- Niacin deficiency
- Vitamin E deficiency
- Pyridoxine deficiency
- H. pylori infection

Less common

- Amyloidosis
- Sjögren's syndrome

Mechanism/s

It is believed that micronutrient deficiency impedes mucosal proliferation.

As cells of the tongue papillae have a high turnover, deficiencies in micronutrients needed for cell proliferation or cell membrane stabilisation may lead to depapillation.[2]

Nutritional deficiency is also thought to change the pattern of microbial flora, thus contributing to glossitis.[3]

Sign value

There is growing evidence that atrophic glossitis is a marker for malnutrition and decreased muscle function.[1] In one large-scale study,[1] atrophic glossitis was found in 13.2% of men and 5.6% of women at home and in 26.6% of men and 37% of women in hospital. It was also correlated with decreased weight, decreased BMI, poor anthropometry measurements and decreased vitamin B12.

In one study[4] of patients with atrophic glossitis, 22.2% of patients had a haemoglobin deficiency, 26.7% were iron deficient, 7.4% were vitamin B12 deficient and 21.6% had raised homocysteine or gastric parietal cell antibodies.

Other smaller case reports[2,5] have also found atrophic glossitis useful in identifying micronutrient deficiencies.

4

Bone tenderness/bone pain

Description

Pain experienced in any part of the skeletal system. Pain may be present with or without tenderness on palpation.

Condition/s associated with

Many different malignancies may cause bone pain.

More common

- Prostate cancer
- Breast cancer
- Multiple myeloma
- Hodgkin's and non-Hodgkin's lymphoma
- Lung cancer
- Ovarian cancer

General mechanism/s

The mechanism involves both elements of neuropathic and inflammatory pain, with modification of the tissues and nerves as well as neurochemical changes in the spinal cord.[6] Conceptualisation of the mechanisms of cancer-induced bone pain can be seen in Figures 4.2 and 4.3.

Cancer-induced bone pain can be caused by:

- direct malignant invasion
- malignancy-induced osteoclast/osteoblast imbalance
- alteration of normal pain pathways.

Complication of direct malignant invasion

As tumour cells invade tissue and bone, they destroy normal architecture. This can result in nerve damage, vascular occlusion, inflammatory responses[6] and/or distension of the pain-sensitive periosteum, bone marrow and mineralised bone[6] – all of which will stimulate nerve afferents and produce pain.[7-9] Direct invasion of the peripheral nerves can also occur, stimulating pain pathways.

Cancer has been shown to induce disorganised sprouting of sensory and sympathetic nerve fibres, which may provide an additional stimulus for breakthrough pain.[6]

Malignancy-induced osteoclast/osteoblast imbalance

Malignancy, whether primary or metastatic, changes the osteoblastic/osteoclastic balance. This results in either lytic lesions or abnormally weakened bone that is subject to microfractures.

Increased bone turnover can also produce pain, similar to the 'growing pains' of rapid growth in adolescence.

Osteoclast/osteoblast imbalance causing pain arises from several pathways:

- Paracrine secretion of endothelin 1 and parathyroid hormone-related protein (PTH-rp) increases osteoclastic activity.
- 'Cross-talk' from malignant cells to osteoclastic cells results in increased osteoclast activity.[10]
- When bone matrix is destroyed, more growth factors are released, which increases cell proliferation and, ultimately, tumour burden.
- Inflammation and release of cytokines such as tumour necrosis factor (TNF), interleukins (IL-1 and IL-6) and prostanoids activate pain fibres.[7,8,11]

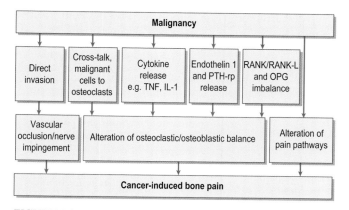

FIGURE 4.2
Mechanisms of cancer-induced bone pain
TNF = tumour necrosis factor; IL-1 = Interleukin 1; PTH-rp = parathyroid hormone-related protein; RANK = receptor activator of nuclear factor kappa; RANK-L = receptor activator of nuclear ligand.

4

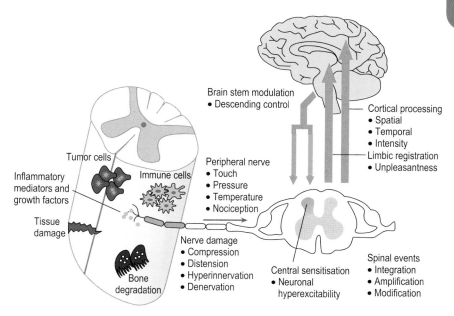

FIGURE 4.3
Mechanisms of cancer-induced bone pain
This figure illustrates the basic mechanisms of pain processes at peripheral, spinal and supraspinal sites and influences of various peripheral mechanisms, including tumour cell- and immune cell–mediated release of pronociceptive factors, direct tissue damage and bone degradation through osteoclast activation. Because of peripheral events, central excitability changes are enacted. Combination of these events produces the final pain experience at the highest brain centres.

Adapted from Falk S, Dickensen AH. Pain and nociception: mechanisms of cancer-induced bone pain. Journal of Clinical Oncology 2014; 32(16): Fig 2.

- Alteration of the receptor activator of nuclear factor kappa (RANK) pathway[8] – RANK is expressed on osteoclasts. RANK ligand (RANK-L) is expressed on a number of cell types including osteoblasts. The RANK to RANK-L interaction is central to maintaining a normal osteoclast activation.[8]

  Activated T cells and cancer cells secrete RANK-L and sequester OPG (a cytokine that limits osteoclast activity), resulting in more osteoclast activation.

- The Wnt (wingless-type) pathway – recent research has unearthed a new family of glycoproteins that influence the bone formation and resorption[12] process directly and also via some of the mechanisms previously described. Its exact influence in cancer-induced bone pain is still to be ascertained.

Alteration of normal pain pathways

Studies have shown that metastatic malignancies in bone can cause alterations in the pain pathway.[7,8,13] These changes lower the pain threshold and increase the likelihood a pain impulse will be triggered. Alterations include:

- reorganisation of the dorsal horn and sensitisation of pain afferents to substance P (which stimulates pain pathways)[10,11]
- increased expression of c-FOS and dynorphin in lamina of dorsal horn

- astrocyte hypertrophy[8] and decreased glutamate reuptake transporters, causing increased glutamate and excitotoxicity[10,11]
- an increase in glial proteins found in the spinal cord which increase pain transmission[10]
- the acidic environment produced by osteoclasts can stimulate pain receptors[7,11]
- an increase in the receptive field for neurons and a change in the ratio of types of neurons present in the dorsal horn, leading to a higher likelihood of neuronal response to low-level stimuli.[6]

It is believed that these changes, among others, contribute to pain directly as well as to hyperexcitability of neurons to stimuli.[6]

Pain itself can alter normal descending pain control mechanisms from the brain, which influence spinal cord impulses and construal of pain.[6]

Sign value

New-onset bone pain is an important sign to recognise in both the cancer-naïve patient and those with a known malignancy. Bone pain is the most frequent complication of metastatic bone disease,[14,15] reported in 50–90% of patients with skeletal metastases and in 70–95% of patients with multiple myeloma. Indeed, in patients with underlying metastases, bone pain or tenderness may be the initial presenting complaint, especially in multiple myeloma.

Chipmunk facies

Description

Abnormality of the craniofacial bones resulting in prominent frontal and parietal bones, a depressed nasal bridge and protruding upper teeth (similar to a chipmunk).

Condition/s associated with

- Beta-thalassaemia
- Parotid gland enlargement

Beta thalassaemia mechanism/s

Extramedullary haematopoiesis (EMH) is the cause of the facies in this setting.

Beta-thalassaemia (decreased or absent production of beta chains) results in abnormal haemoglobin (Hb). This leads to decreased normal haemoglobin synthesis and increased red blood cell destruction. To compensate for the low Hb, the bone marrow increases activity (hyperplasia) and haematopoiesis also takes place outside the bone marrow.[16]

Some bones are affected more than others by expansion and invasion of marrow. In beta-thalassaemia, extramedullary haematopoiesis (EMH) causes skull and facial bone irregularities that alter facial structure. Other sites can also be affected by EMH in beta thalassaemia, including the ribs, limbs, extremities and spine.

4

Compensatory extramedullary haematopoiesis

Extramedullary haematopoiesis (EMH) is an unusual irregularity that is most commonly seen in disorders that lead to the destruction of the normal bone marrow, including myelofibrosis, myeloproliferative disorders and infiltrating tumours, or in situations where the marrow cannot keep up with the demand for new cells (e.g. haemoglobinopathies). In a compensatory effort to maintain erythrogenesis and red blood cell levels, other tissues and sites begin production of red blood cells. EMH may originate from the release of stem cells from the bone marrow into the circulation.[17]

Common sites of EMH include liver, spleen, adrenal glands, kidneys and lymph nodes,[18] but it has also been seen in a number of other locations, including the epidural space, bones, synovium, dermis, pleura, paravertebral and retroperitoneal spaces.

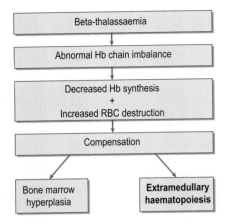

FIGURE 4.4
Extramedullary haematopoiesis

*Based on Swanson TA, Kim SI, Flomin OE,
Underground Clinical Vignettes Step 1:
Pathophysiology I, Pulmonary, Ob/Gyn,
ENT, Hem/Onc, 5th edn, Lippincott,
Williams & Wilkins, 2007: Fig 95-1.*

Conjunctival pallor

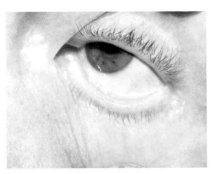

Description

When the lower eyelid is gently pulled down for inspection, the mucosal surface of the inner eyelid is noticeably whiter or paler than the pink-red of health.

Condition/s associated with

• Anaemia

Mechanism/s

Anaemic patients have a deficiency of oxyhaemoglobin (which gives blood its normal red colour). Hence, capillaries and venules appear pale, as does the conjunctiva.

Sign value

A number of studies have appraised the validity of conjunctival pallor in the assessment of anaemia. It has some value as a sign, with sensitivity of 25–62%, specificity of 82–97% and positive likelihood ratio (PLR) of 4.7.[19-23]

Anterior conjunctival rim pallor has been shown to have substantially more specificity than total conjunctival pallor. Sensitivity 10%, specificity 99% with a positive likelihood ratio of 16.7 if present.[24]

4

Ecchymoses, purpura and petechiae

Description

Ecchymoses, purpura and petechiae all refer to different sizes of subcutaneous haematomas. It is important to remember that any one condition can cause a range of stigmata. That is, a petechiae-causing pathology may also produce ecchymoses. In reality, the origins will often overlap (see Table 4.1), and it is more important to have an understanding of the general mechanisms rather than the numerous disorders leading to them.

General mechanism/s

A subcutaneous haematoma of any size can be the result of a disruption of:

- the blood vessel wall
- the normal coagulation/clotting process
- the number or function of platelets.

The consequent subcutaneous bleeding (where haemoglobin produces the initial red/blue discolouration) can then be further classified by size.

Thrombocytopenia

A significant thrombocytopenia will result in inadequate control and clotting of any bleed. This is due to the lack of platelet activation and 'plugging'. Trauma from any cause, no matter how minor, may precipitate mucocutaneous bleeding and, without adequate clotting, petechiae, purpura

TABLE 4.1
Causes of petechiae, purpura and ecchymoses

Petechiae	Purpura	Ecchymoses
Description		
Small (1–2 mm) haemorrhages into mucosal or serosal surfaces	>3 mm haemorrhages, or when ecchymoses and petechiae form in groups[25]	Subcutaneous haematoma >10–20 mm
Condition/s associated with		
Thrombocytopenia of any cause (e.g. autoimmune, heparin-induced, hypersplenism) Bone marrow failure (e.g. malignancy) Defective platelet function (rare) (e.g. Glanzmann's thromboasthenia uraemia) Disseminated intravascular coagulation Infection Bone marrow defects Factor deficiencies	Diseases associated with: As for petechiae: • Trauma • Vasculitis – particularly *palpable* purpura • Amyloidosis • Over-anticoagulation • Factor deficiencies	As for petechiae and purpura: • Trauma – common Diseases causing: • Defective platelet action • Vasculitis – *palpable* purpura • Amyloidosis • Hereditary haemorrhagic telangiectasia • Scurvy • Cushing's syndrome • Over-anticoagulation • Factor deficiencies (e.g. haemophilia)

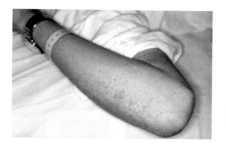

FIGURE 4.6
Petechiae in a patient with thrombocytopenia

Reproduced, with permission, from Little JW, Falace DA, Miller CS, Rhodus NL, Dental Management of the Medically Compromised Patient, *7th edn, St Louis: Mosby Elsevier, 2008: Fig 25-9.*

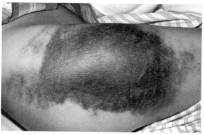

FIGURE 4.7
Ecchymoses in a patient with haemophilia

Reproduced, with permission, from Little JW, Falace DA, Miller CS, Rhodus NL, Dental Management of the Medically Compromised Patient, *7th edn, St Louis: Mosby Elsevier, 2008: Fig 25-16.*

or ecchymoses may develop before the bleed is controlled. It is rare to see spontaneous bleeding with thrombocytopenia until platelets are below $20\,000 \times 10^9/L$. Easy bruising can occur with minor trauma if platelets are between $20\,000 \times 10^9/L$ and $50\,000 \times 10^9/L$.

Vasculitis
Inflammation of the small arterioles or venules in the skin, associated with immune complex deposition, produces inflammation with punctate oedema and haemorrhage and, thus, palpable purpura.[25]

Cushing's
Ecchymoses in Cushing's syndrome are related to a lack of connective tissue support in vessel walls, due to corticosteroid-induced reduction in collagen synthesis.[26]

Mechanism of colour changes
Once under the skin, erythrocytes are phagocytosed and degraded by macrophages, with haemoglobin converted to bilirubin, thus creating blue–green discolouration. Bilirubin is eventually broken down into haemosiderin (which is golden brown)

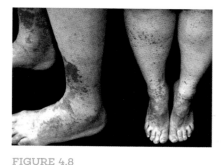

FIGURE 4.8
Palpable purpura
In a patient with Henoch–Schönlein purpura (left) and hepatitis C and cryoglobulinaemia (right).

Reproduced, with permission, from Libby P, Bonow R, Zipes R, Mann D, Braunwald's Heart Disease: A Textbook of Cardiovascular Medicine, *8th edn, Philadelphia: Saunders, 2007: Fig 84-1.*

at the end of the process before skin returns to its normal hue.

Sign value
Although there is limited evidence for the value of these lesions as clinical signs and the specificity is low, given the numerous potentially pathological causes, healthy patients rarely produce these signs and therefore they should be investigated if seen.

4

Gum hypertrophy (gingival hyperplasia)

Description

Excessive growth or expansion of the gingival tissue.

Condition/s associated with

- Leukaemia
- Drug-induced (e.g. phenytoin, cyclosporin)
- Scurvy (uncommon)

Leukaemia mechanism/s

Thought to be due to the invasion of leukaemic cells into the gingival tissues.[27]

Drug-induced mechanism/s

The mechanism is unclear. Believed to be an interaction between the offending drug and epithelial keratinocytes, fibroblasts and collagen, causing an overgrowth of tissue in susceptible individuals.[28]

Phenytoin has been shown to be active in stimulating a group of sensitive fibroblasts, whereas cyclosporin may affect the metabolic function of fibroblasts. A cofactor (e.g. inflammation) may be required to be present in order for the sign to occur.

Sign value

A relatively uncommon sign, seen mostly in acute myelogenous leukaemia, but only in about 3–5% of cases.[29]

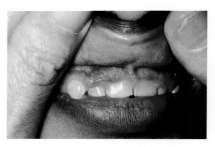

FIGURE 4.9
Gum hypertrophy

Reproduced, with permission, from Sidwell RU et al., J Am Acad Dermatol 2004; 50(2, Suppl 1): 53–56.

Haemolytic/pre-hepatic jaundice

Description

Yellowing of the skin, sclera and mucous membranes.

Condition/s associated with

Pre-hepatic jaundice encompasses jaundice that is a result of any disease or process preceding liver metabolism, such as:

- reabsorption of a large haematoma
- haemolytic causes.

In pre-hepatic jaundice, *red blood cell (RBC) destruction causes excess haem* to be released, which then passes on to the liver to be metabolised. The liver is overwhelmed and unable to conjugate and excrete all the bilirubin, leading to hyperbilirubinaemia and jaundice.

Haemolytic anaemias can be categorised in a number of ways. In Table 4.2 they are divided by the site of red blood cell destruction.

General mechanism/s

The common end point in the development of jaundice is a build-up of *excess bilirubin, which is then deposited in the skin and mucous membranes*. Jaundice is not clinically evident until bilirubin exceeds 3 mg/L. The two main mechanisms of haemolysis leading to hyperbilirubinaemia and jaundice are intravascular and extravascular.

Intravascular haemolysis occurs when red blood cells are destroyed in the circulation, caused by mechanical trauma from a damaged endothelium, complement/antibody-mediated processes (autoimmune), infection (e.g. malaria),[30] oxidative stress (low G6PD) or physical shearing (by going through a dysfunctional aortic valve) or fibrin strands deposited in small vessels (e.g. microangiopathic anaemias).

Extravascular haemolysis is more common, consisting of the removal and destruction of RBCs by macrophages in the spleen or liver (e.g. hereditary spherocytosis or sickle cell anaemia).

It should be noted that some conditions, including G6PD deficiency and immunological-mediated haemolytic anaemia, may have elements of intravascular and extravascular destruction.

The basis for removal of cells from the circulation depends on the underlying pathophysiology of the disorder. The mechanism behind a variety of disorders is summarised in Table 4.2.

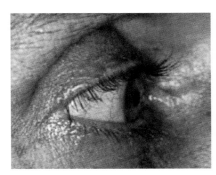

FIGURE 4.10
Jaundice with scleral icterus

Reproduced, with permission, from Stern TA, Rosenbaum JF, Fava M, Biederman J, Rauch SL, Massachusetts General Hospital Comprehensive Clinical Psychiatry, *1st edn, Philadelphia: Mosby, 2008: Fig 21-17.*

4

Drug-induced mechanism/s

Drugs are a common cause of haemolytic or pre-hepatic jaundice. Three principal mechanisms exist:[30]

1 drug absorption or hapten (immunoactive molecules which require a carrier) induced – drug attaches to the RBC membrane and stimulates IgG antibody production, leading to extravascular haemolysis

TABLE 4.2
Mechanisms behind haemolytic anaemias

Factor	Mechanism
Intravascular haemolytic anaemias	
Metallic aortic valve	Shear stress, usually through a dysfunctional valve, leads to mechanical destruction of RBCs
Microangiopathic anaemia	Fibrin strands and platelets are deposited in small vessels causing shearing of circulating RBCs
Immune mediated	Antibodies arising from either a primary or secondary autoimmune disorder, malignancy or drugs attack RBCs, enabling complement fixation and destruction
Malaria	Parasitic, destructive invasion of red blood cells
Glucose-6-phosphate dehydrogenase (G6PD) deficiency	Lack of anti-oxidative enzyme → RBCs susceptible to insult (e.g. hypoxia) → oxidative stress destroys RBCs. Also, damage to haemoglobin and its precipitation into Heinz bodies can impair the cell membrane sufficiently to cause intravascular haemolysis
Paroxysmal nocturnal haemoglobinuria	A genetic or acquired abnormality leads to the absence of key enzymes that protect the RBC from the intravascular complement system. Without these proteins and enzymes present the complement system is able to bind to and destroy the cell
Extravascular haemolytic anaemias	
Hereditary spherocytosis	Genetic abnormality leading to fragile, irregular-shaped RBCs which the spleen removes and destroys
Glucose-6-phosphate dehydrogenase (G6PD) deficiency	Lack of anti-oxidative enzyme – oxidative stress can damage haemoglobin, causing precipitation into Heinz bodies, which are taken out by macrophages within the spleen. Damaged and altered RBCs may also be removed by the spleen
Sickle cell anaemia	Abnormal haemoglobin (RBCs clump together and are more fragile), increased cell stress and breakdown
Immune	Antibodies (either primary or secondary to autoimmune disorder or malignancy) attack RBCs and mark them for removal by the spleen
Malaria	Parasitic, destructive invasion of RBCs
Haemolytic disease of newborn	Maternal antibodies cross the placenta and attack foetal red blood cells

TABLE 4.3
Selected drugs that cause immune-mediated haemolysis

Mechanism	DAT
	Site of haemolysis
	Drugs
Drug absorption (hapten)	Positive anti–IgG
	Extravascular
	Penicillin
	Ampicillin
	Methicillin
	Carbenicillin
	Cephalothin (Keflin)★
	Cephaloridine (Loridine)★
Immune complex	Positive anti–C3
	Intravascular
	Quinidine
	Phenacetin
	Hydrochlorothiazide
	Rifampin (Rifadin)
	Sulfonamides
	Isoniazid
	Quinine
	Insulin
	Tetracycline
	Melphalan (Alkeran)
	Acetaminophen
	Hydralazine (Apresoline)
	Probenecid
	Chlorpromazine (Thorazine)
	Streptomycin
	Fluorouracil (Adrucil)
	Sulindac (Clinoril)
Autoantibody	Positive anti–IgG
	Extravascular
	Alpha-methyldopa
	Mefenamic acid (Ponstel)
	L-dopa
	Procainamide
	Ibuprofen
	Diclofenac (Voltaren)
	Interferon alfa

DAT = direct antiglobulin test.
★Not available in the United States.
Dhaliwal, G et al. Hemolytic Anaemia. American Family Physician 2004; (69)11: Table 2. Adapted, with permission, from Schwartz RS, Berkman EM, Silberstein LE, Autoimmune hemolytic anemias. In: Hoffman R, Benz EJ Jr, Shattil SJ, Furie B, Cohen HJ, Silberstein LE, et al. (eds), Hematology: Basic Principles and Practice, 3rd edn, Philadelphia: Churchill Livingstone, 2000: p. 624.

2 IgM antibody production
  – causing complement activation
  leading to intravascular haemolysis
3 anti-erythrocyte antibody
  induction – drug induces
  antibodies directed against red
  blood cells, causing extravascular
  haemolysis.

Table 4.3 shows examples of
drugs causing these three types of
reactions.

Sign value

Jaundice is pathological and requires
diagnostic work-up to determine
whether it is hepatic or pre-hepatic.
For a review of other causes of
jaundice, see Chapter 6,
'Gastroenterological signs'.

Koilonychia

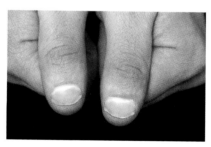

FIGURE 4.11
Koilonychia – spoon-shaped nails

Reproduced, with permission, from Grandinetti LM, Tomecki KJ, Chapter: Nail abnormalities and systemic disease. In: Carey WD, Cleveland Clinic: Current Clinical Medicine, 2nd edn, Philadelphia: Saunders, 2010: Fig 4.

Description

Described as the loss of longitudinal and lateral convexity of the nail, with thinning and fraying of the distal portion. Or put simply – spoon-shaped nails. The name derives from the Greek words for 'hollow' and 'nail'.

Condition/s associated with

More common

- Physiological variant of normal
- Soft nails with occupational damage

Less common

- Iron deficiency anaemia
- Haemochromatosis – rare
- Raynaud's syndrome

Mechanism/s

The exact mechanism is not known. Koilonychia is associated with a soft nail bed and matrix, but the reason for this is unclear.[31]

Sign value

There is little evidence for koilonychia as a sign in iron deficiency anaemia.

4

Leser–Trélat sign

Description

The sudden onset of large numbers of seborrhoeic keratoses with an associated malignant process.

Condition/s associated with

More common

- Adenocarcinoma: stomach, liver, pancreas, colorectal
- Breast cancer
- Lung cancer

Less common

- Urinary tract cancers
- Melanoma

Mechanism/s

Most likely due to paraneoplastic secretion of *different growth factors*, including epidermal growth factor (EGF), growth hormone and transforming growth factor, which *alter the extracellular matrix, promote keratinocyte proliferation* and stimulate the development of seborrhoeic keratoses.[32-34]

Sign value

The value of this sign with regard to internal cancers is controversial. While more associated with adenocarcinoma of the stomach, colon and breast, it has been seen in a variety of other malignancies.[34]

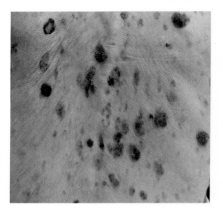

FIGURE 4.12
Leser–Trélat sign

Reproduced, with permission, from Ho ML, Girardi PA, Williams D, Lord RVN, J Gastroenterol Hepatol 2008; 23(4): 672.

Leucoplakia

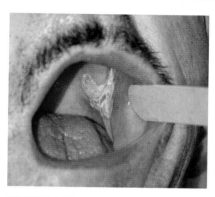

FIGURE 4.13
Leucoplakia

Reproduced, with permission, from World Articles in Ear, Nose and Throat website. Available: http://www.entusa.com/oral_photos.htm [9 Feb 2011].

Description

A fixed white lesion in the oral cavity that cannot be removed by rubbing and does not disappear spontaneously.

Condition/s associated with

Squamous cell carcinoma (SCC) of the head or neck.

Mechanism/s

The reason why leucoplakia develops is not completely clear.

It is often described as a *pre-malignant lesion* with some features of dysplasia. Risk factors for leucoplakia include cigarette smoking and cigarette products, *Candida* infection, previous malignancy or pre-malignancy and human papilloma virus (HPV).[35] It is assumed that all of these risk factors can somehow cause changes in the DNA and/or tumour suppressor genes of cells that result in a disposition to produce cancerous lesions.

Sign value

The overall prevalence of leucoplakia is approximately 0.2–5%.

2–6% of lesions represent dysplasia or early invasive SCC,[36] and 50% of oral SCCs will present with leucoplakia. It is recommended that all patients diagnosed with leucoplakia be evaluated for cancer.

4

Lymphadenopathy

Description
Enlarged lymph nodes able to be palpated or identified on imaging.

Condition/s associated with
Numerous disorders can present with lymphadenopathy as part of their clinical picture. The acronym MIAMI may help the clinician recall the broad causes (see Table 4.4): **M**alignancy, **I**nfectious, **A**utoimmune, **M**iscellaneous and **I**atrogenic.[37]

General mechanism/s
In general, most of the conditions that result in lymphadenopathy do so either via:

1 propagation of an inflammatory response, whether it be systemic, regional or direct[38]
2 invasion and/or proliferation of abnormal or malignant cells.[38,39]

Malignancy
Malignancy causes lymphadenopathy through invasion or infiltration of malignant cells *into* the lymph node or direct proliferation of malignant cells *within* the lymph node.

The lymphatic system provides the predominant mechanism for distant metastatic spread of cells for a variety of solid-tumour cancers (e.g. colorectal, ovarian, prostate). Tumour cells move from the main tumour site via the lymphatic system to lymph nodes, where they accumulate and/or proliferate, enlarging the lymph node.

In lymphoma there is an abnormal proliferation of lymphocytes within the lymph node with associated hyperplasia of normal structures, producing lymphadenopathy.

Infectious causes
The lymphatic system is central to effective functioning of the immune system. Macrophages and other antigen-presenting cells migrate to the lymph nodes in order to present antigens to T and B cells. On recognition of an antigen, T and B cells proliferate within the lymph node in order to generate an effective immune response. The lymphadenopathy seen with infection (local or systemic) is a consequence of this proliferation.

Where *direct invasion* occurs, a solitary lymph node becomes infected with a bacterium or other type of antigen. The resulting immune response results in hyperplasia of the lymph node structures, T and B cell proliferation and infiltration of other immune cells to address the infection. This results in inflammation and swelling of the node.

In the presence of *systemic infection*, reactive hyperplasia can occur. An antigenic (intracellular or extracellular) stimulus is brought to the lymph node and presented to T and B cells, lymphocytes and other cells resident in the node, causing their proliferation.[40]

Autoimmune
Autoimmune causes of lymphadenopathy are similar to infectious causes of lymphadenopathy, except that the antigen is a *self*-antigen and the *inflammatory response* is an *inappropriate* one. B cell proliferation is often seen within the lymph nodes of patients with rheumatoid arthritis whereas T cell proliferation is seen in systemic lupus erythematosus.[40]

TABLE 4.4
Causes of lymphadenopathy – MIAMI acronym

M Malignancy	I Infectious	A Autoimmune	M Miscellaneous	I Iatrogenic
Lymphoma	Tonsillitis	Sarcoidosis	Kawasaki's disease	Serum sickness
Leukaemia	Epstein–Barr virus	SLE	Sarcoidosis	Drugs
Multiple myeloma	Tuberculosis	Rheumatoid arthritis		
Skin cancer	HIV			
Breast cancer	CMV			
	Streptococcal and staphylococcal infection			
	Cat scratch disease			

Based on McGee S, Evidence Based Physical Diagnosis, 2nd edn, Philadelphia: Saunders, 2007: Box 24.1; with permission.

4

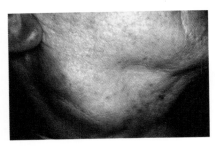

FIGURE 4.14
Cervical lymphadenopathy

Reproduced, with permission, from Little JW, Falace DA, Miller CS, Rhodus NL, Dental Management of the Medically Compromised Patient, 7th edn, St Louis: Mosby, 2008: Fig 24-6.

TABLE 4.5
Values of lymph node characteristics in the diagnosis of malignancy or serious underlying disease

Feature	Value
Hard texture	Sensitivity 48–62%, specificity 83–84%, PLR 3.2, NLR 0.6
Fixed lymph nodes	Sensitivity 12–52%, specificity 97%, PLR 10.9
Lymph node size >9 cm²	Sensitivity 37–38%, specificity 91–98%, PLR 8.4

Sign value

With so many potential causes for lymphadenopathy, its specificity as a sign is limited. The main issue for the clinician is to determine whether it is arising from a malignant cause or something more benign, such as infection.

Several characteristics are said to make a node more suggestive of malignancy. A review[24] of studies regarding these characteristics in the diagnosis of malignancy or serious underlying disease found that the features listed in Table 4.5 generally had higher specificity than sensitivity. That is, if the characteristic was present, it was suggestive of a serious underlying cause but, if it was not present, malignancy or another serious cause could not be ruled out. Evidence of supraclavicular lymphadenopathy

is said to be more indicative of malignancy.

Time course of the development of lymphadenopathy is also used as an indicator of malignancy, with a shorter duration more likely due to an acute infective cause, and a longer time course suggestive of malignancy.

In one study of 457 children presenting with lymphadenopathy, in 98.2% of cases acute lymphadenopathy was due to benign causes. Malignancies were most often associated with chronic and generalised lymphadenopathy.[41]

Painful versus painless nodes

It is generally believed that painful nodes are more likely to be reactive or related to an inflammatory process than painless nodes, which are more likely to be malignant. However, evidence for this assumption is limited.

Lymphadenopathy: location – location – location

The site of lymphadenopathy may help identify the origin of the underlying conditions. Detailed explanations of the anatomy of the lymph system can be found in any anatomy textbook. The drainage areas associated with various lymph nodes are given in brief in Table 4.6.

Using these anatomical landmarks, clinicians can narrow their search for the primary malignancy.

Generalised lymphadenopathy

Generalised lymphadenopathy is usually described as the enlargement of two or more groups of lymph nodes. It is caused by systemic disorders that by their nature affect more than just a localised region of the body. Such conditions include lymphoma, leukaemia, tuberculosis, HIV/AIDS, syphilis, other infectious diseases and some connective tissue disorders (e.g. rheumatoid arthritis). Although this principle is not absolute, it does help shorten the differential diagnosis list.

4

TABLE 4.6
Location of lymphadenopathy

Lymph node	Anatomical drainage area
Cervical	All of the head and neck
Supraclavicular	Thorax, abdominal organs (see Virchow's node)
Epitrochlear	Ulnar aspect or arm and hand[42]
Axillary	Ipsilateral arm, breast and chest
Inguinal – horizontal group	Lower anterior wall, lower anal canal
Inguinal – vertical group	Lower limb, penis, scrotum and gluteal area

Virchow's node – not just gastrointestinal malignancy

Virchow's node refers to supraclavicular lymphadenopathy and has classically been taught as a sign of gastrointestinal malignancy only, but recent research has shown broader associations.

Mechanism/s
Virchow's node is located at the end of the thoracic duct.[43] Accepted theory is that lymph and malignant cells from the gastrointestinal system travel through the thoracic duct and are deposited in Virchow's node.

Condition/s associated with
Studies[44] have now shown Virchow's node to be present with:
- lung cancer – most common[44]
- pancreatic cancer
- oesophageal cancer
- renal cancer
- ovarian cancer
- testicular cancer[45,46]
- stomach cancer
- prostate cancer
- uterine and cervical cancer
- gallbladder cancer – rare
- liver cancer
- adrenal cancer
- bladder cancer.

Neoplastic fever

Description

Typically, a diagnosis of exclusion made only in a patient with cancer, after other possible causes of fever have been ruled out.

Condition/s associated with

Most forms of cancer.

Differential diagnoses include all other common causes of fever.

Mechanism/s

The mechanism is not clear. Suggested theories include:[47]

- pyrogenic cytokines released by cancer cells (e.g. IL-1, IL-6, TNF-alpha and interferon)

- tumour necrosis contributing to release of TNF and other pyrogens

- bone marrow necrosis causing a release of toxins and cytokines from damaged cells.

Sign value

There is limited information as to the value of neoplastic fever as a sign.

Cancer has been shown to be the cause of fever of unknown origin in 20% of cases.[48]

There is value in identifying neoplastic fever, as treatment with NSAIDs (Naproxen) has been shown to alleviate symptoms, unlike the blind use of antibiotics.[47]

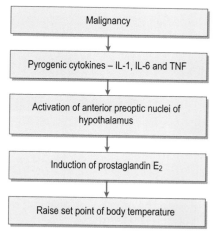

FIGURE 4.15
Neoplastic fever

4

Peau d'orange

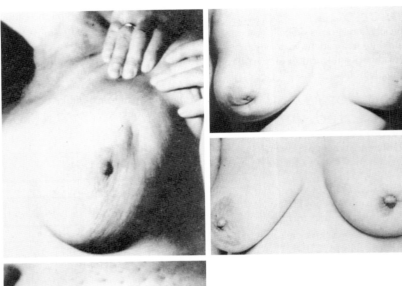

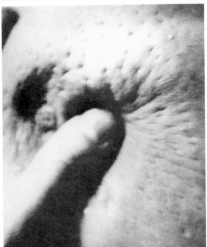

FIGURE 4.16
Peau d'orange

Reproduced, with permission, from Katz JW, Falace DA, Miller CS, Rhodus NL, Comprehensive Gynecology, 5th edn, Philadelphia: Mosby, 2007: Fig 15-13B.

Description

From the French, literally meaning 'skin of an orange', it is a term used to describe a dimpled appearance of the breast skin.

Condition/s associated with

More common

- Breast cancer
- Breast abscess

Less common

- Myxoedema

General mechanism/s

Inflammation and/or oedema that accentuates the depressions at the base of the hair follicles of the breast.

Breast cancer

Cancerous tissue causes the destruction and or/blockage of lymphatics. Skin drainage is compromised and lymphoedema develops, along with thickening and swelling of the skin. Accentuation of the depressions of the skin at the site of the hair follicles produces the dimples.

Tethering of the thickened skin to the underlying *Cooper's ligaments* creates the orange peel appearance.[49]

Sign value

Although there are few studies on the prevalence of peau d'orange in breast cancer, if present on examination further investigation is mandatory.

4

Prostate (abnormal)

Description

While performing a digital rectal examination (DRE), the prostate can be felt and assessed. It is normally described as rubbery and walnut-sized on palpation. Abnormalities which may be found are:

- hard, irregular and/or enlarged nodular prostate
- boggy tenderness – prostatitis.

Condition/s associated with

- Prostate cancer
- Benign prostatic hypertrophy (BPH)
- Prostatitis

Prostate cancer mechanism/s

The mass (tumour or benign) expands the prostate in an irregular fashion creating nodules and alterations in size and shape. Most prostate cancers originate in the peripheral zones of the prostate and, in theory, should be easier to palpate. The underlying cause of prostate cancer is still being researched.

Prostatitis mechanism/s

Anything that can cause inflammation of the gland can cause a tender, boggy-feeling prostate.

The most frequent causes of inflammation of the prostate are bacterial infections, which can be idiopathic, sexually transmitted or arise from recurrent urinary tract infections.

Infection leads to inflammation, oedema (hence the bogginess) and stimulation of pain fibres, causing tenderness.

Prostate cancer screening

At the time of publication, prostate cancer screening (in conjunction with prostate-specific antigen [PSA]) is under intense review. However, there is some evidence of the value of an expertly performed digital rectal examination (DRE):

- Prior to PSA screening, DRE is said to identify 40–50% of biopsy-detected cancers.[50]
- With PSA screening, the number of patients detected on DRE alone has declined – the predictive accuracy of PSA outperforms that of DRE.[51]
- However, potentially aggressive cancers are more prevalent in men who have an abnormal DRE.[51,52]
- A substantial proportion of patients with aggressive cancers were found on DRE alone.[53]

Given the low cost of DRE, despite the discomfort to the patient (and often the examiner), there is still value to the maxim 'if you don't put your finger in it, you put your foot in it'.

Rectal mass

Description
Palpation of an irregular/unexpected mass in the rectum on digital rectal examination (DRE).

Condition/s associated with
- Rectal cancer

Colorectal cancer screening
There are limited studies regarding the true value of DRE findings in surveillance for colorectal cancer. The available evidence for detection of palpable tumour is not strong:

- One meta-analysis[54] showed sensitivity of 64%, specificity of 97% and PPV of 0.47.
- Another more recent study[55] showed sensitivity of 76.2%, specificity of 93% and a low PPV of 0.3.

Based on the above results, it is suggested that, in the primary care setting, palpation of a mass on DRE is an inaccurate and poor predictor of colorectal cancer and holds a high risk of false positive findings, resulting in inappropriate referral for investigation.

4

Trousseau's sign of malignancy

Description

Initially described in the mid-19th century by Dr Armand Trousseau as a *migratory thrombophlebitis preceding diagnosis of occult malignancy*, over time it has been used to describe virtually any thrombotic event associated with malignancy.

In the modern setting, it is most easily thought of as any unexplained thrombotic event that precedes identification of occult visceral malignancy.[56]

N.B. Not to be confused with Trousseau's sign in hypocalcaemia — see Chapter 7, 'Endocrinological signs'.

Condition/s associated with

More common

- Lung cancer
- Pancreatic cancer

Less common

- Gastric cancer
- Colon cancer
- Prostate cancer

Mechanism/s

The exact mechanism of thrombotic events due to occult malignancy is multifaceted and, as such, not fully understood or proven. However, all of the proposed pathways ultimately end in activation of the coagulation system.

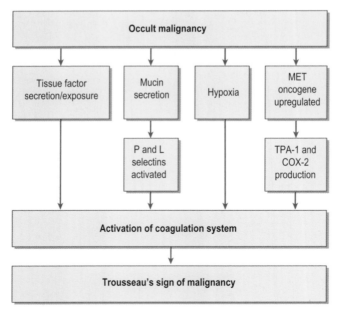

FIGURE 4.17
Mechanism of Trousseau's sign of malignancy

Contributing factors/theories are discussed under the following headings.

Tissue factor

Evidence has shown that some carcinomas:

- expose and/or cause expression of endothelium-based tissue factor (TF)[57,58]
- lead to increased TF levels via expression of tumour oncogenes and inactivation of tumour suppressor genes
- may produce TF in microvesicles
- are constituently TF[58] (e.g. breast and gliomas).

All of the above factors can, in turn, activate the clotting cascade and platelet aggregation at sites distant from the local tumour.[57]

Carcinoma mucins

Mucins are large, heavily glycosylated molecules. Some tumours produce large amounts of mucins, which then interact with P and L selectins to activate tissue multiple pathways to produce platelet plugs, microthrombi and, thus, thrombophlebitis.

Oncogene activation

More recently, activation of the MET oncogene has been postulated to activate tissue plasminogen activator 1 and cyclooxygenase 2, which influence coagulation and haemorrhagic pathways.[59]

Tissue hypoxia

Tissue hypoxia causing increased expression of genes that facilitate coagulation (e.g. plasminogen activator inhibitor-1 [PAI-1]) has also been proposed as a contributing factor.[60] Definitive research on this is lacking.

Other causes

- Cancer procoagulant (CP) is another enzyme which has been shown to activate Factor X independently of Factor VII. It is synthesised by malignant cells.[58]
- Microparticles are small membrane vesicles containing lipids, proteins and nucleic acids which have also been shown to be procoagulant and released by tumours.[58]
- Tumour-induced inflammatory cytokines and angiogenic factors may induce a procoagulant phenotype.[58]

Sign value

Direct studies regarding the sensitivity and specificity of Trousseau's sign are minimal. 11% of all cancer patients will develop thrombophlebitis,[61] whereas 23% of patients may have evidence of it at autopsy.[62] From another perspective, patients with any type of malignancy have a seven-fold risk of venous thromboembolism, and up to 28 times more with some neoplasms.[63] Though robust evidence of Trousseau's sign in malignancy is lacking, in patients who have multiple thrombotic events without identifiable cause, cancer must always be considered.

4

References

1. Bohmer T, Mowe M. The association between atrophic glossitis and protein – calorie malnutrition in old age. *Age Ageing* 2000;**29**:47–50.

2. Drinka PJ, Langer E, Scott L, Morrow F. Laboratory measurements of nutritional status as correlates of atrophic glossitis. *J Gen Intern Med* 1991;**6**:137–40.

3. Sweeney MP, Bagg J, Fell GS, Yip B. The relationship between micronutrient depletion and oral health in geriatrics. *J Oral Pathol Med* 1994;**23**:168–71.

4. Sun A, et al. Significant association with deficiency of haemoglobin, iron, vitamin B12, high homocysteine level and gastric parietal cell antibody positivity with atrophic glossitis. *J Oral Pathol Med* 2012;**41**:500–4.

5. Lehman JS, Bruce AJ, Rogers RS. Atrophic glossitis from vitamin B12 deficiency: a case misdiagnosed as burning mouth disorder. *J Periodontol* 2006;**77**(12):2090–2.

6. Falk S, Dickensen AH. Pain and nociception: mechanisms of cancer-induced bone pain. *J Clin Oncol* 2014;**32**(16):1647–54.

7. Jimenez-Andrade JM, et al. Bone cancer pain. *Ann NY Acad Sci* 2010;**1198**:173–81.

8. Urch C. The pathophysiology of cancer-induced bone pain: current understanding. *Palliat Med* 2004;**18**:267–74.

9. Ripamonti C, Fulfaro F. Pathogenesis and pharmacological treatment of bone pain in skeletal metastases. *Q J Nucl Med* 2001;**45**(1):65–77.

10. von Moos R, Strasser F, Gillessan S, Zaugg K. Metastatic bone pain: treatment options with an emphasis on bisphosphonates. *Support Care Cancer* 2008;**16**:1105–15.

11. Sabino MAC, Mantyh PW. Pathophysiology of bone cancer pain. *J Support Oncol* 2005;**3**(1):15–22.

12. Goldring SR, Goldring MB. Eating bone or adding it: the WNT pathway decides. *Nature Med* 2007;**13**(2):133–4.

13. Gobrilirsch MJ, Zwolak PP, Clohisy DR. Biology of bone cancer pain. *Clin Cancer Res* 2006;**12**(20 Suppl.):6231a–6235a.

14. Coleman RE. Bisphosphonates: clinical experience. *Oncologist* 2004;**9**:14–27.

15. Diel IJ. Bisphosphonates in the prevention of bone metastases: current evidence. *Semin Oncol* 2001;**28**(4):75–80.

16. Fleisher GR, Ludwig S. *Textbook of Pediatric Emergency Medicine*. 6th ed. Philadelphia: Lippincott Williams & Wilkins; 2010.

17. Rodak BF, Fritsma GA, Doig K. *Haematology Clinical Principles and Applications*. St Louis: Saunders; 2007.

18. Aessopos A, et al. Extramedullary hematopoiesis-related pleural effusion: the case of beta-thalassemia. *Ann Thorac Surg* 2006;**81**:2037–43.

19. Nardone DA, Roth KM, Mazur DJ, Mcafee JH. Usefulness of physical examination in detecting the presence or absence of anaemia. *Arch Internal Med* 1990;**150**:201–4.

20. Stolfftzfus RJ, Edward-Raj A, Dreyfuss ML, et al. Clinical pallor is useful in detecting severe anaemia in populations where anaemia is prevalent and severe. *J Nutr* 1999;**129**:1675–81.

21. Kent AR, Elsing SH, Herbert RL. Conjunctival vasculature in the assessment of anaemia. *Ophthalmology* 2000;**107**:274–7.

22. Van de broek NR, Ntonya C, Mhango E, White SA. Diagnosing anaemia in pregnancy in rural clinics. Assessing the potential of haemoglobin colour scale. *Bull World Health Org* 1999;**77**:15–21.

23. Ekunwe EO. Predictive value of conjunctival pallor in the diagnosis of anaemia. *West Afr J Med* 1997;**16**(4):246–50.

24. McGee S. *Evidence Based Physical Diagnosis*. 3rd ed. St Louis: Elsevier; 2012.

25. LeBlond RF, Brown DD, DeGowin RL. Chapter 6: The skin and nails. In: LeBlond RF, Brown DD, DeGowin RL, editors. *DeGowin's Diagnostic Examination*. 9th ed. Available: http://proxy14.use.hcn.com.au/content.aspx?aID=3659565 [2 Aug 2010].

26. Yanovski JA, Cutler GB Jr. Glucocorticoid action and the clinical features of Cushing's syndrome. *Endocrinol Metab Clin North Am* 1994;**23**:487–509.

27. Weckx LL, Tabacow LB, Marcucci G. Oral manifestations of leukemia. *Ear Nose Throat J* 1990;**69**:341–2.

28. Meija LM, Lozada-Nur F. *Drug-induced Gingival Hyperplasia*. Available: http://emedicine.medscape.com/article/1076264-overview [23 Oct 2009].

29. Dreizen S, McCredie KB, Keating MJ, Luna MA. Malignant gingival and skin 'infiltrates' in adult leukemia. *Oral Surg Oral Med Oral Pathol* 1983;**55**:572–9.

30. Dhaliwall G, et al. Hemolytic anaemia. *Am Fam Physician* 2004;**69**(11).

31. Hogan GR, Jones B. The relationship of koilonychias and iron deficiency in infants. *J Paediatr* 1970;**77**(6):1054–7.

32. Rampen HJ, Schwengle LE. The sign of Leser–Trélat: does it exist? *J Acad Dermatol* 1989;**21**:50–5.

33. Hindeldorf B, Sigurgeirsson B, Melander S. Seborrheic keratosis and cancer. *J Academic Dermatol* 1992;**26**:947–50.

34. Yamamoto T. Leser Trelat sign: current observations. *Expert Rev Dermatol* 2013;**October**:541.

35. *Leukoplakia & Erythroplakia. Quick Answers to Medical Diagnosis and Therapy*. Available: http://proxy14.use.hcn.com.au/quickam.aspx [4 Aug 2010].

36. Duncan KO, Geisse JK, Leffell DJ. Chapter 113: Epithelial precancerous lesions. In: Wolff K, Goldsmith LA, Katz SI, Gilchrest B, Paller AS, Leffell DJ, editors. *Fitzpatrick's Dermatology in General Medicine*. 7th ed. Available: http://proxy14.use.hcn.com.au/content.aspx?aID=2981340 [15 Sep 2010].

37. Henry PH, Longo DL. Chapter 60: Enlargement of lymph nodes and spleen. In: Fauci AS, Braunwald E, Kasper DL, et al., editors. *Harrison's Principles of Internal Medicine*. 17th ed. Available: http://proxy14.use.hcn.com.au/content.aspx?aID=2875326 [18 Sep 2010].

38. LeBlond RF, Brown DD, DeGowin RL. Chapter 5: Non-regional systems and diseases. In: LeBlond RF, Brown DD, DeGowin RL, editors. *DeGowin's Diagnostic Examination*. 9th ed. Available: http://proxy14.use.hcn.com.au/content.aspx?aID=3659310. – lymphatic system [18 Sep 2010].

39. Bazemore AW, Smucker DR. Lymphadenopathy and malignancy. *Am Fam Phys* 2002;**66**(11):2103–10.

40. Jung W, Trumper L. Differential diagnosis and diagnostic strategies of lymphadenopathy. *Internist* 2008;**49**(3):305–18, quiz 319–20.

41. Oguz A, Temel EA, Citak EC, Okur FV. Evaluation of peripheral lymphadenopathy in children. *Pediatr Hematol Oncol* 2006;**23**:549–51.

42. Selby CD, Marcus HS, Toghill PJ. Enlarged epitrochlear lymphnodes: an old sign revisited. *J R Coll Phys London* 1992;**26**(2):159–61.

43. Mitzutani M, Nawata S, Hirai I, Murakami G, Kimura W. Anatomy and histology of Virchow's node. *Anat Sci Int* 2005;**80**:193–8.

44. Viacava EP. Significance of supraclavicular signal node in patients with abdominal and thoracic cancer. *Arch Surg* 1944;**48**:109–19.

45. Lee YTN, Gold RH. Localisation of occult testicular tumour with scrotal thermography. *JAMA* 1976;**236**:1975–6.

46. Slevin NJ, James PD, Morgan DAL. Germ cell tumours confined to the supraclavicular fossa: a report of two cases. *Eur J Surg Oncol* 1985;**11**:187–90.

47. Zell JA, Chang JC. Neoplastic fever: a neglected paraneoplastic syndrome. *Support Care Cancer* 2005;**13**:870–7.

48. Jacoby GA, Swartz MN. Fever of undetermined origin. *N Engl J Med* 1973;**289**:1407–10.

49. Kumar V, Abbas AK, Fausto N, et al., editors. *Robbins and Cotran Pathologic Basis of Disease*. 7th ed. Philadelphia: Elsevier; 2005.

4

50. Chodak GW, Keller P, Schoenberg HW. Assessment of screening for prostate cancer using digital rectal examination. *J Urol* 1989;**141**:1136–8.

51. Yossepowitch O. Digital rectal examination remains an important screening tool for prostate cancer. *Eur J Urol* 2009;**54**:483–4.

52. Gosselaar C, Roobol MJ, Roemeling S, Schroder FH. The role of digital rectal examination in subsequent screening visits in the European Randomised Study of Screening for Prostate Cancer (ERSPC), Rotterdam. *Eur Urol* 2008;**54**:581–8.

53. Okotie OT, Roehl KA, Misop H, et al. Characteristics of prostate cancer detected by digital rectal examination only. *Urology* 2007;**70**(6):1117–20.

54. Hoogendam A, Buntinx F, De Vet HCW. The diagnostic value of digital rectal examination in the primary care screening for prostate cancer: a meta-analysis. *Fam Pract* 1999;**16**:621–6.

55. Ang CW, Dawson R, Hall C, Farmer M. The diagnostic value of digital rectal examination in primary care for palpable rectal tumour. *Colorectal Dis* 2007;**10**:789–92.

56. DeWitt CA, Buescher LS, Stone SP. Chapter 154: Cutaneous manifestations of internal malignant disease: cutaneous paraneoplastic syndromes. In: Wolff K, Goldsmith LA, Katz SI, Gilchrest B, Paller AS, Leffell DJ, editors. *Fitzpatrick's Dermatology in General Medicine*. 7th ed. Available: http://proxy14.use.hcn.com.au/content.aspx?aID=2961164 [20 Sep 2010].

57. Varki A. Trousseau's syndrome: multiple definitions and multiple mechanisms. *Blood* 2007;**110**(6):1723–9.

58. Falanga A, Russo L, Verzeroli C. Mechanisms of thrombosis in cancer. *Thromb Res* 2013;**131**(supp1):S59–62.

59. Boccaccio C, Sabatino G, Medico E, et al. The MET oncogene drives a genetic programme linking cancer to haemostasis. *Nature* 2005;**434**:396–400.

60. Denko NC, Giacca AJ. Tissue hypoxia, the physiological link between Trousseau's syndrome and metastasis. *Cancer Res* 2001;**61**:795–8.

61. Walsh-McMonagle D, Green D. Low-molecular-weight heparin in the management of Trousseau's syndrome. *Cancer* 1997;**80**:649.

62. Ogren M. Trousseau's syndrome – what is the evidence? A population-based autopsy study. *Thromb Haemost* 2006;**95**(3):541.

63. Dammacco F, et al. Cancer-related coagulopathy (Trousseau's syndrome): review of the literature and experience of a single center of internal medicine. *Clin Exp Med* 2013;**13**:85–97.

CHAPTER 5

NEUROLOGICAL SIGNS

Understanding the clinical significance of neurological signs poses several challenges that require pre-requisite knowledge of:

- neuroanatomy and topographical anatomy (relevant adjacent structures)

- pathophysiology of neurological disorders and relevant adjacent structures

- pattern recognition of multiple clinical signs

Guide to the 'Relevant neuroanatomy and topographical anatomy' boxes

Key to the symbols used in the 'Relevant neuroanatomy and topographical anatomy' boxes

- Primary neuroanatomical structures in the pathway(s)
⇒ Significant topographical anatomical structure(s)
→ Associated neuroanatomical pathway(s)
Ø Decussation (i.e. where the structure crosses the midline)
× An effector (e.g. muscle)
⊗ A sensory receptor
↔ Structure receives bilateral innervation

This chapter includes additional sections in boxes titled 'Relevant neuroanatomy and topographical anatomy' depicting the neural pathways and associated non-neural structures. Symbols have been used to signify important components of the relevant anatomical pathways.

For example, the most common mechanism of bitemporal hemianopia is compression of the optic chiasm by an enlarging pituitary macroadenoma.

The pituitary gland is located directly inferior to the optic chiasm (i.e. the relevant topographical anatomy). The nerve fibres of the optic chiasm supply each medial hemiretina (i.e. the relevant neuroanatomy), and transmit visual information from each temporal visual hemifield. Dysfunction of these nerve fibres causes impaired vision in bilateral lateral visual hemifields (called bitemporal hemianopia).

See the example below.

Relevant neuroanatomy and topographical anatomy

Neurological structures
PRECHIASMAL STRUCTURES
- Retinal epithelium

$\downarrow$

- Optic nerve
⇒ Orbital apex
⇒ Cavernous sinus
⇒ Optic canal, sphenoid bone

$\downarrow$

CHIASMAL STRUCTURES
- Optic chiasm
⇒ Pituitary gland

$\downarrow$

POSTCHIASMAL STRUCTURES
- Optic tracts

$\downarrow$

- Lateral geniculate nucleus (LGN), thalamus

$\downarrow$

- Superior optic radiation ('Baum's loop'), parietal lobe

$\downarrow$

- Inferior optic radiation ('Meyer's loop'), temporal lobe

$\downarrow$

- Optic cortex, occipital lobe

5

Abducens nerve (CNVI) palsy

Description

There is ipsilateral impaired abduction, and mild esotropia (i.e. medial axis deviation) in the primary gaze position.[1] Dysconjugate gaze worsens when the patient looks towards the side of the lesion (see Figure 5.1B).

Condition/s associated with[1-3]

Common

- Diabetic mononeuropathy/ microvascular infarction
- Elevated intracranial pressure (called a 'false localising sign')

Relevant neuroanatomy and topographical anatomy[1,2]

- Abducens nuclei, dorsal pons
→ Facial nerve fascicles
  ↓
- Abducens fascicles
  ↓
- Abducens nerve
→ Medial longitudinal fasciculus (MLF)
⇒ Subarachnoid space
⇒ Clivus
⇒ Petrodinoid ligament in Dorello's canal
⇒ Cavernous sinus
⇒ Cavernous segment, internal carotid artery
⇒ Superior orbital fissure
⇒ Orbital apex
  ↓
× Lateral rectus muscle

Less common

- Wernicke's encephalopathy
- Cavernous sinus syndrome
- Cavernous carotid artery aneurysm
- Giant cell arteritis
- Cerebellopontine angle tumour

Mechanism/s

Abducens nerve dysfunction causes ipsilateral lateral rectus muscle weakness (see Table 5.1). Abducens nerve palsy is caused by a peripheral lesion of the abducens nerve. Lesions of the abducens nuclei typically result in horizontal gaze paresis (i.e. ipsilateral abduction paresis and contralateral adduction weakness) due to an impaired coordination of conjugate eye movements with the oculomotor motor nuclei, via the medial longitudinal fasciculus (MLF).

Causes of abducens nerve palsy include:

- disorders of the subarachnoid space
- diabetic mononeuropathy, microvascular infarction, and metabolic disorders
- elevated intracranial pressure
- cavernous sinus syndrome – typically multiple cranial nerve abnormalities
- orbital apex syndrome – typically multiple cranial nerve abnormalities.

Disorders of the subarachnoid space

Mass lesions (e.g. aneurysm, tumour, abscess) may compress the abducens nerve as it traverses the subarachnoid space. The abducens nerve emerges from the brainstem adjacent to the basilar and vertebral arteries, and the

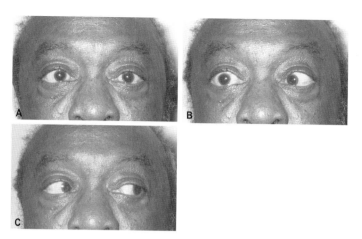

FIGURE 5.1
Right abducens nerve (CNVI) palsy
A Primary gaze position with mild esotropia (right eye deviates nasally); **B** right gaze with impaired abduction; **C** normal left gaze.

Reproduced, with permission, from Daroff RB, Bradley WG et al., Neurology in Clinical Practice, *5th edn, Philadelphia: Butterworth-Heinemann, 2008: Fig 74-7.*

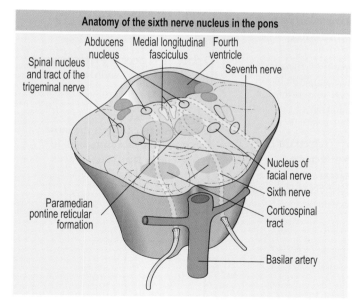

FIGURE 5.2
Anatomy of the abducens nuclei and facial nerve fascicles

Reproduced, with permission, from Yanoff M, Duker JS, Ophthalmology, *3rd edn, St Louis: Mosby, 2008: Fig 9-14-4.*

TABLE 5.1

Mechanisms of clinical features in abducens nerve palsy

Clinical features	Mechanism
• Impaired abduction	→ Lateral rectus muscle weakness
• Esotropia	→ Unopposed medial rectus muscle

clivus. Aneurysmal dilation of these vessels and/or infectious or inflammatory conditions of the clivus can compress the abducens nerve.[1] Often, multiple cranial nerve abnormalities (e.g. CNVI, VII, VIII) coexist since these structures lie in close proximity to one another upon exiting the brainstem.[1]

Diabetic mononeuropathy and microvascular infarction

Diabetic vasculopathy of the vasa nervorum (i.e. disease of the blood supply of the nerve) may result in microvascular infarction of the abducens nerve.[3]

Elevated intracranial pressure, the 'false localising sign'

Due to the relatively fixed nature of the abducens nerve at the pontomedullary sulcus and at the point of entry into Dorello's canal, it is vulnerable to stretch and/or compression injury secondary to elevated intracranial pressure.[1,2] In this setting, abducens nerve palsy is referred to as a 'false localising sign' as the clinical findings are not solely due to an isolated peripheral lesion of the abducens nerve. Causes of elevated intracranial pressure include mass lesions (e.g. tumour, abscess), hydrocephalus, idiopathic intracranial hypertension (IIH; formerly called pseudotumour cerebri) and central venous sinus thrombosis.

Cavernous carotid artery aneurysm and cavernous sinus syndrome

The cavernous segment of the abducens nerve is located adjacent to the cavernous carotid artery, and is prone to compression by aneurysmal dilation of the vessel. See 'Cavernous sinus syndrome' in this chapter.

Orbital apex syndrome

See 'Orbital apex syndrome' in this chapter.

Sign value

Abducens nerve palsy is the most common 'false localising sign' in elevated intracranial pressure.

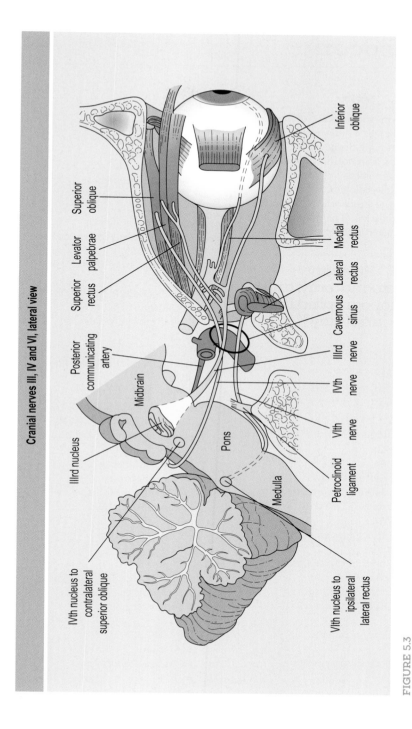

Cranial nerves III, IV and VI, lateral view

Labels: IIIrd nucleus · IVth nucleus to contralateral superior oblique · Posterior communicating artery · Midbrain · Superior rectus · Levator palpebrae · Superior oblique · Inferior oblique · Medial rectus · Lateral rectus · Cavernous sinus · IIIrd nerve · IVth nerve · VIth nerve · Pons · Petroclinoid ligament · Medulla · VIth nucleus to ipsilateral lateral rectus

FIGURE 5.3

Lateral view of the abducens nerve (CNVI) and extraocular structures

Reproduced, with permission, from Yanoff M, Duker JS, Ophthalmology, 3rd edn, St Louis: Mosby, 2008: Fig 9-15-1.

5

Anisocoria

Description

Anisocoria is the presence of unequal pupils. There is a difference of at least 0.4 mm in pupil diameter.[4]

Anisocoria in normal individuals without neurological or ocular disease is termed physiological anisocoria. Physiological anisocoria occurs in 38% of the population. The difference in pupil diameter is rarely greater than 1.0 mm.[5]

Relevant neuroanatomy and topographical anatomy[6,7]

Pupillary constriction/ parasympathetic pathway

EFFERENT LIMB
- Edinger–Westphal nucleus midbrain
  ↓
- Oculomotor nerve (CNIII)
- ⇒ Posterior communicating artery (PComm), circle of Willis
- ⇒ Uncus, medial temporal lobe
- ⇒ Superior orbital fissure, sphenoid bone
- ⇒ Cavernous sinus
- ⇒ Orbital apex
  ↓
- Ciliary ganglion
  ↓
- Short ciliary nerves
  ↓
- × Pupillary constrictor muscles
- × Levator palpebrae muscle
- × Iris

Pupillary dilation/ sympathetic pathway

FIRST-ORDER NEURON
- Hypothalamus
  ↓
- Sympathetic fibres, brainstem
  ↓
- Sympathetic fibres, intermediate horn, spinal cord
- ⇒ Central canal spinal cord
  ↓
SECOND-ORDER NEURON (PREGANGLIONIC FIBRE)
- Sympathetic trunk
- ⇒ Lung apex
  ↓
- Superior cervical ganglion (C2)
  ↓
THIRD-ORDER NEURON (POSTGANGLIONIC FIBRE)
- Superior cervical ganglion (C2)
- ⇒ Carotid sheath
- ⇒ Carotid artery
- ⇒ Superior orbital fissure
- ⇒ Cavernous sinus
- ⇒ Orbital apex
  ↓
- Ciliary body
  ↓
- × Pupillary radial muscles
- × Superior tarsal muscle
- × Sweat glands

Eye structures
- ⇒ Cornea
- ⇒ Anterior chamber
- ⇒ Iris
- × Pupillary constrictor muscles
- × Pupillary radial muscles

Condition/s associated with[4,7,8]

Common

- Physiological anisocoria
- Oculomotor nerve (CNIII) palsy (e.g. uncal herniation, posterior communicating artery aneurysm)

Less common

- Horner's syndrome
- Acute angle closure glaucoma
- Anterior uveitis
- Adie's tonic pupil

Mechanism/s

Physiological anisocoria may result from asymmetrical inhibition of the Edinger–Westphal nuclei in the midbrain.[9]

Pathological anisocoria is caused by:

- pupillary constrictor muscle weakness – mydriasis
- pupillary dilator muscle weakness – miosis
- pupillary constrictor muscle spasm – miosis.

Disorders of the afferent limb of the pupillary light reflex (CNII) do not cause anisocoria because the optic nerves form bilateral and symmetric connections with each oculomotor nucleus, such that pupillary responses to changes in ambient light are equal.[4]

At first glance, it may not be obvious which eye is the abnormal one. The abnormal eye typically has a decreased or absent pupillary light response. To identify the abnormal eye, the degree of anisocoria is assessed in dim light (i.e. in the dark) and reassessed in bright light.[8] If the magnitude of anisocoria increases in the dark (i.e. the normal pupil dilates appropriately), then the abnormal eye has the smaller pupil diameter. If the magnitude of anisocoria increases in bright light (i.e. the normal pupil constricts appropriately), the abnormal eye has the larger pupil.

Anisocoria more prominent in the dark

Anisocoria that worsens in the dark is caused by an abnormally small pupil (i.e. miosis). For bilateral small pupils, see 'Pinpoint pupils' and 'Argyll Robertson pupils' in this chapter. Causes of an abnormally small pupil include:[6]

- Horner's syndrome
- pupillary constrictor muscle spasm
- drug effects.

Horner's syndrome[10–12]

Horner's syndrome is caused by a lesion of the sympathetic pathway at one of three levels: 1) first-order neuron, 2) second-order neuron or 3) third-order neuron. Horner's syndrome is a triad of miosis, ptosis with apparent enophthalmos and anhydrosis (see 'Horner's syndrome' in this chapter).

Pupillary constrictor muscle spasm

Inflammation of the iris and/or anterior chamber may irritate the pupillary constrictor muscle resulting in spasm and miosis. Associated features may include visual acuity loss, photophobia, a red eye and a pupil with an irregular margin. Causes of pupillary constrictor muscle spasm include traumatic iritis and anterior uveitis.

Drugs

Systemic drug toxicity generally causes symmetrical changes in the pupils. Drug-induced anisocoria is more likely to be caused by unilateral topical drug exposure (may be unintentional or iatrogenic). Muscarinic agonists (e.g. pilocarpine), adrenergic antagonists (e.g. timolol) and opioids (e.g. morphine) cause pupil constriction (see 'Pinpoint pupils' in this chapter).

5

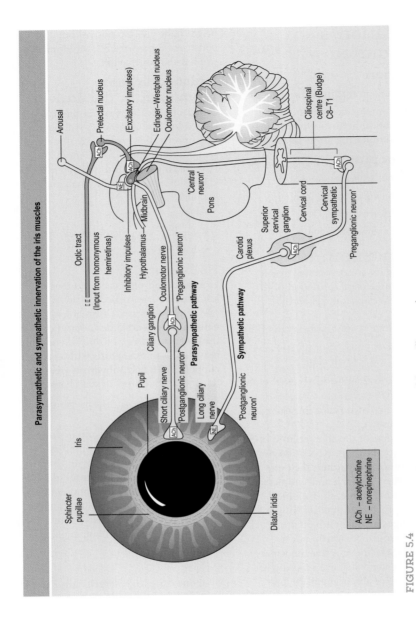

Parasympathetic and sympathetic innervation of the iris muscles

FIGURE 5.4

Parasympathetic and sympathetic innervation of the pupillary muscles

Reproduced, with permission, from Yanoff M, Duker JS, Ophthalmology, 3rd edn, St Louis: Mosby, 2008: Fig 9-19-5.

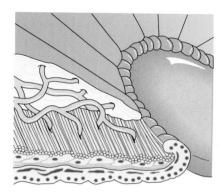

FIGURE 5.5
Circumferential distribution of the pupillary
constrictor muscles and radial distribution of
the pupillary dilator muscles

*Based on Dyck PJ, Thomas PK, Peripheral
Neuropathy, 4th edn, Philadelphia: Saunders,
2005: Fig 9-1.*

Anisocoria more prominent in bright light

Anisocoria that increases in bright light
is caused by an abnormally large pupil
(i.e. mydriasis). Causes of an
abnormally large pupil include:[6]

- oculomotor nerve (CNIII) palsy
- Adie's tonic pupil
- damage to the neuromuscular
  structures of the iris
- drugs.

Oculomotor nerve (CNIII) palsy

The oculomotor nerve innervates the
pupillary constrictor muscle, levator
palpebrae muscle and all extraocular
muscles, except the superior oblique
and lateral rectus muscles. Oculomotor
nerve palsy results in ipsilateral
mydriasis due to weakness of the
pupillary constrictor muscle.
Oculomotor nerve palsy may be
'complete' (i.e. gaze palsy, ptosis and
mydriasis), 'pupil sparing' (gaze palsy
and ptosis) or limited to the pupil
(mydriasis only). Causes include

posterior communicating (PCOM)
artery aneurysm, diabetic
mononeuropathy/microvascular
infarction, uncal herniation,
ophthalmoplegic migraine, cavernous
sinus syndrome and orbital apex
syndrome[7,13] (see 'Oculomotor nerve
(CNIII) palsy' in this chapter).

Adie's tonic pupil

The four characteristics of Adie's tonic
pupil are:[4,14–16]

1. unilateral mydriasis
2. decreased or absent pupillary light
   response
3. light–near dissociation (see
   'Light–near dissociation' in this
   chapter)
4. pupillary constrictor muscle
   sensitivity to pilocarpine.

Adie's tonic pupil is caused by
injury to the ciliary ganglion and/or
postganglionic fibres and results in
abnormal regrowth of the short ciliary
nerves.[4] Normally, the ciliary ganglion
sends 30 times more nerve fibres to the
ciliary muscle than the pupillary
constrictor muscle. Aberrant regrowth
of the ciliary nerves (a random process)
favours reinnervation of the pupillary
sphincter, rather than the ciliary
muscle.[14–16] It is associated with
vermiform movements of the iris
sphincter. Causes of Adie's tonic pupil
include orbital trauma, orbital tumours
and varicella zoster infection in the
ophthalmic division of the trigeminal
nerve (CNV V1).

Damage to the neuromuscular structures of the iris

Traumatic injury, inflammation or
ischaemia of the neuromuscular
structures of the iris may result in a
poorly reactive, mid-range dilated
pupil.[9] Associated features may include
an irregular pupillary margin,
photophobia, decreased visual acuity
and decreased pupillary light response.

5

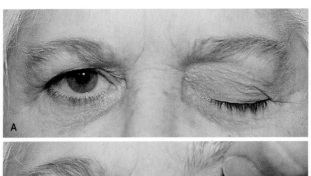
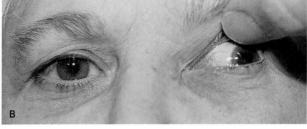

FIGURE 5.6
Complete left oculomotor nerve palsy
A Complete ptosis; **B** left exotropia and left hypotropia.
Reproduced, with permission, from Yanoff M, Duker JS, Ophthalmology, *3rd edn, St Louis: Mosby, 2008: Fig 11-10-2.*

Causes include ocular trauma, endophthalmitis and acute angle closure glaucoma.

Drugs
Systemic drug toxicity typically results in symmetrical changes in pupil diameter. Anisocoria is more likely to be caused by unilateral topical exposure (unintentional or iatrogenic). For example, unilateral ocular exposure can occur during the administration of nebulised salbutamol in a patient with a loosely fitting mask. Causes include cholinergic antagonists (e.g. atropine, ipratropium) and adrenergic agonists (e.g. cocaine, salbutamol).[9]

Sign value
Anisocoria may be a sign of a potentially life-threatening condition (e.g. uncal herniation) or an acute eye-threatening condition (e.g. acute angle closure glaucoma). Identify the abnormal eye, and whether mydriasis or miosis is present. Interpret the findings in the context of the overall clinical setting. Is the patient obtunded? Does the patient have ocular pain, no pain, a red eye, ptosis, gaze paresis?

Anosmia

Neuroanatomy and topographical anatomy[6,18]

- Olfactory neuroepithelium
  ↓
- Olfactory nerves
⇒ Cribriform plate, ethmoid bone
  ↓
- Olfactory bulb
⇒ Olfactory sulcus, inferior frontal lobe
  ↓
- Olfactory tracts
  ↓
- Olfactory cortex, medial temporal lobe
  ↓
- Thalamus, entorhinal cortex, hippocampus, amygdala

Description

Anosmia is absence of the sense of smell. Hyposmia is a decreased ability to recognise smells. Disorders of olfaction may be unilateral or bilateral.[17] Olfaction is assessed with familiar scents such as coffee or mint. Noxious substances stimulate sensory fibres of the trigeminal nerve and may confound the evaluation.[17]

Condition/s associated with[17,19,20]

Common

- Upper respiratory tract infection (URTI)
- Chronic allergic or vasomotor rhinitis
- Trauma
- Cigarette smoking
- Normal ageing
- Alzheimer's disease

Less common

- Tumour – meningioma
- Iatrogenic
- Drugs
- Kallman's syndrome

Mechanism/s

Aetiologies of anosmia are either intranasal or neurogenic in origin.[17] Causes of anosmia include:[17,19,20]

- olfactory cleft obstruction
- inflammatory disorders of the olfactory neuroepithelium
- traumatic injury of the olfactory nerves
- olfactory bulb or tract lesion
- degenerative disease of the cerebral cortex
- normal ageing.

Olfactory cleft obstruction

Mechanical airway obstruction impairs the transmission of odoriferous substances to the olfactory receptor cells on the olfactory neuroepithelium. Causes include nasal polyposis, tumour, foreign body and excess secretions.[21]

Inflammatory disorders of the olfactory neuroepithelium

Inflammation of the olfactory mucosa can cause dysfunction of the olfactory neuroepithelium.[21] Alterations in nasal

5

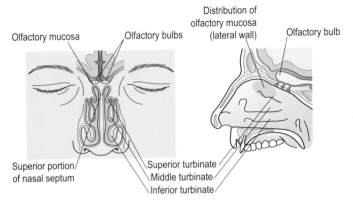

FIGURE 5.7
Functional anatomy of the peripheral olfaction pathway
Reproduced, with permission, from Bromley SM, Am Fam Physician 2000; 61(2): 427–436: Fig 2A.

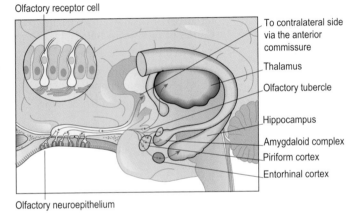

FIGURE 5.8
Functional anatomy of the central olfaction pathway
Reproduced, with permission, from Bromley SM, Am Fam Physician 2000; 61(2): 427–436: Fig 2B.

air flow, mucociliary clearance, secretory product obstruction, polyps or retention cysts likely contribute to olfactory neuroepithelium dysfunction.[21,22] Causes include URI, allergic or vasomotor rhinitis and cigarette smoking.

Traumatic injury of the olfactory nerves

Stretching and shearing of the olfactory nerves may occur in rapid acceleration–deceleration-type injuries (e.g. motor vehicle collision) as the olfactory nerves are fixed in the cribriform plate of the ethmoid bone. Direct penetrating or blunt injury to the olfactory system may impair function.[23]

Olfactory bulb or tract lesion

Intracranial masses at the base of the frontal lobes can cause dysfunction of the olfactory bulbs and/or olfactory tracts due to mass effect. Causes include meningioma, metastases, complicated meningitis and sarcoidosis.[6,17] Diseases of the ethmoid bone may result in compression of the olfactory neurons as they traverse the cribriform plate. Causes include Paget's disease, osteitis fibrosa cystica, bony metastases and trauma.

Neurodegenerative disease of the cerebral cortex

In Alzheimer's disease, there is degeneration of the medial temporal lobe and other cortical areas involved in olfactory processing.[24] Other neurodegenerative cortical diseases associated with anosmia include Lewy body dementia, Parkinson's disease and Huntington's disease.[17]

Normal ageing

Age-related olfactory changes include reduced olfactory sensitivity, intensity, identification and discrimination. These changes may be due to dysfunction at the receptor or neuron level secondary to underlying disease states, pharmacological agents or changes in neurotransmitter levels.[17]

Sign value

Anosmia is most commonly caused by benign intranasal disorders such as allergic rhinitis or URTI. Although much less common, anosmia may be the presenting symptom of a mass compressing the olfactory bulb.

In a study of 278 consecutive patients with anosmia or hyposmia evaluated in an ENT clinic, the aetiology was upper respiratory tract infection in 39%, sinonasal disease in 21%, idiopathic in 18%, trauma in 17% and congenital in 3% of patients.[25]

5

Argyll Robertson pupils and light-near dissociation

Description

Arygll Robertson pupils are characterised by:[4,9]

- miosis (small pupils)
- absence of the pupillary light response
- brisk accommodation reaction
- bilateral involvement.

Light-near dissociation is defined as:[4,9]

- a normal accommodation response
- a sluggish or absent pupillary light response.

Light-near dissociation is present if the near pupillary response (tested in moderate light) exceeds the best pupillary response with a bright light source.[9]

Condition/s associated with[6,9,26,27]

- Multiple sclerosis
- Neurosarcoidosis
- Tertiary syphilis

Mechanism/s

Argyll Roberston pupils and light-near dissociation are caused by a pretectal lesion in the dorsal midbrain affecting the fibres of light reflex, which spare the fibres of the accommodation pathway that innervate the Edinger–Westphal nuclei (see Figure 5.10).[26]

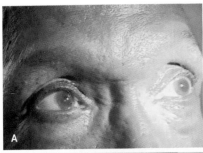
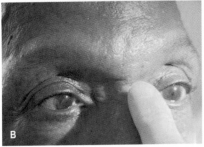

FIGURE 5.9
Argyll Robertson physical findings
A Lack of pupillary constriction to light;
B pupillary constriction to accommodation.

Reproduced, with permission, from Aziz TA, Holman RP, Am J Med 2010; 123(2): 120–121.

Sign value

Argyll Robertson pupils are classically associated with tertiary syphilis. Historically, clinicians referred to this condition as the 'prostitute's pupil'.

Relevant neuroanatomy and topographical anatomy[6]

Accommodation and pupillary light pathways

AFFERENT STRUCTURES

- Retinal neuroepithelium

  ↓

- Optic nerve (CNII)

  ↓

- Pretectal nucleus midbrain

  ↓

- ↔ Bilateral innervation of Edinger–Westphal nuclei

  ↓

EFFERENT STRUCTURES

- Visual cortex (accommodation only)

  ↓

- Accommodation area, visual cortex (accommodation only)

  ↓

- Pretectal nuclei, midbrain

  ↓

- Edinger–Westphal nuclei, midbrain

  ↓

- Oculomotor nerve (CNIII)

  ↓

- Ciliary ganglion

  ↓

- Short ciliary nerves

  ↓

- × Pupillary constrictor muscles
- × Ciliary muscle
- × Medial rectus muscles

5

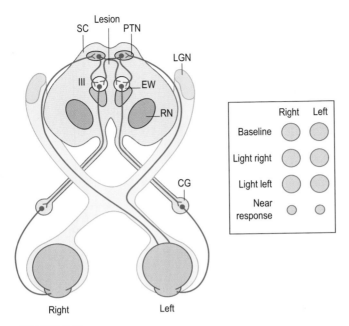

FIGURE 5.10

Pupillary response associated with light–near dissociation due to lesion in the pretectum
CG = ciliary ganglion; EW = Edinger–Westphal nucleus; LGN = lateral geniculate nucleus;
PTN = pretectal nucleus; RN = red nucleus; SC = superior colliculus.

Reproduced, with permission, from Goldman L, Ausiello D, Cecil Medicine, 23rd edn, Philadelphia: Saunders, 2007: Fig 450-2.

Ataxic gait

> ## Relevant neuroanatomy and topographical anatomy[6]
>
> CEREBELLUM
> - Vermis and flocculonodular lobe
>   - → Anterior corticospinal tract
>   - → Reticulospinal tract
>   - → Vestibulospinal tract
>   - → Tectospinal tract
> - Paravermal (intermediate) hemisphere
>   - → Lateral corticospinal tract
>   - → Rubrospinal tract
> - Lateral hemisphere
>   - → Lateral corticospinal tract

Description

An ataxic gait has a 'drunken' or staggering quality and is characterised by a wide-based stance to accommodate instability.[28] It becomes more pronounced on a narrow base, during heel-to-toe walking and during rapid postural adjustments.[28]

Condition/s associated with[6,28,29]

Common

- Intoxication – alcohol
- Drug toxicity – lithium, phenytoin, benzodiazepine

Less common

- Cerebellar infarction
- Vertebral artery dissection
- Cerebellar mass lesion – tumour, abscess, AVM
- Multiple sclerosis
- HSV cerebellitis
- Hereditary cerebellar degeneration (Freidreich's ataxia)
- Paraneoplastic cerebellar degeneration

Mechanism/s

Ataxic gait may be present with midline and/or lateral cerebellar dysfunction. Dysfunction of the midline cerebellar structures (e.g. vermis, flocculonodular lobes, intermediate lobe) results in impaired trunk coordination, disequilibrium and increased body sway.[28] Causes of ataxic gait include:

- central cerebellar structure dysfunction: vermis, flocculonodular lobe, intermediate hemisphere
- lateral hemisphere lesion.

Cerebellar vermis lesion

Isolated dysfunction of the cerebellar vermis may cause pure truncal ataxia with paucity of hemispheric cerebellar signs (e.g. dysmetria, dysdiadochokinesis, intention tremor).[28] Lower limb coordination during the heel-to-shin test may be relatively normal during supine

5

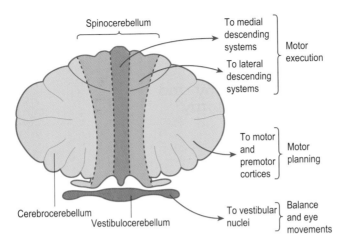

FIGURE 5.11
Functional anatomy of the cerebellum (see also Table 5.2)

From Barrett KE, Barman SM, Boitano S et al., Ganong's Review of Medical Physiology,
23rd edn. Modified from Kandel ER, Schwartz JH, Jessell TM (eds), Principles of Neural Science,
4th edn, McGraw Hill, 2000.

TABLE 5.2
Functional anatomy of the cerebellum and associated motor pathways

Cerebellar anatomy	Function	Associated motor pathways
Vermis and flocculonodular lobe	• Proximal limb and trunk coordination • Vestibulo-ocular reflexes	• Anterior corticospinal tract • Reticulospinal tract • Vestibulospinal tract • Tectospinal tract
Intermediate hemisphere	• Distal limb coordination	• Lateral corticospinal tracts • Rubrospinal tracts
Lateral hemisphere	• Motor planning, distal extremities	• Lateral corticospinal tracts

Adapted from Blumenfeld H, Neuroanatomy Through Clinical Cases, *Sunderland: Sinauer, 2002.*

examination.[28] Lesions of the flocculonodular lobe are characterised by multidirectional truncal instability, disequilibrium and severe impairment of trunk coordination.[28] This pattern is seen in lithium and phenytoin toxicity.

Lateral hemisphere lesion
Hemispheric lesions usually cause ipsilateral abnormalities in coordinated leg movements, and stepping is irregular in timing, length and direction.[28,29] Stepping is typically slow and careful, and instability is accentuated during heel-to-toe walking.[28,29] Associated features include dysmetria, dysdiadochokinesis and intention tremor. This pattern is often seen in cerebellar infarction and mass lesions.

Sign value

Ataxic gait is associated with midline and lateral cerebellar dysfunction. Gait assessment in patients with suspected cerebellar dysfunction is a critical physical examination component. In multiple studies of 444 patients with unilateral cerebellar lesions, ataxic gait was present in 80–93% of patients.[4,30]

5

Atrophy (muscle wasting)

Description

There is decreased muscle mass. Moderate-to-severe unilateral muscle wasting is typically apparent on gross inspection and comparison with the unaffected side. Comparison of axial limb circumference is a reliable method for identifying subtle asymmetrical muscle wasting.[4,18]

Condition/s associated with

Common

- Muscle disuse – fracture, arthritis, prolonged immobility
- Radiculopathy
- Peripheral neuropathy
- Peripheral vascular disease

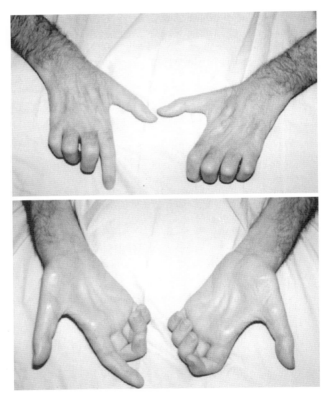

FIGURE 5.12
Muscle wasting in the intrinsic hand muscles in a patient with amyotrophic lateral sclerosis
Reproduced, with permission, from Daroff RB, Bradley WG et al., Neurology in Clinical Practice, 5th edn, Philadelphia: Butterworth-Heinemann, 2008: Fig 78-4.

Less common

- Motor neuron disease
- Poliomyelitis

Mechanism/s

Muscle atrophy is caused by:
- lower motor neuron (LMN) disorders
- disuse atrophy
- myopathy
- peripheral vascular disease.

Lower motor neuron disorders

Muscle denervation results in profound muscle atrophy and is associated with fasciculations. Loss of lower motor neuron input at the neuromuscular junction causes breakdown of actin and myosin, resulting in a decrease in cell size and involution of myofibrils.[31,32] Causes include radiculopathy, compression peripheral neuropathy (e.g. carpal tunnel syndrome) and hereditary peripheral neuropathy (e.g. Marie–Charcot–Tooth disease), and motor neuron disease (e.g. amyotrophic lateral sclerosis).[31,33–36]

Disuse atrophy

Disuse atrophy is caused by decreased muscle utilisation following trauma (e.g. fracture and immobilisation) or in chronic painful conditions (e.g. arthritis). Muscle wasting is present in the distribution of immobilised muscles. Disuse atrophy is a physiological response to decreased muscle use, resulting in a reduction in muscle fibre size and decreased muscle volume.

Myopathy

Myopathies are an uncommon cause of muscle wasting. Myopathies predominantly affect the proximal muscle groups. In advanced muscular dystrophies (e.g. Duchenne's muscular dystrophy), muscle fibres undergo degeneration and are replaced by fibrofatty tissue and collagen.[31] This may also result in pseudohypertrophy or apparent enlargement. Myotonic dystrophy, unlike other myopathies, is associated with wasting of the distal muscle groups and facial muscles.

Peripheral vascular disease

Inadequate tissue perfusion to meet the metabolic demands of peripheral tissues (e.g. muscles) causes muscle fibre atrophy. The most common cause is atherosclerosis. Evidence of trophic changes due to inadequate tissue perfusion often coexist (e.g. poikilothermia, hair loss, skin ulceration).

5

Sign value

Pronounced muscle atrophy is most commonly a lower motor neuron sign. The distribution of muscle atrophy and associated features (e.g. upper motor neuron signs versus lower motor neuron signs) is important when considering aetiologies of muscle wasting (see also 'Weakness' in this chapter). Refer to Tables 5.3 and 5.4.

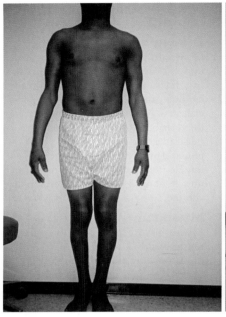
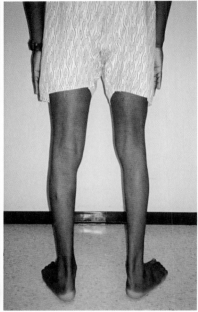

FIGURE 5.13
Left calf atrophy following acute poliomyelitis
Reproduced, with permission, from Bertorini TE, Neuro-muscular Case Studies, 1st edn, Philadelphia: Butterworth-Heinemann, 2007: Fig 76-1.

TABLE 5.3
Clinical utility of thenar atrophy in carpal tunnel syndrome

	Sensitivity	Specificity	Positive LR	Negative LR
Thenar atrophy[33–35]	4–28%	82–99%	NS	NS

Adapted from McGee S, Evidence Based Physical Diagnosis, 2nd edn, St Louis: Saunders, 2007.

TABLE 5.4

Clinical utility of calf wasting in lumbosacral radiculopathy

	Sensitivity	Specificity	Positive LR	Negative LR
Ipsilateral calf wasting[36]	29%	94%	5.2	0.8

Adapted from McGee S, Evidence Based Physical Diagnosis, *2nd edn, St Louis: Saunders, 2007.*

Babinski response

Description

The Babinski response, or upgoing plantar response, is an abnormal cutaneous reflex of the foot associated with upper motor neuron dysfunction.[4] In a positive Babinski response, scratching the lateral plantar surface of the foot causes contraction of the extensor hallucis longus muscle and extension of the great toe.[4] Under normal circumstances the toe goes down.

Relevant neuroanatomy and topographical anatomy

UPPER MOTOR NEURON
- Motor cortex
  ↓
- Corona radiata, subcortical white matter
  ↓
- Posterior limb, internal capsule
  ↓
- Corticospinal tracts, medial brainstem
  ↓
- Ø Pyramidal decussation, medulla
  ↓
- Lateral corticospinal tracts, spinal cord
  ↓
CUTANEOUS REFLEX
  → Inhibitory interneuron
  → Sensory afferent neuron
  → Alpha motor neuron

Condition/s associated with[4]

Common
- Cerebral infarction
- Cerebral haemorrhage
- Spinal cord injury

Less common
- Lacunar infarction, posterior limb internal capsule
- Multiple sclerosis
- Mass lesion – tumour, abscess, AVM

Mechanism/s

Before 1 or 2 years of age, a stimulus applied to the lower extremities, such as pressure or stroking of the plantar aspect of the foot, causes involuntary ankle dorsiflexion and great toe extension.[4] The response is a primitive reflex that disappears later in life.[4] After 1 or 2 years of age, normal development of the central nervous system extinguishes this response.[4,37] In a positive Babinski response, upper motor neuron dysfunction disrupts the normal plantar cutaneous reflex and the primitive response re-emerges.[4] Other upper motor neuron signs may coexist (e.g. spasticity, weakness, hyperreflexia). In the hyperacute period following upper motor neuron dysfunction, the Babinski response (as with spasticity and hyperreflexia) may be absent. It may take hours or days for these signs to emerge.[38,39]

Sign value

The Babinski sign is an upper motor neuron sign. It may be absent initially in the hyperacute period following upper motor neuron dysfunction. Refer to Table 5.5.

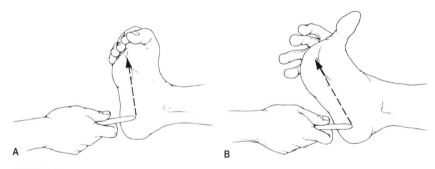

FIGURE 5.14
Babinski test
A Downgoing or negative, normal; **B** upgoing or positive Babinski response, abnormal.

Reproduced, with permission, from Benzon H et al., Raj's Practical Management of Pain, *4th edn, Philadelphia: Mosby, 2008: Fig 10-1.*

TABLE 5.5
Clinical utility of the Babinski test in patients with unilateral cerebral hemisphere lesion[38]

	Sensitivity	Specificity	Positive LR	Negative LR
Babinski response[40]	45%	98%	19.0	0.6

Adapted from McGee S, Evidence Based Physical Diagnosis, *2nd edn, St Louis: Saunders, 2007.*

5

Bradykinesia

Relevant neuroanatomy and topographical anatomy

BASAL GANGLIA
- Globus pallidus interna
- Globus pallidus externa
- Putamen
- Caudate nucleus
- Substantia nigra
- Subthalamic nuclei
- Striatum

Description

Bradykinesia is a slowness or poverty of movement. Hypokinesia is a decreased ability to initiate a movement. Bradykinesia and hypokinesia are associated with disorders of the basal ganglia. Weakness is not typically a prominent feature.[40,41]

Condition/s associated with[42]

Common

- Parkinson's disease
- Dopamine antagonists – haloperidol, metoclopramide

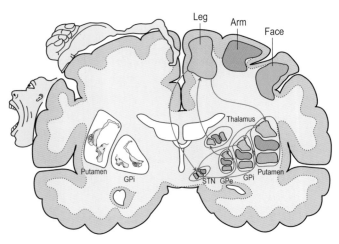

FIGURE 5.15
Basal ganglia motor circuit and somatotopic organisation
GPe = globus pallidus pars externa; GPi = globus pallidus pars interna; STN = subthalamic nucleus.

Reproduced, with permission, from Rodriguez-Oroz MC, Jahanshahi M, Krack P et al., Initial clinical manifestations of Parkinson's disease: features and pathophysiological mechanisms. Lancet Neurol 2009; 8: 1128–1139: Fig 2.

Less common

- Diffuse white matter disease – lacunar infarction(s)
- Multisystem atrophy
- Progressive supranuclear palsy
- Corticobasilar degeneration

Mechanism/s

The exact mechanism of bradykinesia is unknown. The direct and indirect pathways are theoretical models of the functional organisation of the basal ganglia. The direct pathway mediates initiation and maintenance of movement, and the indirect pathway functions to inhibit superfluous movement. In general, degeneration of the substantia nigra or dopamine receptor antagonism causes inhibition of the direct pathway and potentiation of the indirect pathway. This results in net inhibition effects on the cortical pyramidal pathways and

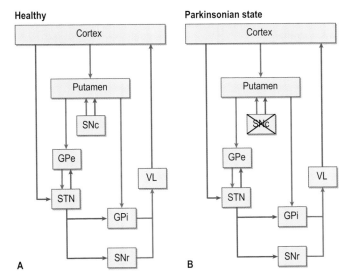

FIGURE 5.16

Classic pathophysiological model in parkinsonism

A Cortical motor areas project glutamatergic axons to the putamen, which sends gamma-aminobutyric acid (GABA)ergic projections to the GPi and the SNr by two pathways: the monosynaptic GABAergic 'direct pathway' (putamen–GPi) and the trisynaptic (putamen–GPe–STN–GPi/SNr) 'indirect pathway'. Dopamine from the SNc facilitates putaminal neurons in the direct pathway and inhibits those in the indirect pathway. Activation of the direct pathway causes reduced neuronal firing in the GPi/SNr and movement facilitation. Activation of the indirect pathway suppresses movements. The STN is also activated by an excitatory projection from the cortex called the 'hyperdirect pathway'. **B** Functional deficiency of dopamine also causes increased activity in the indirect pathway and hyperactivity of the STN. Functional dopamine deficiency also results in decreased activity of the indirect pathway. Together, these result in increased GPi/SNr output inhibition of the VL nucleus of the thalamus and reduced activation of cortical and brainstem motor regions. GPe = globus pallidus pars externa; GPi = globus pallidus pars interna; SNc = substantia nigra pars compacta; SNr = substantia nigra pars reticulata; STN = subthalamic nucleus; VL = ventrolateral nucleus, thalamus.

Reproduced, with permission, from Rodriguez-Oroz MC, Jahanshahi M, Krack P et al., Initial clinical manifestations of Parkinson's disease: features and pathophysiological mechanisms. Lancet Neurol 2009; 8: 1128–1139: Fig 3.

bradykinesia.[40,43,44] Associated signs of parkinsonism include resting tremor, rigidity and postural instability. Causes of bradykinesia include:

- Parkinson's disease and the Parkinson's plus syndromes
- dopamine antagonists.

Parkinson's disease and the Parkinson's plus syndromes

Parkinson's disease and the Parkinson's plus syndromes (multisystem atrophy, progressive supranuclear palsy, corticobasilar degeneration) are neurodegenerative diseases that affect the basal ganglia, as well as other neurological structures. Degeneration of the substantia nigra results in a deficiency of dopaminergic neurons supplying the putamen and causes a relative imbalance between the direct and indirect pathways.[44]

Dopamine antagonists

Central-acting dopamine antagonists block the effect of dopamine in the putamen. Blocking dopaminergic receptors in the putamen causes dysfunction of the direct and indirect pathways.

Sign value

Wenning GK et al. reported a sensitivity of 90% and specificity of 3% of bradykinesia in the diagnosis of Parkinson's disease confirmed on post mortem examination.[45]

Broca's aphasia (expressive aphasia)

Relevant neuroanatomy and topographical anatomy[46]
• Broca's area – posterior inferior frontal gyrus, dominant hemisphere ⇒ Superior division, middle cerebral artery (MCA)

Description

Broca's aphasia, or expressive aphasia, is a disorder of speech fluency (i.e. word production). Comprehension is less affected (compare this with receptive aphasia or Wernicke's aphasia; see 'Wernicke's aphasia' in this chapter). Patients demonstrate speech that is laboured and short, lacks normal intonation, and is grammatically simple and monotonous.[6] Typically, phrase length is decreased and the number of nouns is out of proportion to the use of prepositions and articles.[6,46]

Condition/s associated with

Common

- MCA territory infarction, dominant hemisphere
- Cerebral haemorrhage, dominant hemisphere
- Vascular dementia

Less common

- Alzheimer's disease
- Mass lesion – tumour, abscess, AVM
- Trauma
- Migraine, complicated
- Primary progressive aphasia

Mechanism/s

Broca's aphasia is typically caused by a lesion in the posterior inferior frontal gyrus of the dominant hemisphere.[46,47] This region is supplied by branches of the superior division of the middle cerebral artery (MCA).[46] The most common cause is superior division MCA territory infarction. Patient hand dominance (i.e. being left or right handed) correlates with the side of the dominant cerebral hemisphere, and therefore has potential localising value (see also 'Hand dominance' in this chapter). Larger lesions may affect the motor and sensory cortex resulting in contralateral motor and sensory findings.[47] Associated motor and sensory findings are more commonly associated with Broca's aphasia, due to the proximity of the motor cortex to the vascular distribution of the superior division of the middle cerebral artery (see Table 5.6).[46]

Sign value

Broca's aphasia, or expressive aphasia, is a dominant cortical localising sign. Acute onset aphasia should be considered a sign of stroke until proven otherwise.

5

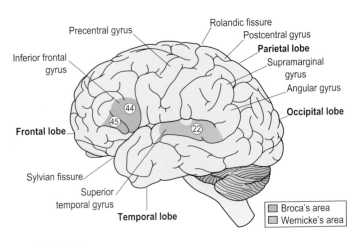

FIGURE 5.17
Broca's area: the posterior inferior frontal gyrus, dominant hemisphere
22 = Brodmann's area 22; 44 = Brodmann's area 44; 45 = Brodmann's area 45.

Reproduced, with permission, from Daroff RB, Bradley WG et al., Neurology in Clinical Practice, 5th edn, Philadelphia: Butterworth-Heinemann, 2008: Fig 12A-1.

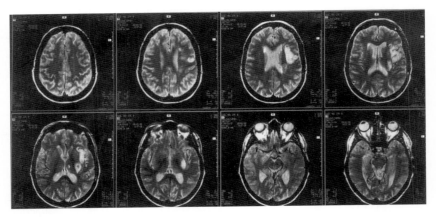

FIGURE 5.18
MRI imaging study in a patient with Broca's aphasia caused by infarction of Broca's area, subcortical white matter and the insula

Reproduced, with permission, from Daroff RB, Bradley WG et al., Neurology in Clinical Practice, 5th edn, Philadelphia: Butterworth-Heinemann, 2008: Fig 12A-3.

TABLE 5.6
Clinical features of Broca's aphasia

Clinical feature	Abnormality in Broca's aphasia
Spontaneous speech	• Nonfluent, mute or telegraphic • Dysarthria usually present
Naming	• Impaired
Comprehension	• Intact (mild difficulty with complex grammatical phrases)
Repetition	• Impaired
Reading	• Often impaired
Writing	• Impaired, dysmorphic, dysgrammatical
Associated signs	• Contralateral motor and sensory findings

Adapted from Kirshner HS, Language and speech disorders: aphasia and aphasiac syndromes. In: Bradley WG, Daroff RB, Fenichel G et al., Neurology in Clinical Practice, *5th edn, Philadelphia: Butterworth-Heinemann, 2008.*

5

Brown-Séquard syndrome

Relevant neuroanatomy and topographical anatomy

Spinal cord
DORSAL COLUMN PATHWAY
- Ø Medial lemniscus, medulla
  - Dorsal columns

SPINOTHALAMIC TRACTS
- Spinothalamic tracts
  - Ø White ventral commissure, spinal cord

MOTOR
- Ø Pyramidal decussation medulla
- Lateral corticospinal tract
- Anterior horn grey matter

Description

Brown-Séquard syndrome is a rare clinical syndrome caused by spinal cord hemisection and is characterised by:[48,49]

- ipsilateral weakness below the lesion
- ipsilateral loss of light touch, vibration, proprioception and sensation below the lesion
- contralateral loss of temperature and pain sensation below the lesion
- a narrow band of ipsilateral complete sensory loss at the level of the lesion.

Condition/s associated with

Common
- Penetrating trauma

Less common
- Multiple sclerosis
- Mass lesion – tumour, abscess, AVM

Mechanism/s

The mechanisms of clinical findings in Brown-Séquard syndrome are listed in Table 5.7 (see also Figure 5.21).

Sign value

Brown-Séquard syndrome is a rare clinical syndrome associated with spinal cord hemisection.

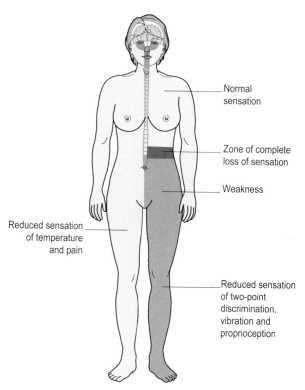

FIGURE 5.19

Distribution of motor and sensory findings in left-sided spinal cord hemisection (i.e. Brown-Séquard syndrome at approximately T8 spinal level)

Reproduced, with permission, from Purves D, Augustine GJ, Fitzpatrick D et al. (eds), Neuroscience, 2nd edn, Sunderland (MA): Sinauer Associates, 2001: Fig 10.4.

5

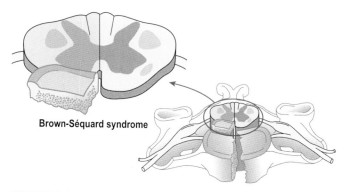

FIGURE 5.20

Schematic diagram of a lesion associated with Brown-Séquard syndrome due to burst fracture

Reproduced, with permission, from Daroff RB, Bradley WG et al., Neurology in Clinical Practice, 5th edn, Philadelphia: Butterworth-Heinemann, 2008: Fig 54C-8.

TABLE 5.7
Neuroanatomical mechanisms of Brown-Séquard syndrome

Clinical signs	Mechanism
• Ipsilateral weakness below the lesion • Upper motor neuron signs	→ Corticospinal tract lesion
• Ipsilateral loss of light touch, vibration, proprioception below the lesion	→ Dorsal column lesion
• Ipsilateral narrow band complete sensory loss at the level of the lesion, and 'sensory level'	→ Spinothalamic tract, dorsal column +/− posterior horn cells and sensory nerve root lesion
• Contralateral loss of pain and temperature sensation below the lesion	→ Spinothalamic tract lesion (*Note*: Lesion is above decussation at each spinal level, thus deficits are contralateral below the lesion)

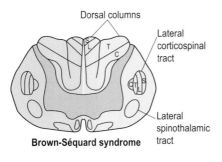

Dorsal columns
Lateral corticospinal tract
Lateral spinothalamic tract
Brown-Séquard syndrome

FIGURE 5.21
Neuroanatomy of the spinal cord long tracts and grey matter in Brown-Séquard syndrome

Reproduced, with permission, from Browner BD, Skeletal Trauma, 4th edn, Philadelphia: Saunders, 2008: Fig 25-7.

Brudzinski sign

Relevant neuroanatomy and topographical anatomy

• Meninges: dura mater
⇒ Spinal nerves

Description

With the patient in the supine position, passive neck flexion results in active hip flexion and knee flexion. Dr Josef Brudzinski first described this clinical sign in children with bacterial meningitis.

Condition/s associated with

• Meningitis, bacterial
• Meningitis, viral
• Meningitis, fungal
• Meningitis, aseptic
• Subarachnoid haemorrhage, aneurysmal

Mechanism/s

Passive neck flexion results in mechanical stress on the spinal nerves and the arachnoid mater, which may be somewhat alleviated by active hip flexion and knee flexion. When the subarachnoid space is inflamed, as with meningitis, mechanical forces on the arachnoid mater result in tenderness and an attempt to alleviate pain (hip flexion, knee flexion).[50]

Sign value

Thomas KE et al. reported a sensitivity of 5%, a positive likelihood ratio of 0.97, and a negative likelihood ratio of 1.0 in the diagnosis of bacterial meningitis.[51] Brudzinski sign has very limited utility to exclude or identify meningitis.

A lumbar puncture should be performed in patients with suspected meningitis.

5

Cavernous sinus syndrome

Relevant neuroanatomy and topographical anatomy[6]

CAVERNOUS SINUS CONTENTS:
- Oculomotor nerve (CNIII)
- Trochlear nerve (CNIV)
- Ophthalmic division (V1) trigeminal nerve (CNV)
- Maxillary division (V2) of trigeminal nerve (CNV)
- Abducens nerve (CNVI)
- Sympathetic plexus
  ⇒ Venous plexus
  ⇒ Carotid artery
  ⇒ Pituitary gland
  ⇒ Sphenoid sinus
  ⇒ Ethmoid sinus

the cavernous sinus: oculomotor nerve (CNIII), trochlear nerve (CNIV), ophthalmic division of the trigeminal nerve (CNV V1), maxillary division of the trigeminal nerve (CNV V2), abducens nerve (CNVI) and sympathetic fibres.[6]

Condition/s associated with[6,52]

Common
- Septic thrombosis
- Aseptic thrombosis

Less common
- Tolosa–Hunt syndrome
- Cavernous carotid artery aneurysm
- Mucormycosis
- Pituitary apoplexy
- Cavernous–carotid sinus fistula

Description

Cavernous sinus syndrome is a clinical syndrome of multiple cranial nerve abnormalities affecting the contents of

Mechanism/s

The cavernous sinus contains neural and vascular structures (see Table 5.8) and is located in close proximity to the

TABLE 5.8
Neuroanatomical mechanism of cavernous sinus syndrome

Clinical signs	Nerve dysfunction
• Extraocular muscle weakness – all muscles except SO, LR • Mydriasis and poorly reactive pupil • Ptosis	→ Oculomotor nerve (CNIII)
• Superior oblique muscle weakness	→ Trochlear nerve (CNIV)
• Hyperaesthesia or anaesthesia in the distribution of the ophthalmic nerve and/or maxillary nerve • Decreased corneal sensation • Decreased corneal reflex	→ Ophthalmic branch trigeminal nerve (CNV V1) → Maxillary branch trigeminal nerve (CNV V2)
• Lateral rectus muscle weakness	→ Abducens nerve (CNVI)
• Horner's syndrome	→ Sympathetic fibres

SO = superior oblique muscle; LR = lateral rectus muscle.

pituitary gland and ethmoid and sphenoid sinuses. Associated findings include unilateral periorbital oedema, photophobia, proptosis, papilloedema, retinal haemorrhages and decreased visual acuity.[52] Causes of cavernous sinus syndrome include:[1,52,53]

- septic thrombosis
- aseptic thrombosis
- cavernous internal carotid artery aneurysm
- pituitary apoplexy
- disorders of the sphenoid and ethmoid sinuses.

Septic thrombosis

The most common sources of septic thrombosis are infective foci of the sphenoid or ethmoid sinuses.[52] Other sources include dental infection, central facial cellulitis and otitis media.[52] Infectious organisms enter the cavernous sinus through venous and lymphatic vessels from the surrounding ocular and facial structures or via direct spread from adjacent tissues.

Aseptic thrombosis

Aseptic thrombosis is less common than septic thrombosis and is associated with hypercoagulable states (e.g. polycythaemia, sickle cell disease, trauma, pregnancy, oral contraceptive use).[52]

Cavernous internal carotid artery aneurysm

Expansion of a cavernous internal carotid artery aneurysm can result in injury due to mass effect. The abducens nerve (CNVI) is typically affected first, due to its close proximity to the cavernous segment of the internal carotid artery.[1]

Pituitary apoplexy

Pituitary apoplexy is acute haemorrhage into a pre-existing pituitary macroadenoma, which causes local mass effect and injury to the surrounding tissues. Pituitary apoplexy is also associated with bitemporal hemianopia due to compression of the optic chiasm. Risk factors include hypotension, stimulation of gland growth (e.g. pregnancy), anticoagulation and hyperaemia.[52]

Disorders of the sphenoid and ethmoid sinuses

Acute and chronic erosive inflammatory conditions of the sphenoid and ethmoid sinuses may lead to contiguous spread of an infectious or inflammatory process to the adjacent cavernous sinus (refer to Figure 5.22).

5

Optic chiasm and cavernous sinuses (coronal section)

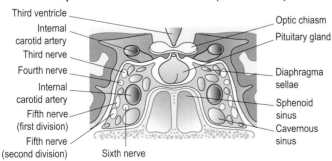

FIGURE 5.22
Contents of the cavernous sinus

Reproduced, with permission, from Yanoff M, Duker JS, Ophthalmology, 3rd edn, St Louis: Mosby, 2008: Fig 9-11-3.

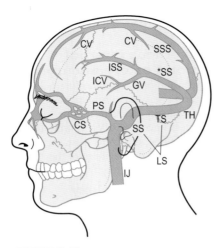

Causes include bacterial sinusitis, mucormycosis, Tolosa–Hunt syndrome and tumours.[52,53]

Sign value

Cavernous sinus syndrome is a medical emergency with high morbidity and mortality. Mucormycosis is a surgical emergency requiring debridement of infected devitalised tissues and intravenous antifungal therapy.

FIGURE 5.23
Venous drainage of the intracranial structures
CS = cavernous sinus; CV = cortical veins; GV = great vein of Galen; ICV = internal cerebral vein; IJ = internal jugular vein; ISS = inferior sagittal sinus; LS = lateral sinus; PS = petrosal sinus; SS = sigmoid sinus; *SS = straight sinus; SSS = superior sagittal sinus; TH = torcular Herophili; TS = transverse sinus.

Reproduced, with permission, from Goldman L, Ausiello D, Cecil Medicine, 23rd edn, Philadelphia: Saunders, 2007: Fig 430-6.

Clasp-knife phenomenon

Description

Clasp-knife phenomenon is characterised by brisk relaxation of hypertonic muscle groups during tone assessment.[54] The name arises from the similarity of the phenomenon to opening and closing the blade of a pocket knife due to the action of the spring.[4]

Relevant neuroanatomy and topographical anatomy

UPPER MOTOR NEURON
- Motor cortex
  ↓
- Corona radiata, subcortical white matter
  ↓
- Posterior limb, internal capsule
  ↓
- Corticospinal tracts, medial brainstem
  ↓
- Ø Pyramidal decussation, medulla
  ↓
- Corticospinal tracts, spinal cord
- ⇒ Central canal, spinal cord
  ↓
MONOSYNAPTIC STRETCH REFLEX
- → Inhibitory interneuron
- → Sensory afferent neuron
- → Alpha motor neuron

Condition/s associated with

Common
- Cerebral infarction
- Cerebral haemorrhage
- Cerebral palsy

Less common
- Multiple sclerosis
- Myelopathy
- Mass lesion – tumour, abscess, AVM

Mechanism/s

The mechanism of clasp-knife phenomenon is unknown. It is associated with upper motor neuron dysfunction and spasticity. It is thought to arise due to inappropriate activity of muscle spindles and extrafusal muscle fibres due to loss of inhibitory supraspinal pathways.[55]

Sign value

Clasp-knife phenomenon is an upper motor neuron sign and is present in approximately 50% of patients with spasticity.[56,57]

5

Clonus

Description
Clonus is a rhythmic, sustained muscular contraction initiated with a brisk stretching force in a muscle group.[4] Clonus is most commonly elicited in the ankle by abrupt passive dorsiflexion. It can also be assessed in other locations, such as the quadriceps, finger flexors, jaw and other muscle groups.[4]

Relevant neuroanatomy and topographical anatomy

UPPER MOTOR NEURON
- Motor cortex
  ↓
- Corona radiata, subcortical white matter
  ↓
- Posterior limb, internal capsule
  ↓
- Corticospinal tracts, medial brainstem
  ↓
- Ø Pyramidal decussation, medulla
  ↓
- Corticospinal tracts, spinal cord
  ⇒ Central canal, spinal cord
  ↓

MONOSYNAPTIC STRETCH REFLEX
  → Inhibitory interneuron
  → Sensory afferent neuron
  → Alpha motor neuron

Condition/s associated with

Common
- Cerebral infarction
- Cerebral haemorrhage
- Lacunar infarction, posterior limb internal capsule
- Multiple sclerosis
- Spinal cord injury

Less common
- Mass lesion – tumour, abscess, AVM
- Serotonin syndrome

Mechanism/s
Clonus is an upper motor neuron sign. Essentially it is a result of pronounced hyperreflexia. Clonus is caused by a self-sustaining, oscillating, monosynaptic stretch reflex.[58] Causes of clonus include:
- upper motor neuron lesion
- serotonin syndrome.

Upper motor neuron lesion
See 'Hyperreflexia' in this chapter.

Serotonin syndrome
Serotonin syndrome is characterised by altered mental status, autonomic dysfunction, fever and neuromuscular excitability.[59] The mechanism of clonus in serotonin syndrome is not known. Clonus likely results from an excessive agonism of 5-HT receptors in the peripheral nervous system, resulting in sensitisation of monosynaptic stretch reflexes.[60]

Sign value

Clonus is most commonly a sign of longstanding upper motor neuron dysfunction. In the setting of altered mental status, fever, hypertension, tachycardia and tremor, serotonin syndrome should be considered.

5

Cogwheel rigidity

<table>
<tr><td>

Relevant neuroanatomy and topographical anatomy

BASAL GANGLIA
- Globus pallidus pars interna
- Globus pallidus pars externa
- Putamen
- Caudate nucleus
- Substantia nigra
- Subthalamic nuclei
- Striatum

</td></tr>
</table>

Description

Cogwheel rigidity is resistance during passive range of movement, which intermittently gives way like a lever pulling over a ratchet.[61] It is a sign of extrapyramidal dysfunction.

Rigidity has three characteristics:[4,61]

1 Resistance is velocity-independent (i.e. the degree of resistance to passive movement is constant with slow or fast movement).

2 Flexor and extensor tone are equal.

3 There is no associated weakness.
See also 'Rigidity' in this chapter.

Condition/s associated with

Common
- Parkinson's disease
- Dopamine antagonists – haloperidol, metoclopramide

Less common
- Multisystem atrophy
- Progressive supranuclear palsy
- Corticobasal degeneration
- Diffuse white matter disease – lacunar infarction(s)

Mechanism/s

Cogwheel rigidity is associated with extrapyramidal disorders.[6,61] The mechanism of cogwheel rigidity is poorly understood. Cogwheel rigidity has been attributed to the combined effects of rigidity and tremor (see also 'Bradykinesia' and 'Parkinsonian tremor' in this chapter).[6,61] Rigidity likely results from changes in extrapyramidal regulation of supraspinal motor neurons and changes in spinal cord motor neuron activity in response to peripheral stimulation in stretch reflexes (see also 'Rigidity' in this chapter).[44]

Sign value

Cogwheel rigidity is a sign of extrapyramidal dysfunction. It is most commonly associated with Parkinson's disease.

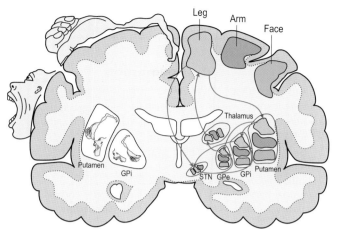

FIGURE 5.24
Basal ganglia motor circuit and somatotopic organisation
GPe = globus pallidus pars externa; GPi = globus pallidus pars interna; STN = subthalamic nucleus.

Reproduced, with permission, from Rodriguez-Oroz MC, Jahanshahi M, Krack P et al., Initial clinical manifestations of Parkinson's disease: features and pathophysiological mechanisms. Lancet Neurol 2009; 8: 1128–1139: Fig 2.

5

Corneal reflex

Description

When the cornea is stimulated with a wisp of cotton, there is a reflexive blinking response in both eyes (a normal response). An abnormal corneal reflex is either an:

- afferent defect – absence of bilateral blinking, due to ophthalmic division of the trigeminal nerve (CNV V1) dysfunction

  or

- efferent defect – absence of unilateral blinking, due to facial nerve (CNVII) palsy.

In the clinical test, a wisp of cotton is applied from the side to prevent a 'blink to threat' response, which is mediated by visual cues (CNII) and thus may confound the examination.

Condition/s associated with

Common

- Bell's palsy (idiopathic facial nerve palsy)
- Facial nerve palsy

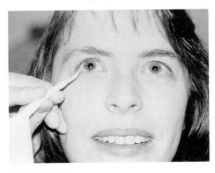

FIGURE 5.25
Corneal reflex

Reproduced, with permission, from University of California, San Diego, A Practical Guide to Clinical Medicine. Available: http://meded.ucsd. edu/clinicalmed/neuro2.htm [8 Dec 2010].

Less common

- Brain death
- Cerebellopontine angle tumour – acoustic schwannoma, glomus tumour
- Cavernous sinus syndrome

Mechanism/s

The afferent limb of the corneal reflex is supplied by the ophthalmic division of the trigeminal nerve (CNV V1). The efferent motor limb is supplied by the facial nerve (CNVII), which innervates the orbicularis oculi muscles. Absence of the corneal reflex may be due to a defect in the afferent or efferent pathway. Lesions of the afferent pathway result in a bilateral absence of the blinking response when the abnormal eye is tested with cotton wool. Lesions of the efferent limb will cause an absent blinking response on the affected side, with preservation of the blinking response on the contralateral side. Causes of an absent corneal reflex include:

- facial nerve palsy
- disorders of the ophthalmic division of the trigeminal nerve (CNV V1)
- disorders of the cornea.

Facial nerve palsy

See 'Facial muscle weakness' in this chapter.

Disorders of the ophthalmic division of the trigeminal nerve (CNV V1)

Disorders of the ophthalmic division of the trigeminal nerve include orbital apex syndrome, cavernous sinus syndrome, superior orbital fissure stenosis and mass lesions (e.g. tumour,

Relevant neuroanatomy and topographical anatomy[1]

AFFERENT LIMB
⊗ Light touch receptor, cornea
↓
• Long ciliary nerves
↓
• Ophthalmic division (VI) trigeminal nerve (CNV)
⇒ Orbital apex
⇒ Cavernous sinus
⇒ Superior orbital fissure
↓
• Trigeminal (gasserian) ganglion
⇒ Meckel's cave, petrous bone
↓
• Trigeminal sensory nucleus, pons
↓
↔ Bilateral innervation efferent structures
↓
EFFERENT LIMB
• Facial nuclei

↓
• Facial nerve
⇒ Cerebellopontine angle
⇒ Internal acoustic meatus
⇒ Mastoid sinus
⇒ Geniculate ganglion
⇒ Stylomastoid foramen
↓
× Orbicularis oculi muscles

abscess) affecting the nerve segment spanning the subarachnoid space. See also 'Orbital apex syndrome' and 'Cavernous sinus syndrome' in this chapter.

Disorders of the cornea

Disorders of the cornea causing dysfunction of the neurosensory elements of the long ciliary nerves may result in an afferent defect in the corneal reflex. Causes include trauma, contact lens desensitisation, globe rupture and topical analgesia.

Sign value

Corneal reflex testing may be useful in unilateral sensorineural hearing loss and unilateral facial weakness, and in the assessment of brainstem function. The corneal reflex has been reported to be absent in 8% of normal elderly patients in one study.[4,62] In a single study, the sensitivity of an efferent abnormality of the corneal reflex in the detection of acoustic neuroma (i.e. acoustic schwannoma) was 33%.[4,63]

5

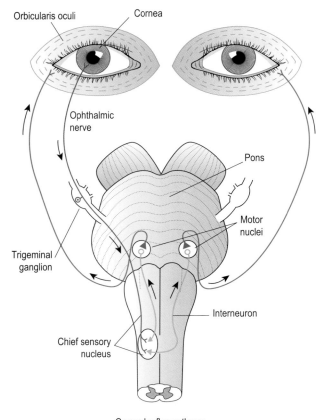

Corneal reflex pathway

FIGURE 5.26

Corneal reflex pathway

Normally, lightly touching the cornea results in bilateral blinking. The afferent limb is the ophthalmic division of the trigeminal nerve (CNV V1). The efferent limb is the facial nerve (CNVII), which innervates the orbicularis oculi muscles.

Reproduced, with permission, from O'Rahilly R, Muller F, Carpenter F, Basic Human Anatomy: A Study of Human Structure, *Philadelphia: Saunders, 1983: Fig 46-8.*

Crossed-adductor reflex

Relevant neuroanatomy and topographical anatomy

UPPER MOTOR NEURON
- Motor cortex

    ↓
- Corona radiata, subcortical white matter

    ↓
- Posterior limb, internal capsule

    ↓
- Corticospinal tracts, medial brainstem

    ↓
- Ø Pyramidal decussation, medulla

    ↓
- Corticospinal tracts, spinal cord
- ⇒ Central canal, spinal cord

    ↓

MONOSYNAPTIC STRETCH REFLEX
- → Inhibitory interneuron

    ↓
- → Sensory afferent neuron
- → Alpha motor neuron

Description

Adductor muscle contraction of the leg occurs following percussion of the contralateral medial femoral condyle, patella or patella tendon.[4,64] It is a sign of hyperreflexia.

Condition/s associated with

Common

- Cerebral infarction
- Cerebral haemorrhage

Less common

- Lacunar infarction, posterior limb internal capsule
- Multiple sclerosis
- Spinal cord injury
- Mass lesion – tumour, abscess, AVM

Mechanism/s

The force of the reflex hammer is conducted through bone and soft tissues to distant hyperreflexic muscles, eliciting a stretch–reflex–mediated contraction of the adductor muscles on the opposite side (see 'Hyperreflexia' in this chapter).[4]

Sign value

The cross-adductor reflex, like other radiating reflexes, is a sign of hyperreflexia in upper motor neuron disorders.

5

Dysarthria

TABLE 5.9
Characteristics of dysarthria subtypes

Dysarthria subtype	Characteristics
Flaccid dysarthria	• Speech may sound nasal or slurred[65,66]
Spastic dysarthria	• Speech may sound as if patient is squeezing out words from a pursed mouth[65,66]
Ataxic dysarthria	• Speech is uncoordinated; range, timing and direction may be inaccurate; rate is slow; may be explosive in quality[65,66]
Hypokinetic dysarthria	• Speech may sound monotonous or slow-paced; rate may vary; rigidity may be present[65,66]
Hyperkinetic dysarthria	• Involuntary disruptions in sounds and/or movements[65,66]

Description

Dysarthria is a disorder of speech articulation. Comprehension and speech content are not affected. There are several types of dysarthria that vary in the rate, volume, rhythm and sound of the patient's speech (see Table 5.9).[65–67]

Condition/s associated with

Common

- Intoxication (e.g. alcohol, benzodiazepine)
- Drug toxicity (e.g. lithium, phenytoin)

Relevant neuroanatomy and topographical anatomy

- Cerebellum
- Upper motor neuron
- Lower motor neuron

Less common

- Cerebellar infarction
- Vertebral artery dissection
- Cerebellar mass lesion – tumour, abscess, AVM
- Multiple sclerosis
- HSV cerebellitis
- Hereditary cerebellar degeneration (Freidreich's ataxia)
- Paraneoplastic cerebellar degeneration

Mechanism/s

Dysarthria is caused by disorders of the:

- cerebellum
- upper motor neuron
- lower motor neuron
- oral cavity and oropharynx.

Disorders of the cerebellum

Cerebellar dysfunction disrupts coordination of the muscles of articulation resulting in slurred speech, explosive speech or speech that is broken up into syllables with noticeable pauses (i.e. staccato speech or scanning speech).[67] Common causes include alcohol intoxication, cerebellar infarction and phenytoin toxicity.

Disorders of the upper motor neuron

Dysarthria may occur following MCA distribution cerebral infarction or in diffuse bilateral upper motor neuron disorders (e.g. vascular dementia, MS). Spasticity of the muscles of speech articulation disrupts the normal mechanical properties of the oropharyngeal structures during speech.

Disorders of the lower motor neuron

Dysfunction of the facial nerve may result in hypotonia and weakness of the muscles of speech articulation.

Disorders of the oral cavity and oropharynx

Local disorders of the oral cavity and oropharynx disrupt the transmission of sound waves through the oral cavity, resulting in 'slurred' speech. The rate and rhythm of speech are typically not affected. Common causes include trauma and neck neoplasia and iatrogenic causes (e.g. local anaesthesia).

Sign value

Dysarthria is typically a sign of cerebellar dysfunction, but may be present in a variety of other conditions. In a group of 444 patients with unilateral cerebellar lesions, dysarthria was found in approximately 10–25% of cases.[4,29,30]

5

Dysdiadochokinesis

Relevant neuroanatomy and topographical anatomy

CEREBELLUM
- Intermediate cerebellar hemisphere
  - → Lateral corticospinal tract
  - → Rubrospinal tract
- Lateral cerebellar hemisphere
  - → Lateral corticospinal tract

BASAL GANGLIA
- Globus pallidus interna
- Globus pallidus externa
- Putamen
- Substantia nigra
- Striatum

Description

Dysdiadochokinesis is difficulty in performing rapid alternating movements. The patient's movements may be slow and/or clumsy.

Condition/s associated with

Common

- Alcohol intoxication
- Drug toxicity – lithium, phenytoin, benzodiazepine

Less common

- Cerebellar infarction
- Vertebral artery dissection
- Cerebellar mass lesion – tumour, abscess, AVM
- Multiple sclerosis
- HSV cerebellitis
- Hereditary cerebellar degeneration (Freidreich's ataxia)
- Paraneoplastic cerebellar degeneration

Mechanism/s

Dysdiadochokinesis is a cerebellar sign. The intermediate and lateral hemispheres of the cerebellum mediate coordinated movements of the distal extremities (see Table 5.10). Lesions of the intermediate and lateral cerebellar hemispheres cause slow, uncoordinated and clumsy movements of the ipsilateral distal extremities during attempted rapid alternating movements.[4,6,29,68] Intermediate and lateral hemisphere dysfunction results in delays of motor initiation and movement termination at the end of movement (i.e. dysmetria). This, combined with abnormalities of movement force and acceleration, contribute to dysdiadochokinesis.[68]

Sign value

In a group of 444 patients with unilateral cerebellar lesions, dysdiadochokinesis was present in 47–69% of patients.[4,29,30]

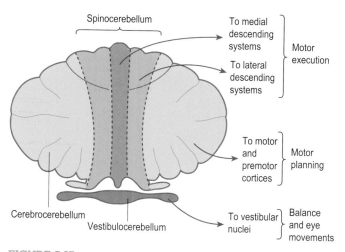

FIGURE 5.27
Functional anatomy of the cerebellum

From Barrett KE, Barman SM, Boitano S et al., Ganong's Review of Medical Physiology, *23rd edn. Modified from Kandel ER, Schwartz JH, Jessell TM (eds),* Principles of Neural Science, *4th edn, McGraw Hill, 2000.*

TABLE 5.10
Functional anatomy of the cerebellum and associated motor pathways

Cerebellar anatomy	Function	Associated motor pathways
Intermediate hemisphere	• Distal limb coordination	• Lateral corticospinal tracts • Rubrospinal tracts
Lateral hemisphere	• Motor planning, distal extremities	• Lateral corticospinal tracts

Adapted from Blumenfeld H, Neuroanatomy Through Clinical Cases, *Sunderland: Sinauer, 2002.*

Dysmetria

Relevant neuroanatomy and topographical anatomy

- Intermediate cerebellar hemisphere
  - → Lateral corticospinal tract
  - → Rubrospinal tract
- Lateral cerebellar hemisphere
  - → Lateral corticospinal tract

Description

Dysmetria is a disturbance of the rate, range and force of movement of the extended limb as it approaches a target.[4,6,69] Dysmetria is elicited during the finger-to-nose and heel-to-shin tests.[6]

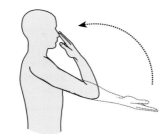

A   Finger-to-nose test

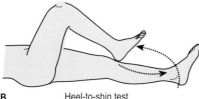

B   Heel-to-shin test

FIGURE 5.28
A Finger-to-nose test; **B** heel-to-shin test
Reproduced, with permission, from LeBlond RF, DeGowin RL, Brown DD, DeGowin's Diagnostic Examination, *10th edn: Fig 14.13. Available: http://www.accessmedicine. com [8 Dec 2010].*

Condition/s associated with

Common

- Alcohol intoxication
- Drug toxicity – lithium, phenytoin, benzodiazepine

Less common

- Cerebellar infarction
- Vertebral artery dissection
- Cerebellar mass lesion – tumour, abscess, AVM
- Multiple sclerosis
- HSV cerebellitis
- Hereditary cerebellar degeneration (Freidreich's ataxia)
- Paraneoplastic cerebellar degeneration

Mechanism/s

Dysmetria is a cerebellar sign. The intermediate and lateral hemispheres of the cerebellum facilitate coordinated movement of the distal extremities (see Table 5.11). Lesions of the intermediate and lateral cerebellar hemispheres may cause slow, uncoordinated and clumsy movements of the ipsilateral distal extremity during attempted target localisation tasks.[4] Delays in motor

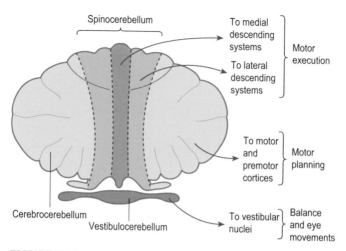

FIGURE 5.29
Functional anatomy of the cerebellum

From Barrett KE, Barman SM, Boitano S et al., Ganong's Review of Medical Physiology, *23rd edn. Modified from Kandel ER, Schwartz JH, Jessell TM (eds),* Principles of Neural Science, *4th edn, McGraw Hill, 2000.*

TABLE 5.11
Functional anatomy of the cerebellum and associated motor pathways

5

Cerebellar anatomy	Function	Associated motor pathways
Intermediate hemisphere	• Distal limb coordination	• Lateral corticospinal tracts • Rubrospinal tracts
Lateral hemisphere	• Motor planning, distal extremities	• Lateral corticospinal tracts

Adapted from Blumenfeld H, Neuroanatomy Through Clinical Cases, *Sunderland: Sinauer, 2002.*

initiation and movement termination, and abnormalities of movement force and acceleration, contribute to dysmetria.[68]

Sign value

In a group of 444 patients with unilateral cerebellar lesions, dysmetria was present in 71–86% of patients.[4,29,30]

Dysphonia

Description

Dysphonia is a disorder of phonation (sound production) due to dysfunction of the larynx and/or vocal cords.[70] The patient's voice may sound hoarse, weak, excessively breathy, harsh or rough.[70]

Condition/s associated with[6,70,71]

Common

- Viral laryngitis
- Vocal cord polyp
- Iatrogenic – prolonged endotracheal intubation

Less common

- Tumour – squamous cell carcinoma
- Recurrent laryngeal nerve palsy – iatrogenic, Pancoast's tumour, penetrating neck trauma, thoracic aortic aneurysm

- Laryngospasm
- Lateral medullary syndrome (Wallenberg's syndrome)
- Angioedema

Mechanism/s

Dysphonia is due to an abnormality within the larynx, vocal cords or the nerves that innervate these structures, which results in disruption of sound production due to changes in the mechanical function of the larynx and vocal cords.

Causes of dysphonia include:

- local disorders of the vocal cords and larynx
- disorders of the glossopharyngeal nerve, vagus nerve and recurrent laryngeal nerve
- brainstem lesion.

Local disorders of the vocal cords and larynx

Mechanical disruption of vocal cord opposition, vibration or movement causes a change in sound generation. Causes include viral laryngitis, vocal cord polyp, neoplasia (e.g. squamous cell carcinoma), trauma, angioedema and iatrogenic (e.g. prolonged endotracheal intubation).

Disorders of glossopharyngeal nerve, vagus nerve and recurrent laryngeal nerve

The recurrent laryngeal nerve follows a long intrathoracic course and is vulnerable to compression or injury at several sites (e.g. Pancoast's tumour, penetrating neck trauma, thoracic aortic aneurysm, left atrial dilatation, iatrogenic injury in thyroidectomy).[6] Disorders of the glossopharyngeal nerve and vagus nerve may result in

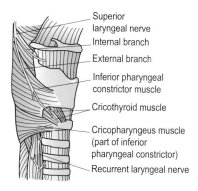

- Superior laryngeal nerve
- Internal branch
- External branch
- Inferior pharyngeal constrictor muscle
- Cricothyroid muscle
- Cricopharyngeus muscle (part of inferior pharyngeal constrictor)
- Recurrent laryngeal nerve

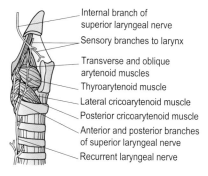

- Internal branch of superior laryngeal nerve
- Sensory branches to larynx
- Transverse and oblique arytenoid muscles
- Thyroarytenoid muscle
- Lateral cricoarytenoid muscle
- Posterior cricoarytenoid muscle
- Anterior and posterior branches of superior laryngeal nerve
- Recurrent laryngeal nerve

FIGURE 5.30
Anatomy and innervation of the laryngeal muscles and vocal cords

Reproduced, with permission, from Townsend CM, Beauchamp RD, Evers BM, Mattox K, Sabiston Textbook of Surgery, 18th edn, Philadelphia: Saunders, 2008: Fig 41-13.

hoarseness due to a lesion involving cranial nerve nuclei or nerve fascicles (e.g. lateral medullary syndrome) or a lesion of the cranial nerve at the brainstem exit point (e.g. glomus tumour). See also 'Hoarseness' in this chapter.

Disorders of the brainstem

See 'Wallenberg's syndrome' in this chapter.

Sign value

Dysphonia can be an important sign of recurrent laryngeal nerve, vagus nerve (CNX) or nucleus ambiguus dysfunction, but is most commonly associated with viral laryngitis.

Dysphonia should be interpreted in the context of the overall clinical findings. Isolated dysphonia that lasts longer than 2 weeks is unlikely to be caused by viral laryngitis and should prompt further evaluation.[71]

5

Essential tremor

Relevant neuroanatomy and topographical anatomy

CEREBELLUM
- Vermis and flocculonodular lobe
  - → Anterior corticospinal tract
  - → Reticulospinal tract
  - → Vestibulospinal tract
  - → Tectospinal tract
- Paravermal (intermediate) hemisphere
  - → Lateral corticospinal tract
  - → Rubrospinal tract
- Lateral hemisphere
  - → Lateral corticospinal tract

Description

Essential tremor is a 4–12 Hz symmetric tremor of the upper limbs, with postural (seen in the outstretched arm) and/or kinetic (during movement) components.[4,41] It may also affect the jaw, tongue, and head and neck muscles, leading to a characteristic 'nodding yes' or 'shaking no' tremor.[4]

Condition/s associated with[4,41]

Common

- Familial essential tremor

Less common

- Sporadic essential tremor

Mechanism/s

The mechanism of essential tremor is not known. Essential tremor may originate from dysfunction of the cerebellum.[41] Approximately two-thirds of patients have a positive family history of tremor, and first-degree relatives of patients with essential tremor are 5 to 10 times more likely to develop the disease.[41] Several genetic loci have been identified in hereditary essential tremor.[41]

Sign value

Essential tremor has a relatively benign natural history and should be differentiated from other forms of tremor.

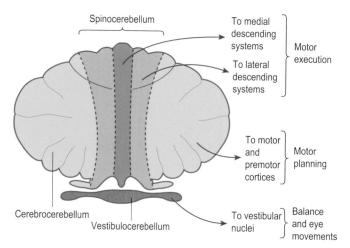

FIGURE 5.31
Functional anatomy of the cerebellum

From Barrett KE, Barman SM, Boitano S et al., Ganong's Review of Medical Physiology, *23rd edn. Modified from Kandel ER, Schwartz JH, Jessell TM (eds),* Principles of Neural Science, *4th edn, McGraw Hill, 2000.*

5

Facial muscle weakness (unilateral)

Description

The facial muscles appear asymmetrical due to unilateral weakness. There are two distinct patterns of facial weakness: upper motor neuron and lower motor neuron.

Condition/s associated with

Upper motor neuron

Common

- Cerebral infarction, MCA territory
- Cerebral haemorrhage

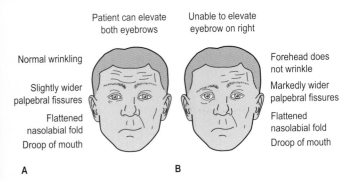

Patient can elevate both eyebrows

Unable to elevate eyebrow on right

Normal wrinkling

Slightly wider palpebral fissures

Flattened nasolabial fold

Droop of mouth

Forehead does not wrinkle

Markedly wider palpebral fissures

Flattened nasolabial fold

Droop of mouth

A

B

FIGURE 5.32
Typical appearance of: **A** upper motor neuron (central) facial weakness; **B** lower motor neuron (peripheral) facial weakness

Reproduced, with permission, from Stern TA et al., Massachusetts General Hospital Comprehensive Clinical Psychiatry, *1st edn, Elsevier Health Sciences, 2008: Fig 72-7.*

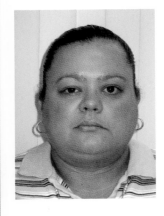

FIGURE 5.33
Left facial nerve (peripheral) palsy

Reproduced, with permission, from Daroff RB, Bradley WG et al., Neurology in Clinical Practice, *5th edn, Philadelphia: Butterworth-Heinemann, 2008: Fig 74–9.*

CLINICAL PEARL

<table>
<tr><td>

Relevant neuroanatomy and topographical anatomy[6]

UPPER MOTOR NEURON
• Motor cortex
↓
• Corona radiata, subcortical white matter
↓
• Posterior limb, internal capsule
↓
• Pyramidal tracts, brainstem
↓
∅ Decussation
↓
↔ Bilateral supranuclear innervation (upper facial muscles)
↓
LOWER MOTOR NEURON
• Facial nerve nuclei pons
↓
• Facial nerve fascicle
⇒ Abducens nuclei
↓
• Facial nerve
⇒ Cerebellopontine angle
⇒ Internal acoustic meatus
↓
• Geniculate ganglion
↓
× Lacrimal gland
⇒ Mastoid sinus
× Stapes
× Tongue
× Submandibular glands
⇒ Stylomastoid foramen
× Facial muscles

</td></tr>
</table>

Less common
• Lacunar infarction, posterior limb internal capsule
• Mass lesion – tumour, abscess, AVM

Lower motor neuron (facial nerve palsy)[1,6,72,73]

Common
• Bell's palsy (idiopathic facial nerve palsy) – 65%[73]
• Trauma – 25%[73]

Less common
• Tumour – acoustic schwannoma, cholesteatoma – 5%[73]
• Diabetic mononeuropathy/ microvascular infarction
• Ramsay Hunt syndrome
• HIV infection
• Lyme disease
• Sarcoidosis

Mechanism/s
Unilateral facial weakness is caused by:
• upper motor neuron weakness
• lower motor neuron weakness (facial nerve palsy).

Upper motor neuron weakness
Upper motor neuron facial weakness is characterised by weakness, limited to the lower contralateral facial muscles (i.e. sparing the forehead), due to bilateral supranuclear innervation and bilateral upper facial cortical representation in the motor cortex (see Figure 5.35A).[74] Upper motor neuron facial weakness may be associated with arm and/or leg weakness, and dominant or non-dominant cortical localising signs.

5

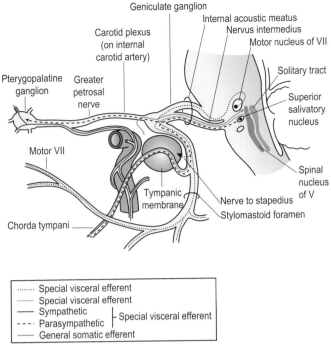

Geniculate ganglion

Internal acoustic meatus
Nervus intermedius
Motor nucleus of VII

Carotid plexus
(on internal
carotid artery)

Solitary tract

Pterygopalatine   Greater
ganglion   petrosal
nerve

Superior
salivatory
nucleus

Motor VII

Spinal
nucleus
of V

Tympanic
membrane

Nerve to stapedius

Chorda tympani

Stylomastoid foramen

⋯⋯ Special visceral efferent	
―――― Special visceral efferent	
―― Special visceral efferent	
―― Sympathetic	⎱ Special visceral efferent
- - - Parasympathetic	⎰
―― General somatic efferent	

FIGURE 5.34
Functional anatomy of the facial nerve

Reproduced, with permission, from Dyck PJ, Thomas PK, Peripheral Neuropathy, *4th edn,
Philadelphia: Saunders, 2005: Fig 50-4.*

Lower motor neuron weakness (facial nerve palsy)

Lower motor neuron facial weakness is characterised by ipsilateral upper and lower facial muscle weakness.[6,72] The facial nerve is the final common pathway of facial muscle innervation. Lesions of the peripheral nerve result in complete unilateral facial muscle weakness (see Figure 5.35B). Associated features include hyperacusis, abnormal taste sensation in the anterior two-thirds of the tongue, efferent abnormality of the corneal reflex and a dry irritated eye. See Table 5.12 for mechanisms of clinical findings in facial nerve palsy.[75,76]

Sign value

Unilateral facial muscle weakness should be evaluated rapidly to determine whether an upper motor neuron pattern (e.g. acute stroke) or lower motor neuron pattern is present.

The epidemiology of lower motor neuron facial weakness is listed in Table 5.13.

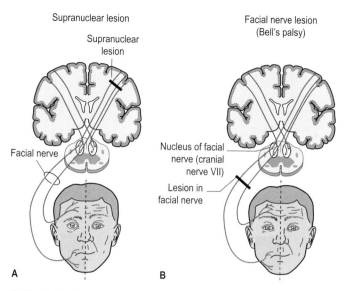

FIGURE 5.35

Schematic representation of innervation of the facial muscles

A Upper motor neuron (central) weakness results in limited lower facial muscle weakness with sparing of the upper facial muscles. **B** Lower motor neuron (peripheral) weakness results in complete unilateral facial muscle weakness.

Reproduced, with permission, from Timestra JD, Khatkhate N, Am Fam Phys *2007; 76(7): 997–1002.*

5

TABLE 5.12

Mechanisms of clinical findings in facial nerve palsy

Clinical finding	Mechanism
Complete facial muscle weakness	→ Facial nerve innervates ipsilateral upper and lower facial muscles
Hyperacusis	→ Ipsilateral stapedius muscle weakness
Dysgeusia, anterior two-thirds of tongue	→ Facial nerve supplies ipsilateral anterior two-thirds of tongue
Dry irritated eye	→ Orbicularis oculi muscle weakness results in incomplete eye closure → Lacrimal gland dysfunction
Abnormal corneal reflex (efferent)	→ Facial nerve forms efferent limb of the corneal reflex
Abnormal sensation, oropharynx or external auditory meatus	→ Facial nerve branches innervate ipsilateral oropharynx and external auditory meatus
Vesicular eruption, oropharynx or external auditory meatus	→ Ramsey Hunt syndrome, or reactivation herpes zoster infection of geniculate ganglion, results in vesicular eruption in distribution of cutaneous nerve branches

TABLE 5.13

Causes of facial nerve (CNVII) palsy[75,76]

Cause	Prevalence
Bell's palsy (idiopathic facial nerve palsy)	50–87%
Surgical or accidental trauma	5–22%
Ramsay Hunt syndrome	7–13%
Tumours (e.g. cholesteatoma or parotid tumours)	1–6%
Miscellaneous	8–11%

Fasciculations

<table>
<tr><td>

Relevant neuroanatomy and topographical anatomy

LOWER MOTOR NEURON
- Anterior horn, spinal cord
  ↓
- Nerve root
  ⇒ Intervertebral disc
  ⇒ Intervertebral foramen
  ↓
- Nerve plexus (e.g. brachial plexus)
  ↓
- Peripheral nerve
  ⇒ Potential sites of nerve entrapment (e.g. carpal tunnel)
  ↓
→ Neuromuscular junction
  ↓
× Motor unit, skeletal muscle

</td></tr>
</table>

Description
Fasciculations are involuntary, nonrhythmic contractions of small muscle groups caused by spontaneous firing of motor units.[4] They appear on the surface of the muscle as fine, rapid, flickering contractions, irregular in timing and location.[58]

Condition/s associated with[4,58,77]

Common
- Benign fasciculations
- Motor neuron disease (amyotrophic lateral sclerosis)
- Radiculopathy

Less common
- Depolarising paralytic agent – succinylcholine
- Cholinergic toxicity – organophosphate toxicity
- Funnel–web spider envenomation
- Thyrotoxicosis
- Poliomyelitis
- Spinal muscular atrophy

Mechanism/s
Fasciculations are typically a lower motor neuron sign caused by spontaneous firing of motor units.[58,77] Mechanisms of fasciculations include:
- lower motor neuron disorders
- toxins and drugs
- benign fasciculations.

Lower motor neuron disorders
Denervation and reinnervation of muscle fibres secondary to lower motor neuron disease causes the spontaneous excitation of individual motor units.[31] Pathological fasciculations are most common in disorders of the anterior horn cells (e.g. motor neuron disease, poliomyelitis), radiculopathy and, less commonly, in entrapment mononeuropathy and peripheral neuropathy.[77] The distribution of fasciculations (e.g. nerve root, peripheral nerve, hands, tongue) and the presence of lower motor neuron signs (e.g. muscle wasting, hypotonia, weakness, hyporeflexia) are important when considering potential aetiologies. Fasciculations of the tongue are associated with motor neuron disease (e.g. amyotrophic lateral sclerosis).

5

Toxins and drugs

Cholinergic toxicity

Cholinergic toxicity (e.g. organophosphate poisoning) causes fasciculations due to potentiation of acetylcholine at the neuromuscular junction. Associated features of the cholinergic toxidrome include diarrhoea, urination, miosis, bradycardia, bronchorrhoea, lacrimation, salivation and sweating.

Funnel-web spider venom

The funnel-web spider produces a toxin that inhibits the inactivation of sodium channels, resulting in neurotransmitter release and prolonged alpha motor neuron depolarisation, causing spontaneous excitation of skeletal muscle groups.[78]

Benign fasciculations

Fasciculations in the setting of an otherwise normal neurological exam are termed benign fasciculations. Benign fasciculations may be exacerbated by mental or physical fatigue, caffeine, smoking or sympathomimetic agents.[58]

Sign value

Fasciculations in the setting of an otherwise normal neurological examination are likely to be benign.[79,80]

Fasciculations in addition to lower motor neuron signs (e.g. hypotonia, weakness, hyporeflexia) are evidence of lower motor neuron dysfunction until proven otherwise. Fasciculations of the tongue occur in approximately one-third of patients with amyotrophic lateral sclerosis.[81]

Gag reflex

Relevant neuroanatomy and topographical anatomy[1,82,83]

CENTRAL PATHWAYS
- Vomiting centre, brainstem
- Cortical areas

AFFERENT LIMB – GLOSSOPHARYNGEAL NERVE (CNIX)
- ⊗ 'Trigger zones' – palatoglossal and palatopharyngeal folds, base of tongue, palate, uvula, posterior pharyngeal wall
  ↓
- Glossopharyngeal nerve fibres
  ↓
- Petrosal ganglion
- ⇒ Jugular foramen
  ↓
- Solitary nucleus, medulla
  ↓

EFFERENT LIMB – GLOSSOPHARYNGEAL NERVE (CNIX)
- Nucleus ambiguus, medulla
- ⇒ Jugular foramen
  ↓
- Petrosal ganglion
  ↓
- × Stylopharyngeus and superior pharyngeal constrictor muscles

EFFERENT LIMB – VAGUS NERVE (CNX)
- Nucleus ambiguus and dorsal motor nucleus, medulla
  ↓
- Vagus nerve
- ⇒ Jugular foramen
- ⇒ Nodose ganglion
  ↓
- × Palatal constrictors and intrinsic laryngeal muscles

5

Description

Absence of stylopharyngeus muscle and superior pharyngeal muscle constriction following stimulation of the posterior tongue and/or oropharynx.[1] Absence of the gag reflex can be unilateral or bilateral.

Condition/s associated with[1]

Common

- Normal variant
- Coma
- Drugs – ethanol, benzodiazepine, opioid
- Lateral medullary syndrome (Wallenberg's syndrome)

Less common

- Cerebellopontine tumour – acoustic schwannoma, glomus tumour
- Internal carotid artery dissection

Mechanism/s

The afferent limb of the gag reflex is mediated by the glossopharyngeal nerve (CNIX), whereas the efferent limb is mediated by the glossopharyngeal nerve (CNIX) and the vagus nerve (CNX).[1] External factors, such as nausea or chronic emesis, may confound the evaluation of the gag reflex, as they may sensitise or desensitise the gag response. Visual, auditory and olfactory stimuli may also sensitise the gag response.[84,85] The gag reflex is absent in a significant percentage of normal individuals.[86] Causes of an absent gag reflex include:

- normal variant
- generalised CNS depression
- glossopharyngeal nerve (CNIX) lesion

- vagus nerve (CNX) lesion
- lateral medullary syndrome (Wallenberg's syndrome).

Normal variant

The gag reflex is absent in a significant proportion of the population. Absence of the gag reflex is likely caused by suppression of the reflex by higher cortical centres and/or desensitisation of the reflex response with ageing.

Generalised CNS depression

The obtunded or comatose patient may have an absent gag reflex due to generalised central nervous system dysfunction.

Glossopharyngeal nerve lesion

Glossopharyngeal nerve palsy causes ispilateral loss of the gag reflex, decreased pharyngeal elevation, dysarthria and dysphagia.[1] Causes of glossopharygneal nerve dysfunction include cerebellopontine angle tumours, Chiari I malformations, jugular foramen syndrome, neoplasia and iatrogenic injury following laryngoscopy or tonsillectomy.[1]

Vagus nerve lesion

Vagus nerve dysfunction causes ipsilateral loss of pharyngeal and laryngeal sensation, unilateral loss of sensation in the external ear, dysphagia, hoarseness, unilateral paresis of the uvula and soft palate, and deviation of the uvula away from the side of the lesion.[1] Causes of vagus nerve dysfunction include internal carotid artery dissection, neoplasia and trauma.

Lateral medullary syndrome (Wallenberg's syndrome)

Lateral medullary syndrome most commonly results from posterior inferior cerebellar artery (PICA) territory infarction due to vertebral artery insufficiency. Infarction of the solitary nucleus and/or nucleus ambiguus in the medulla may result in an absent ipsilateral gag reflex.

Sign value

An absent gag reflex occurs in a significant percentage of the normal population. In a study of 140 healthy subjects at various ages, the gag reflex was absent in 37% of subjects.[86]

5

Gerstmann's syndrome

Relevant neuroanatomy and topographical anatomy
• Angular gyrus, dominant parietal lobe ⇒ Subcortical white matter, parietal lobe[88]

Description

Gerstmann's syndrome is a disorder of higher visuospatial function.[87] Gerstmann's syndrome is a tetrad:[6]

1 acalculia – difficulty with simple addition and subtraction
2 agraphia – difficulty with writing a sentence
3 left/right confusion – difficulty identifying left- and right-sided body parts
4 finger agnosia – difficulty correctly identifying each finger.

Typically, other deficits coexist (e.g. aphasia, apraxia, amnesia and intellectual impairment).[6]

Condition/s associated with[89]

Common

- Cerebral infarction, MCA territory
- Cerebral haemorrhage
- Vascular dementia

Less common

- Alzheimer's disease
- Mass lesion – tumour, abscess, AVM

Mechanism/s

Gertsmann's syndrome is typically associated with a lesion in the angular gyrus of the dominant parietal lobe.[87,90] Each component of Gertsmann's syndrome, individually, has poor localising value and can occur with a variety of lesions. It is unclear whether the four components of Gerstmann's syndrome truly share a common neural pathway or whether they cluster together in large, dominant parietal lesions.[87,90] A recent study, using structural and functional neuroimaging in normal subjects, mapped cortical activation patterns of the brain associated with components of Gerstmann's tetrad. Each component of Gerstmann's syndrome was associated with a variety of cortical and subcortical regions. Gerstmann's syndrome likely results from damage to a focal region of subcortical white matter resulting in intraparietal disconnection.[88]

Sign value

Gerstmann's syndrome is a dominant cortical localising sign.

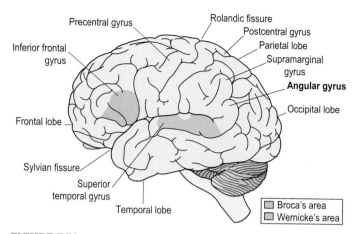

FIGURE 5.36
Angular gyrus, dominant parietal lobe in Gerstmann's syndrome

Reproduced, with permission, from Daroff RB, Bradley WG et al., Neurology in Clinical Practice, *5th edn, Philadelphia: Butterworth-Heinemann, 2008: Fig 12A-1.*

5

Glabellar tap (Myerson's sign)

Relevant neuroanatomy and topographical anatomy
• Frontal lobes

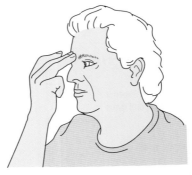

FIGURE 5.37
Glabellar tap

Description

Tapping the glabella (between the patient's eyebrows) causes blinking, which typically ceases after several taps. Persistent blinking (i.e. more than 4 or 5 blinks) in response to glabellar tapping is abnormal (called Myerson's sign).[4]

Condition/s associated with

Common

- Parkinson's disease
- Alzheimer's dementia
- Vascular dementia

Less common

- Frontotemporal dementia
- Lewy Body dementia
- Advanced HIV/AIDS dementia

Mechanism/s

The mechanism of Myerson's sign is not known. The reflex is likely mediated by nonprimary motor cortical areas, which exert an inhibitory control of the blink to threat reflex.[91] Damage to these areas may result in disinhibition and thus 'release' the reflex.[91] The mechanism of Myerson's sign in Parkinson's disease is not known.

Sign value

Myerson's sign has been described in normal subjects. The prevalence varies significantly between studies.[92-95]

Myerson's sign is classically associated with Parkinson's disease.

Global aphasia

Description

Global aphasia is a disturbance of speech with expressive and receptive components (i.e. a combination of Broca's and Wernicke's aphasia).[46] Speech is nonfluent or nonexistent, and comprehension is impaired. Naming, repetition, reading and writing are all affected.[46] See 'Wernicke's aphasia' and 'Broca's aphasia' in this chapter.

Condition/s associated with[6,96]

Common

- Cerebral infarction, MCA territory
- Cerebral haemorrhage
- Alzheimer's disease
- Vascular dementia

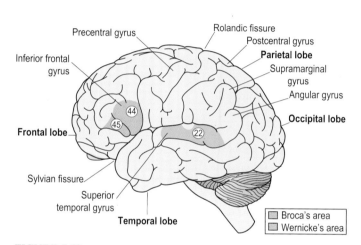

FIGURE 5.38
Broca's area and Wernicke's area
22 = Brodmann's area 22; 44 = Brodmann's area 44; 45 = Brodmann's area 45.

Reproduced, with permission, from Daroff RB, Bradley WG et al., Neurology in Clinical Practice, 5th edn, Philadelphia: Butterworth-Heinemann, 2008: Fig 12A-1.

Relevant neuroanatomy and topographical anatomy

- Broca's area – posterior inferior frontal gyrus, dominant hemisphere
- Wernicke's area – posterior superior temporal gyrus, dominant hemisphere
⇒ Superior and inferior divisions, middle cerebral artery (MCA)

Less common

- Mass lesion – tumour, abscess, AVM
- Primary progressive aphasia

Mechanism/s

Global aphasia (refer to Table 5.14 for clinical features) is caused by a lesion of the posterior inferior frontal gyrus (i.e. Broca's area), the posterior superior temporal gyrus of the dominant hemisphere (i.e. Wernicke's area) and/or the adjacent subcortical white matter.[46] This region is typically supplied by branches of the middle cerebral artery (MCA). The most common cause is MCA territory infarction. Most patients will have contralateral motor and sensory findings, and contralateral hemianopia.[46]

Sign value

Global aphasia is a dominant cortical localising sign.[96]

TABLE 5.14
Clinical features of global aphasia

Clinical feature	Abnormality in global aphasia
Spontaneous speech	• Mute or nonfluent
Naming	• Impaired
Comprehension	• Impaired
Repetition	• Impaired
Reading	• Impaired
Writing	• Impaired
Associated signs	• Contralateral motor findings • Contralateral sensory findings • Contralateral hemianopia

Adapted from Kirshner HS, Language and speech disorders: aphasia and aphasiac syndromes. In: Bradley WG, Daroff RB, Fenichel G et al., Neurology in Clinical Practice, *5th edn, Philadelphia: Butterworth-Heinemann, 2008.*

Grasp reflex

<table>
<tr><td>

Relevant neuroanatomy and topographical anatomy

• Frontal lobes

</td></tr>
</table>

Description

The patient involuntarily grasps the examiner's fingers when the examiner strokes the patient's thenar eminence.[4] The grasp reflex is a primitive reflex present in infancy, which normally disappears later in life.[4,97]

Condition/s associated with

Common

• Alzheimer's dementia
• Vascular dementia

Less common

• Frontotemporal dementia
• Lewy body dementia (LBD)
• Advanced HIV/AIDS

Mechanism/s

The grasp reflex is present in normal infants from approximately 25 weeks to 6 months of age.[91] The reflex is likely controlled by nonprimary motor cortical areas, which exert an inhibitory control of the spinal reflex following normal central nervous system development.[91] Frontal lobe disease may result in disinhibition of the reflex, and thus 'release' the reflex.

Sign value

In a study of patients admitted to a neurology service, a positive grasp reflex predicted lesions in the frontal lobe, deep nuclei or subcortical white matter with a sensitivity of 13%, specificity of 99% and a positive likelihood ratio of 20.2.[98]

5

Hand dominance

TABLE 5.15
Dominant and non-dominant cortical localising signs

Dominant cortical localising signs	Non-dominant cortical localising signs
• Aphasia • Gerstmann's syndrome	• Hemineglect syndrome • Anosognosia • Apraxia

Description/ mechanism/s

Hand dominance is clinically significant in the context of dominant cortical localising signs (see Table 5.15). The side of hand dominance correlates with the side of the dominant cerebral hemisphere and therefore has potential localising value.

- Right-hand dominant:
  - 96% of patients have left-sided dominant cerebral hemisphere[99]
  - 4% of patients have right-sided dominant cerebral hemisphere[99]

- Left-hand dominant:
  - 73% of patients have left-sided dominant cerebral hemisphere[99]
  - 27% of patients have right-sided dominant cerebral hemisphere[99]

Sign value

In patients with dominant or non-dominant cortical localising signs, hand dominance has potential localising value.

Hearing impairment

Description

Hearing is evaluated at the bedside with the whispered voice test (note that this is a poor screening test), Weber test and Rinne test. Clinically, significant hearing loss (i.e. >30 dB) will be missed roughly 50% of the time without formal evaluation (e.g. audiometry).[100]

Relevant neuroanatomy and topographical anatomy[18,101,102]

⇒ External ear canal
↓
⇒ Tympanic membrane
↓
⇒ Malleus, incus, stapes bones
↓
⇒ Middle ear
↓
⊗ Cochlea
↓
• Vestibulocochlear nerve (CNVIII)
⇒ Mastoid sinus
⇒ Internal acoustic meatus
⇒ Cerebellopontine angle
↓
• Brainstem nuclei
↓
• Brainstem ascending sensory fibres
↓
• Inferior colliculi
↓
• Medical geniculate nuclei, thalamus
↓
• Auditory cortex, transverse gyri of Heschl, temporal lobe

Condition/s associated with[101,102]

Common
- Impacted cerumen
- Presbyacusis (age-related hearing loss)
- Otitis media with effusion
- Tympanic membrane perforation
- Otosclerosis
- Drugs – gentamicin, furosemide, aspirin

Less common
- Ménière's disease
- Vestibular neuritis
- Acoustic schwannoma
- Meningitis
- Cholesteatoma

Mechanism/s

Mechanisms of hearing loss include:
- conductive hearing loss
- sensorineural hearing loss
- central hearing loss (rare).

Conductive hearing loss

In conductive hearing loss, sound waves are not transmitted to the sensorineural structures of the auditory system. Conductive hearing loss can result from a disorder of the external ear canal, tympanic membrane, ossicles or middle ear.[101,102] The most common cause of conductive hearing loss is cerumen or 'wax' impaction in the external canal.[102] Causes include otitis media with effusion, tympanic

5

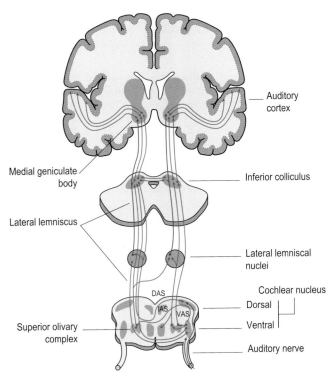

FIGURE 5.39

Central auditory pathways

DAS = dorsal acoustic stria; IAS = intermediate acoustic stria; VAS = ventral acoustic stria.

Reproduced, with permission, from Flint PW et al., Cummings Otolaryngology: Head and Neck Surgery, *5th edn, Mosby, 2010: Fig 128-6.*

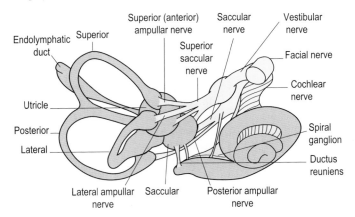

FIGURE 5.40

The vestibular system and peripheral auditory components

Reproduced, with permission, from Flint PW et al., Cummings Otolaryngology: Head and Neck Surgery, *5th edn, Mosby, 2010: Fig 163-1.*

membrane perforation, otosclerosis and cholesteatoma.

Sensorineural hearing loss

Sensorineural hearing loss results from dysfunction of the cochlea, the auditory division of the acoustic nerve and/or the vestibulocochlear nerve.[101] Different frequencies of sound are detected in different segments of the spiral-shaped cochlea. In cochlear lesions, hearing levels for varying frequencies are typically unequal.[101] Causes include Ménière's disease, cerebellopontine angle tumours (e.g. acoustic schwannoma), vestibular neuritis and ototoxic drugs (e.g. gentamicin, furosemide, aspirin).

Central hearing loss (rare)

Bilateral sensorineural hearing loss may result from bilateral lesions of the primary auditory cortex in the transverse gyri of Heschl.[101]

Sign value

Asymmetrical sensorineural hearing loss is concerning for a focal neurological lesion (e.g. a tumour in the internal auditory meatus or cerebellopontine area).[101] In a study of patients with >15 dB hearing loss in two or more frequencies, or ≥15% asymmetry in speech discrimination scores, approximately 10% of patients had an identifiable tumour on MRI.[103]

5

Hemineglect syndrome

TABLE 5.16
Clinical features of hemineglect syndrome[6,104]

Clinical feature	Characteristics
Sensory neglect	Patient ignores visual, tactile or auditory stimuli in the contralateral hemispace
Motor neglect	Patient performs fewer movements in the contralateral hemispace
Combined sensory/motor neglect	Combination of the features above
Conceptual neglect	Patient's internal representation of own body and/or external environment exhibits neglect

Description

Hemineglect syndrome is a disorder of conscious perception, characterised by a lack of awareness of the contralateral visual hemispace and contralateral body (refer to Table 5.16 for clinical features).[6] The patient may be completely unaware of their own body or objects in the neglected space (i.e. anosognosia). The presence of hemineglect is typically evaluated with clock face drawing, search/cancellation and/or line bisection tests.[104]

Condition/s associated with

Common

- Cerebral infarction
- Cerebral haemorrhage

Less common

- Mass lesion – tumour, abscess, AVM

Mechanism/s

The most common cause of hemineglect syndrome is a lesion at the temporoparietal junction of the non-dominant hemisphere.[105,106] These areas of the brain mediate conscious representation of sensation, motor

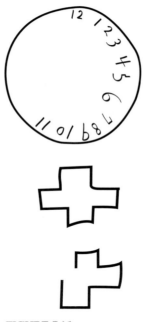

FIGURE 5.41
Results of clock face drawing in hemineglect syndrome

Reproduced, with permission, from Daroff RB, Bradley WG et al., Neurology in Clinical Practice, 5th edn, Philadelphia: Butterworth-Heinemann, 2008: Fig 6-3.

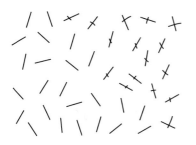

FIGURE 5.42
Results of search/cancellation task in
hemineglect syndrome

Albert ML, Articles, Neurology *1973;*
23(6): 658. doi:10.1212/WNL.23.6.658;
doi:10.1212/WNL.23.6.658 1526-632X.

Relevant neuroanatomy and topographical anatomy

• Temporo-parietal
junction, non-dominant
hemisphere

---

activities such as visual scanning and
limb exploration, and motivational
relevance.[107] The exact location
responsible for hemineglect syndrome
is unclear. Several areas have been
implicated and include the angular
gyrus of the posterior parietal cortex in
the right hemisphere, right superior
temporal cortex, right inferior parietal
lobule, cingulate gyrus, thalamus and
basal ganglia.[108]

Sign value
Hemineglect syndrome is a non-
dominant cortical localising sign. In a
study of 140 consecutive patients
admitted with right hemisphere stroke,
visual hemineglect syndrome was
present in 56% of patients.[109]

5

High stepping gait

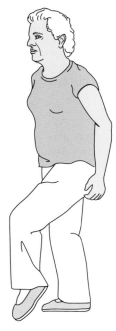

FIGURE 5.43
High stepping gait
Based on Neurocenter. Available: http://neurocenter.gr/N-S.html [5 Apr 2011].

Description

A high stepping gait is characterised by pronounced hip and knee flexion, in order to clear the lower limb or limb(s) with foot drop during leg swing.[28,43]

Condition/s associated with[3]

Common

- Common peroneal nerve neuropathy
- L5 radiculopathy

Relevant neuroanatomy and topographical anatomy

- Nerve root (L5)
- ⇒ Intervertebral disc
- ⇒ Intervertebral foramina
  ↓
- Peripheral nerve (sciatic nerve, common peroneal nerve)
- ⇒ Potential sites of nerve injury (e.g. trauma, head of fibula)
  ↓
- × Muscles of the anterior compartment, leg

Less common

- Sciatic nerve palsy
- Length-dependent peripheral neuropathy – alcohol, diabetes mellitus
- Hereditary peripheral neuropathy – Marie–Charcot–Tooth disease
- Myopathy – scapuloperoneal muscular dystrophy

Mechanism/s

High stepping gait is associated with foot drop. Foot drop is caused by weakness of the anterior compartment muscles of the leg (e.g. tibialis anterior, extensor hallicus longus, extensor hallicus brevis muscles). Causes of high stepping gait include:

- L5 radiculopathy
- common peroneal nerve palsy
- sciatic nerve palsy

- length-dependent peripheral neuropathy
- Charcot–Marie–Tooth disease
- scapuloperoneal muscular dystrophy.

L5 radiculopathy

The L5 nerve root nerve fibres supply the muscles of the anterior compartment of the leg. The most common causes of L5 radiculopathy are intervertebral disc or intervertebral foramen disease (e.g. osteoarthritis). Other causes of radiculopathy include neoplasia, epidural abscess and trauma. Associated features of L5 radiculopathy include ankle dorsiflexor weakness and sensory abnormalities (e.g. pain, sensory loss) in the L5 dermatome (i.e. lateral aspect of the foot).

Common peroneal nerve palsy

The common peroneal nerve branches into the deep and superficial peroneal nerves, which innervate the muscles of the anterior and lateral compartments of the leg, respectively. The common peroneal nerve is vulnerable to traumatic injury due to its superficial location adjacent to the fibular head (see Figure 5.44). Common causes of peroneal nerve palsy include penetrating or blunt trauma at the fibular head and chronic compression secondary to immobility. Associated features include ankle dorsiflexion weakness (anterior compartment muscle weakness), ankle eversion weakness (lateral compartment muscle weakness) and sensory loss of lateral

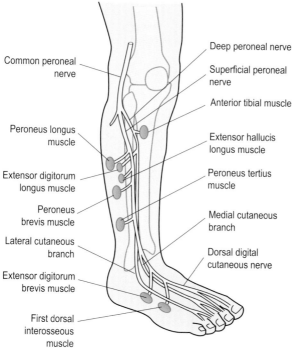

Common peroneal nerve

Peroneus longus muscle

Extensor digitorum longus muscle

Peroneus brevis muscle

Lateral cutaneous branch

Extensor digitorum brevis muscle

First dorsal interosseous muscle

Deep peroneal nerve

Superficial peroneal nerve

Anterior tibial muscle

Extensor hallucis longus muscle

Peroneus tertius muscle

Medial cutaneous branch

Dorsal digital cutaneous nerve

FIGURE 5.44

Anatomy of the common, superficial and deep peroneal (fibular) nerves

Reproduced, with permission, from Canale ST, Beaty JH, Campbell's Operative Orthopaedics, 11th edn, St Louis: Mosby, 2007: Fig 59-39.

aspect of the leg (dysfunction of lateral sural cutaneous nerve).

Sciatic nerve palsy
Sciatic nerve palsy results in evidence of common peroneal nerve dysfunction (e.g. dorsiflexion weakness, ankle eversion weakness) and tibial nerve dysfunction (e.g. plantarflexion weakness, decreased/absent ankle jerk reflex). The most common causes are posterior hip dislocation, fracture and penetrating injury of the buttock.[3]

Length-dependent peripheral neuropathy
Causes of length-dependent peripheral neuropathy include diabetes mellitus, alcohol and inherited neuropathies.[3] A wide range of metabolic abnormalities in the peripheral nerve result in axonal degeneration, which starts in the most distal portion of the nerve and progressively affects more proximal fibres.[3] Associated features include a progressive glove-and-stocking pattern of motor deficits and sensory deficits, distal muscle weakness, muscle atrophy, trophic changes and loss of ankle reflexes.[3]

Charcot–Marie–Tooth disease
Charcot–Marie–Tooth (CMT) disease is a form of hereditary motor and sensory neuropathy that results in bilateral peroneal muscular atrophy.[3] Charcot–Marie–Tooth disease is the most common inherited neuropathy.

Scapuloperoneal muscular dystrophy
Scapuloperoneal muscular dystrophy is a rare primary disorder of muscle that affects the anterior compartment muscles.

Sign value
High stepping gait is most commonly due to a lower motor neuron disorder of the peripheral nerve or nerve root.

Hoarseness

Relevant neuroanatomy and topographical anatomy

UPPER MOTOR NEURON
↔ Bilateral upper motor neuron

LOWER MOTOR NEURON
• Nucleus ambiguus medulla
↓
• Vagus nerve (CNX)
⇒ Jugular foramen
↓

• Right recurrent laryngeal nerve ⇒ Thoracic cavity	↓ • Left recurrent laryngeal nerve ⇒ Thoracic cavity ⇒ Arch aorta ⇒ Left atria
↓ × Vocal cord muscles	↓ × Vocal cord muscles

5

Description

Hoarseness is the sound produced with asymmetrical contraction or incongruent apposition of the vocal cords.

Condition/s associated with

Common

• Viral laryngitis
• Iatrogenic – traumatic or prolonged endotracheal intubation
• Iatrogenic – recurrent laryngeal nerve injury

Less common

• Vocal cord polyps
• Recurrent laryngeal nerve palsy – Pancoast's tumour, thoracic aortic aneurysm
• Lateral medullary syndrome (Wallenberg's syndrome)
• Ortner's syndrome

Mechanism/s

Hoarseness is caused by:

• recurrent laryngeal nerve palsy
• nucleus ambiguus lesion
• local disorders of the vocal cords
• disorders of the cricoarytenoid joint.

Recurrent laryngeal nerve palsy

The recurrent laryngeal nerve, a branch of the vagus nerve, undertakes a long, convoluted course after exiting the medulla, going through the neck and thoracic cavity, under and around the aortic arch (left recurrent laryngeal nerve only), past the left atrium and then up along the trachea to the muscles of the vocal cords. It is susceptible to a diverse variety of insults along its pathway. Causes include Pancoast's tumour, atrial enlargement (i.e. Ortner's syndrome), thoracic aortic aneurysm and iatrogenic injury following thyroidectomy.[110,111]

Nucleus ambiguus lesion (e.g. lateral medullary syndrome)

Damage to the nucleus ambiguus in the medulla can cause hoarseness. This can be caused by posterior inferior cerebellar artery (PICA) territory

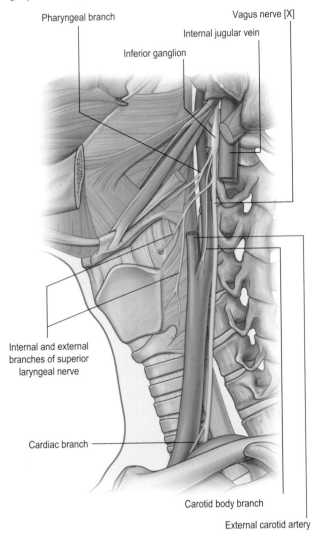

Pharyngeal branch

Vagus nerve [X]

Internal jugular vein

Inferior ganglion

Internal and external branches of superior laryngeal nerve

Cardiac branch

Carotid body branch

External carotid artery

FIGURE 5.45
Anatomy of the vagus nerve

Reproduced, with permission, from Drake R, Vogl AW, Mitchell AWM, Gray's Anatomy for Students, 2nd edn, Philadelphia: Churchill Livingstone, 2009: Fig 8-164.

infarction in lateral medullary syndrome (see 'Wallenberg's syndrome' in this chapter).

Local disorders of the vocal cords

Local vocal cord swelling or a mass lesion causing poor vocal cord opposition can lead to asynchronous vibratory contractions of the vocal cords. The most common cause is viral laryngitis. Other causes include vocal cord polyps, tumours (e.g. squamous cell carcinoma) and iatrogenic trauma (e.g. endotracheal intubation).

Disorders of the cricoarytenoid joint[112,113]

Rheumatoid arthritis affecting the cricoarytenoid joint (a synovial joint) may impair the coordinated movement of the vocal cords, resulting in hoarseness.

Sign value

Hoarseness is most commonly associated with viral laryngitis but can be an important sign of neurological disease. Hoarseness should be interpreted in the context of the overall clinical findings. Isolated hoarseness that lasts longer than 2 weeks is unlikely to be caused by viral laryngitis and should prompt further evaluation.[71]

5

Hoffman's sign

Relevant neuroanatomy and topographical anatomy
UPPER MOTOR NEURON • Motor cortex ↓ • Corona radiata, subcortical white matter ↓ • Posterior limb, internal capsule ↓ • Pyramidal tracts, medial brainstem ↓ Ø Pyramidal decussation, medulla ↓ • Lateral corticospinal tracts, spinal cord ↓ MONOSYNAPTIC STRETCH REFLEX → Inhibitory intemeuron → Alpha motor neuron → Sensory afferent

Condition/s associated with

Common

- Normal variant
- Cerebral infarction, MCA territory
- Cerebral haemorrhage
- Lacunar infarction, posterior limb internal capsule

Less common

- Multiple sclerosis
- Spinal cord injury
- Central mass lesion – tumour, abscess, AVM

Mechanism/s

Hoffman's sign is caused by activation of a monosynaptic stretch reflex. Exaggeration of the reflex is caused by hyperreflexia in the setting of upper motor neuron dysfunction (see also 'Hyperreflexia' in this chapter).[58]

Sign value

Hoffman's sign is a sign of hyperreflexia. It may be present in some normal individuals.

Description

Sudden stretch of the finger flexors causes involuntary finger flexor contraction due to activation of a monosynaptic stretch reflex.[4]

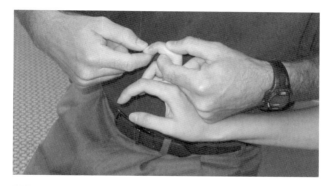

FIGURE 5.46
Hoffman's sign

Reproduced, with permission, from Fernandez-de-las-Penas C, Cleland J, Huijbregts P (eds), Neck and Arm Pain Syndromes, *1st edn, London: Churchill Livingstone, 2011: Fig 9-1.*

5

Horner's syndrome

Relevant neuroanatomy and topographical anatomy

Sympathetic pathway
FIRST-ORDER NEURON
- Hypothalamus

$\downarrow$

- Sympathetic fibres, brainstem

$\downarrow$

- Sympathetic fibres, intermediate horn, spinal cord

$\downarrow$

SECOND-ORDER NEURON (PREGANGLIONIC FIBRE)
- Sympathetic trunk
- ⇒ Lung apex

$\downarrow$

- Superior cervical ganglion C2

$\downarrow$

THIRD-ORDER NEURON (POSTGANGLIONIC FIBRE)
- Superior cervical ganglion C2
- ⇒ Carotid sheath
- ⇒ Carotid artery
- ⇒ Superior orbital fissure
- ⇒ Cavernous sinus
- ⇒ Orbital apex

$\downarrow$

- Ciliary body

$\downarrow$

- × Pupillary dilator muscles
- × Superior tarsal muscle
- × Sweat glands

Description
Horner's syndrome is a triad of unilateral:[4,10,11]

1. miosis
2. ptosis with apparent enophthalmos
3. anhydrosis.

Condition/s associated with[4,10–12]

Common
- Lateral medullary syndrome (Wallenberg's syndrome)
- Pancoast's tumour
- Idiopathic
- Iatrogenic – complication of carotid endarterectomy

Less common

- Spinal cord lesion above T1
- Thoracic aortic aneurysm
- Carotid artery dissection
- Complicated migraine
- Cavernous sinus syndrome

Mechanism/s

Causes of Horner's syndrome are divided into:

- first-order sympathetic neuron lesion
- second-order sympathetic neuron lesion
- third-order sympathetic neuron lesion.

First-order sympathetic neuron lesion

The first-order sympathetic neuron travels from the hypothalamus to the C8–T1 level of the spinal cord. Causes of lesions in the first-order sympathetic neuron include hypothalamic lesions (e.g. infarct, tumour), lateral medullary syndrome (Wallenberg's syndrome) and syringomyelia.[8,114]

Second-order sympathetic neuron lesion

The second-order sympathetic neuron travels a long intrathoracic course from the C8–T1 level of the spinal cord to the superior cervical ganglion at the level of C2. Associated findings in

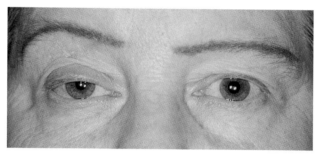

FIGURE 5.47
Right Horner's syndrome
Reproduced, with permission, from Yanoff M, Duker JS, Ophthalmology, 3rd edn, St Louis: Mosby, 2008: Fig 12-5-4.

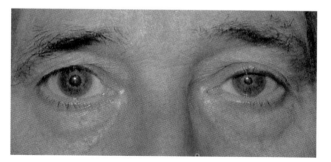

FIGURE 5.48
Left Horner's syndrome in a patient with syringomyelia
Reproduced, with permission, from Goldman L, Ausiello D, Cecil Medicine, 23rd edn, Philadelphia: Saunders, 2007: Fig 450-5.

5

second-order causes of Horner's syndrome include C8 or T1 nerve roots signs or significant findings in the chest.[8,114] Causes of lesions in the second-order sympathetic neuron include thoracic aortic aneurysm, lower brachial plexus injury (e.g. Klumpke's palsy), Pancoast's tumour, carotid artery dissection and iatrogenic injury following carotid endarterectomy.

Third-order sympathetic neuron lesion

The third-order sympathetic neuron travels from the cervical ganglion at the level of C2 to the pupillary dilator muscle and the superior tarsal muscle.

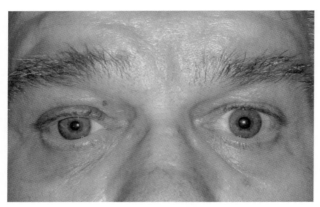

FIGURE 5.49
Right Horner's syndrome following right neck dissection

Reproduced, with permission, from Flint PW, Haughey BH, Lund VJ et al., Cummings Otolaryngology: Head & Neck Surgery, *5th edn, Philadelphia: Mosby, 2010: Fig 122-8.*

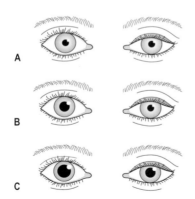

FIGURE 5.50
Left Horner's syndrome
A Mild upper lid ptosis and miosis in room light. **B** Anisocoria is increased 5 seconds after the lights are dimmed due to dilation lag of the left pupil. **C** Fifteen seconds after the lights are dimmed, the left pupil exhibits increased dilation compared to the image in **B**.

Reproduced, with permission, from Daroff RB, Bradley WG et al., Neurology in Clinical Practice, *5th edn, Philadelphia: Butterworth-Heinemann, 2008: Fig 17-6.*

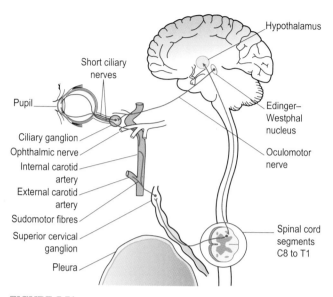

FIGURE 5.51
Sympathetic and parasympathetic innervation of the pupil

Reproduced, with permission, from Duong DK, Leo MM, Mitchell EL, Emerg Med Clin N Am *2008; 26: 137–180, Fig 3.*

5

Causes include head and neck trauma and local eye pathology.[4,10,11]

Sign value

In the hospital setting, causes of Horner's syndrome vary depending on the admitting service. On a neurology service, 70% of patients with Horner's syndrome have lesions in the first-order neuron (e.g. brainstem stroke is the most common cause).[4,115] On a medicine service, 70% of patients have a lesion of the second-order neuron caused by tumours (e.g. lung and thyroid malignancies) or trauma (e.g. trauma of the neck, chest, spinal nerves, subclavian or carotid arteries).[4,116] On an ophthalmology service, patients are more likely to have second- or third-order neuron lesions (e.g. complicated migraine, skull fracture or cavernous sinus syndrome).[4,10–12]

Hutchinson's pupil

Description

Hutchinson's pupil is a non-reactive dilated pupil caused by oculomotor nerve compression secondary to uncal herniation. Other signs of oculomotor nerve palsy (e.g. extraocular muscle weakness, ptosis) may also be present (see also 'Oculomotor nerve palsy' in this chapter).

Relevant neuroanatomy and topographical anatomy

Pupillary constriction/ parasympathetic pathway

EFFERENT LIMB

- Edinger–Westphal nucleus midbrain
  ↓
- Oculomotor nerve (CNIII)
  ⇒ Uncus, medial temporal lobe
  ↓
- Ciliary ganglion
  ↓
- Short ciliary nerves
  ↓
× Pupillary constrictor muscles
× Levator palpebrae muscle
× Iris

Condition/s associated with

- Uncal herniation
  » Intracranial haemorrhage – epidural, subdural, parenchymal haemorrhage
  » Cerebral infarction, MCA/ICA territory (severe oedema)
  » Mass lesion – tumour, abscess, AVM

Mechanism/s

Uncal herniation most commonly results from an expanding extra-axial intracranial haematoma or mass.[117] Increasing intracranial volume and intracranial pressure result in cerebral herniation when the expanding intracranial contents (e.g. a mass) exceed the capacity of the cerebral tissue and intracranial contents to accommodate such a change.[117] Cerebral tissue moves in the direction of the pressure gradient (i.e. caudally towards the foramen magnum). Herniation of the medial temporal lobe and uncus may result in compression of the midbrain and oculomotor nerve, resulting in a non-reactive dilated pupil.[6,9,117] See 'Oculomotor nerve palsy' in this chapter.

Sign value

Hutchinson's pupil is a catastrophic sign of oculomotor nerve compression due to uncal herniation. When present, mortality approaches 100% without emergent medical intervention and surgical decompression.[117]

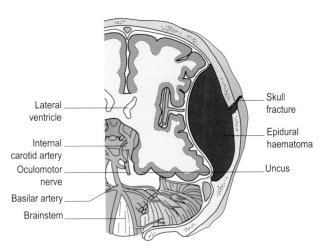

Lateral ventricle

Internal carotid artery

Oculomotor nerve

Basilar artery

Brainstem

Skull fracture

Epidural haematoma

Uncus

FIGURE 5.52
Schematic representation of uncal herniation caused by an epidural haematoma, resulting in oculomotor nerve (CNIII) compression

Reproduced, with permission, from Marx JA, Hockberger RS, Walls RM et al., Rosen's Emergency Medicine, *7th edn, Philadelphia: Mosby, 2010: Fig 38-5.*

5

Hutchinson's sign

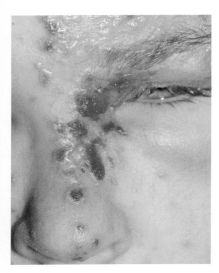

FIGURE 5.53
Hutchinson's sign
Herpes zoster reactivation involving the nasociliary nerve.

Reproduced, with permission, from Palay D, Krachmer J, Primary Care Ophthalmology, 2nd edn, Philadelphia: Mosby, 2005: Fig 6-9.

Relevant neuroanatomy and topographical anatomy

⊗ Sensory receptors light touch/pain/temperature
 ↓
• Ophthalmic division (V1) trigeminal nerve (CNV)
 ⇒ Cavernous sinus
 ⇒ Superior orbital fissure
 ↓
• Trigeminal (Gasserian) ganglion, Meckel's cave petrous bone

Description

Hutchinson's sign is a vesicular eruption on the tip of the nose due to a reactivation of varicella zoster virus (VZV) infection involving the nasociliary nerve, a branch of the ophthalmic division of the trigeminal nerve (CNV V1).

Condition/s associated with[1]

Common

• Varicella zoster virus (VZV) – 'shingles'

Mechanism/s

Herpes zoster reactivation involving the nasociliary branch of the ophthalmic division of the trigeminal nerve typically pre-empts ocular involvement (i.e. herpes zoster ophthalmicus).

Sign value

Early identification of Hutchinson's sign strongly predicts eye involvement (i.e. herpes zoster ophthalmicus).[118]

Hyperreflexia

Description

Stretch reflexes are more brisk than normal. Hyperreflexia is an upper motor neuron sign. Hyperreflexia is significant in the following clinical scenarios:[4]

- hyperreflexia PLUS upper motor neuron signs (e.g. spasticity, weakness, clonus, Babinski sign)
- reflex amplitude is asymmetric
- reflex is brisk compared with reflexes from a higher spinal level, signifying potential spinal cord disease.

The National Institute of Neurological Disorders and Stroke (NINDS) describes a standardised method of grading reflexes (see Table 5.17).[4]

TABLE 5.17
NINDS Muscle Stretch Reflex Scale[4]

Grade	Findings
0	Reflex absent
1	Reflex small, less than normal
	Includes a trace response or a response brought out only by reinforcement
2	Reflex in lower half of normal range
3	Reflex in upper half of normal range
4	Reflex enhanced, more than normal
	Includes clonus if present, which optionally can be noted in an added verbal description of the reflex

Adapted from McGee S, Evidence Based Physical Diagnosis, 2nd edn, St Louis: Saunders, 2007.

Condition/s associated with

Common

- Normal variant
- Cerebral infarction, MCA territory
- Cerebral haemorrhage
- Lacunar infarction, posterior limb internal capsule

Relevant neuroanatomy and topographical anatomy

UPPER MOTOR NEURON
- Motor cortex
  ↓
- Corona radiata, subcortical white matter
  ↓
- Posterior limb, internal capsule
  ↓
- Corticospinal tracts, medial brainstem
  ↓
Ø Pyramidal decussation, medulla
  ↓
- Lateral corticospinal tracts, spinal cord
  ↓
MONOSYNAPTIC STRETCH REFLEX
  → Inhibitory interneuron
  → Alpha motor neuron
  → Sensory afferent

5

Less common

- Multiple sclerosis
- Spinal cord injury
- Brainstem lesion (medial medullary syndrome)
- CNS mass lesion – tumour, abscess, AVM
- Serotonin syndrome
- Strychnine toxicity
- *Clostridium tetani* infection (tetanus)

Mechanism/s

Upper motor neuron lesion

Upper motor neuron lesions cause an increase in gamma motor neuron activity and a decrease in inhibitory interneuron activity, resulting in a state of hyperexcitability of alpha motor neurons.[119] Associated findings in upper motor neuron disease include spasticity, weakness, pronator drift, and Babinski sign. Upper motor neuron lesions cause contralateral hyperreflexia if present above the pyramidal decussation (e.g. pons, medulla, posterior limb internal capsule, motor cortex) and ipsilateral hyperreflexia if the lesion is present below the pyramidal decussation (e.g. spinal cord). The distribution of hyperreflexia and associated upper motor neuron signs is important when considering a potential aetiology (see Tables 5.16, 5.18, 5.19).

Serotonin syndrome

See 'Clonus' in this chapter.

Strychnine toxicity

See 'Spasticity' in this chapter.

Clostridium tetani infection (tetanus)

See 'Spasticity' in this chapter.

Sign value

Unilateral hyperreflexia is most commonly an upper motor neuron sign. Diffuse hyperreflexia is a key finding in serotonin syndrome and strychnine toxicity.

Refer to Table 5.18 for clinical utility.

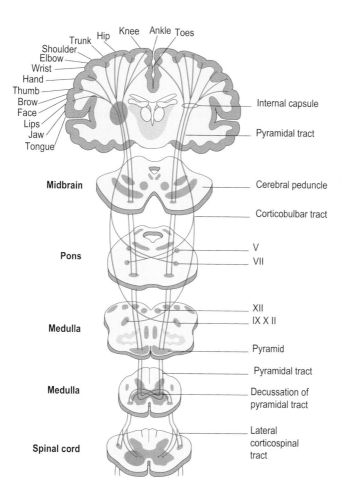

FIGURE 5.54
Upper motor neuron anatomy

Reproduced, with permission, from Clark RG, Manter and Gatz's Essential Neuroanatomy and Neurophysiology, *5th edn, Philadelphia: FA Davis Co, 1975.*

TABLE 5.18
Clinical utility of hyperreflexia in unilateral hemisphere lesions[119]

	Sensitivity	Specificity	Positive LR	Negative LR
Hyperreflexia[119]	69%	88%	5.8	0.4

Adapted from McGee S, Evidence Based Physical Diagnosis, *2nd edn, St Louis: Saunders, 2007.*

Hyporeflexia and areflexia

Description

Stretch reflexes are decreased (hyporeflexia) or absent (areflexia) despite reinforcement manoeuvres (e.g. Jendrassik manoeuvre). Hyporeflexia is significant in the following clinical scenarios:[4]

- hyporeflexia PLUS lower motor neuron signs (e.g. fasciculations, hypotonia, weakness)
- hyporeflexia PLUS suspected hyperacute upper motor neuron disorder (e.g. stroke, spinal cord injury [called spinal shock])
- asymmetric reflex amplitude.

The NINDS Muscle Stretch Reflex Scale describes a standardised method of grading reflexes (see Table 5.17).[48,120]

Condition/s associated with

Common

- Hyperacute upper motor neuron disorder – CVA, spinal cord injury
- Radiculopathy – intervertebral disc herniation, spondylosis

Less common

- Peripheral neuropathy
- Myasthenia gravis
- Guillain–Barré syndrome
- Poliomyelitis
- Botulism
- Tick paralysis

Mechanism/s

Hyporeflexia and areflexia are caused by:

- peripheral neuropathy
- radiculopathy
- Guillain–Barré syndrome

Relevant neuroanatomy and topographical anatomy

UPPER MOTOR NEURON
→ Upper motor neuron
↓
→ Inhibitory interneuron

AFFERENT LIMB
⊗ Muscle spindle
↓
• Sensory afferent nerve
↓
• Nerve root
↓
• Dorsal horn grey matter
→ Inhibitory interneuron
↓
EFFERENT LIMB
• Anterior horn grey matter
↓
• Nerve root
⇒ Intervertebral foramen
⇒ Intervertebral disc
↓
• Peripheral nerve
⇒ Potential site of vulnerability
↓
× Muscle

- disorders of the anterior horn cells
- disorders of the neuromuscular junction: myasthenia gravis, botulism, tick paralysis
- hyperacute upper motor neuron injury
- normal variant.

Peripheral neuropathy

Compression mononeuropathy (e.g. carpal tunnel syndrome) results in a pattern of neurological deficits distal to the site of nerve injury. Common causes include carpal tunnel syndrome, common peroneal nerve palsy and radial nerve palsy (see Table 5.19). Length-dependent peripheral neuropathy is associated with the classic 'glove-and-stocking' distribution of sensory, motor and reflex findings. Sensory, motor and reflex abnormalities progressively increase as more proximal nerve fibres are affected. Common causes include diabetes mellitus, alcohol and drugs.

Radiculopathy

In disorders of the nerve root, hyporeflexia or areflexia often coexist with positive or negative sensory findings in a dermatomal distribution. Diminished reflexes are largely due to dysfunction of the afferent limb of the reflex arc.[121] In patients less than 45 years of age, the most common cause is intervertebral disc disease. In older patients, the most common cause is spondylosis and osteophyte formation (see Table 5.20).[121]

Flaccid paresis: Guillain–Barré syndrome

Acute inflammatory demyelinating polyradiculopathy, or Guillain–Barré syndrome, causes areflexia in the distribution of the affected nerve roots. An ascending pattern of lower motor neuron findings is characteristic (e.g. hypotonia, weakness, areflexia). It may be preceded by an infectious illness (e.g. *Campylobacter jejuni*, Cytomegalovirus, Epstein-Barr virus, *Mycoplasma pneumonia*).

Disorders of the anterior horn cells

Disorders of the anterior horn cells cause diminished reflexes due to dysfunction of the efferent limb of the reflex. Lower motor neuron findings are characteristic (e.g. wasting, fasciculations, hypotonia, weakness). Causes include motor neuron disease (e.g. amyotrophic lateral sclerosis), poliomyelitis and spinal muscular atrophy.

Disorders of the neuromuscular junction: myasthenia gravis, botulism, tick paralysis

Myasthenia gravis results in autoimmune destruction of the post-synaptic acetylcholine receptor and disruption of the normal reflex arc.

Botulinum toxin inhibits the proteins responsible for the normal docking of granules containing acetylcholine (Ach), preventing acetylcholine from reaching post-synaptic Ach receptors.

Tick paralysis is caused by a neurotoxin release in the tick's saliva during a blood meal. The exact mechanism is thought to be inhibition of Ach release at the neuromuscular junction.

Hyperacute upper motor neuron injury

Acute spinal cord injury in the cervical and upper thoracic cord may result in areflexia, flaccid paralysis, complete sensory loss and sympathetic autonomic dysfunction below the level of the injury, resulting in a clinical syndrome known as spinal shock.[48] In the first 24 hours following spinal cord injury, spinal cord neurons are less excitable, likely due to decreased muscle spindle excitability and segmental input from afferent pathways caused by loss of tonic facilitation by gamma motor neurons.[48]

A similar temporal pattern of hyporeflexia occurs in the hyperacute period following acute hemispheric stroke.

5

TABLE 5.19
Reflex, motor and sensory findings in disorders of the peripheral nerves

Peripheral nerve	Reflex	Muscles/ movement	Sensory	Causes of dysfunction
Axillary	None	Deltoid	Over deltoid	Anterior shoulder dislocation Fractured neck of humerus
Musculo–cutaneous	Biceps jerk	Biceps Brachialis	Lateral forearm	Rare
Radial	Triceps jerk and supinator jerk	Triceps Wrist extensors Brachioradialis Supinator	Lateral dorsal forearm and back of thumb and index finger	Crutch palsy 'Saturday night palsy' Fractured humerus Entrapment in supinator muscle
Median	Finger jerk	Long finger flexors 1st, 2nd, 3rd digits Wrist flexors Pronator forearm Abductor pollicis brevis	Lateral palm, thumb and lateral 2 fingers, lateral half of 4th digit	Carpal tunnel syndrome Direct traumatic injury
Ulnar	None	Intrinsic hand muscles except abductor pollicis brevis, lateral 2 lumbicals, opponens policis, flexor policis brevis Flexor carpi ulnaris Long flexors 4th and 5th digits	Median palm, 5th digit, and medial half of 4th digit	Trauma Prolonged bed rest Olecranon fracture Ganglion of wrist joint
Obturator	Adductor reflex	Adductor	Medial surface thigh	Pelvic neoplasm Pregnancy
Femoral	Knee jerk	Knee extension	Antero-medial surface thigh and leg to medial malleolus	Femoral hernia Pregnancy Pelvic haematoma Psoas abscess
Sciatic, peroneal division	None	Ankle dorsiflexion and eversion	Anterior leg, dorsum ankle and foot	Trauma at neck of fibula Hip fracture or dislocation
Sciatic, tibial division	Ankle jerk	Plantarflexion and inversion	Posterior leg, sole and lateral border foot	Rare

Adapted from Patten J, Neurological Differential Diagnosis, *New York: Springer-Verlag, 1977; p. 211.*

TABLE 5.20

Reflex, motor and sensory findings in disorders of the cervical and lumbosacral nerve roots

Nerve root	Reflex	Muscles/ movement	Sensory	Causes of dysfunction
C5	Biceps jerk	Deltoid Supraspinatus Infraspinatus Rhomboids	Lateral border upper arm	Brachial neuritis Cervical spondylosis Upper brachial plexus avulsion
C6	Supinator jerk	Brachioradialis Brachialis	Lateral forearm including thumb	Intervertebral disc lesion Cervical spondylosis
C7	Triceps jerk	Latissimus dorsi Pectoralis major Triceps Wrist extensors Wrist flexors	Over triceps, mid-forearm and middle finger	Intervertebral disc lesion Cervical spondylosis
C8	Finger jerk	Finger flexors Finger extensors Flexor carpi ulnaris	Medial forearm and little finger	Rare in disk lesions or spondylosis
T1	None	Intrinsic hand muscles	Axilla to olecranon	Cervical rib Thoracic outlet syndrome Pancoast's tumour Metastatic carcinoma
L2	None	Hip flexors	Across upper thigh	
L3	Adductor and knee jerk	Quadriceps and adductor	Across lower thigh	Neurofibroma Meningioma Metastases
L4	Knee jerk	Ankle inverters	Across to knee to medial malleolus	
L5	None	Ankle dorsiflexors	Leg to dorsum and sole of foot	Disk prolapse Metastases Neurofibroma
S1	Ankle jerk	Ankle plantarflexor and everters	Behind lateral malleolus to lateral foot	Disk prolapse Metastases Neurofibroma

Adapted from Patten J, Neurological Differential Diagnosis, *New York: Springer-Verlag, 1977; p. 211.*

Normal variant

Diffuse hyporeflexia, in isolation, does not necessarily represent neurological disease.[122,123] Decreased or absent reflexes are significant when accompanied by lower motor neuron signs (e.g. wasting, fasciculations, hypotonia, weakness), in instances of asymmetrical reflexes or with other focal neurological signs.

Sign value

In several studies of patients without known pre-existing neurological disease, 6–50% of patients lack bilateral ankle jerk reflexes despite reinforcement manoeuvres, and a small proportion of the population has generalised hyperreflexia.[4,122–126]

The clinical utility of reflex examination findings in detecting cervical and lumbosacral radiculopathy is presented in Table 5.21.[127–132]

Hyporeflexia and weakness is associated with several inflammatory and toxin-mediated diseases.

TABLE 5.21

Clinical utility of reflex findings in cervical and lumbosacral nerve root dysfunction

Reflex examination	Sensitivity, %	Specificity, %	Positive LR	Negative LR
Decreased biceps or brachioradialis reflex, detecting C6 radiculopathy[127]	53	96	14.2	0.5
Decreased triceps reflex, detecting C7 radiculopathy[127,128]	15–65	81–93	3.0	NS
Asymmetric quadriceps reflex, detecting L3 or L4 radiculopathy[129–131]	30–57	93–96	8.7	0.6
Asymmetric ankle jerk reflex, detecting S1 radiculopathy[36]	45–91	53–94	2.9	0.4

Adapted from McGee S, Evidence Based Physical Diagnosis, *2nd edn, St Louis: Saunders, 2007.*

Hypotonia

Relevant neuroanatomy and topographical anatomy

LOWER MOTOR NEURON
- Anterior horn grey matter, spinal cord
$$\downarrow$$
- Nerve root
⇒ Intervertebral disc
⇒ Intervertebral foramen
$$\downarrow$$
- Nerve plexus (e.g. brachial plexus)
$$\downarrow$$
- Peripheral nerve
⇒ Potential sites of nerve entrapment (e.g. carpal tunnel)

CEREBELLUM
- Vermis and flocculonodular lobe
→ Anterior corticospinal tract
→ Reticulospinal tract
→ Vestibulospinal tract
→ Tectospinal tract
- Paravermal (intermediate) hemisphere
→ Lateral corticospinal tract
→ Rubrospinal tract
- Lateral hemisphere
→ Lateral corticospinal tract

5

Description

Hypotonia is decreased resistance to passive movement due to decreased resting muscle tone. The limb may feel 'floppy', the outstretched arm when tapped may demonstrate wider than normal excursions, and the knee jerk may be abnormally pendular (i.e. swings more).[4,18]

Condition/s associated with

Less common
- Peripheral neuropathy
- Myasthenia gravis
- Guillain–Barré syndrome
- Poliomyelitis
- Botulism
- Tick paralysis

Mechanism/s

Hypotonia is caused by:

- lower motor neuron disorders
- cerebellar disorders
- hyperacute upper motor neuron disorders
- disorders of the neuromuscular junction: myasthenia gravis, botulism, tick paralysis.

Lower motor neuron disorders

Muscle denervation results in decreased resting muscle tone and flaccid paresis. Causes include radiculopathy, peripheral neuropathy and Guillain–Barré syndrome. Associated features of lower motor neuron disorders include wasting, fasciculations, weakness and hyporeflexia or areflexia.

Cerebellar disorders

The mechanism of hypotonia in cerebellar lesions is not known. Hypotonia in cerebellar disease may result from a relative paucity of neural input to the descending motor tracts (e.g. anterior corticospinal tract, reticulospinal tract, vestibulospinal tract, tectospinal tracts). Associated features of cerebellar disease include dysdiadochokinesis, intention tremor, dysmetria, nystagmus and dysarthria.

Hyperacute upper motor neuron disorders

Acute stroke and/or spinal cord injury may result in hypotonia and flaccid paresis immediately following injury. Spasticity and spastic paresis develop days to weeks later.[56] Acute spinal cord injury in the cervical and upper thoracic cord may cause hypotonia, areflexia, flaccid paralysis, complete sensory loss and autonomic dysfunction below the level of the injury, resulting in a clinical syndrome known as spinal shock.[48] The exact mechanism of spinal shock is unknown. In the first 24 hours following spinal cord injury, spinal cord neurons are less excitable, likely due to decreased muscle spindle excitability and segmental input from afferent pathways caused by loss of tonic facilitation by gamma motor neurons.[48]

Disorders of the neuromuscular junction: myasthenia gravis, botulism, tick paralysis

Botulism is caused by the bacterium *Clostridium botulinum*, which produces a toxin that blocks the release of acetylcholine at the motor terminal.[133]

See mechanisms in 'Hyporeflexia'.

Sign value

Hypotonia is most commonly a lower motor neuron sign.

Diffuse hypotonia and weakness is associated with several inflammatory and toxin-mediated diseases.

In a group of 444 patients with unilateral cerebellar lesions, hypotonia was present in 76% of patients.[4,29,30]

Intention tremor

Relevant neuroanatomy and topographical anatomy

CEREBELLUM
- Vermis and flocculonodular lobe
  - → Anterior corticospinal tract
  - → Reticulospinal tract
  - → Vestibulospinal tract
  - → Tectospinal tract
- Paravermal (intermediate) hemisphere
  - → Lateral corticospinal tract
  - → Rubrospinal tract
- Lateral hemisphere
  - → Lateral corticospinal tract

Description

Intention tremor is a slow (2–4 Hz) tremor during voluntary movement that develops as the limb approaches the target.[41] Tests to assess target seeking, such as the finger-to-nose test and heel-to-shin test, are performed to detect intention tremor.[41]

Condition/s associated with

Common

- Intoxication – alcohol, benzodiazepine
- Cerebellar infarction
- Multiple sclerosis

Less common

- Vertebral artery dissection
- Cerebellar mass lesion – tumour, abscess, AVM
- HSV cerebellitis
- Hereditary cerebellar degeneration (Freidreich's ataxia)
- Paraneoplastic cerebellar degeneration

Mechanism/s

Intention tremor is an ipsilateral cerebellar sign. Lesions of the intermediate and lateral cerebellar hemispheres may cause slow, uncoordinated and clumsy movements of the ipsilateral distal extremity that are aggravated during attempted target localisation tasks (see Table 5.22).[4] The oscillations result from uncoordinated contractions predominantly of the proximal limb musculature perpendicular to the axis of motion.[41] Delays in motor initiation and movement termination, and abnormalities of movement force and acceleration, contribute to intention tremor.[68]

Sign value

Intention tremor is an ipsilateral hemispheric cerebellar sign.

In two studies of patients with unilateral cerebellar lesions, intention tremor was present in 29%.[4,29,30]

5

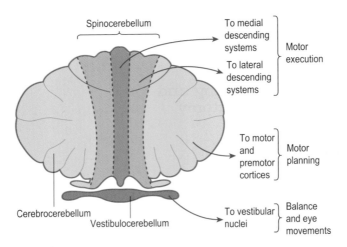

FIGURE 5.55
Functional anatomy of the cerebellum

From Barrett KE, Barman SM, Boitano S et al., Ganong's Review of Medical Physiology, *23rd edn. Modified from Kandel ER, Schwartz JH, Jessell TM (eds),* Principles of Neural Science, *4th edn, McGraw Hill, 2000.*

TABLE 5.22
Functional anatomy of the cerebellum and associated motor pathways

Cerebellar anatomy	Function	Associated motor pathways
Intermediate hemisphere	Distal limb coordination	Lateral corticospinal tracts Rubrospinal tracts
Lateral hemisphere	Motor planning, distal extremities	Lateral corticospinal tracts

Adapted from Blumenfeld H, Neuroanatomy Through Clinical Cases, *Sunderland: Sinauer, 2002.*

Internuclear ophthalmoplegia (INO)

<table>
<tr><td>

Relevant neuroanatomy and topographical anatomy

- Abducens nuclei, pons
↓
- Ø Medial longitudinal fasciculus (MLF)
↓
- Oculomotor nuclei, midbrain

</td></tr>
</table>

Description

Internuclear ophthalmoplegia (INO) is characterised by impaired adduction of the eye on the abnormal side and horizontal jerk nystagmus in the opposite eye upon lateral gaze away from the side of the lesion. The remainder of the extraocular movements, including convergence, are normal.[4,134]

Condition/s associated with[134–138]

- Multiple sclerosis
- Dorsal pontine infarction

Mechanism/s

INO is caused by a lesion in the medial longitudinal fasciculus (MLF). The MLF connects the abducens nerve (CNVI) nuclei to the oculomotor nerve (CNIII) nuclei and facilitates conjugate eye movements during lateral gaze by coordinating adduction with abduction.[134] INO should be differentiated from peripheral causes of isolated medial rectus paresis (this is called pseudo–internuclear ophthalmoplegia) including partial oculomotor nerve palsy, myasthenia gravis, Miller Fisher's syndrome and disorders of the medial rectus muscle.[134–138]

5

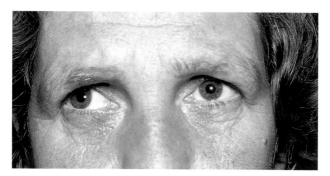

FIGURE 5.56
Right lateral gaze with evidence of left adduction paresis in a patient with internuclear ophthalmoplegia

Reproduced, with permission, from Miley JT, Rodriguez GJ, Hernandez EM et al., Neurology *2008; 70(1): e3–e4, Fig 1.*

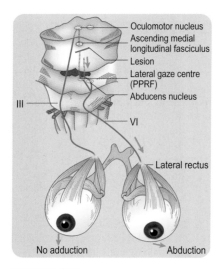

FIGURE 5.57
Schematic representation of the abducens nuclei, medial longitudinal fasciculus (MLF) and oculomotor nuclei pathways involved in internuclear ophthalmoplegia
PPRF = paramedian pontine reticular formation.

Adapted from Medscape, Overview of vertebrobasilar stroke. Available: http://emedicine. medscape.com/article/323409-media [5 Apr 2011]. Courtesy B D Decker Inc.

Sign value

In a study of patients with bilateral INO, multiple sclerosis was present in 97% of patients. The most common cause of unilateral INO was vertebrobasilar territory infarction.[139]

Jaw jerk reflex

Relevant neuroanatomy and topographical anatomy[6]

AFFERENT LIMB
⊗ Muscle spindle
↓
• Mandibular branch trigeminal nerve (CNV V3)
⇒ Foramen ovale
↓
• Trigeminal (Gasserian) ganglion
⇒ Meckel's cave, petrous bone
↓
• Mesencephalic trigeminal nucleus
↓

EFFERENT LIMB
• Motor trigeminal nucleus, pons
↓
• Trigeminal (Gasserian) ganglion
⇒ Meckel's cave, petrous bone
⇒ Foramen ovale
↓
• Mandibular branch trigeminal nerve (CNV V3)
↓
× Masseter muscle

Description

Percussion of the chin causes contraction of the masseter muscles due to activation of a monosynaptic stretch reflex.[6,58] The jaw jerk reflex may be present in the absence of neurological disease.

Condition/s associated with[6,58,107,140]

Common

• Normal variant
• Diffuse white matter disease – lacunar infarction(s)
• Vascular dementia

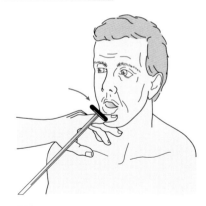

FIGURE 5.58
Jaw jerk reflex

Reproduced, with permission, from Walker HK, Hall WD, Hurst JW, Clinical Methods: The History, Physical, and Laboratory Examinations, *3rd edn, Boston: Butterworths, 1990: Fig 50.2.*

5

Less common

- Motor neuron disease (amyotrophic lateral sclerosis)
- Bilateral cerebral infarction
- Multiple sclerosis
- Progressive multifocal leucoencephalopathy (PML)
- Central pontine myelinolysis

Mechanism/s

A brisk jaw jerk reflex is a sign of bilateral upper motor neuron disease. Loss of supranuclear innervation of the motor trigeminal nucleus causes hyperexcitability of alpha motor neurons innervating the masseter muscles (see 'Hyperreflexia' in this chapter).[107]

Sign value

A brisk jaw jerk reflex is a sign of bilateral upper motor neuron disease above the pons.

Jolt accentuation

Description

Rapid horizontal rotation of the neck (2–3 Hz) in a patient with suspected meningeal irritation results in exacerbation of pre-existing headache.

Condition/s associated with

- Meningitis, bacterial
- Meningitis, viral
- Meningitis, fungal
- Meningitis, aseptic

Mechanism/s

Rotational and centrifugal forces upon inflamed meninges are thought to exacerbate cephalgia when meningeal irritation is present.

Sign value

A study of 197 patients who underwent lumbar puncture with suspected meningitis reported a sensitivity of 21% and a specificity of 82% for CSF pleocytosis (i.e. meningitis of any aetiology). Based upon the most recent data, jolt accentuation is inadequately sensitive to rule out suspected meningitis and has limited utility to predict meningitis.[141]

A lumbar puncture should be performed in patients with suspected meningitis.

5

Kernig's sign

Relevant neuroanatomy and topographical anatomy
• meninges: dura mater ⇒ spinal nerves

Description

With the patient lying supine with the hip flexed to 90°, the examiner attempts to passively extend the knee from 90°. Resistance to passive knee extension at less than 135° is considered a positive sign.[4]

Condition/s associated with

- Meningitis, bacterial
- Meningitis, viral
- Meningitis, fungal
- Meningitis, aseptic

Mechanism/s

Passive extension of the knee with the hip at 90° results in mechanical stress on the spinal nerves, arachnoid mater and subarachnoid space. When the subarachnoid space is inflamed, as in meningitis, mechanical forces on the arachnoid mater result in resistance to further movement to prevent worsening discomfort.[50]

Sign value

Thomas et al. reported a sensitivity of 5%, a positive likelihood ratio of 0.95 and a negative likelihood ratio of 1.0.[51] Nakao JH et al. reported a sensitivity of 2% and specificity of 97%. Kernig's sign is inadequately sensitive to use as a screening manoeuvre for suspected meningitis.[141] Kernig's sign has limited utility.

In patients with suspected meningitis (i.e. overall history and physical examination), a lumbar puncture should be performed.

Light—near dissociation

<table>
<tr><td>

Relevant neuroanatomy and topographical anatomy[9]

Accommodation and pupillary light pathways

AFFERENT STRUCTURES
- Retinal neuroepithelium
  ↓
- Optic nerve (CNII)
  ↓
- Pretectal nucleus midbrain
  ↓
↔ Bilateral innervation of Edinger—Westphal nuclei
  ↓

EFFERENT STRUCTURES
- Visual cortex (accommodation only)
  ↓
- Accommodation area, visual cortex (accommodation only)
  ↓
- Pretectal nuclei, midbrain ⇒ Pineal gland
  ↓
- Edinger—Westphal nuclei, midbrain
  ↓
- Oculomotor nerve (CNIII)
  ↓
- Ciliary ganglion
  ↓
- Short ciliary nerves
  ↓
× Pupillary constrictor muscles
× Ciliary muscle
× Medial rectus muscles

</td></tr>
</table>

Description

Light—near dissociation is characterised by:[9]
- normal accommodation response (pupils constrict to near stimuli)
- sluggish or absent pupillary light response.

Light—near dissociation is present if the near pupillary response (tested in moderate light) exceeds the best pupillary response with a bright light source.[9] Light—near dissociation is associated with Argyll Robertson pupils (see 'Argyll Robertson pupils' in this chapter).

Condition/s associated with[4,9]

Common
- Dorsal midbrain lesion
- Argyll Robertson pupils

Less common
- Pinealoma
- Hydrocephalus
- Multiple sclerosis
- Neurosarcoidosis
- Adie's tonic pupil

Mechanism/s

Causes of light—near dissociation include:
- dorsal midbrain lesion
- Adie's tonic pupil
- Argyll Robertson pupils.

Dorsal midbrain lesion

Loss of pretectal light input to oculomotor nuclei, due to a lesion in the tectum of the midbrain, results in impaired pupillary response with preservation of the accommodation

5

pathways. Dorsal midbrain syndrome (called Parinaud's syndrome) is a clinical syndrome associated with a lesion of the posterior commissure and interstitial nucleus characterised by:[7,13,142]

- vertical gaze palsy
- normal to large pupils with light—near dissociation
- convergence—retraction nystagmus
- eyelid retraction.

Adie's tonic pupil

The five characteristics of Adie's tonic pupil are:[4,14-16]

1 unilateral mydriasis
2 decreased or absent pupillary light reaction

3 delayed near—light reaction in pupillary constriction and accommodation
4 pupillary constrictor sensitivity to pilocarpine
5 vermiform movements of iris sphincter.

Adie's tonic pupil is caused by injury to the ciliary ganglion and/or postganglionic fibres and results in abnormal regrowth of the short ciliary nerves.[4] Normally, the ciliary ganglion sends 30 times more nerve fibres to the ciliary muscle than to the pupillary constrictor muscle.[14-16] Adie's tonic pupil is mostly commonly idiopathic and benign. Other aetiologies include orbital trauma, orbital tumours and varicella zoster infection in the

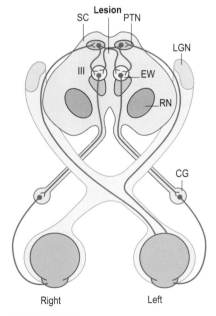
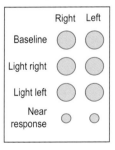

FIGURE 5.59
Pupillary response associated with light—near dissociation due to lesion in the pretectum
CG = ciliary ganglion; EW = Edinger—Westphal nucleus; LGN = lateral geniculate nucleus; PTN = pretectal nucleus; RN = red nucleus; SC = superior colliculus.

Reproduced, with permission, from Goldman L, Ausiello D, Cecil Medicine, 23rd edn, Philadelphia: Saunders, 2007: Fig 450-2.

ophthalmic division of the trigeminal nerve.[4]

Argyll Robertson pupils

See 'Argyll Robertson pupils' in this chapter.

Sign value

Light–near dissociation is associated with a dorsal midbrain lesion. It is classically associated with Argyll Robertson pupils in tertiary syphilis.

5

Myotonia – percussion, grip

Description

Percussion myotonia is a sustained muscle contraction following percussion of a muscle.[4] Grip myotonia is a sustained muscle contraction following forceful contraction of the hand muscles.[4]

Relevant neuroanatomy and topographical anatomy[143–145]
× Muscle ion channels

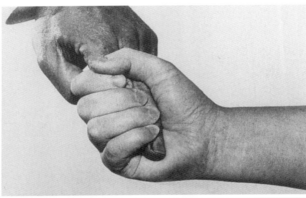

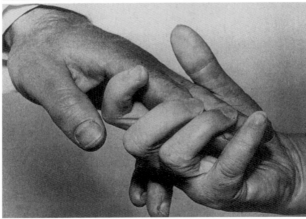

FIGURE 5.60
Grip myotonia

Reproduced, with permission, from Libby P, Bonow RO, Mann DL, Zipes DP, Braunwald's Heart Disease: A Textbook of Cardiovascular Medicine, *8th edn, Philadelphia: Saunders, 2007: Fig 87-7.*

Condition/s associated with

Common

- Myotonic dystrophy

Less common

- Myotonia congenita
- Paramyotonia congenita

Mechanism/s

Myotonia results from electrical instability of the sarcolemmal membrane causing prolonged depolarisation of the muscle fibres. Causes include:

- myotonia congenita
- myotonic dystrophy
- paramyotonia congenita.

Myotonia congenita

In myotonia congenita, abnormal sarcolemmal chloride channels cause prolonged depolarisation of the sarcolemmal membrane and muscle hyperexcitability.[143]

Myotonic dystrophy

Myotonic dystrophy is a trinucleotide repeat disorder, which is thought to arise from abnormal gene transcription of the genes adjacent to the myotonic dystrophy protein kinase (MDPK) gene on chromosome 19q13.3.[144] Studies have shown that abnormally transcribed mRNA is directly toxic and causes abnormal splicing variants in various mRNA transcripts, including a muscle chloride ion channel.[145] Disease progression causes progressive muscle weakness. Myotonia may eventually disappear in severely affected muscle groups.[144]

Paramyotonia congenita

Paramyotonia congenita is a form of potassium-sensitive myotonia. It is caused by a mutation in a gene on chromosome 17q which encodes a sodium channel protein. The myotonia typically affects the muscles of the face and hands and is exacerbated by repetitive exercise and cold temperatures.[143,144]

Sign value

Myotonia is associated with ion channel disorders (channelopathies).

5

Oculomotor nerve (CNIII) palsy

Description

Oculomotor nerve (CNIII) palsy is characterised by the following findings in the primary gaze position:[4]

- hypotropia (eye deviated down)
- exotropia (eye deviated out)
- ptosis
- mydriasis.

There is impaired elevation, depression, adduction and extorsion of the affected eye.

Oculomotor nerve palsy can be complete (gaze paresis, ptosis, mydriasis), pupillary sparing (gaze paresis, ptosis) or with isolated pupil involvement (mydriasis only).

Condition/s associated with[1,146–151]

Common

- Diabetic mononeuropathy/ microvascular infarction
- Uncal herniation

Less common

- Posterior communicating (PCOM) artery aneurysm
- Ophthalmoplegic migraine (transient)
- Mass lesion – tumour, abscess, AVM

Mechanism/s

Complete oculomotor nerve palsy

The oculomotor nerve innervates all of the extraocular muscles except the

---

Relevant neuroanatomy and topographical anatomy

- Edinger–Westphal nuclei, midbrain
  ↓
- Oculomotor nuclei, midbrain
  ↓
- Oculomotor nerve
⇒ Posterior communicating (PComm) artery, circle of Willis
⇒ Uncus, medial temporal lobe
⇒ Subarachnoid space
⇒ Superior orbital fissure
⇒ Cavernous sinus
⇒ Orbital apex
  ↓
x EOMs: medial rectus, superior rectus, inferior rectus, inferior oblique muscles
x Pupillary constrictor muscle
x Levator palpebrae muscle

---

superior oblique and lateral rectus muscles (i.e. superior rectus, medial rectus, inferior rectus, inferior oblique). Weakness of the pupillary constrictor muscles and levator palpebrae muscle causes mydriasis and ptosis, respectively. Mechanisms of clinical findings in oculomotor nerve palsy are listed in Table 5.23.

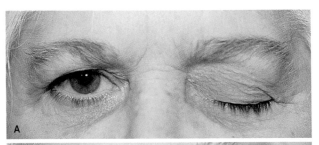

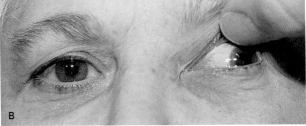

FIGURE 5.61
Complete oculomotor nerve (CNIII) palsy
A Complete left ptosis; **B** left exotropia and hypotropia.
Reproduced, with permission, from Yanoff M, Duker JS, Ophthalmology, 3rd edn, St Louis: Mosby, 2008: Fig 11-10-2.

5

TABLE 5.23
Mechanisms of the clinical features of oculomotor nerve (CNIII) palsy

Feature of oculomotor nerve palsy	Mechanism
Hypotropia	→ Unopposed superior oblique muscle
Exotropia	→ Unopposed lateral rectus muscle
Ptosis	→ Levator palpebrae weakness
Mydriasis	→ Pupillary constrictor muscle weakness
Impaired elevation	→ Superior rectus muscle weakness
Impaired depression	→ Inferior rectus muscle weakness
Impaired adduction	→ Medial rectus muscle weakness
Impaired extorsion	→ Inferior oblique muscle weakness

Oculomotor nerve palsy with pupil sparing

The central fibres of the oculomotor nerve are more vulnerable to microvascular infarction. A lesion limited to the central fibres of the oculomotor nerve may result in oculomotor nerve palsy with pupillary sparing.

Oculomotor nerve palsy with isolated pupil involvement

The fibres of the oculomotor nerve innervating the pupillary constrictor muscle are located superomedially near the nerve surface and are particularly prone to compressive lesions.[1,150] Compressive peripheral lesions of the oculomotor nerve may initially manifest with isolated pupil involvement.

In general, causes of oculomotor nerve (CNIII) palsy include:

- disorders of the nerve segment in the subarachnoid space
- diabetic mononeuropathy and microvascular infarction
- cavernous sinus syndrome (multiple cranial nerve abnormalities)
- orbital apex syndrome (multiple cranial nerve abnormalities)

Disorders of the nerve segment in the subarachnoid space

Compression of the oculomotor nerve spanning the subarachnoid space is caused by mass lesions (e.g. tumour, abscess), posterior communicating (PCOM) artery aneurysm and uncal herniation.

Posterior communicating (PCOM) artery aneurysm

The oculomotor nerve exits the midbrain adjacent to the posterior communicating (PCOM) artery, posterior cerebral artery (PCA) and superior cerebellar arteries (SCAs). Aneurysms of any of these arteries can cause oculomotor nerve palsy. Aneurysms of the PCOM artery are the most common.[148] Early diagnosis is potentially life-saving, as there is a risk of aneurysm rupture and death.

Uncal herniation (Hutchinson's pupil)

See 'Hutchinson's pupil' in this chapter.

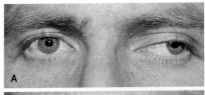
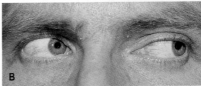
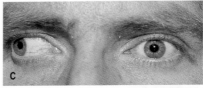
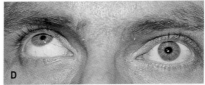
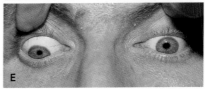

FIGURE 5.62

Partial left oculomotor nerve (CNIII) palsy **A** Primary gaze position, with mild ptosis, exotropia, hypotropia, mild mydriasis of left eye; **B** normal left gaze; **C** right gaze with impaired adduction left eye; **D** upward gaze with poor elevation left eye; **E** downward gaze with impaired depression left eye.

Reproduced, with permission, from Yanoff M, Duker JS, Ophthalmology, 3rd edn, St Louis: Mosby, 2008: Fig 11-10-1.

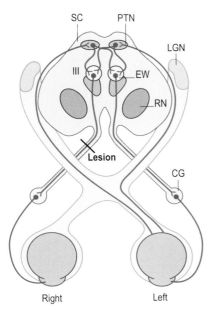

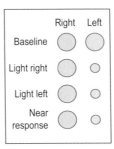

FIGURE 5.63
Pupillary response associated with oculomotor nerve palsy
CG = ciliary ganglion; EW = Edinger–Westphal nucleus; LGN = lateral geniculate nucleus;
PTN = pretectal nucleus; RN = red nucleus; SC = superior colliculus.

*Reproduced, with permission, from Goldman L, Ausiello D, Cecil Medicine, 23rd edn, Philadelphia:
Saunders, 2007: Fig 450-2.*

5

Diabetic mononeuropathy and microvascular infarction

Diabetes mellitus causes various cranial mononeuropathies due to diabetic vasculopathy of the vasa nervorum (i.e. disease of the blood supply of the peripheral nerve), resulting in microvascular infarction of the nerve.[3]

Cavernous sinus syndrome

See 'Cavernous sinus syndrome' in this chapter.

Orbital apex syndrome

See 'Orbital apex syndrome' in this chapter.

Sign value

In a group of patients with oculomotor nerve palsy due to aneurysmal compression, 95% had abnormal pupil findings (e.g. mydriasis, abnormal light reflex). 73% of patients with microvascular infarction of the oculomotor nerve demonstrated a pupil-sparing oculomotor nerve (CNIII) palsy.[150–157] Refer to Table 5.24 for the causes of oculomotor nerve palsy.

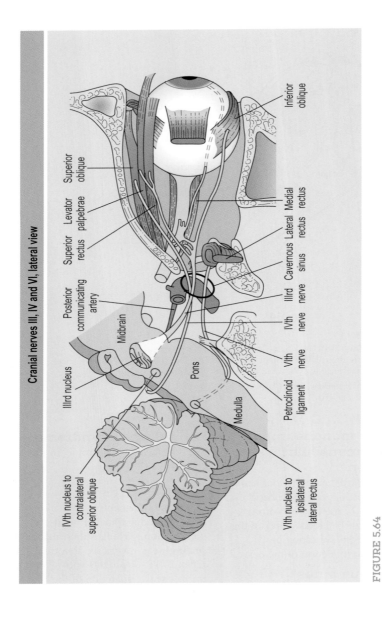

Cranial nerves III, IV and VI, lateral view

IIIrd nucleus

IVth nucleus to contralateral superior oblique

VIth nucleus to ipsilateral lateral rectus

Midbrain

Pons

Medulla

Posterior communicating artery

Superior rectus

Levator palpebrae

Superior oblique

Inferior oblique

Petroclinoid ligament

VIth nerve

IVth nerve

IIIrd nerve

Cavernous sinus

Lateral rectus

Medial rectus

FIGURE 5.64

Anatomy of the oculomotor nerve (CNIII), lateral view

Reproduced, with permission, from Yanoff M, Duker JS, Ophthalmology, 3rd edn, St Louis: Mosby, 2008: Fig 9-15-1.

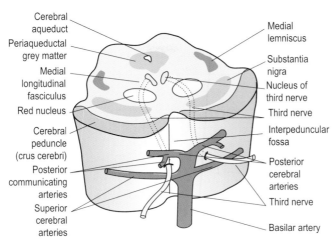

Anatomy of midbrain at the level of the third nerve nucleus

FIGURE 5.65

Neuroanatomy of the oculomotor nerve brainstem exit points, including the posterior cerebral arteries, posterior communicating arteries and superior cerebellar arteries

Reproduced, with permission, from Yanoff M, Duker JS, Ophthalmology, 3rd edn, St Louis: Mosby, 2008: Fig 9-14-2.

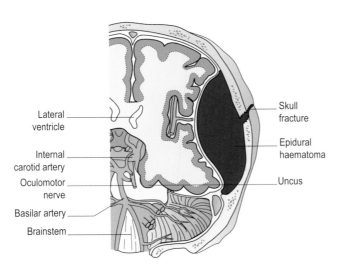

FIGURE 5.66

Schematic representation of uncal herniation resulting in oculomotor nerve compression

Reproduced, with permission, from Marx JA, Hockberger RS, Walls RM et al., Rosen's Emergency Medicine, 7th edn, Philadelphia: Mosby, 2010: Fig 38-5.

TABLE 5.24
Causes of acquired third nerve palsy

Cause(s)	Adults (%)
Trauma	14
Neoplasm	11
Aneurysm	12
Vascular/diabetic	23
Other	16
Idiopathic	24

Adapted from Kodsi SR, Younge BR, Acquired oculomotor, trochlear, and abducent cranial nerve palsies in pediatric patients. Am J Ophthalmol *1992; 114: 568–574.*

Optic atrophy

Description
The optic disc appears asymmetrical, smaller in size, and pale white in colour.[18]

Relevant neuroanatomy and topographical anatomy
• Optic nerve ⇒ Orbital apex ⇒ Optic canal ⇒ Subarachnoid space

Condition/s associated with[158,159]

Common
- Anterior ischaemic optic neuropathy (AION)
- Multiple sclerosis

Less common
- Chronic optic neuritis
- Glaucoma
- Tumour
- Thyroid eye disease
- Leber's hereditary optic neuropathy

5

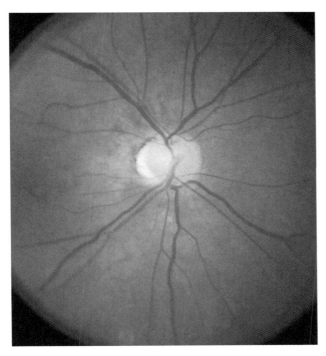

FIGURE 5.67
Optic atrophy

Reproduced, with permission, from Isaacson RS, Optic atrophy. In: Ferri FF, Clinical Advisor 2011. Philadelphia: Mosby, 2011: Fig 1-220.

Mechanism/s

Optic atrophy is caused by a long-standing lesion of the optic nerve or by increased intracranial pressure. The patient may have associated bedside clinical evidence of optic nerve dysfunction (e.g. decreased visual acuity, central scotoma).[159]

Sign value

Optic atrophy is caused by degeneration of the fibres of the optic nerve due to a lesion of the optic nerve of at least 4–6 weeks duration.[159,160]

Orbital apex syndrome

Relevant neuroanatomy and topographical anatomy

ORBITAL APEX CONTENTS
• Optic nerve (CNII)
• Oculomotor nerve (CNIII)
• Trochlear nerve (CNIV)
• Ophthalmic division (V1) trigeminal nerve (CNV)
• Abducens nerve (CNVI)
• Sympathetic plexus
    ⇒ Venous plexus
    ⇒ Periorbital soft tissue

Description

Orbital apex syndrome is a cranial nerve syndrome associated with proptosis, involving the contents of the orbital apex:[6,49]

- optic nerve (CNII)
- oculomotor nerve (CNIII)
- trochlear nerve (CNIV)
- ophthalmic division of the trigeminal nerve (CNV V1)
- abducens nerve (CNVI)
- sympathetic fibres.

Condition/s associated with[6,49]

Common

- Tolosa–Hunt syndrome
- Orbital granuloma

Less common

- Mucormycosis
- Retrobulbar haemorrhage
- Graves' ophthalmopathy

Mechanism/s

Typically, an enlarging infectious or inflammatory mass at the orbital apex leads to proptosis and pain. Proptosis is related to mass effect on the orbital contents.[49] Unlike in cavernous sinus syndrome, patients typically have early involvement of the optic nerve (CNII) with evidence of visual loss or an afferent pupillary defect.[6,49] The mechanisms of clinical features in orbital apex syndrome are listed in Table 5.25.

Sign value

Orbital apex syndrome is an emergency and has a high morbidity.

5

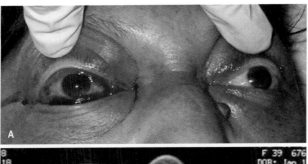

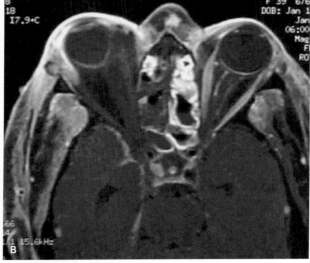

FIGURE 5.68
Patient with rhinocerebral mucormycosis resulting in orbital apex syndrome
A Patient with prominent right proptosis and ophthalmoplegia; **B** MRI of right retro-orbital infectious mass.

Reproduced, with permission, from Yanoff M, Duker JS, Ophthalmology, 3rd edn, St Louis: Mosby, 2008: Fig 9-23-1.

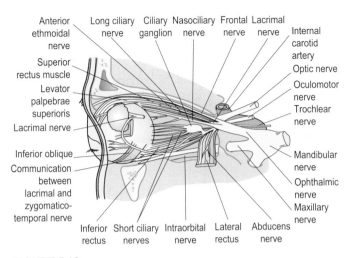

FIGURE 5.69
Anatomy of the contents of the orbital apex

Reproduced, with permission, from Daroff RB, Bradley WG et al., Neurology in Clinical Practice, *5th edn, Philadelphia: Butterworth-Heinemann, 2008: Fig 74-1.*

TABLE 5.25
Mechanisms of clinical signs in orbital apex syndrome

Clinical signs and sequelae	Cranial nerve dysfunction
Decreased visual acuity, afferent pupillary defect, decreased colour vision, decreased brightness sense	→ Optic nerve (CNII)
Extraocular muscle paresis Mydriasis and poorly reactive pupil Ptosis	→ Oculomotor nerve (CNIII)
Superior oblique muscle paresis	→ Trochlear nerve (CNIV)
Hypoaesthesia or anaesthesia distribution ophthalmic nerve Decreased corneal sensation	→ Ophthalmic branch, trigeminal nerve (CNV V1)
Abducens muscle paresis	→ Abducens nerve (CNVI)

5

Palmomental reflex

Relevant neuroanatomy and topographical anatomy
• Frontal lobes

Description

The palmomental reflex is characterised by ipsilateral contraction of the mentalis muscle (lower lip protrusion or wrinkling) when the examiner strokes the patient's thenar eminence.[4] The palmomental reflex is a primitive reflex that is normally present in infancy.[4] The reflex may reappear later in life due to frontal lobe disease or normal ageing.[97]

Condition/s associated with

Common

- Normal variant
- Alzheimer's dementia
- Frontotemporal dementia
- Vascular dementia

Less common

- Parkinson's disease
- Advanced HIV/AIDS

Mechanism/s

The mechanism of re-emergence of the palmomental reflex is unknown. The reflex is likely controlled by nonprimary motor cortical areas, which exert an inhibitory control of the spinal reflex.[161] Damage to these areas may result in disinhibition and thus 'release' the reflex.[91,161]

Sign value

In a study of 39 patients with a unilateral palmomental reflex, an ipsilateral cerebral hemisphere lesion was found in 44%, a contralateral lesion in 36%, bilateral lesions in 10% and no lesions were found in 10%.[162] The side of the reflex does not always correlate with the side of the lesion.[162] The palmomental sign may be present in approximately 3–70% of normal subjects.[4,92–94,163–166]

Papilloedema

Relevant neuroanatomy and topographical anatomy

- Optic disc
  ↓
- Optic nerve
  ⇒ Optic canal
  ⇒ Orbital apex
  ⇒ Cavernous sinus
  ⇒ Subarachnoid space
  ⇒ Midbrain

Description

Papilloedema is swelling and blurring of the optic disc margins.

Condition/s associated with

Common

- Optic neuritis
- Elevated intracranial pressure, any cause

Less common

- Drugs – ethambutol, chloramphenicol
- Idiopathic intracranial hypertension (IIH)
- Optic nerve lesion – tumour, AVM
- Hydrocephalus

Mechanism/s

Papilloedema is caused by increased intracranial pressure or a compression lesion of the optic nerve. Disc swelling papilloedema results from blockage of axoplasmic flow in neurons of the optic nerve, resulting in swelling of the axoplasm of the optic disc.[160] Papilloedema is associated with other signs of optic nerve dysfunction (e.g. decreased visual acuity, relative afferent pupillary defect [RAPD], monocular vision loss). The most common visual defects in acute papilloedema are enlargement of the physiological blind spot, concentric constriction and inferior nasal field loss.[160]

Sign value

Papilloedema is a sign of optic nerve (CNII) swelling due to increased intracranial pressure or a compressive optic nerve lesion.

5

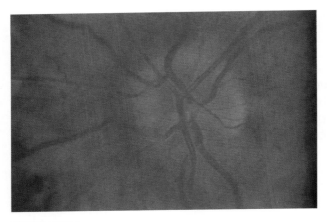

FIGURE 5.70
Swollen optic disc in early papilloedema

Reproduced, with permission, from Daroff RB, Bradley WG et al., Neurology in Clinical Practice, *5th edn, Philadelphia: Butterworth-Heinemann, 2008: Fig 15-9.*

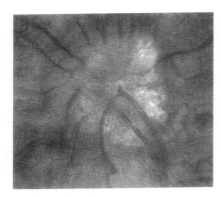

FIGURE 5.71
Chronic papilloedema with marked disc elevation and gliosis

Reproduced, with permission, from Daroff RB, Bradley WG et al., Neurology in Clinical Practice, *5th edn, Philadelphia: Butterworth-Heinemann, 2008: Fig 15-11.*

Parkinsonian gait

<table>
<tr><td>

Relevant neuroanatomy and topographical anatomy

BASAL GANGLIA
- Globus pallidus pars Interna
- Globus pallidus pars externa
- Putamen
- Caudate nucleus
- Substantia nigra
- Subthalamic nuclei
- Striatum

</td></tr>
</table>

Description

The parkinsonian gait is characterised by a reduced arm swing, increased tremor of the upper extremity during walking, turning en bloc and slow, shuffling gait on a narrow base.[28,43] Patients may initiate walking with a series of rapid, short, shuffling steps prior to breaking into a normal stepping pattern (i.e. start hesitation).[28] Once walking is initiated, it may be interrupted by short shuffling steps or cessation of movement (i.e. freezing) if an obstacle is encountered.[28]

Condition/s associated with[4,28,41,43,45]

Common
- Parkinson's disease
- Dopamine antagonists – haloperidol, metoclopramide

Less common
- Lacunar infarction, basal ganglia
- Basal ganglia haemorrhage
- Multisystem atrophy
- Progressive supranuclear palsy
- Corticobasilar degeneration

Mechanism/s

Postural changes in parkinsonism (e.g. stooped posture, shoulder flexion) move the patient's centre of gravity forward, worsening balance during locomotion. During initiation of movement, patients may take a series of small, rapid steps (i.e. festination) to accommodate for balance disequilibrium caused by the generalised flexion posture.[28] See also 'Bradykinesia' in this chapter.

Sign value

Parkinsonian gait is associated with Parkinson's disease, the Parkinson's plus syndromes and anti–dopaminergic drug effects.

5

Parkinsonian tremor

Relevant neuroanatomy and topographical anatomy

BASAL GANGLIA
- Globus pallidus pars interna
- Globus pallidus pars externa
- Putamen
- Caudate nucleus
- Substantia nigra
- Subthalamic nuclei
- Striatum

Description

The parkinsonian tremor is a 4–6 Hz 'pill-rolling' tremor of the fingertips, hand and forearm that is more pronounced at rest (i.e. a resting tremor).[4]

Condition/s associated with[4,41]

Common

- Parkinson's disease
- Drugs – dopamine antagonists (e.g. haloperidol, metoclopramide)

Less common

- Lacunar infarction, basal ganglia
- Basal ganglia haemorrhage
- Multisystem atrophy
- Progressive supranuclear palsy
- Corticobasilar degeneration

Mechanism/s

The mechanism of parkinsonian tremor is controversial. Rhythmic and synchronous excitation of neurons in the subthalamic nucleus and globus pallidus pars interna correlates with tremor in the limbs of patients with Parkinson's disease and monkeys treated with MPTP.[44,167] The underlying pathophysiology may be due to one or more central pacemakers or circuits of oscillating neuronal activity in the basal ganglia.[168]

Sign value

Refer to Table 5.26.

TABLE 5.26
Clinical utility of resting tremor in Parkinson's disease[167]

	Sensitivity	Specificity	Positive LR	Negative LR
Resting tremor[45]	76%	39%	NS	NS

Adapted from McGee S, Evidence Based Physical Diagnosis, *2nd edn, St Louis: Saunders, 2007.*

Photophobia

Relevant neuroanatomy and topographical anatomy
⇒ Cornea ⇒ Uvea
↓   ↓ • Non-image-forming retinal neuroepithelium   • Ophthalmic division (VI) trigeminal nerve (CNV) and C2, C3 sensory nerve cells, optic nerve   • Meninges ↓   ↓   ↓ • Region posterior thalamus, pain pathway

Description

Photophobia is light-induced ocular and/or cephalic discomfort.[169] The patient exhibits discomfort and aversion to light stimuli, resulting in involuntary eye closure and/or gaze deviation.

Condition/s associated with[169,170]

Common

- Migraine headache
- Corneal abrasion
- Keratitis – UV, contact lens

Less common

- Glaucoma
- Subarachnoid haemorrhage, aneurysmal
- Meningitis – bacterial, viral, fungal, aseptic
- Anterior uveitis
- HSV keratitis

Mechanism/s

The mechanism of photophobia is controversial.[169,171] Photophobia may be a protective mechanism that protects the central retina from potentially damaging short wavelength visible light.[169,171]

Causes of photophobia include:

- inflammation of the meninges
- migraine
- corneal injury
- anterior uveitis.

Inflammation of the meninges

Meningeal irritation is caused by infection, non-infectious inflammation, chemical inflammation and subarachnoid haemorrhage. Associated signs of meningeal irritation include nuchal rigidity, Kernig's sign, Brudzinski's sign and jolt accentuation.

Migraine

Non-image-forming retinal neuroepithelial cells project to an area in the posterior thalamus that also receives input from the dura mater. The cells in the posterior thalamus respond to input from both the non-image-forming retinal

5

neuroepithelial cells and trigeminal and cervical nerves innervating the dura mater. In migraine, it has been suggested that input from the retinal neuroepithelial cells potentially augments migraine pain, resulting in photophobia.[171]

Corneal injury

Traumatic and inflammatory disorders of the cornea cause photophobia. The cornea is densely innervated, and light exacerbates ocular discomfort. Causes include contact lens acute red eye and corneal abrasion.

Anterior uveitis

Inflammation or mechanical irritation of the iris, pupillary sphincter muscle and radial muscle cause photophobia. Discomfort is likely exacerbated by mechanical stress due to the change in pupil size during the pupillary light response and hippus.[170]

Sign value

Photophobia is a sign of meningeal irritation, but is also associated with several other neurological and ocular disorders.

Photophobia occurs in more than 80% of patients with migraine.[170]

Physiological tremor

<table>
<tr><td>Relevant neuroanatomy and topographical anatomy</td></tr>
</table>

→ Sympathetic nervous system
× Agonist and antagonist muscle groups

Description

Physiological tremor is a 7–12 Hz tremor, typically more pronounced in the outstretched arm (i.e. a postural tremor).[4,18,172] Physiological tremor occurs in all normal subjects, although it may not be visible to the naked eye. Enhanced physiological tremor (i.e. the tremor becomes more prominent) is caused by a provoking factor such as hyperthyroidism, hypoglycaemia, drug withdrawal states, anxiety or fear.

Condition/s associated with

Common

• Normal

Less common (i.e. enhanced physiological tremor)

• Hyperthyroidism
• Hypoglycaemia

• Withdrawal states
• Sympathomimetic agents
• Fatigue
• Anxiety
• Fear

Mechanism/s

Physiological tremor is mechanical in origin and results from oscillation of agonist and antagonist muscle groups due to the combined effect of firing motor neurons, synchronisation of muscle spindle feedback and mechanical properties of the limbs.[172] Enhanced physiological tremor is caused by increases in circulating catecholamines (e.g. adrenaline, noradrenaline) and/or catecholamine receptor upregulation (e.g. hyperthyroidism), which increase the twitch force of motor units.[173]

Sign value

Uncomplicated physiological tremor is present in many normal individuals. Enhanced physiological tremor may be associated with an underlying disorder (e.g. hyperthyroidism, sympathomimetic agent toxicity, withdrawal state).[174]

5

Pinpoint pupils

Relevant neuroanatomy and topographical anatomy

Central pathways
- Kappa-1 (κ_1) receptor
- Alpha-2 (α_2) receptor

Sympathetic pathway
FIRST-ORDER NEURON
- Hypothalamus

  ↓

- Sympathetic fibres, brainstem

  ↓

- Sympathetic fibres, intermediate horn, spinal cord

  ↓

SECOND-ORDER NEURON (PREGANGLIONIC FIBRE)
- Sympathetic trunk

  ↓

- Superior cervical ganglion C2

  ↓

THIRD-ORDER NEURON (POSTGANGLIONIC FIBRE)
- Superior cervical ganglion C2

  ↓

- Ciliary body

  ↓

- × Pupillary dilator muscles

Parasympathetic pathway
- Edinger–Westphal nucleus, midbrain

  ↓

- Oculomotor nerve (CNIII)

  ↓

- Ciliary ganglion

  ↓

- Short ciliary nerves

  ↓

- Neuromuscular junction

  ↓

- × Pupillary constrictor muscle
- ⇒ Iris

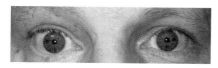

FIGURE 5.72
Bilateral pinpoint pupils, less than 2 mm in diameter and symmetric

Murphy SM et al., Neuromuscular Disorders *2011; 21(3): 223–226, Copyright © 2010 Elsevier B.V.*

Description

Pinpoint pupils are symmetric, constricted pupils with a diameter <2 mm.

Condition/s associated with[175–178]

Common
- Opioid – morphine, heroin
- Senile miosis

Less common
- Pontine haemorrhage
- Cholinergic toxicity – organophosphate poisoning
- Upward transtentorial herniation
- Central α-2 agonist – clonidine, dexmedetomidine
- Beta-adrenergic antagonist – carvedilol, timolol

Mechanism/s

The causes of pinpoint pupils are:
- opioid effect
- pontine haemorrhage
- cholinergic toxicity
- α-2 agonist effect
- cerebral herniation with pontine compression
- beta-blocker effect
- senile miosis in normal ageing.

Opioid effect

Binding of opioids at central kappa-1 (κ_1) receptors causes miosis.[175] Not all opioids cause pupillary constriction due to heterogenous binding affinity at κ_1 receptors. Patients taking meperidine, propoxyphene and pentazocine may not have pupillary constriction.[175,176]

Pontine haemorrhage

Pontine haemorrhage disrupts the descending sympathetic fibres in the pons, resulting in unopposed parasympathetic input and bilateral miosis.[177] Associated features include profound bilateral cranial nerve signs (e.g. facial nerve palsy, abducens nerve palsy), motor long tract signs, coma and cerebral herniation.

Cholinergic toxicity

Cholinergic toxicity causes bilateral miosis due to potentiation of muscarinic receptors at the neuromuscular junction. Muscarinic stimulation also results in diarrhoea, urination, bradycardia, bronchorrhoea, bronchospasm, excitation of skeletal muscle, lacrimation and gastrointestinal distress.[178] Causes of cholinergic toxicity include organophosphate and carbamate toxicity (e.g. insecticide poisoning).

α-2 agonist effect

Clonidine is a central alpha-2 (α_2) receptor agonist that inhibits central sympathetic outflow. Inhibition of norepinephrine release causes decreased sympathetic outflow, resulting in bilateral miosis.[179–181]

Cerebral herniation with pontine compression

Central transtentorial herniation, cerebellotonsillar herniation and upward transtentorial herniation cause bilateral miosis due to compression of

5

the pons.[117] Central transtentorial herniation is typically caused by an expanding vertex, frontal lobe or occipital lobe lesion.[117] Cerebellotonsillar herniation is most commonly caused by a cerebellar mass or rapid displacement of the brainstem.[117,182] Upward transtentorial herniation typically results from an expanding posterior fossa lesion.[117]

Beta-blocker effect

Beta-adrenergic antagonism relaxes the pupillary dilator muscle and results in miosis.

Senile miosis in normal ageing

With normal ageing, the pupils decrease in size and have a decreased mydriatic response in low light conditions.[183]

Sign value

Pinpoint pupils are associated with several toxicological and neurological disorders. The most common rapidly reversible cause of coma with pinpoint pupils is opioid toxicity.

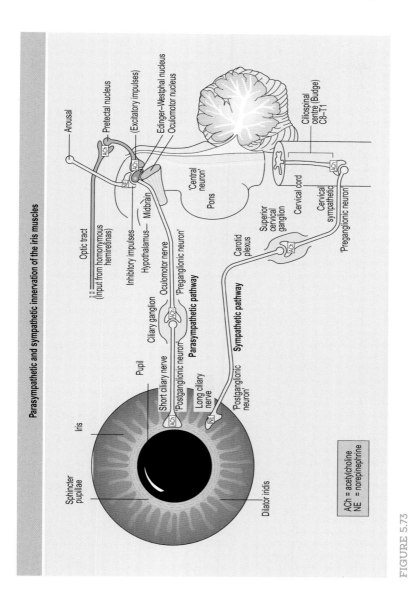

FIGURE 5.73

Parasympathetic and sympathetic pathways innervating the iris muscles

Reproduced, with permission, from Yanoff M, Duker JS, Ophthalmology, 3rd edn, St Louis: Mosby, 2008: Fig 9-19-5.

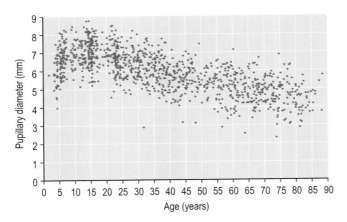

FIGURE 5.74

Changes in pupillary size (horizontal diameter) in darkness at various ages

Reproduced, with permission, from Dyck PJ, Thomas PK, Peripheral Neuropathy, *4th edn, Philadelphia: Saunders, 2005: Fig 9-5.*

Pronator drift

Relevant neuroanatomy and topographical anatomy

UPPER MOTOR NEURON
• Motor cortex
↓
• Corona radiata, subcortical white matter
↓
• Posterior limb, internal capsule
↓
• Corticospinal tracts, medial brainstem
↓
Ø Pyramidal decussation, medulla
↓
• Lateral corticospinal tracts, spinal cord

Description
There is asymmetric pronation and downward arm drift when the patient is instructed to extend both arms with palms straight facing the ceiling. Downward arm drift, forearm pronation and flexion of the wrist and elbow typically begin distally and progress proximally.[18]

Condition/s associated with

Common
• Cerebral infarction, MCA territory
• Lacunar infarction, posterior limb internal capsule

Less common
• Cerebral haemorrhage, parenchymal

• Mass lesion – tumour, abscess, AVM
• Subdural haematoma

Mechanism/s
It is a sign of unilateral upper motor lesion, typically of the contralateral cerebral hemisphere. When visual cues are removed, subtle upper motor neuron weakness causes the weak upper limb to pronate and drift downwards.

Sign value
Pronator drift is the most sensitive sign to detect subtle upper motor neuron weakness.[4,18]

Refer to Table 5.27 for clinical utility.

5

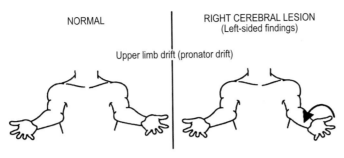

NORMAL

RIGHT CEREBRAL LESION
(Left-sided findings)

Upper limb drift (pronator drift)

FIGURE 5.75
Pronator drift: the left arm drifts outwards and rotates inwards

Based on McGee S, Evidence Based Physical Diagnosis, *2nd edn, Philadelphia: Saunders, 2007: Fig 57.1.*

TABLE 5.27
Clinical utility of pronator drift in unilateral cerebral hemisphere lesions

	Sensitivity	Specificity	Positive LR	Negative LR
Pronator drift[40,119]	79–92%	90–98%	10.3	0.1

Adapted from McGee S, Evidence Based Physical Diagnosis, *2nd edn, St Louis: Saunders, 2007.*

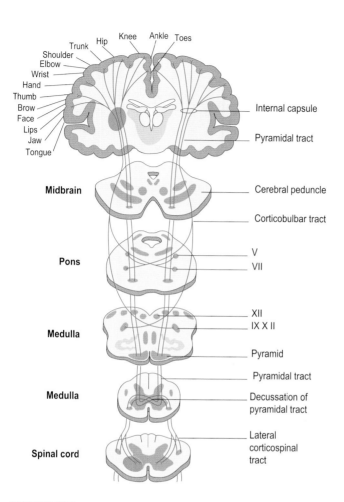

FIGURE 5.76
Upper motor neuron anatomy

Reproduced, with permission, from Clark RG, Manter and Gatz's Essential Neuroanatomy and Neurophysiology, 5th edn, Philadelphia: FA Davis Co, 1975.

Ptosis

Relevant neuroanatomy and topographical anatomy[7]

Superior tarsal muscle and sympathetic pathway

FIRST-ORDER NEURON

- Hypothalamus

↓

- Sympathetic fibres, brainstem

↓

- Sympathetic fibres, intermediate horn, spinal cord T1

↓

SECOND-ORDER NEURON (PREGANGLIONIC FIBRE)

- Sympathetic trunk
⇒ Lung apex

↓

- Superior cervical ganglion C2

↓

THIRD-ORDER NEURON (POSTGANGLIONIC FIBRE)

- Superior cervical ganglion C2
⇒ Carotid sheath
⇒ Carotid artery
⇒ Superior orbital fissure
⇒ Cavernous sinus
⇒ Orbital apex

↓

× Superior tarsal muscle

Levator palpebrae muscle and parasympathetic pathway

- Edinger–Westphal nucleus, midbrain

↓

- Oculomotor nerve (CNIII)

↓

- Posterior communicating artery, circle of Willis
⇒ Cavernous sinus
⇒ Superior orbital fissure, sphenoid bone
⇒ Orbital apex

↓

- Ciliary ganglion

↓

× Levator palpebrae muscle

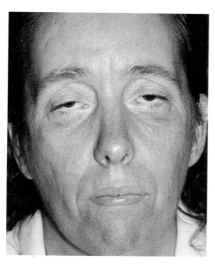

FIGURE 5.77
Patient with myotonic dystrophy with the characteristic 'hatchet facies' and bilateral ptosis

Reproduced, with permission, from Yanoff M, Duker JS, Ophthalmology, *3rd edn, St Louis: Mosby, 2008: Fig 9-17-4.*

Description

Ptosis is an abnormally droopy eyelid. It can be unilateral or bilateral. Normally, the upper eyelid covers the upper 1–2 mm of the iris, and the lower eyelid just touches the lower border of the iris.[7]

Condition/s associated with[7,184]

Common

- Levator aponeurosis dehiscence
- Dermatochalasis

Less common

- Horner's syndrome
- Oculomotor nerve (CNIII) palsy
- Myasthenia gravis (bilateral)
- Myotonic dystrophy (bilateral)

Mechanism/s

Causes of ptosis include:[7,185,186]

- Horner's syndrome
- oculomotor nerve (CNIII) palsy
- disorders of the neuromuscular junction
- myotonic dystrophy
- mechanical disorders of the periorbital connective tissue.

Horner's syndrome

Horner's syndrome is caused by a lesion in the sympathetic pathway, which innervates the superior tarsal muscle (i.e. Müller's muscle), radial muscle of the iris and sweat glands in the face. Superior tarsal muscle weakness causes ptosis in Horner's syndrome. See 'Horner's syndrome' in this chapter.

Oculomotor nerve (CNIII) palsy

The levator palpebrae muscle is innervated by the parasympathetic fibres of the oculomotor nerve. Oculomotor nerve palsy results in ptosis due to weakness of the levator palpebrae muscle.[7] See 'Oculomotor nerve (CNIII) palsy' in this chapter.

Disorders of the neuromuscular junction

Myasthenia gravis is an autoimmune disorder characterised by antibodies against post-synaptic acetylcholine receptors of the neuromuscular junction. The extraocular muscles and facial muscles are predominantly affected. In myasthenia gravis, muscle weakness increases with use (i.e. fatiguability). In addition, muscle weakness may resolve if the temperature of the muscle is decreased, which can be demonstrated with the 'ice-on-eyes' test at the bedside.[186]

Myotonic dystrophy

Unlike most other primary disorders of muscle (i.e. myopathies), myotonic dystrophy causes weakness predominantly in the facial and

5

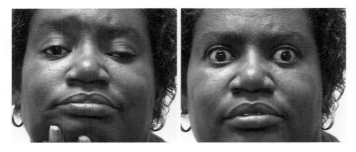

FIGURE 5.78
Patient with myasthenia gravis before and after the edrophonium test showing bilateral ptosis, more prominent on the left

Reproduced, with permission, from Daroff RB, Bradley WG et al., Neurology in Clinical Practice, *5th edn, Philadelphia: Butterworth-Heinemann, 2008: Fig 82-4.*

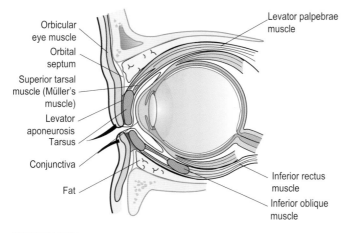

FIGURE 5.79
Anatomy of the eyelid muscles

Reproduced, with permission, from Flint PW et al., Cummings Otolaryngology: Head and Neck Surgery, *5th edn, Philadelphia: Mosby, 2010: Fig 30-9.*

peripheral muscle groups. Other features of myotonic dystrophy include percussion and grip myotonia.[184]

Mechanical disorders of the periorbital connective tissue

Levator aponeurosis dehiscence is caused by dissociation of the levator muscle and connective tissue from the tarsal insertion site. Focal swelling or degenerative changes in the skin and soft tissues of the eyelid can cause ptosis. Dermatochalasis is characterised by redundant tissue in the upper eyelid causing the upper lid to droop.

Sign value

Ptosis is a sign of primary eyelid muscle weakness, a neurological disorder or a disorder of the connective tissue of the eyelid.

Complete unilateral ptosis should prompt rapid pupillary examination to identify possible life-threatening oculomotor nerve (CNIII) palsy due to aneurysm.

Relative afferent pupillary defect (RAPD) (Marcus Gunn pupil)

Description

Relative dilation of both pupils occurs when a torch is moved from the normal side to the abnormal side (i.e. the side with the afferent pupillary defect) during the swinging torch test.[4] An afferent pupillary defect is a disorder of the afferent limb of the pupillary light response pathway (e.g. optic nerve, retinal neuroepithelium).

Relevant neuroanatomy and topographical anatomy

AFFERENT LIMB
  • Retinal neuroepithelium
    ↓
  • Optic nerve (CNII)
    ↓
  • Pretectal nucleus, midbrain
    ↓
  ↔ Bilateral innervation of Edinger–Westphal nuclei
    ↓
EFFERENT LIMB
  • Edinger–Westphal nucleus, midbrain
    ↓
  • Oculomotor nerve (CNIII)
    ↓
  • Ciliary ganglion
    ↓
  • Short ciliary nerves
    ↓
  × Pupillary constrictor muscle

Condition/s associated with[4,187]

Common

- Optic neuritis
- Anterior ischaemic optic neuropathy (AION)

Less common

- Vitreal haemorrhage
- Retinal detachment
- Retinoblastoma
- Mass lesion – tumour, abscess, AVM

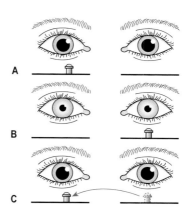

FIGURE 5.80
Schematic depiction of a right relative afferent pupillary defect identified using the swinging torch test
A Right eye illuminated; poor direct and consensual reaction; **B** excellent direct and consensual response with illumination of the left eye; **C** light swung from left to right with redilatation of both pupils.

Reproduced, with permission, from Daroff RB, Bradley WG et al., Neurology in Clinical Practice, *5th edn, Philadelphia: Butterworth-Heinemann, 2008: Fig 39-3.*

Mechanism/s

A relative afferent pupillary defect is caused by asymmetrical input to the Edinger–Westphal nuclei from the optic nerve (CNII) or retinal neuroepithelium.[4,187] Symmetrical disorders (i.e. symmetric disease in both optic nerves) will not produce a relative afferent pupillary defect. The swinging torch test is only able to detect relative differences between the two afferent pathways. Mechanisms of RAPD include:

- optic nerve disorders
- retinal neuroepithelium disorders (uncommon).

Optic nerve disorders

Asymmetric disorders of the optic nerve are the most common cause of an afferent pupillary defect. The patient may have associated clinical evidence of optic nerve dysfunction (e.g. papilloedema, decreased visual acuity, visual field defects, decreased colour vision).[159] Causes include optic neuritis, anterior ischaemic optic neuropathy (AION) and tumours of the optic nerve (e.g. optic nerve glioma). Idiopathic intracranial hypertension and other causes of elevated intracranial pressure may cause an RAPD only rarely if optic nerve dysfunction is asymmetrical.

Retinal neuroepithelium disorders (uncommon)

Severe asymmetric retinal disease is a less common cause of an afferent pupillary defect. Typically, the degree of paradoxical dilation is more subtle than in optic nerve dysfunction.[188,189] Causes include age-related macular

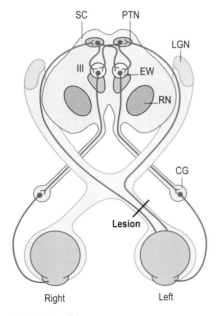

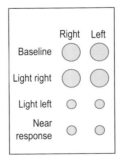

FIGURE 5.81
Pupillary response associated with RAPD
CG = ciliary ganglion; EW = Edinger–Westphal nucleus; LGN = lateral geniculate nucleus; PTN = pretectal nucleus; RN = red nucleus; SC = superior colliculus.

Reproduced, with permission, from Goldman L, Ausiello D, Cecil Medicine, 23rd edn, Philadelphia: Saunders, 2007: Fig 450-2.

degeneration, diabetic retinopathy, hypertensive retinopathy and central retinal artery occlusion.

Sign value

The sensitivity of an RAPD in the detection of unilateral optic nerve disease is 92–98%.[190,191] The relative afferent pupillary defect or Marcus Gunn pupil is an important sign classically associated with optic neuritis.

5

Rigidity

Description

Rigidity is increased resistance to passive movement due to an abnormal increase in resting muscle tone. There are three defining characteristics:[4]

1 resistance independent of the velocity of muscle stretch (i.e. the magnitude of resistance during passive movement is the same with slow or fast movement)

2 equal flexor and extensor tone

3 no associated weakness.

Rigidity is a sign of extrapyramidal disease. It is sometimes referred to as plastic, waxy or lead-pipe rigidity.[6] Rigidity may worsen with active movements of the patient's contralateral limb, a phenomenon known as activated rigidity.[61]

Relevant neuroanatomy and topographical anatomy

BASAL GANGLIA
- Globus pallidus pars interna
- Globus pallidus pars externa
- Putamen
- Caudate nucleus
- Substantia nigra
- Subthalamic nuclei
- Striatum

Condition/s associated with

Common

- Parkinson's disease
- Dopamine antagonists – haloperidol, metoclopramide

Less common

- Diffuse white matter disease – lacunar infarction(s)
- Multisystem atrophy
- Progressive supranuclear palsy
- Corticobasilar degeneration

Mechanism/s

The mechanism of rigidity in parkinsonism is not known.[44] Rigidity may result from changes in extrapyramidal regulation of supraspinal motor neurons and changes in spinal cord motor neuron activity.[44] Cogwheel rigidity is a type of rigidity associated with Parkinson's disease in which ratchet-like interruptions in muscle tone occur during passive range of motion.[61] Cogwheel rigidity has been attributed to the combined effects of rigidity and tremor.[61]

Sign value

Rigidity is a sign of an extrapyramidal disorder and neuroleptic malignant syndrome (NMS). (Table 5.28)

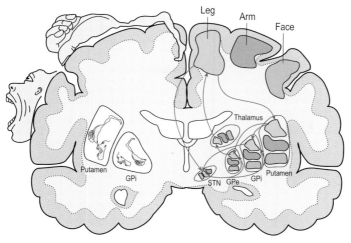

FIGURE 5.82
Basal ganglia motor circuit and somatotopic organisation
GPe = globus pallidus pars externa; GPi = globus pallidus pars interna; STN = subthalamic nucleus.

Reproduced, with permission, from Rodriguez-Oroz MC, Jahanshahi M, Krack P et al., Initial clinical manifestations of Parkinson's disease: features and pathophysiological mechanisms. Lancet Neurol *2009; 8: 1128–1139, Fig 2.*

TABLE 5.28
Clinical utility of rigidity in Parkinson's disease

Prominent rigidity on initial examination in detecting Parkinson's disease[45]	
	Sensitivity
Rigidity[45]	96%

Adapted from McGee S, Evidence Based Physical Diagnosis, *2nd edn, St Louis: Saunders, 2007.*

5

Romberg's test

Relevant neuroanatomy and topographical anatomy
• Vestibular system • Proprioceptive pathways • Visual pathways

Description

The patient is asked to stand with feet together, close both eyes and maintain the posture for 60 seconds. If the patient cannot maintain a stable stance the test is positive.[4]

Condition/s associated with

Common

- Intoxication – alcohol, benzodiazepine
- Vestibulotoxic drugs – furosemide, gentamicin

Less common

- Subacute combined degeneration of the cord (Vitamin B12 deficiency)
- Tabes dorsalis (tertiary syphilis)
- Vestibular neuritis

Mechanism/s

Three things maintain postural stability when standing: visual information, cerebellar and vestibular function, and proprioception (refer to Table 5.29). Note that the majority of patients with cerebellar lesions are unable to maintain balance despite visual cues and thus are not amenable to Romberg testing.[4,69] A positive Romberg test is caused by:

- proprioceptive dysfunction
- vestibular dysfunction.

Proprioceptive dysfunction

In patients with mild proprioceptive loss, visual cues may be sufficient to compensate for the deficit to maintain postural stability. Thus, when visual input is removed, compensation is no

TABLE 5.29
Functional anatomy of the cerebellum and associated motor pathways

Cerebellar anatomy	Function	Associated motor pathways
Vermis and flocculonodular lobe	• Proximal limb and trunk coordination • Vestibulo-ocular reflexes	• Anterior corticospinal tract • Reticulospinal tract • Vestibulospinal tract • Tectospinal tract

Adapted from Blumenfeld H, Neuroanatomy Through Clinical Cases, *Sunderland: Sinauer, 2002.*

longer sufficient to maintain postural stability, resulting in a positive Romberg's test. Causes include sensory peripheral neuropathy and dorsal column dysfunction (e.g. tabes dorsalis, subacute combined degeneration of the cord).

Vestibular dysfunction

In patients with vestibular dysfunction (e.g. vestibular neuritis), visual cues may be sufficient to accommodate disequilibrium to maintain postural stability. When visual information is removed, vertigo and/or disequilibrium result in postural instability.

Sign value

Notermans NC et al., in a study of 153 patients assessed with the Romberg test, reported that all control subjects had a negative test. Half of the patients with proprioceptive loss lasted only 10 seconds before having a positive test.[192]

Dr Moritz Romberg originally described the manoeuvre in patients with tabes dorsalis (tertiary syphilis affecting the spinal cord posterior columns). A positive Romberg test suggests proprioceptive loss or vestibular dysfunction.

5

Sensory level

Relevant neuroanatomy and topographical anatomy

Spinal cord
DORSAL COLUMN PATHWAY
- Dorsal columns
    - Ø Medial lemniscus, medulla

SPINOTHALAMIC TRACTS
- Spinothalamic tracts
    - Ø White ventral commissure, spinal cord

Description
A sensory level is a spinal level at which there is an abrupt sensory loss.[121]

Condition/s associated with

Common
- Spinal cord injury, trauma

Less common
- Transverse myelitis
- Multiple sclerosis
- Mass lesion – tumour, epidural abscess, AVM

Mechanism/s
A spinal cord lesion results in positive sensory deficits (i.e. paraesthesias, dysaesthesia) at the level of the lesion, and negative sensory deficits (i.e. anaesthesia) below the lesion. Sensory pathways above the lesion are not affected and, thus, sensation remains intact in the spinal levels above the lesion.

Sign value
Identification of a sensory level has localising value in spinal cord lesions. In a patient with traumatic spinal cord injury, a sensory level above T6 is associated with the development of neurogenic shock.

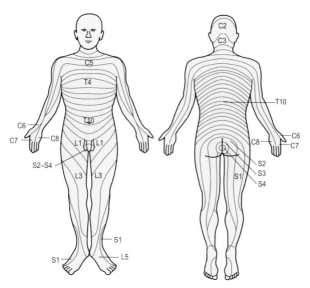

FIGURE 5.83
Dermatomes

Reproduced, with permission, from Daroff RB, Bradley WG et al., Neurology in Clinical Practice, *5th edn, Philadelphia: Butterworth-Heinemann, 2008: Fig 30-3.*

5

Sensory loss

Description

Sensory loss is characterised by
modality (light touch, vibration and
proprioception; pain and temperature)
and anatomical distribution (see
Table 5.30).

Light touch, vibration and proprioception

Light touch, vibration and
proprioception sensation is
predominantly mediated via the dorsal
column tract and medial lemniscus
pathway.

Pain and temperature

Pain and temperature sensation is
mediated by the spinothalamic tract
pathway.

Condition/s associated with

Common

- Compression mononeuropathy
  – carpal tunnel syndrome
- Peripheral neuropathy – diabetic
  neuropathy
- Cerebral infarction
- Cerebral haemorrhage
- Spinal cord injury
- Radiculopathy

Less common

- Transverse myelitis
- Lateral medullary syndrome
  (Wallenberg's syndrome)
- Compartment syndrome
- Syringomyelia
- Mass lesion – tumour, abscess,
  AVM

Mechanism/s

Causes of sensory loss include:

- sensory cortex lesion
- anterior limb of the internal capsule
  lesion
- thalamus lesion
- brainstem lesion
- spinal cord lesion
- radiculopathy
- peripheral neuropathy.

Sensory cortex lesion

Unilateral lesions of the sensory cortex
cause contralateral complete
hemisensory loss in the distribution of
structures of the sensory homunculus.
Isolated lesions of the post-central
gyrus may result in more sensory loss
than motor loss.[121]

Anterior limb, internal capsule lesion

A lesion in the anterior limb of the
internal capsule typically causes pure
contralateral complete hemisensory loss
of the face, arm and leg due to the
dense distribution of sensory fibres in
this region.[121] Muscle weakness may
coexist if there is involvement of the
posterior limb of the internal capsule.
The most common cause is a lacunar
infarction.

Thalamus lesion

The most common cause of pure
hemisensory loss (contralateral face,
arm, body and leg) in the absence of
motor findings is thalamic infarction.[121]
Causes of thalamic lesions include
lacunar infarction, cerebral
haemorrhage and tumours.

Brainstem lesion

Brainstem lesions are characterised by crossed motor sensory and/or motor deficits. Cranial nerve nuclei dysfunction in the region of the lesion causes ipsilateral cranial nerve abnormalities. Long tract dysfunction (e.g. pyramidal tracts, medial lemniscus, spinothalamic tract) results in contralateral motor and sensory abnormalities below the lesion. The prototypical brainstem syndrome with crossed sensory findings is Wallenberg's syndrome. See also 'Wallenberg's syndrome' in this chapter.

Spinal cord lesion

Spinal cord lesions cause ipsilateral loss of light touch, vibration and proprioception sensation because the dorsal column pathway decussates in the medulla (above the lesion). Contralateral loss of pain and temperature sensation will result because the spinothalamic tract decussates at each spinal level (below the lesion). In cord hemisection, or Brown-Séquard syndrome, there will also be a narrow band of complete sensory loss at the level of the lesion. In complete cord lesions a sensory level (a discrete loss of sensation below a certain dermatomal level) is characteristic.

Radiculopathy

Disorders of the nerve root typically cause positive (dysaesthesia or burning, paraesthesias, pain) and negative (anaesthesia or numbness) sensory findings in the distribution of the affected dermatome. Sensory abnormalities typically occur prior to motor abnormalities. The most common causes are intervertebral disc disease and spondylosis (see Table 5.30).

Peripheral neuropathy

The most common mechanisms of peripheral neuropathy are: 1) length-dependent peripheral neuropathy and 2) compression mononeuropathy.

Length-dependent peripheral neuropathy

Length-dependent peripheral neuropathy is caused by axonal degeneration in the most distal portion of the nerve and progresses towards the cell body.[3,121] Causes of length-dependent peripheral neuropathy include diabetes mellitus, alcohol, inherited neuropathies and heavy metal toxicity.

Compression mononeuropathy

Compression peripheral neuropathy is caused by mechanical injury that leads to degeneration of the axons and myelin distal to the site of injury (Wallerian degeneration). Motor and sensory deficits in the distribution of the affected peripheral nerve are characteristic.[3] Peripheral nerves susceptible to compression or traumatic injury are most commonly affected (e.g. median nerve, common peroneal nerve, radial nerve).

Sign value

The modality or modalities of sensory loss, anatomical distribution and associated signs are critical when considering the aetiologies of sensory loss.

5

<table>
<tr><td>

Relevant neuroanatomy and topographical anatomy[4,6]

DORSAL COLUMN AND MEDIAL LEMNISCUS PATHWAY (LIGHT TOUCH, VIBRATION AND PROPRIOCEPTION)

- Sensory cortex
  ↓
- Anterior limb, internal capsule
  ↓
- Ventral posterior lateral nuclei, thalamus
  ↓
- Medial lemniscus, brainstem
  ↓
- Ø Medial lemniscus, medulla
  ↓
- Nucleus gracilis and nucleus cuneatus, medulla
  ↓
- Dorsal columns, spinal cord
  ↓
- Dorsal horn grey matter, spinal cord
  ↓
- Nerve root
- ⇒ Intervertebral disc
- ⇒ Intervertebral foramina
  ↓
- Peripheral nerve
- ⇒ Potential sites of nerve compression (e.g. carpal tunnel)
  ↓
- ⊗ Various sensory receptors

</td><td>

SPINOTHALAMIC TRACT (PAIN AND TEMPERATURE)

- Sensory cortex
  ↓
- Anterior limb internal, capsule
  ↓
- Ventral posterior lateral nuclei, thalamus
  ↓
- Spinothalamic tract, brainstem
  ↓
- Spinothalamic tract, spinal cord
  ↓
- Ø Ventral white commissure (anterior commissure)
- ⇒ Central canal, spinal cord
  ↓
- Posterior horn grey matter
  ↓
- Posterior nerve root
- ⇒ Intervertebral disc
- ⇒ Intervertebral foramen
  ↓
- Peripheral nerve
- ⇒ Potential sites of nerve entrapment (e.g. carpal tunnel)
  ↓
- ⊗ Nociceptor, temperature receptor

</td></tr>
</table>

TABLE 5.30

Mechanisms of patterns of sensory loss

Pattern of sensory loss	Mechanism(s)
Face and arm 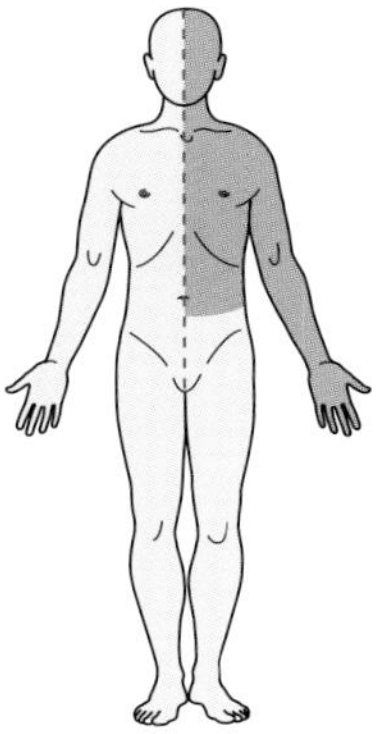 Figure 5.84	• MCA territory infarction • Mass lesion, sensory cortex
Leg 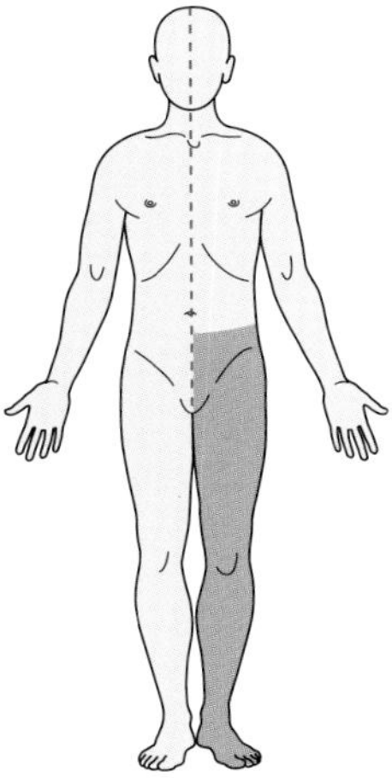 Figure 5.85	• Mass lesion, sensory cortex • ACA territory infarction

5

TABLE 5.30
Mechanisms of patterns of sensory loss—cont'd

Pattern of sensory loss	Mechanism(s)
Face, arm, leg 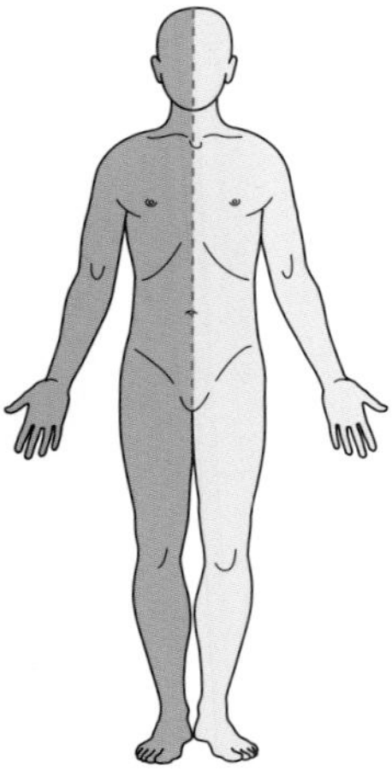 Figure 5.86	• Thalamic lesion • Anterior limb, internal capsule lesion • ICA (ACA + MCA) territory infarction
Ipsilateral face + contralateral arm and leg 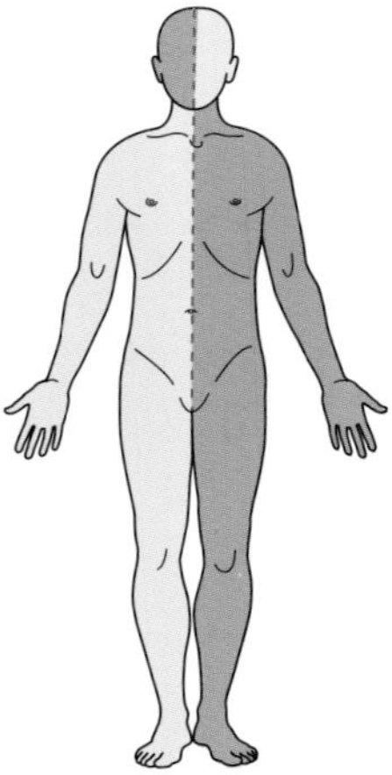 Figure 5.87	• Lateral medullary syndrome (Wallenberg's syndrome)

TABLE 5.30
Mechanisms of patterns of sensory loss—cont'd

Pattern of sensory loss	Mechanism(s)
Loss of pain and temperature in both arms in cape distribution 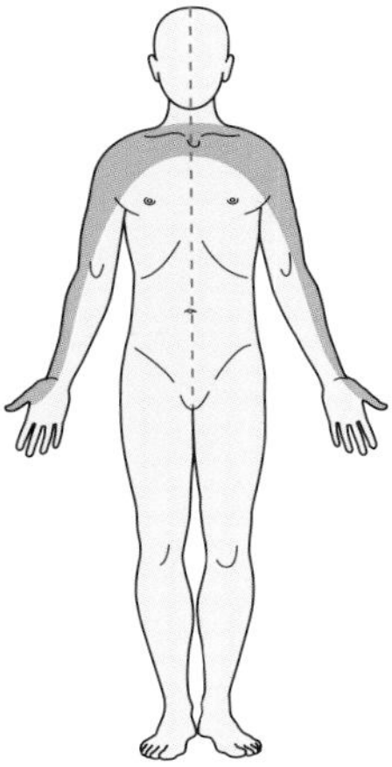 Figure 5.88	• Central cord syndrome, cervical spinal cord
Upper and lower limbs 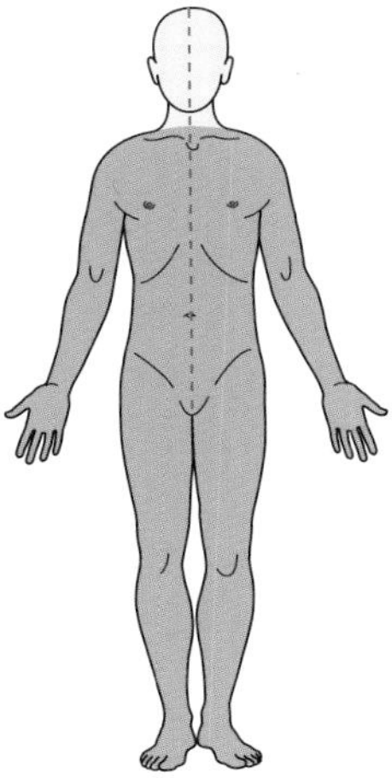 Figure 5.89	• Cervical spinal cord lesion

5

TABLE 5.30
Mechanisms of patterns of sensory loss—cont'd

Pattern of sensory loss	Mechanism(s)
Lower limbs 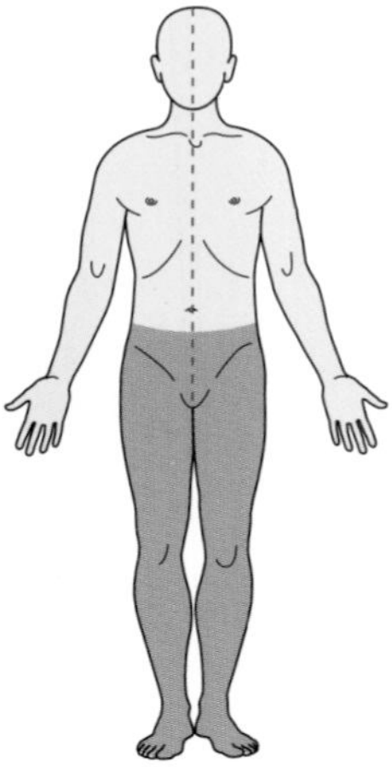 Figure 5.90	• Spinal cord lesion below T1, above L1/L2
Peripheral nerve distribution 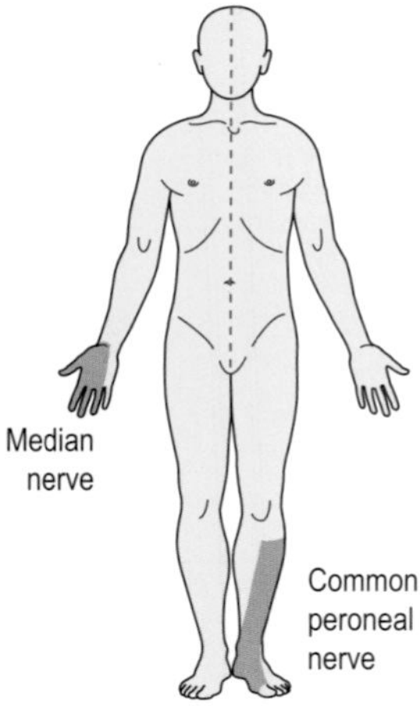 Median nerve Common peroneal nerve Figure 5.91	• Compression peripheral mononeuropathy

TABLE 5.30
Mechanisms of patterns of sensory loss—cont'd

Pattern of sensory loss	Mechanism(s)
Glove-and-stocking distribution 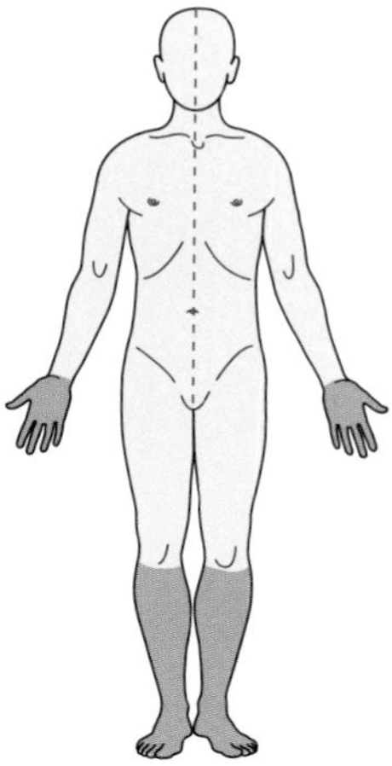 Figure 5.92	• Length-dependent peripheral neuropathy
Dermatomal distribution 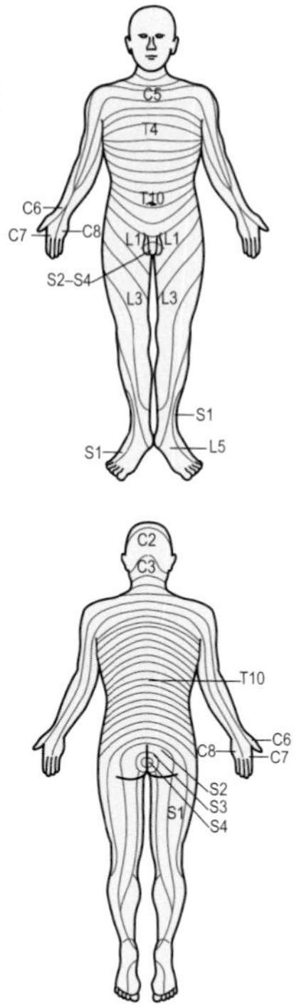 Figure 5.93	• Radiculopathy

5

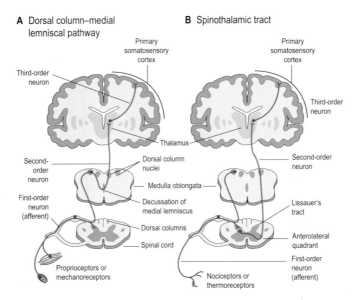

A Dorsal column–medial lemniscal pathway

B Spinothalamic tract

FIGURE 5.94
Relevant pathways in sensory loss
A Dorsal column–medial lemniscal pathway; **B** spinothalamic tract pathway.

Based on http://virtual.yosemite.cc.ca.us/rdroual/Course%20Materials/Physiology%20101/Chapter%20 Notes/Fall%202007/chapter_10%20Fall%202007.htm [5 Apr 2011].

Spasticity

Description

Spasticity is increased resistance to passive movement due to an abnormal increase in resting muscle tone. There are three distinct features:[4,193]

1 Resistance is velocity-dependent (i.e. muscle tone increases with the velocity of passive movement).
2 There is flexor–extensor tone dissociation (i.e. increased tone in flexors of the arms and extensors of the lower limbs).
3 Weakness is present.

Relevant neuroanatomy and topographical anatomy

UPPER MOTOR NEURON
• Motor cortex
↓
• Corona radiata, subcortical white matter
↓
• Posterior limb, internal capsule
↓
• Corticospinal tracts, medial brainstem
↓
Ø Pyramidal decussation, medulla
↓
• Lateral corticospinal tracts, spinal cord
↓
MONOSYNAPTIC STRETCH REFLEX
→ Inhibitory interneuron
→ Sensory afferent neuron
→ Alpha motor neuron

Condition/s associated with

Common

• Normal variant
• Cerebral infarction, MCA territory
• Cerebral haemorrhage
• Lacunar infarction, posterior limb internal capsule

Less common

• Multiple sclerosis
• Spinal cord injury
• Brainstem lesion (medial medullary syndrome)
• CNS mass lesion – tumour, abscess, AVM
• Serotonin syndrome
• Strychnine toxicity
• *Clostridium tetani* infection (tetanus)

Mechanism/s

Spasticity is caused by:

• upper motor neuron disorder
• toxicological and infectious disorders (rare).

Upper motor neuron disorder

Upper motor neuron dysfunction causes a decrease in inhibitory interneuron activity and an increase in gamma motor neuron activity, resulting in a state of hyperexcitability of alpha motor neurons.[58] Hyperexcitability of alpha neurons results in increased resting muscle tone and increased resistance during passive movement. In the hyperacute period following upper motor neuron injury, spasticity is often absent. It takes days to weeks for spasticity to develop

5

following acute upper motor neuron injury.[39]

Toxicological and infectious disorders

Clostridium tetani produces a toxin that inhibits the release of GABA from inhibitory interneurons in the spinal cord, causing prolonged excitation of the alpha motor neuron, resulting in spastic paresis.[194] Strychnine blocks the uptake of glycine at post-synaptic spinal cord motor neurons, causing prolonged excitation of the alpha motor neuron and spastic paresis.[195]

Sign value

Spasticity is a sign of upper motor neuron dysfunction but is also associated with several toxicological disorders.

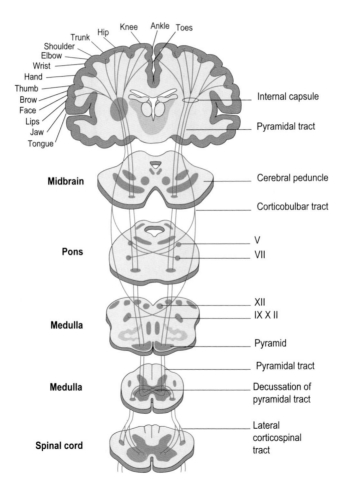

FIGURE 5.95

Upper motor neuron anatomy

Based on Clark RG, Manter and Gatz's Essential Neuroanatomy and Neurophysiology, *5th edn, Philadelphia: FA Davis Co, 1975.*

Sternocleidomastoid and trapezius muscle weakness (accessory nerve [CNXI] palsy)

Relevant neuroanatomy and topographical anatomy

UPPER MOTOR NEURON
- Motor cortex
  ↓
- Corona radiata, subcortical white matter
  ↓
- Posterior limb, internal capsule
  ↓
- Pyramidal tracts, brainstem
  ↓
Ø Decussation 1
  ↓
Ø Decussation 2
  ↓
LOWER MOTOR NEURON
- Accessory nucleus, medulla
  ↓
- Accessory nerve
⇒ Foramen magnum
⇒ Posterior triangle, neck
  ↓
× Sternocleidomastoid muscle

Description

Accessory nerve (CNXI) palsy results in sternocleidomastoid and/or trapezius muscle weakness.

Sternocleidomastoid weakness is performed via resistance testing against head turning:

- weakness head turn left → right sternocleidomastoid weakness
- weakness head turn right → left sternocleidomastoid weakness.

Trapezius weakness is performed by resistance testing against shoulder shrugging. The levator scapulae muscle also plays a role in this movement.[6,196]

Condition/s associated with

Common

- Iatrogenic – complication of neck dissection
- Penetrating trauma posterior triangle neck

Less common

- Mass lesion – tumour, abscess, AVM

Mechanism/s

Accessory nerve palsy is most commonly caused by peripheral nerve lesions secondary to trauma or mass lesions. Accessory nerve palsies may spare the sternocleidomastoid muscle because its branches diverge early from the main nerve trunk.[197]

5

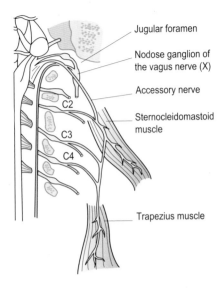

Jugular foramen

Nodose ganglion of
the vagus nerve (X)

Accessory nerve

C2

Sternocleidomastoid
muscle

C3

C4

Trapezius muscle

FIGURE 5.96
Innervation of the sternocleidomastoid and
trapezius muscles by the accessory nerve
(CNXI)

*Reproduced, with permission, from Daroff RB,
Bradley WG et al., Neurology in Clinical
Practice, 5th edn, Philadelphia: Butterworth-
Heinemann, 2008: Fig 74-13.*

Tongue deviation (hypoglossal nerve [CNXII] palsy)

Relevant neuroanatomy and topographical anatomy
UPPER MOTOR NEURON • Motor cortex ↓ • Corona radiata, subcortical white matter ↓ • Posterior limb, internal capsule ↓ • Pyramidal tracts, brainstem ↓ Ø Decussation ↓ LOWER MOTOR NEURON • Hypoglossal nucleus, medulla ↓ • Hypoglossal nerve ⇒ Hypoglossal canal ⇒ Carotid artery ↓ × Genioglossus muscle

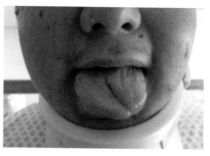

FIGURE 5.97
Patient with left hypoglossal nerve palsy with tongue deviation towards the side of the lesion

Rué V. et al., Delayed hypoglossal nerve palsy following unnoticed occipital condyle fracture. Neurochirurgie 2013; 59(6): 221–223. Copyright © 2013 Elsevier Masson SAS.

5

Description
The tongue deviates towards the side of the lesion.

Condition/s associated with

Common
- Iatrogenic – complication of carotid endarterectomy
- Penetrating neck trauma

Less common
- Carotid artery aneurysm
- Mass lesion – tumour, abscess
- Carotid artery dissection

Mechanism/s

The genioglossus muscle is innervated by the ipsilateral hypoglossal nerve and moves the tongue medially and forwards. Normally, the medial forces of each genioglossus muscle are balanced and the tongue is protruded in the midline. If genioglossus weakness is present, the tongue deviates towards the side of weakness, due to loss of the medial force on the affected side.[4,6,198]

Hypoglossal nerve (CNXII) palsy

Hypoglossal nerve palsies are often accompanied by other cranial nerve findings.[199] Causes include hypoglossal canal stenosis, internal carotid artery aneurysm, internal carotid artery dissection, iatrogenic injury following carotid endarterectomy and penetrating neck injury.[200–202]

Sign value

The hypoglossal nerve is the most common cause of tongue deviation. The tongue deviates towards the side of the lesion.

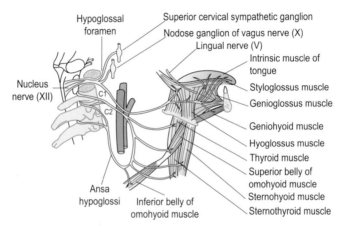

FIGURE 5.98
Neuroanatomy and topographical anatomy of the hypoglossal nerve (CNXII)

Reproduced, with permission, from Daroff RB, Bradley WG et al., Neurology in Clinical Practice, 5th edn, Philadelphia: Butterworth-Heinemann, 2008: Fig 74-16.

Trochlear nerve (CNIV) palsy

Relevant neuroanatomy and topographical anatomy

- Trochlear nuclei, dorsal midbrain
  ↓
- Ø Decussation
  ↓
- Trochlear nerve
  ⇒ Subarachnoid space
  ⇒ Superior orbital fissure
  ⇒ Cavernous sinus
  ⇒ Orbital apex
  ↓
- × Superior oblique muscle

Description

Trochlear nerve (CNIV) palsy is characterised by (findings in the primary gaze position):[1]

- hypertropia (upward deviation)
- extorsion (external rotation)
- head tilt, in the direction opposite to the side of the affected eye.

Dysconjugate gaze worsens when the patient looks down and away from the side of the affected eye (such as when going down a spiral staircase).

Condition/s associated with[1,203–205]

Common

- Blunt head trauma
- Diabetic mononeuropathy/ microvascular infarction

Less common

- Midbrain lesion – tumour, multiple sclerosis, AVM
- Hydrocephalus
- Pinealoma
- Cavernous sinus syndrome (multiple cranial nerve abnormalities)

Mechanism/s

The trochlear nerve (CNIV) innervates the contralateral superior oblique muscle and crosses the midline immediately after exiting the dorsal midbrain. Lesions of the trochlear nerve result in contralateral findings. The mechanisms of features of trochlear nerve palsy are described in Table 5.31.

TABLE 5.31
Mechanisms of features of trochlear nerve (CNIV) palsy

Feature of trochlear nerve palsy	Mechanism
Hypertropia	→ Unopposed inferior oblique and superior rectus muscles
Extorsion	→ Unopposed inferior oblique muscle
Head tilt	→ Patient accommodates extorted eye
Impaired depression	→ Superior oblique weakness
Impaired intorsion	→ Inferior oblique weakness

5

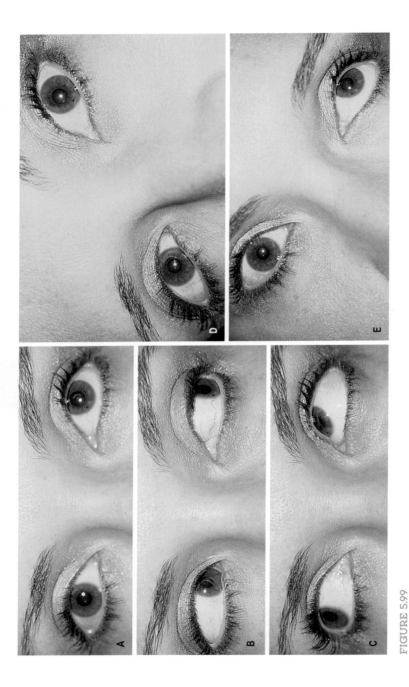

FIGURE 5.99
Patient with trochlear nerve (CNIV) palsy
A Primary position with left hypertropia and extorsion; **B** relatively normal left gaze away from fields of action of left superior orbital oblique muscle; **C** right gaze; **D** no vertical deviation of the left eye during contralateral head tilt, due to reflex excyclotorsion accomplished by the inferior rectus and inferior oblique muscles; **E** pronounced left hypertropia on ipsilateral head tilt, following reflex incyclotorsion recruitment of superior rectus muscle and weak superior oblique muscle (due to inability to compensate superior rectus muscle contraction by the weak superior oblique muscle).

Reproduced, with permission, from Yanoff M, Duker JS, Ophthalmology: 3rd edn, St Louis: Mosby, 2008: Fig 11-10-4.

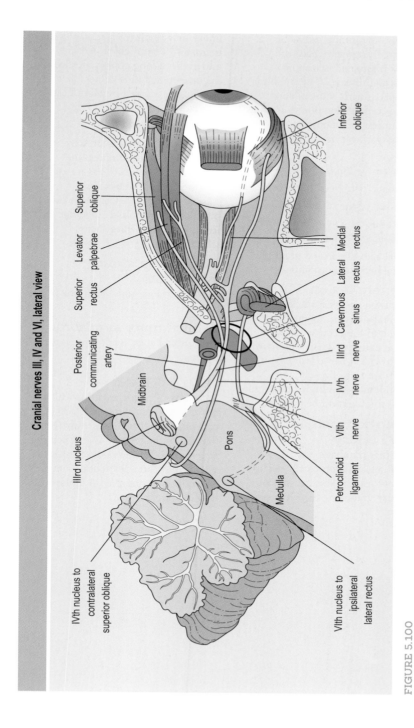

Cranial nerves III, IV and VI, lateral view

IIIrd nucleus

IVth nucleus to contralateral superior oblique

Posterior communicating artery

Superior rectus

Levator palpebrae

Superior oblique

Inferior oblique

Midbrain

Pons

Medulla

Petroclinoid ligament

VIth nerve

IVth nerve

IIIrd nerve

Cavernous sinus

Lateral rectus

Medial rectus

VIth nucleus to ipsilateral lateral rectus

FIGURE 5.100
Lateral view of the trochlear nerve (CNIV)

Reproduced, with permission, from Yanoff M, Duker JS, Ophthalmology, 3rd edn, St Louis: Mosby, 2008: Fig 9-15-1.

5

The most common causes of isolated trochlear nerve palsy are traumatic injury and ischaemic microvascular disease.[1] The trochlear nerve is particularly vulnerable to traumatic compression due to its long course outside the brainstem.[1,205] Causes of trochlear nerve (CNIV) palsy include:

- brainstem lesion
- traumatic peripheral nerve injury
- disorders of the subarachnoid space
- cavernous sinus syndrome (multiple cranial nerve abnormalities)
- orbital apex syndrome (multiple cranial nerve abnormalities).

Brainstem lesion

Lesions of the trochlear nuclei cause contralateral superior oblique muscle paresis due to the decussation of the nerve as it exits the dorsal midbrain. Isolated trochlear nerve lesions in the brainstem are rare. Typically, in brainstem lesions, multiple brainstem localising findings will be present.[203,204]

Traumatic trochlear nerve (CNIV) injury

Unlike other traumatic cranial neuropathies, which typically occur secondary to severe mechanisms of head injury, traumatic trochlear nerve injury may result from relatively minor trauma.[205] The trochlear nerve undertakes a long course after exiting the brainstem and is vulnerable to compression caused by blunt head trauma.

Disorders of the subarachnoid space

Mass lesions may compress the trochlear nerve (CNIV) as it exits the brainstem and traverses the subarachnoid space. Causes include infectious or neoplastic meningeal irritation and trochlear nerve schwannoma.[204]

Cavernous sinus syndrome

See 'Cavernous sinus syndrome' in this chapter.

Orbital apex syndrome

See 'Orbital apex syndrome' in this chapter.

Sign value

In a study of patients with trochlear nerve palsy, approximately 45% of patients tilted their heads away from the side of the lesion.[206–208] When the patients tilted their heads towards the side of the lesion, 96% of patients experienced worsening in diplopia and hypertropia.[206,208]

Truncal ataxia

<table>
<tr><td>

Relevant neuroanatomy and topographical anatomy

CEREBELLUM
- Vermis and flocculonodular lobe
  - → Anterior corticospinal tract
  - → Reticulospinal tract
  - → Vestibulospinal tract
  - → Tectospinal tract

</td></tr>
</table>

Description

Postural instability due to incoordination of the proximal muscles groups of the body assessed while sitting upright and/or oscillatory movements of head and neck (i.e. titubation).[69] Patients may require assistance to maintain an upright posture.

Condition/s associated with[6,69]

Common

- Alcohol intoxication
- Drug toxicity – lithium, phenytoin, benzodiazepine

Less common

- Cerebellar infarction
- Basilar artery territory infarction
- Multiple sclerosis
- Mass – tumour, abscess, AVM
- HSV cerebellitis
- Hereditary cerebellar degeneration (Freidreich's ataxia)
- Paraneoplastic cerebellar degeneration

Mechanism/s

Midline structures of the cerebellum (vermis and flocculonodular lobe) coordinate movements in the axial musculature via the descending axial motor pathways.[6,69] Lesions in these structures cause truncal ataxia and titubation. Refer to Table 5.32 for motor pathways associated with the cerebellum.

Sign value

Truncal ataxia is a midline cerebellar sign.

5

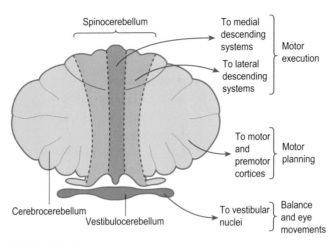

FIGURE 5.101
Functional anatomy of the cerebellum

From Barrett KE, Barman SM, Boitano S et al., Ganong's Review of Medical Physiology, *23rd edn. Modified from Kandel ER, Schwartz JH, Jessell TM (eds),* Principles of Neural Science, *4th edn, McGraw Hill, 2000.*

TABLE 5.32
Functional anatomy of the cerebellum and associated motor pathways

Cerebellar anatomy	Function	Associated motor pathways
Vermis and flocculonodular lobe	• Proximal limb and trunk coordination • Vestibulo–ocular reflexes	• Anterior corticospinal tract • Reticulospinal tract • Vestibulospinal tract • Tectospinal tract
Intermediate hemisphere	• Distal limb coordination	• Lateral corticospinal tracts • Rubrospinal tracts
Lateral hemisphere	• Motor planning, distal extremities	• Lateral corticospinal tracts

Adapted from Blumenfeld H, Neuroanatomy Through Clinical Cases, *Sunderland: Sinauer, 2002.*

Uvular deviation

Description

When a patient says 'ah', there is dynamic deviation of the uvula to one side upon contraction of the palator constrictor muscle.

Relevant neuroanatomy and topographical anatomy[1]

UPPER MOTOR NEURON
• Motor cortex
↓
• Corona radiata, subcortical white matter
↓
• Posterior limb, internal capsule
↓
• Motor long tracts, brainstem
↓
Ø Decussation
↓
GLOSSOPHARYNGEAL NERVE (CNIX) AND VAGUS NERVE (CNX)
• Nucleus ambiguus and dorsal motor nucleus, medulla
⇒ Jugular foramen
↓
• Nodose ganglion
↓
× Palatal constrictors and intrinsic laryngeal muscles

Condition/s associated with[1]

Common

• Diabetic mononeuropathy/microvascular infarction
• Iatrogenic – complication of tonsillectomy

Less common

• Lateral medullary syndrome (Wallenberg's syndrome)
• Cerebellopontine tumour
• Internal carotid artery dissection
• Mass – glomus tumour, AVM
• Trauma – jugular foramen fracture (multiple cranial nerve abnormalities)

Mechanism/s

Uvular deviation is caused by:

• nucleus ambiguus lesion
• glossopharyngeal nerve (CNIX)
• glossopharyngeal nerve (CNIX) and vagus nerve (CNX) palsies.

Nucleus ambiguus lesion

A lesion of the nucleus ambiguus causes ipsilateral weakness of the palatal constrictor muscles, and results in uvular deviation away from the side of the lesion. Causes include lateral medullary syndrome (Wallenberg's syndrome), infectious disorders and multiple sclerosis.[1]

Vagus nerve (CNX) palsy

In vagus nerve palsy, ipsilateral weakness of the uvula and soft palate causes the uvula to deviate away from the affected side. Associated features include unilateral loss of pharyngeal

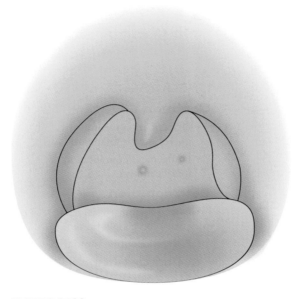

FIGURE 5.102
Uvular deviation to the right following acute stroke affecting the left glossopharyngeal nerve (CNIX)

Based on Scollard DM, Skinsnes OK, Oropharyngeal leprosy in art, history, and medicine. Oral Surg, Oral Med, Oral Pathol, Oral Radiol, Endod *1999; 87(4): 463–470.*

and laryngeal sensation, unilateral loss of sensation in the external ear, dysphagia and hoarseness.[1] Causes include trauma, cerebellopontine angle tumours and iatrogenic injury following tonsillectomy.

Sign value

Dynamic uvular deviation is a sign of glossopharyngeal nerve (CNIX) and vagus nerve (CNX) palsies or a nucleus ambiguus lesion.

Vertical gaze palsy

Relevant neuroanatomy and topographical anatomy[138]

HIGHER CENTRE INPUT
• Cerebral hemisphere
• Superior colliculus
• Vestibular nuclei
• Cerebellum

BRAINSTEM 'GAZE CENTRES'
• Midbrain reticular formation
⇒ Pineal gland
⇒ Third ventricle
↓
• Interstitial nucleus of Cajal
↓
Ø Posterior commissure
↓
• Oculomotor nuclei (CNIII)
• Trochlear nuclei (CNIV)

Description
Vertical gaze palsy is a group of uncommon gaze disorders that include upward gaze palsy, downward gaze palsy and a combined upward and downward gaze palsy.

Condition/s associated with[13,134,138,142]

Common
• Pinealoma
• Hydrocephalus
• Progressive supranuclear palsy (PSP)

Less common
• Multiple sclerosis
• Wernicke's encephalopathy
• Tay–Sachs disease
• HIV/AIDS encephalopathy

Mechanism/s
The midbrain reticular formation (MRF) mediates vertical gaze and vergence eye movements.[138]

Upward gaze paresis is caused by:
• posterior commissure lesion.

Downward gaze paresis and combined upgaze and downgaze paresis are caused by:
• bilateral rostral interstitial medial longitudinal fasciculus (riMLF) lesions.

Posterior commissure lesion
A lesion in the posterior commissure will result in vertical gaze palsy due to a loss of input from the interstitial nucleus of Cajal to the oculomotor nuclei, resulting in weakness of the superior rectus muscle and inferior oblique muscle.

Bilateral riMLF lesions
Bilateral riMLF lesions result in loss of neural input to the oculomotor nuclei and trochlear nuclei, resulting in weakness of the inferior rectus muscle and superior oblique muscles, respectively.[1] In combined upgaze and downgaze palsy there is weakness of the superior rectus muscle, inferior rectus muscle, inferior oblique muscle and superior oblique muscle.

Sign value
Vertical gaze palsy is a sign of a midbrain lesion.

5

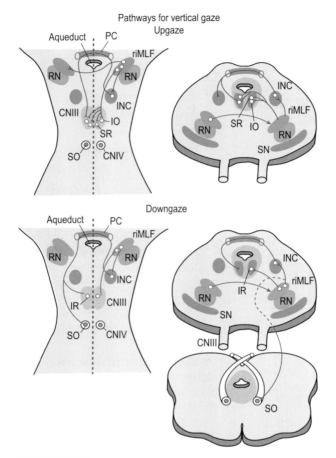

Pathways for vertical gaze

FIGURE 5.103

Neural pathways associated with vertical gaze

Upgaze pathways originate in the rostral interstitial nucleus of the medial longitudinal fasciculus (MLF) and project dorsally to innervate the oculomotor and trochlear nerves, travelling through the posterior commissure. Upgaze paralysis is a feature of the dorsal midbrain syndrome as a result of the lesion's effect on the posterior commissure. Downgaze pathways also originate in the rostral interstitial nucleus of the MLF but probably travel more ventrally. Bilateral lesions are also needed to affect downgaze and usually are located dorsomedial to the red nucleus. INC = interstitial nucleus of Cajal; IO = inferior oblique subnucleus; IR = inferior rectus subnucleus; PC = posterior commissure; riMLF = rostral interstitial nucleus of the medial longitudinal fasciculus; RN = red nucleus; SN = substantia nigra; SO = superior oblique subnucleus; SR = superior rectus subnucleus.

Reproduced, with permission, from Yanoff M, Duker JS, Ophthalmology, 3rd edn, St Louis: Mosby, 2008: Fig 9-13-4.

Visual acuity

Description

Visual acuity is a *vital sign* of the eye. Visual acuity is assessed using the Snellen chart. Decreased visual acuity is characterised by a patient who is unable to read the 6/9 line or has a significant change in visual acuity from baseline. Patients with astigmatism should wear their glasses, or contacts, or use a pinhole refractor during the examination to compensate for refractive error.[209]

(*Note*: this section will focus on neurological conditions associated with visual acuity abnormalities. An ophthalmology text should be consulted for further information.)

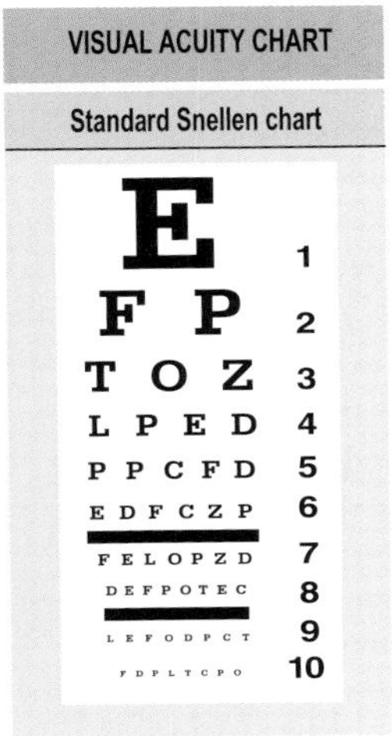

VISUAL ACUITY CHART

Standard Snellen chart

FIGURE 5.104
Snellen chart

Reproduced, with permission, from Yanoff M, Duker JS, Ophthalmology, 3rd edn, St Louis: Mosby, 2008: Fig 2-6-7.

Relevant neuroanatomy and topographical anatomy

Nervous system

PRECHIASMAL STRUCTURES
- Retinal epithelium
  ↓
- Optic nerve
⇒ Orbital apex
⇒ Optic canal, sphenoid bone
  ↓

CHIASMAL STRUCTURES
- Optic chiasm
⇒ Pituitary gland
⇒ Cavernous sinus
  ↓

POSTCHIASMAL STRUCTURES
- Optic tracts
  ↓
- Lateral geniculate nucleus (LGN), thalamus
  ↓
- Superior optic radiation, parietal lobe ('Baum's loop')
  ↓
- Inferior optic radiation, temporal lobe ('Meyer's loop')
  ↓
- Optic cortex, occipital lobe

EYE
- Cornea
- Anterior chamber
- Lens
- Posterior chamber
- Vitreous body
- Retinal epithelium

5

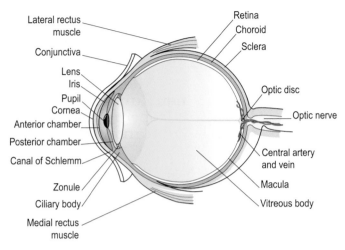

FIGURE 5.105
Anatomy of the eye

Reproduced, with permission, from Goldman L, Ausiello D, Cecil Medicine, 23rd edn, Philadelphia: Saunders, 2007: Fig 449-2.

Condition/s associated with[6,210]

Common

- Bilateral occipital lobe infarction
- Bilateral occipital lobe haemorrhage
- Optic neuritis
- Elevated intracranial pressure, any cause

Less common

- Ocular migraine
- Idiopathic intracranial hypertension (IIH)
- Anterior ischaemic optic neuropathy (AION)
- Orbital apex syndrome
- Mass lesion – tumour, abscess, AVM
- Cerebral venous sinus thrombosis

Mechanism/s

Neurological conditions associated with decreased visual acuity include:

- unilateral or bilateral prechiasmal lesions
- bilateral postchiasmal lesions.

Chiasmal lesions and unilateral postchiasmal lesions are not usually associated with decreased visual acuity. Rather, they typically result in a visual field defect. See 'Visual field defects' in this chapter.

Unilateral or bilateral prechiasmal lesion(s)

Unilateral prechiasmal lesions (e.g. optic glioma, optic neuritis) result in ipsilateral monocular visual loss. Associated features may include papilloedema, optic atrophy and a relative afferent pupillary defect (RAPD). The intracranial segments of the optic nerves are supplied by branches of the anterior cerebral, middle cerebral and anterior communicating arteries. Due to the extensive blood supply of these structures, infarction is rare.[211]

Bilateral postchiasmal lesions

Bilateral occipital lobe lesions (e.g. infarction, haemorrhage) result in a cortical blindness. Patients may be unaware of the abnormality (i.e. anosognosia).

Sign value

In a study of 317 new patients, near visual acuity of 6/12 (i.e. 20/40) or worse had a sensitivity of 75%, specificity of 74% and LR of 2.8 for detection of significant ocular disease.[212] Distance visual acuity testing of 6/9 (i.e. 20/30) or worse had a sensitivity of 74%, specificity of 73% and LR of 2.7 for detection of significant ocular disease.[212]

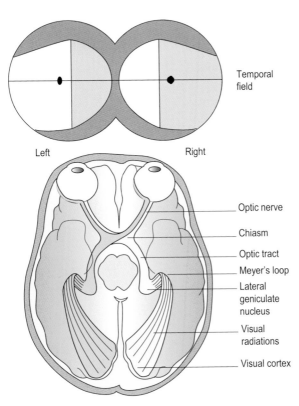

Temporal field

Left   Right

Optic nerve

Chiasm

Optic tract

Meyer's loop

Lateral geniculate nucleus

Visual radiations

Visual cortex

FIGURE 5.106
The visual pathways

Reproduced, with permission, from Daroff RB, Bradley WG et al., Neurology in Clinical Practice, *5th edn, Philadelphia: Butterworth-Heinemann, 2008: Fig 39-1.*

Visual field defects

Description

Visual field defects are partial deficits in the normal field of vision. The extent of the normal visual field is approximately 90° temporally, 50° superiorly, 50° nasally and 60° inferiorly.[140]

Visual field defects are detected at the bedside using the confrontation technique. Simultaneous testing of two

---

Relevant neuroanatomy and topographical anatomy

Eye
- Cornea
- Anterior chamber
- Lens
- Posterior chamber
- Vitreous body
- Retinal epithelium

Neurological structures

PRECHIASMAL STRUCTURES
- Retinal epithelium
↓
- Optic nerve
⇒ Orbital apex
⇒ Cavernous sinus
⇒ Optic canal, sphenoid bone
↓

CHIASMAL STRUCTURES
- Optic chiasm
⇒ Pituitary gland
↓

POSTCHIASMAL STRUCTURES
- Optic tracts
↓
- Lateral geniculate nucleus (LGN), thalamus
↓
- Superior optic radiation ('Baum's loop'), parietal lobe
↓
- Inferior optic radiation ('Meyer's loop'), temporal lobe
↓
- Optic cortex, occipital lobe

quadrants is clinically useful in suspected parietal lobe lesions to detect visual hemineglect. In visual hemineglect, the patient may perceive the moving object in the left visual hemifield in isolation, but may be unable to perceive the object when simultaneous visual stimuli are presented to both visual fields.[4,213]

Condition/s associated with

Common

- PCA territory infarction
- MCA territory infarction
- Occipital lobe haemorrhage
- Age-related macular degeneration

Less common

- Retinitis pigmentosa
- Pituitary macroadenoma
- Craniopharyngioma
- Central retinal artery branch occlusion
- Multiple sclerosis

Mechanism/s

The causes of visual field defects (see Table 5.33) are divided into the following categories:

- disorders of the prechiasmal structures
- disorders of the optic chiasm
- disorders of the postchiasmal structures.

In general, visual field defects that cross the vertical meridian (vertical line dividing each visual hemifield) are due to prechiasmal lesions or primary eye disorders.[4] Visual field defects that do not cross the vertical meridian, such as in homonymous hemianopia, are caused by chiasmal or postchiasmal lesions.[4]

Prechiasmal disorders

Unilateral prechiasmal disorders cause ipsilateral monocular visual field defects that may cross the vertical meridian (i.e. the vertical line 'bisecting' the visual field).[4]

Altitudinal scotoma – branch central retinal artery occlusion

Occlusion of the superior or inferior branch central retinal artery may cause infarction of the superior or inferior half of the retina, resulting in an inferior or superior altitudinal scotoma, respectively.

5

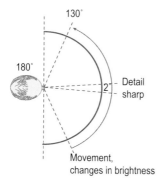
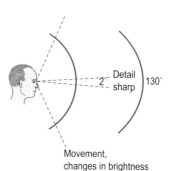

FIGURE 5.107
Extent of the normal visual field

Based on the Scottish Sensory Centre, Functional assessment of vision. Available: http://www.ssc. education.ed.ac.uk/courses/vi&multi/vmay06c.html [5 Apr 2011].

TABLE 5.33
Mechanisms of visual fields defects[4,8,212,214]

Visual field defect	Mechanism(s)
Altitudinal scotoma 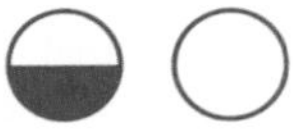 Figure 5.108	• Branch central retinal artery occlusion • Retinal detachment • Partial optic nerve lesion
Central scotoma 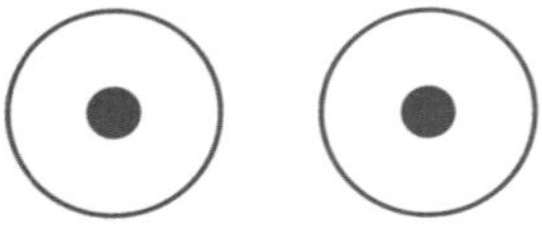 Figure 5.109	• Macular degeneration • Optic nerve lesion
Constricted visual field ('tunnel vision') 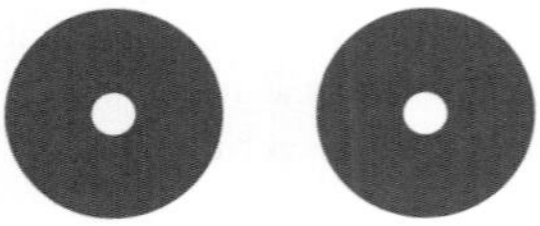 Figure 5.110	• Glaucoma • Retinitis pigmentosa • Central retinal artery occlusion with ciliretinal artery sparing • Chronic papilloedema
Bitemporal hemianopia 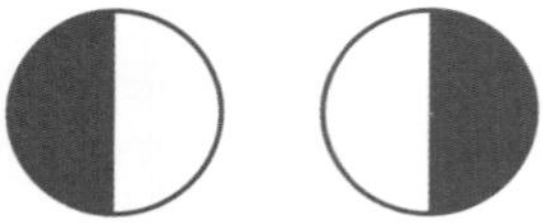 Figure 5.111	• Optic chiasm lesion
Homonymous hemianopia 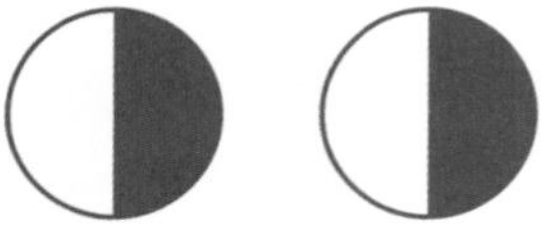 Figure 5.112	• Optic cortex lesion • Superior and inferior optic radiations lesion • LGN, thalamus lesion • Optic tract lesion (least common)
Homonymous hemianopia with macular sparing 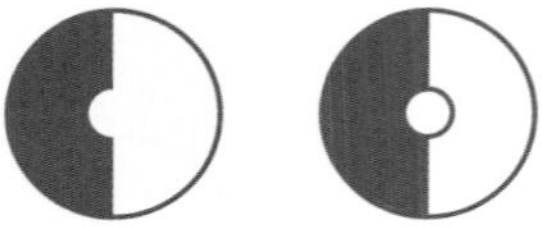 Figure 5.113	• Occipital pole lesion
Homonymous quadrantanopia 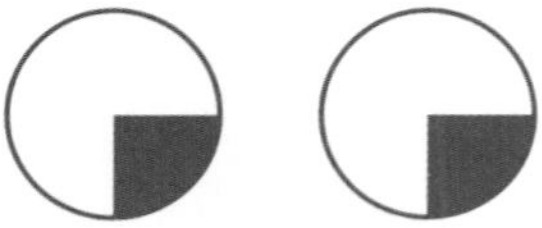 Figure 5.114	• Optic radiation lesion

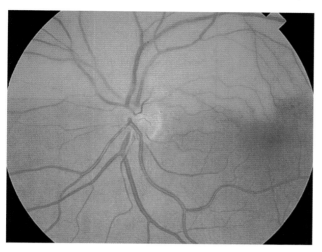

FIGURE 5.115
Superior retinal infarction (pale region) due to branch retinal artery occlusion, resulting in inferior altitudinal scotoma

Reproduced, with permission, from Yanoff M, Duker JS, Ophthalmology, 3rd edn, St Louis: Mosby, 2008: Fig 6-16-6.

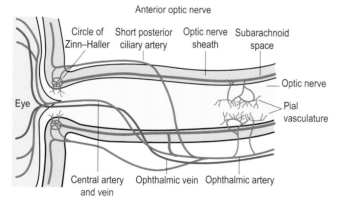

FIGURE 5.116
Anatomy of the vascular supply of the anterior optic nerve

Reproduced, with permission, from Yanoff M, Duker JS, Ophthalmology, 3rd edn, St Louis: Mosby, 2008: Fig 9-2-3.

Constricted visual field – central retinal artery occlusion [CRAO] with cilioretinal artery sparing

The cilioretinal artery supplies the macula and fovea (e.g. the central portions of the visual space). CRAO with cilioretinal artery sparing thus causes infarction of the retinal neuroepithelium, with the exception of the most central region, resulting in a constricted visual field defect.[213]

Constricted visual field – retinitis pigmentosa

The most common form of retinitis pigmentosa causes progressive loss of peripheral retinal rod photoreceptors, resulting in impaired vision in low light and loss of the peripheral vision (i.e. a constricted visual field).[214]

Central scotoma – disorders of the optic nerve

The area where the optic nerve enters the retina corresponds to the location of the physiological blindspot that is due to the absence of retinal photoreceptors in this region. Optic nerve disorders may cause enlargement of the physiological blind spot and/or central scotoma.[3]

Central scotoma – macular degeneration

Disorders of the macula are due to injury to the retina in the foveal and parafoveal regions, resulting in a central scotoma.[213] The fovea represents the region with the largest density of rods and highest visual acuity at the site of fixation (i.e. the most central portion of the visual field).

Optic chiasm lesions

Optic chiasm lesions cause dysfunction of the nerve fibres supplying the medial hemiretinas, and thus result in bitemporal hemianopia. Optic chiasm lesions typically result from compression by an adjacent mass. The most common cause is a pituitary macroadenoma. Other causes include craniopharyngioma and pituitary apoplexy.[212] Associated features of optic chiasm lesions include disruption of the hypothalamic–pituitary axis, headache and hydrocephalus.[211]

Postchiasmal disorders

Postchiasmal disorders cause homonymous visual field defects. Nerve fibres from the optic cortex, optic radiations and lateral geniculate nucleus (LGN) of the thalamus contain fibres that supply the ipsilateral temporal hemiretina and the contralateral medial hemiretina.[4,6] Fibres destined for the contralateral hemiretina cross at the optic chiasm.

Homonymous hemianopia with macular sparing

Occipital lobe lesions sparing the posterolateral striate cortex, which contains the fibres representing the macula and fovea, may result in homonymous hemianopia with macular sparing.[213] The fovea and macula together make up a small percentage of the total area of the retina but are supplied by a relatively large number of nerve fibres. Due to the relatively large representation, incomplete occipital lobe lesions may spare enough of these fibres to preserve central vision.[211,212]

Sign value

In detecting a visual field defect of prechiasmal origin, the confrontation technique has a sensitivity of 11–58%, specificity of 93–99% and positive likelihood ratio of 6.1.[215–219]

In detecting a visual field defect of chiasmal or postchiasmal origin, the confrontation technique has a sensitivity of 43–86%, specificity of 86–95% and positive likelihood ratio of 6.8.[215–219]

Refer to Table 5.34 for clinical utility of hemianopia in unilateral cerebral hemisphere lesions.

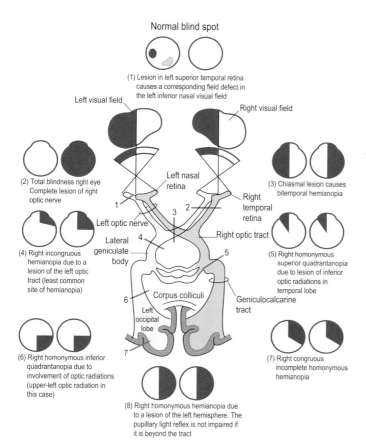

Normal blind spot

(1) Lesion in left superior temporal retina causes a corresponding field defect in the left inferior nasal visual field

Left visual field

Right visual field

(2) Total blindness right eye Complete lesion of right optic nerve

Left nasal retina

(3) Chiasmal lesion causes bitemporal hemianopia

Right temporal retina

Left optic nerve

Right optic tract

(4) Right incongruous hemianopia due to a lesion of the left optic tract (least common site of hemianopia)

Lateral geniculate body

(5) Right homonymous superior quadrantanopia due to lesion of inferior optic radiations in temporal lobe

Corpus colliculi

Geniculocalcarine tract

Left occipital lobe

(6) Right homonymous inferior quadrantanopia due to involvement of optic radiations (upper-left optic radiation in this case)

(7) Right congruous incomplete homonymous hemianopia

(8) Right homonymous hemianopia due to a lesion of the left hemisphere. The pupillary light reflex is not impaired if it is beyond the tract

FIGURE 5.117
Topographical mechanisms of visual field defects

Reproduced, with permission, from Daroff RB, Bradley WG et al., Neurology in Clinical Practice, 5th edn, Philadelphia: Butterworth-Heinemann, 2008: Fig 14-3.

TABLE 5.34
Clinical utility of hemianopia in unilateral cerebral hemisphere lesions[40]

	Sensitivity	Specificity	Positive LR	Negative LR
Hemianopia[40]	30%	98%	NS	0.7

Adapted from McGee S, Evidence Based Physical Diagnosis, 2nd edn, St Louis: Saunders, 2007.

5

Waddling gait (bilateral Trendelenburg gait)

Relevant neuroanatomy and topographical anatomy
× Proximal muscle groups

Description

Exaggerated rotation of the pelvis and pronounced lower limb swing compensate for bilateral proximal leg and hip girdle muscle weakness.[28,43] Pelvic instability results in a characteristic stance of slight hip flexion and exaggerated lumbar lordosis.[28] Weakness of the hip extension also impairs the patient's ability to stand from a squatting position.[28] Patients may use their hands to push themselves up to stand from a squatting position (i.e. Gowers' sign).[28]

Condition/s associated with[220]

Common

- Muscular dystrophy – limb girdle muscular dystrophy, Duchenne's muscular dystrophy
- Metabolic myopathy – thyroid myopathy

Less common

- Polymyositis
- Dermatomyositis
- Mitochondrial myopathy
- Glucocorticoid-induced myopathy

Mechanism/s

A waddling gait is caused by bilateral proximal hip muscle weakness. Proximal muscle weakness is most commonly associated with primary muscle disorders (myopathy).[54] Proximal muscle weakness and pelvic girdle instability result in a characteristic stance of slight hip flexion and exaggerated lumbar lordosis to maintain balance during gait examination.

Sign value

Waddling gait is a sign of proximal muscle weakness.

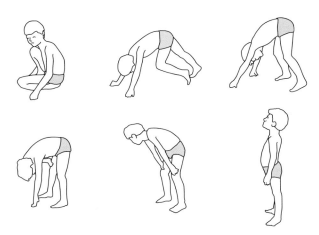

FIGURE 5.118
Gowers' sign in proximal muscle weakness

Reproduced, with permission, from Canale ST, Beaty JH, Campbell's Operative Orthopaedics, 11th edn, St Louis: Mosby, 2007: Fig 32-5.

5

Wallenberg's syndrome (lateral medullary syndrome)

Description

Lateral medullary syndrome is a brainstem vascular syndrome characterised by:

- uvular deviation away from the side of the lesion
- ipsilateral impaired palatal elevation
- dysarthria, dysphagia, hoarseness
- ipsilateral facial sensory loss
- ipsilateral Horner's syndrome
- ipsilateral cerebellar ataxia
- contralateral loss (pain and temperature) below the lesion.

Relevant neuroanatomy and topographical anatomy

BRAINSTEM
- Nucleus ambiguus (CNIX/X)
- Trigeminal sensory nuclei (CNV)
- Descending sympathetic fibres
- Spinocerebellar tract
- Spinothalamic tracts

Condition/s associated with[121]

- Posterior inferior cerebellar artery (PICA) territory infarction
- Vertebral artery insufficiency

Mechanism/s

Posterior inferior cerebellar artery (PICA) territory infarction may result in dysfunction of multiple brainstem nuclei in the lateral medulla. See Table 5.35 for mechanisms of the clinical findings in lateral medullary syndrome.

Sign value

Wallenberg's syndrome is most commonly due to ischemic stroke in the distribution of the posterior inferior cerebellar artery (PICA).

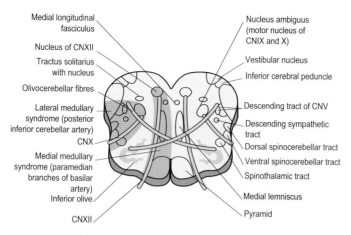

FIGURE 5.119

Affected brainstem nuclei and long tracts in lateral medullary syndrome (lateral shaded area)

Reproduced, with permission, from Flint PW et al., Cummings Otolaryngology: Head and Neck Surgery, *5th edn, Philadelphia: Mosby, 2010: Fig 166-4.*

TABLE 5.35

Mechanisms of features of lateral medullary syndrome

Clinical signs	Nerve dysfunction
• Uvular deviation away from side of lesion • Ipsilateral palatal elevation • Dysarthria • Dysphagia • Hoarseness	→ Nucleus ambiguus (CNIX, X)
• Ipsilateral facial sensory loss	→ Descending tract, CNV
• Ipsilateral Horner's syndrome	→ Descending sympathetic fibres
• Ipsilateral cerebellar ataxia	→ Spinocerebellar tracts
• Contralateral loss (pain and temperature) below lesion	→ Spinothalamic tract

5

Weakness

Description

Muscle weakness is characterised by the grade of weakness, anatomical distribution and associated findings (e.g. lower motor neuron signs, upper motor neuron signs, cortical localising signs).

Muscle weakness is graded according to the system developed by the British Medical Research Council (MRC) during World War II (see Table 5.36).[221]

Condition/s associated with

Common

- MCA territory infarction
- Cerebral haemorrhage

TABLE 5.36
British Medical Research Council System of Grading Muscle Power[221]

Grade	Feature(s)
0/5	No contraction
1/5	Muscle flicker
2/5	Any movement, but not against gravity
3/5	Movement against gravity, no movement against resistance
4–/5	Movement against gravity but barely against resistance
4/5	Movement against gravity and resistance
4+/5	Movement against gravity and almost full power against resistance
5/5	Normal power

Adapted from McGee S, Evidence Based Physical Diagnosis, *2nd edn, St Louis: Saunders, 2007.*

- Lacunar infarction, posterior limb internal capsule
- Myelopathy
- Compression mononeuropathy – carpal tunnel syndrome
- Radiculopathy
- Hypokalaemia

Less common

- Multiple sclerosis
- Peripheral neuropathy
- Guillain–Barré syndrome
- Myasthenia gravis
- Myopathy
- Todd's paralysis
- Hypoglycaemia
- Poliomyelitis

Mechanism/s

Mechanisms of weakness are grouped according to the anatomical distribution and associated findings (e.g. upper motor neuron findings, lower motor neuron findings, cortical localising signs etc.). See Tables 5.37 and 5.38.

The mechanisms of weakness include:

- motor cortex lesion
- posterior limb, internal capsule lesion
- medial brainstem lesion
- spinal cord lesion
- radiculopathy
- Guillain–Barré syndrome
- peripheral neuropathy
- disorders of the neuromuscular junction
- myopathy

Relevant neuroanatomy and topographical anatomy

UPPER MOTOR NEURON
- Motor cortex
  ↓
- Corona radiata, subcortical white matter
  ↓
- Posterior limb, internal capsule
  ↓
- Pyramidal tracts, medial brainstem
  ↓
Ø Pyramidal decussation, medulla
  ↓
- Lateral corticospinal tracts, spinal cord
⇒ Central canal, spinal cord
  ↓
LOWER MOTOR NEURON
- Anterior horn grey matter, spinal cord
  ↓
- Nerve root
⇒ Intervertebral disc
⇒ Intervertebral foramen
  ↓
- Nerve plexus (e.g. brachial plexus)
  ↓
- Peripheral nerve
⇒ Potential sites of nerve entrapment (e.g. carpal tunnel)
  ↓
NEUROMUSCULAR JUNCTION
- Neuromuscular junction
  ↓
MUSCLE
× Muscle

- metabolic, toxicological and infectious disorders
- aortic dissection.

Motor cortex lesion

Results in contralateral hemiparesis in the somatotopic distribution of the motor cortex (i.e. the homunculus).

Associated upper motor neuron signs are characteristic. Immediately following acute ischaemic infarction of the motor cortex hypotonia, flaccid paresis and hyporeflexia or areflexia may be present. Spasticity and hyperreflexia develop days to weeks later.[56]

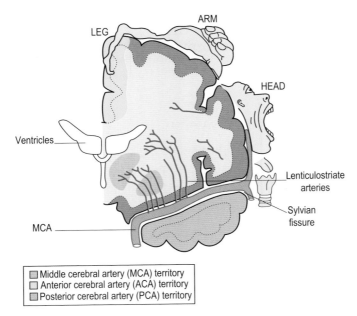

FIGURE 5.120
Anterior circulation and somatotopic organisation, motor cortex
Reproduced, with permission, from Lewandowski CA, Rao CPV, Silver B, Transient ischemic attack: definitions and clinical presentations. Ann Emerg Med *2008; 52(2): S7–S16, Fig 7.*

Posterior limb, internal capsule lesion

Causes contralateral pure motor hemiparesis of the face, arm and leg. Associated upper motor neuron signs are characteristic. Due to the close proximity of motor fibres to one another in the posterior limb of the internal capsule, even small lesions may result in pure hemimotor findings in the face, arm and leg. The most common cause is lacunar infarction.

Medial brainstem lesion

Medial brainstem lesions may affect cranial nerve motor nuclei and/or the descending long tracts of motor fibres.[222] Brainstem lesions are characterised by motor and/or sensory findings that cross the midline (e.g. ipsilateral cranial nerve findings and contralateral long tract findings). Causes include medial brainstem

vascular syndromes, haemorrhagic infarction, multiple sclerosis and tumours.

Spinal cord lesion

Unilateral spinal cord lesions affecting the lateral cortical spinal tract cause ipsilateral weakness. The upper motor neuron fibres have crossed in the pyramidal decussation in the medulla. Associated upper motor neuron signs are characteristic.

Radiculopathy

Motor findings occur in the distribution of a nerve root(s). Lesions of the nerve root typically cause positive (e.g. pain) and negative (e.g. decreased sensation) sensory abnormalities in the distribution of one or more nerve roots. Lower motor neuron signs are characteristic. Mechanical injury to the nerve root causes degeneration of the axons and

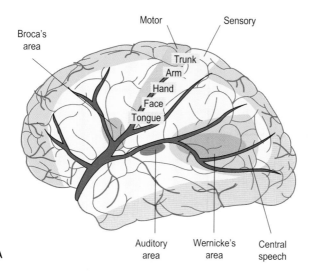

Motor   Sensory

Broca's
area

Trunk
Arm
Hand
Face
Tongue

A

Auditory   Wernicke's   Central
area   area   speech

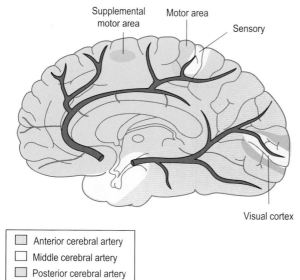

Supplemental   Motor area
motor area
Sensory

5

B

Visual cortex

☐ Anterior cerebral artery
☐ Middle cerebral artery
☐ Posterior cerebral artery

FIGURE 5.121
Vascular territories of the cerebral arteries
A Lateral aspect of the cerebral cortex; **B** medial aspect of the cerebral cortex.

Reproduced, with permission, from Goldman L, Ausiello D, Cecil Medicine, 23rd edn, Philadelphia: Saunders, 2007: Fig 430-3.

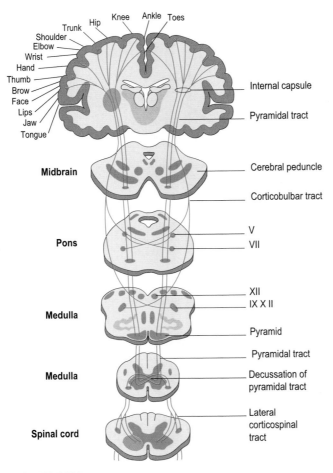

FIGURE 5.122
Upper motor neuron anatomy

Reproduced, with permission, from Clark RG, Manter and Gatz's Essential Neuroanatomy and Neurophysiology, *5th edn, Philadelphia: FA Davis Co, 1975.*

TABLE 5.37
Upper and lower motor neuron signs

Upper motor neuron signs[58]	Lower motor neuron signs[58]
• Spasticity • Clonus • Weakness • Hyperreflexia • Babinski sign	• Fasciculations • Muscle atrophy • Hypotonia • Weakness • Hyporeflexia/areflexia

TABLE 5.38

Mechanisms of weakness based on the pattern of clinical findings

Pattern of weakness	Mechanism(s)
Arm and leg 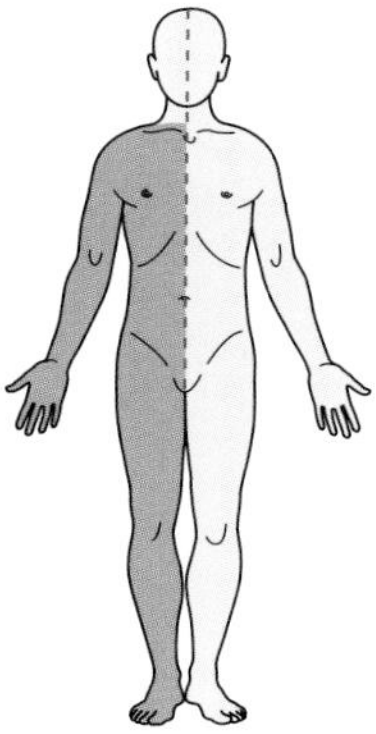 Figure 5.123	• Contralateral motor cortex lesion • Ipsilateral cervical spinal cord lesion • Contralateral posterior limb, internal capsule lesion • Todd's paralysis
Ascending weakness 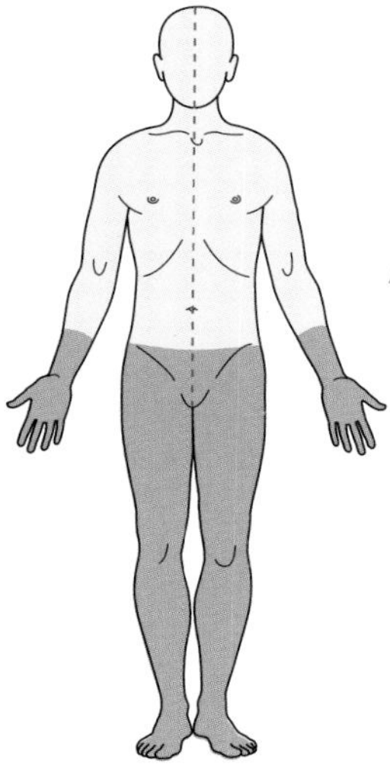 Figure 5.124	• Guillain–Barré syndrome • Tick paralysis

5

TABLE 5.38
Mechanisms of weakness based on the pattern of clinical findings—cont'd

Pattern of weakness	Mechanism(s)
Descending weakness 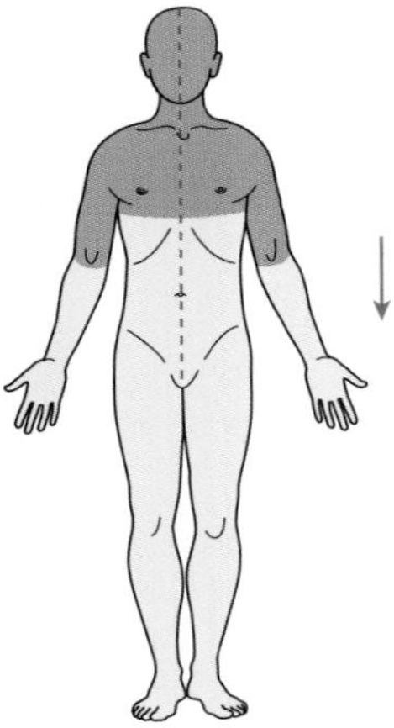 Figure 5.125	• Botulism • Miller Fisher variant Guillain–Barré syndrome • Diphtheria polyneuropathy
Bilateral arms and legs 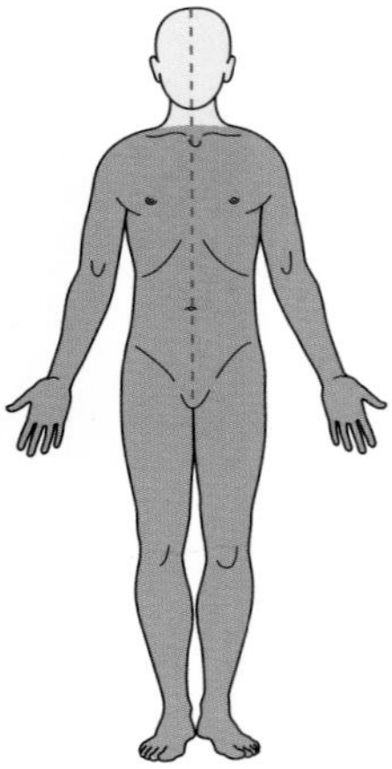 Figure 5.126	• Complete cervical spinal cord lesion • Anterior cord syndrome

TABLE 5.38

Mechanisms of weakness based on the pattern of clinical findings—cont'd

Pattern of weakness	Mechanism(s)
Bilateral upper limbs 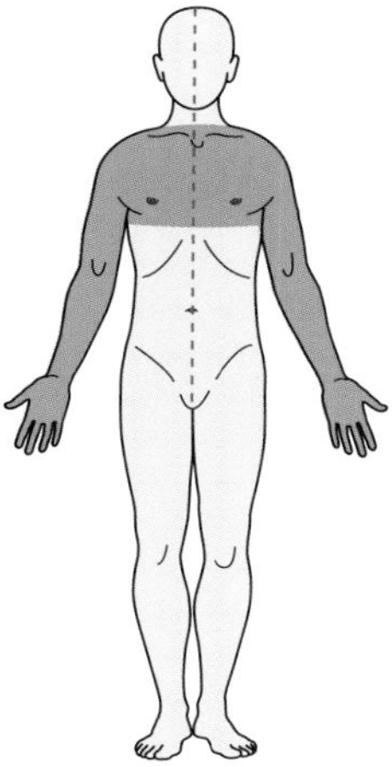 Figure 5.127	• Cervical syringomyelia • Cervical radiculopathy
Distal muscle groups 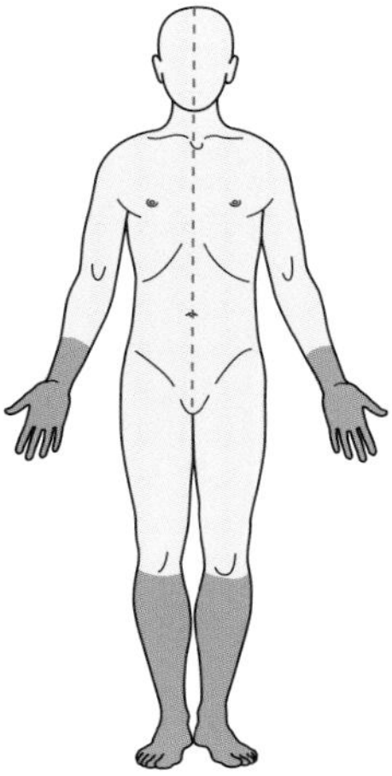 Figure 5.128	• Peripheral neuropathy • Myotonic dystrophy

5

TABLE 5.38
Mechanisms of weakness based on the pattern of clinical findings—cont'd

Pattern of weakness	Mechanism(s)
Face and arm 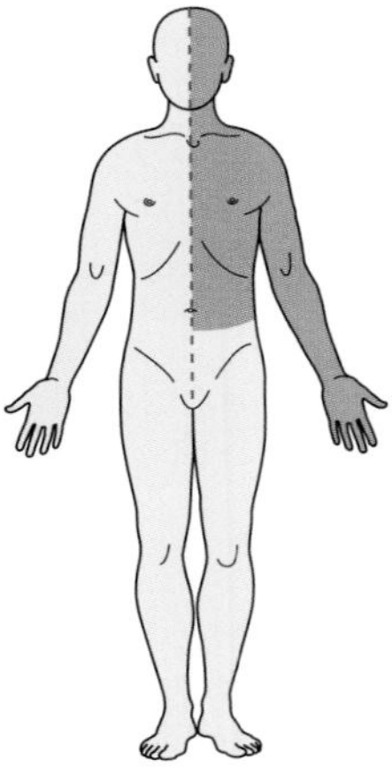 Figure 5.129	• MCA territory infarction
Face, arm and leg 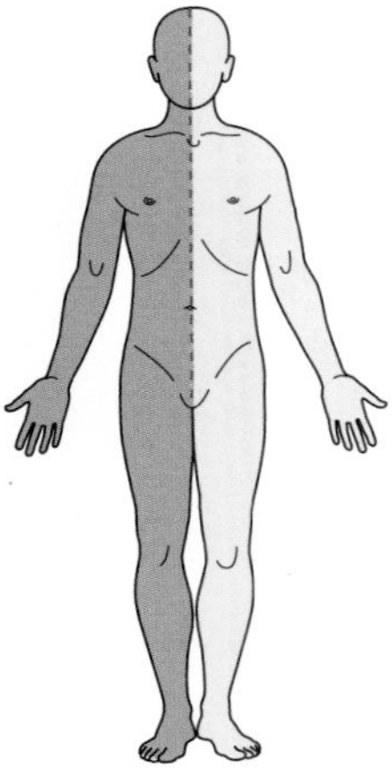 Figure 5.130	• Posterior limb, internal capsule lesion • ICA territory (ACA + MCA) infarction

TABLE 5.38
Mechanisms of weakness based on the pattern of clinical findings—cont'd

Pattern of weakness	Mechanism(s)
Face and contralateral arm and leg 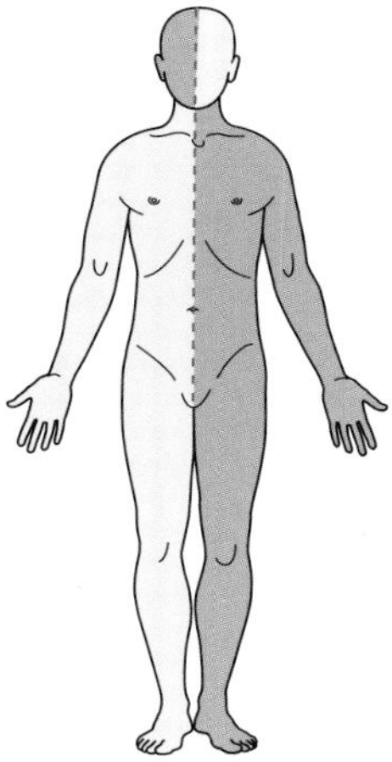 Figure 5.131	• Brainstem lesion
Leg 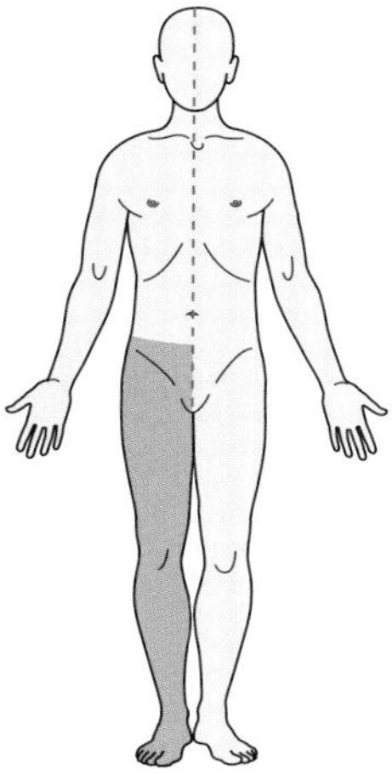 Figure 5.132	• ACA territory infarction

5

TABLE 5.38
Mechanisms of weakness based on the pattern of clinical findings—cont'd

Pattern of weakness	Mechanism(s)
Peripheral nerve distribution	• Compression mononeuropathy
Nerve root distribution	• Radiculopathy
 Figure 5.133	
Proximal muscle groups	• Myopathy
 Figure 5.134	
Distal muscle groups	• Length-dependent peripheral neuropathy

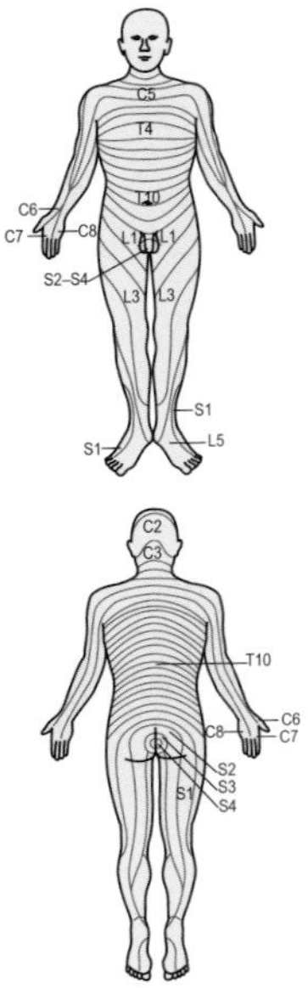

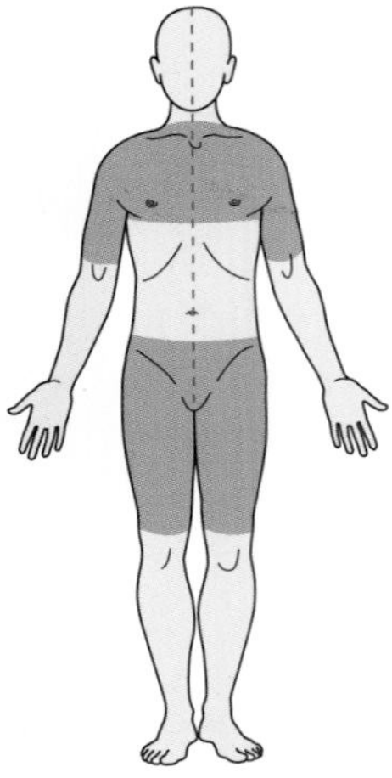

myelin distal to the site of injury (Wallerian degeneration), resulting in sensory and motor deficits in the distribution of the affected nerve root. Common causes include spondylosis, intervertebral disc disease and tumours. See Table 5.38.

Guillain–Barré syndrome (GBS)

Guillain–Barré syndrome (GBS), or acute inflammatory demyelinating polyradiculopathy, is characterised by demyelination with variable axonal degeneration and lymphocytic infiltration and is associated with several preceding infectious illnesses (e.g. *Campylobacter jejuni*, herpes viruses, *Mycoplasma pneumonia*).[223] GBS typically causes ascending flaccid paresis. Lower motor neuron signs are characteristic.

Peripheral neuropathy

Causes include compression mononeuropathy and length-dependent peripheral neuropathy.

Compression mononeuropathy

Mechanical injury causes degeneration of the axons and myelin distal to the site of injury (i.e. Wallerian degeneration), resulting in motor and sensory deficits in the distribution of the affected peripheral nerve.[221] Causes include carpal tunnel syndrome, common peroneal nerve palsy and radial nerve palsy ('Saturday night' palsy).

Length-dependent peripheral neuropathy

Length-dependent peripheral neuropathy may result from failure of the perikaryon to synthesise enzymes or proteins, dysfunction in axonal transport or disturbances in energy metabolism. A variety of metabolic abnormalities within the peripheral nerve result in degeneration of the distal nerve fibres, which progresses proximally. Causes include diabetes mellitus, alcohol and inherited neuropathies.[221]

Disorders of the neuromuscular junction

Myasthenia gravis is caused by antibodies directed against acetylcholine receptors on the postsynaptic neuromuscular membrane. Myasthenia gravis typically involves muscles of the eyes and face, and muscle strength that decreases with activity (fatiguability). Lambert–Eaton syndrome is a paraneoplastic syndrome associated with small-cell lung carcinoma, and is caused by antibodies against presynaptic calcium channels.[224] Characteristics include proximal muscle weakness and weakness that transiently improves with increased activity.[224]

Myopathy

Myopathies typically result in proximal weakness. One exception is myotonic dystrophy, which preferentially affects cranial and distal muscle groups. Causes of myopathy include muscular dystrophy, metabolic myopathy and inflammatory myopathy.

Metabolic, toxicological and infectious disorders

Metabolic and toxic disorders typically cause diffuse muscle weakness due to changes in the excitability (i.e. resting membrane potential) of nerve fibres and/or muscle fibres, or due to direct toxic effects to nerves or muscles. Causes include hypokalaemia, hypocalcaemia, hypoglycaemia, strychnine toxicity, tetanus and botulism.

Clostridium botulinum

Botulism is caused by the bacterium *Clostridium botulinum*, which produces a toxin that blocks the release of acetylcholine at the motor terminal.[133]

5

Tick paralysis

Tick paralysis is caused by a toxin produced by the tick during feeding, which augments axonal sodium flux across the membrane without affecting the neuromuscular junction.[225,226] Motor nerve terminal function rapidly improves after tick removal.[225] Characteristics include ascending flaccid paresis and acute ataxia, which may progress to bulbar involvement and respiratory arrest.[226]

Aortic dissection

Acute aortic dissection may present with weakness in a distribution compatible with acute ischemia stroke, or in a pattern atypical for single neurological lesion. Patients may present with a variety of symptoms and signs including chest pain radiating to the back, abdominal pain, syncope, shortness of breath, hypertension, pulse asymmetry, focal weakness or focal sensory loss.

Sign value

The grade, distribution and progression of weakness, and associated findings (e.g. lower motor neuron signs, upper motor neuron signs, cortical localising signs) are important when considering potential aetiologies of weakness. In patients presenting with weakness in an atypical distribution for a single neurological lesion, acute aortic dissection should be considered.

Wernicke's aphasia (receptive aphasia)

Relevant neuroanatomy and topographical anatomy

- Wernicke's area – posterior superior temporal gyrus, dominant hemisphere
- ⇒ Inferior division, middle cerebral artery (MCA)

Description

Receptive aphasia is a disorder of language comprehension. Speech fluency (word production) is typically not affected. The patient's speech is meaningless or strange and may contain paraphasic errors (inappropriate word substitutions based on meaning or sound).[6,46]

Condition/s associated with[6,67]

Common

- MCA territory infarction
- Cerebral haemorrhage
- Vascular dementia
- Migraine (transient)

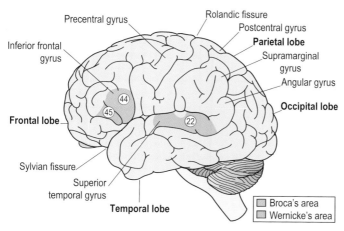

Precentral gyrus
Rolandic fissure
Postcentral gyrus
Parietal lobe
Inferior frontal gyrus
Supramarginal gyrus
Angular gyrus
44
45
Occipital lobe
Frontal lobe
22
Sylvian fissure
Superior temporal gyrus
Temporal lobe
☐ Broca's area
☐ Wernicke's area

FIGURE 5.135
Wernicke's area, posterior superior temporal gyrus, dominant hemisphere
22 = Brodmann's area 22; 44 = Brodmann's area 44; 45 = Brodmann's area 45.

Reproduced, with permission, from Daroff RB, Bradley WG et al., Neurology in Clinical Practice, 5th edn, Philadelphia: Butterworth-Heinemann, 2008: Fig 12A-1.

5

Less common

- Alzheimer's disease
- Mass lesion – tumour, abscess, AVM
- Primary progressive aphasia

Mechanism/s

Wernicke's aphasia is caused by a lesion in the posterior superior temporal gyrus of the dominant hemisphere.[227] This region is supplied by branches of the inferior division of the middle cerebral artery (MCA).[47] The most common cause of Wernicke's aphasia is ischaemic infarction of the inferior division of the MCA. Patient hand dominance (being left or right handed) correlates with the side of the dominant cerebral hemisphere and, therefore, has potential localising value

(see also 'Hand dominance' in this chapter). Larger lesions may affect the motor and sensory cortex and/or optic pathways, resulting in contralateral motor and sensory findings and contralateral homonymous hemianopia.[46] Associated contralateral homonymous hemianopia is more common in Wernicke's aphasia (receptive aphasia), whereas motor and sensory findings are more common in Broca's aphasia (expressive aphasia).[46] Refer to Table 5.39 for clinical features of Wernicke's aphasia.

Sign value

Wernicke's aphasia, or receptive aphasia, is a dominant cortical localising sign. Acute onset aphasia should be considered a sign of stroke until proven otherwise.

TABLE 5.39
Clinical features of Wernicke's aphasia

Clinical feature(s)	Abnormality in Wernicke's aphasia
Spontaneous speech	• Fluent, with paraphasic errors • Dysarthria usually absent
Naming	• Impaired (often bizarre paraphasic misnaming)
Comprehension	• Impaired
Repetition	• Impaired
Reading	• Impaired for comprehension and reading aloud
Writing	• Well formed, paragraphic
Associated signs	• Contralateral hemianopia • Contralateral motor and sensory findings less common

Adapted from Kirshner HS, Language and speech disorders: aphasia and aphasiac syndromes. In: Bradley WG, Daroff RB, Fenichel G et al., Neurology in Clinical Practice, 5th edn, Philadelphia: Butterworth-Heinemann, 2008.

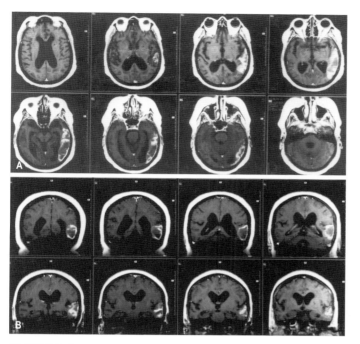

FIGURE 5.136
MRI of a patient with Wernicke's aphasia caused by a temporal lobe lesion
A Axial images; **B** coronal images.

Reproduced, with permission, from Daroff RB, Bradley WG et al., Neurology in Clinical Practice, *5th edn, Philadelphia: Butterworth-Heinemann, 2008: Fig 12A-4.*

5

References

1. Rucker JC. Cranial neuropathies. In: Bradley WG, Daroff RB, Fenichel G, et al., editors. *Neurology in Clinical Practice*. 5th ed. Philadelphia: Butterworth-Heinemann; 2008.

2. Hanson RA, Ghosh S, Gonzalez-Gomez I, et al. Abducens length and vulnerability? *Neurology* 2004;**62**:33–6.

3. Harati Y, Bosch EP. Disorders of the peripheral nerves. In: Bradley WG, Daroff RB, Fenichel G, et al., editors. *Neurology in Clinical Practice*. 5th ed. Philadelphia: Butterworth-Heinemann; 2008.

4. McGee S. *Evidence Based Physical Diagnosis*. 2nd ed. St Louis: Saunders; 2007.

5. Lam BL, Thompson HS, Corbett JJ. The prevalence of simple anisocoria. *Am J Ophthalmol* 1987;**104**:69–73.

6. Blumenfeld H. *Neuroanatomy Through Clinical Cases*. Sunderland: Sinauer; 2002.

7. Rucker JC. Pupillary and eyelid abnormalities. In: Bradley WG, Daroff RB, Fenichel G, et al., editors. *Neurology in Clinical Practice*. 5th ed. Philadelphia: Butterworth-Heinemann; 2008.

8. Thompson HS, Pilley SFJ. Unequal pupils: a flow chart for sorting out the anisocorias. *Surv Ophthalmol* 1976;**21**:45–8.

9. Kardon RH. The pupils. In: Yanoff M, Duker JS, editors. *Ophthalmology*. 3rd ed. St Louis: Mosby; 2008.

10. Cremer SA, Thompson HS, Digre KB, et al. Hydroxyamphetamine mydriasis in Horner's syndrome. *Am J Ophthlamol* 1990;**110**:71–6.

11. Maloney WF, Younge BR, Moyer NJ. Evaluation of the causes and pharmacologic localization in Horner's syndrome. *Am J Ophthalmol* 1980;**90**:394–402.

12. Van der Wiel HL, Van Gijn J. Localization of Horner's syndrome: use and limitations of hydroxyamphetamine test. *J Neurol Sci* 1983;**59**:229–35.

13. Wall M. Brainstem syndromes. In: Bradley WG, Daroff RB, Fenichel G, et al., editors. *Neurology in Clinical Practice*. 5th ed. Philadelphia: Butterworth-Heinemann; 2008.

14. Thompson HS. Segmental palsy of the iris sphincter in Adie's syndrome. *Arch Ophthalmol* 1978;**96**:1615–20.

15. Loewenstein O, Loewenfeld IR. Pupillotonic pseudotabes (syndrome of Markus–Weill and Reys–Holmes–Adie): a critical review of the literature. *Surv Ophthalmol* 1967;**10**:129–85.

16. Loewenfled IR, Thompson HS. The tonic pupil: a re-evaluation. *Am J Ophthalmol* 1967;**63**:46–87.

17. Finelli PF, Mair RG. Disturbances of smell and taste. In: Bradley WG, Daroff RB, Fenichel G, et al., editors. *Neurology in Clinical Practice*. 5th ed. Philadelphia: Butterworth-Heinemann; 2008.

18. Talley NJ, O'Connor S. The nervous system. In: Talley NJ, O'Connor S, editors. *Clinical Examination, A Systematic Guide to Physical Diagnosis*. 5th ed. Sydney: Churchill Livingstone; 2006. pp. 283–368.

19. Deems DA, Doty RL, Settle RG, et al. Smell and test disorders, a study of 750 patients from the University of Pennsylvania smell and taste center. *Arch Otolaryngol Head Neck Surg* 1991;**117**:519–28.

20. Bromley SM. Smell and taste disorders: a primary care approach. *Am Fam Physician* 2000. Available: http://www.aafp.org/afp/20000115/427.html [5 May 2010].

21. Hellings PW, Rombaux P. Medical therapy and smell dysfunction. *B-ENT* 2009;**5**(Suppl. 13):71–5.

22. Li C, Yousem DM, Doty RL, et al. Neuroimaging in patients with olfactory dysfunction. *AJR Am J Roetgenol* 1994;**162**(2):411–18.

23. Wu AP, Davidson T. Post-traumatic anosmia secondary to central nervous system injury. *Am J Rhinol* 2008;**22**(6):606–7.

24. Murphy C, Cerf-Ducastel B, Calhoun-Haney R, et al. ERP, fMRI and functional connectivity studies of brain response to odor in normal aging and Alzheimer's disease. *Chem Senses* 2005;**30**(1):i170–1.

25. Temmel AFP, Quint C, Schickinger-Fischer B, et al. Characteristics of olfactory disorders in relation to major causes of olfactory loss. *Arch Otolaryngol Head Neck Surg* 2002;**128**(6):635–41.

26. Poole CJM. Argyll Robertson pupils due to neurosarcoidosis: evidence for site of a lesion. *Br Med J* 1984;**289**:356.

27. Loewenfeld IE. The Argyll Robertson pupil, 1869–1969: a critical survey of the literature. *Surv Ophthalmol* 1969;**14**:199–299.

28. Thompson PD. Gait disorders. In: Bradley WG, Daroff RB, Fenichel G, et al., editors. *Neurology in Clinical Practice*. 5th ed. Philadelphia: Butterworth-Heinemann; 2008.

29. Gilman S, Bloedel JR, Lechtenberg R. *Disorders of the Cerebellum*. Philadelphia: FA Davis; 1981.

30. Amici R, Avanzini G, Pacini L. *Cerebellar Tumours: Clinical Analysis and Physiopathologic Correlations*. Basel: S. Karger; 1976.

31. Anthony DC, Frosch MP, De Dirolami U. Peripheral nerve and skeletal muscle. In: Kumar V, Abbas AK, Fausto N, editors. *Pathologic Basis of Disease*. 7th ed. Philadelphia: Saunders; 2005. pp. 1347–419.

32. Gomes MD, et al. Atrogin-1, a muscle-specific F-box protein highly expressed during muscle atrophy. *Proc Natl Acad Sci U S A* 2001;**98**(25):14440–5.

33. Gerr F, Letz R. The sensitivity and specificity of tests for carpal tunnel syndrome vary with the comparison subjects. *J Hand Surg [Br]* 1998;**23B**:151–5.

34. Golding DH, Rose DM, Selvarajah K. Clinical tests for carpal tunnel syndrome: an evaluation. *Br J Rheumatol* 1986;**25**:388–90.

35. Katz JN, Larson MG, Sabra A, et al. Carpal tunnel syndrome: diagnostic utility of history and physical examination findings. *Ann Intern Med* 1990;**112**:321–7.

36. Kerr RSC, Cadoux-Hudson TA, Adams CBT. The value of accurate clinical assessment in the surgical management of the lumbar disc protrusion. *J Neurol Neurosurg Psychiatry* 1988;**51**:169–73.

37. van Gijn J. The Babinksi reflex. *Postgrad Med J* 1995;**71**:645–8.

38. Byrne TN, Waxman SG. Paraplegia and spinal cord syndromes. In: Bradley WG, Daroff RB, Fenichel G, et al., editors. *Neurology in Clinical Practice*. 5th ed. Philadelphia: Butterworth-Heinemann; 2008.

39. Misulis KE. Hemiplegia and monoplegia. In: Bradley WG, Daroff RB, Fenichel G, et al., editors. *Neurology in Clinical Practice*. 5th ed. Philadelphia: Butterworth-Heinemann; 2008.

40. Sawyer RN, Hanna JP, Ruff RL, et al. Asymmetry of forearm rolling as a sign of unilateral cerebral dysfunction. *Neurology* 1993;**43**:1596–8.

41. Jankovic J, Shannon KM. Movement disorders. In: Bradley WG, Daroff RB, Fenichel G, et al., editors. *Neurology in Clinical Practice*. 5th ed. Philadelphia: Butterworth-Heinemann; 2008.

42. Heilman KM, Valenstein E, Gonzale Rothi LJ, et al. Upper limb action-intentional and cognitive apraxic motor disorders. In: Bradley WG, Daroff RB, Fenichel G, et al., editors. *Neurology in Clinical Practice*. 5th ed. Philadelphia: Butterworth-Heinemann; 2008.

43. Talley NJ, O'Connor S. *Examination Medicine: A Guide to Physician Training*. 5th ed. Sydney: Churchill Livingstone; 2006.

44. Rodriguez-Oroz MC, Jahanshahi M, Krack P, et al. Initial clinical manifestations of Parkinson's disease: features and pathophysiological mechanisms. *Lancet Neurol* 2009;**8**:1128–39.

45. Wenning GK, Ben-Shlomo Y, Hughes A, et al. What clinical features are most useful to distinguish multiple system atrophy from Parkinson's disease? *J Neurol Neurosurg Psychiatry* 2000;**68**:434–40.

5

46. Kirshner HS. Language and speech disorders: aphasia and aphasiac syndromes. In: Bradley WG, Daroff RB, Fenichel G, et al., editors. *Neurology in Clinical Practice.* 5th ed. Philadelphia: Butterworth-Heinemann; 2008.

47. Kang SY, Kim JS. Anterior cerebral artery infarction: stroke mechanism and clinical imaging in 100 patients. *Neurology* 2008;**70**:2386–93.

48. Goldstein JN, Greer DM. Rapid focused neurological assessment in the emergency department and ICU. *Emerg Med Clin North Am* 2009;**27**:1–16.

49. Gala VC, Voyadizis J-M, Kim D-H, et al. Trauma of the nervous system: spinal cord trauma. In: Bradley WG, Daroff RB, Fenichel G, et al., editors. *Neurology in Clinical Practice.* 5th ed. Philadelphia: Butterworth-Heinemann; 2008.

50. O'Connell JEA. The clinical signs of meningeal irritation. *Brain* 1946;**69**:9–21.

51. Thomas KE, Hasburn R, et al. The diagnostic accuracy of Kernig's sign, Brudzinski's sign, and nuchal rigidity in adults with suspected meningitis. *Clin Infect Dis* 2002;**35**(1):46–62.

52. Quiros PA. Urgent neuro-ophthalmologic pathologies. In: Yanoff M, Duker JS, editors. *Ophthalmology.* 3rd ed. St Louis: Mosby; 2008.

53. Nath A. Brain abscess and parameningeal infections. In: Goldman L, Ausiello D, editors. *Cecil Medicine.* 23rd ed. Philadelphia: Saunders; 2008.

54. Robinson JA, Preston DC, Shapiro BE. Proximal, distal, and generalized weakness. In: Bradley WG, Daroff RB, Fenichel G, et al., editors. *Neurology in Clinical Practice.* 5th ed. Philadelphia: Butterworth-Heinemann; 2008.

55. Young RR. Treatment of spastic patients. *N Engl J Med* 1989;**320**:1553–5.

56. Twitchell TE. The restoration of motor function following hemiplegia in man. *Brain* 1951;**74**:443–80.

57. Burke D, Gillies JD, Lance JW. The quadriceps stretch reflex in human spasticity. *J Neurol Neurosurg Psychiatry* 1970;**33**:216–23.

58. Murray B, Mitsumoto H. Disorders of upper and lower motor neurons. In: Bradley WG, Daroff RB, Fenichel G, et al., editors. *Neurology in Clinical Practice.* 5th ed. Philadelphia: Butterworth-Heinemann; 2008.

59. Brent J, Palmer R. Monoamine oxidase inhibitors and serotonin syndrome. In: Shannon MW, Borron SW, Burns MJ, editors. *Haddad and Winchester's Clinical Management of Poisoning and Drug Overdose.* Philadelphia: Saunders; 2007.

60. Boyer EW, Shannon M. The serotonin syndrome. *N Engl J Med* 2005;**352**(11):1112–20.

61. Jankovic J, Lang AE. Movement disorders: diagnosis and assessment. In: Bradley WG, Daroff RB, Fenichel G, et al., editors. *Neurology in Clinical Practice.* 5th ed. Philadelphia: Butterworth-Heinemann; 2008.

62. Rai GS, Elias-Jones A. The corneal reflex in elderly patients. *J Am Geriatr Soc* 1979;**27**:317–18.

63. Harner SG, Laws ER. Clinical findings in patients with acoustic neuroma. *Mayo Clin Proc* 1983;**58**:721–58.

64. Teasdall RD, van den Ende H. The crossed adductor reflex in humans. An EMG study. *Can J Neurol Sci* 1981;**8**:81–5.

65. Kortte JH, Palmer JB. Speech and language disorders. In: Frontera WR, Silver JK, Rizzo TD, editors. *Essentials of Physical Medicine and Rehabilitation.* 2nd ed. Philadelphia: Saunders; 2008.

66. Duffy JR. *Motor Speech Disorders: Substrates, Differential Diagnosis and Management.* St Louis: Mosby; 1995.

67. Talley NJ, O'Connor S. *Clinical Examination: A Systematic Guide to Physical Diagnosis.* 5th ed. Chatswood: Churchill Livingstone; 2006.

68. Diener HC, Dichagans J. Pathophysiology of cerebellar ataxia. *Mov Disord* 1992;**7**(2):95–109.

69. Subramony SH. Ataxic disorders. In: Bradley WG, Daroff RB, Fenichel G, et al., editors. *Neurology in Clinical Practice*. 5th ed. Philadelphia: Butterworth-Heinemann; 2008.

70. Cohen SM, Elackattu A, Noordzij P, et al. Palliative treatment of dysphonia and dysarthria. *Otolaryngol Clin North Am* 2009;**42**:107–21.

71. Lee A. Hoarseness and laryngitis. In: Bope ET, Rakel RE, Kellerman R, editors. *Conn's Current Therapy 2010*. 1st ed. Philadelphia: Saunders; 2010.

72. Gilden DH. Bell's palsy. *N Eng J Med* 2004;**351**:1323–31.

73. Ward BK, Schaitkin BM. Acute peripheral facial paralysis (Bell's palsy). In: Bope ET, Rakel RE, Kellerman RD, editors. *Conn's Current Therapy 2010*. Philadelphia: Saunders; 2010.

74. Morecraft RJ, Louie JL, Herrick JL, et al. Cortical innervation of the facial nucleus in the non-human primate: a new interpretation of the effects of stroke and related subtotal brain trauma on the muscles of facial expression. *Brain* 2001;**124**:176–208.

75. Park HW, Watkins AL. Facial paralysis: analysis of 500 cases. *Arch Phys Med* 1949;**30**: 749–62.

76. May M, Klein SR. Differential diagnosis of facial nerve palsy. *Otolaryngol Clin North Am* 1991;**24**:613–45.

77. Layzer RB. The origin of muscle fasciculations and cramps. *Muscle Nerve* 1994;**17**(11): 1243–9.

78. Nicholson GM, Walsh R, Little MJ, et al. Characterization of the effects of robustoxin, the lethal neurotoxin from the Sydney funnel-web spider *Atrax robustus*, on sodium channel activation and inactivation. *Pflugers Arch* 1998;**436**:117–26.

79. Blexrud MD, Windebank AJ, Daube JR. Long-term follow-up on 121 patients with benign fasciculations. *Ann Neurol* 1993;**34**:622–5.

80. Reed DM, Kurland LT. Muscle fasciculations in a healthy population. *Arch Neurol* 1963;**9**:363–7.

81. Li TM, Alberman E, Swash M. Clinical features and associations of 560 cases of motor neuron disease. *J Neurol Neurosurg Psychiatry* 1990;**53**:1043–5.

82. Saliba DL. Reliable block of the gag reflex in one minute or less. *J Clin Anesth* 2009;**21**(6):463.

83. Meeker HG, Magalee R. The conservative management of the gag reflex in full denture patients. *N Y State Dent J* 1986;**52**:11–14.

84. Murphy WM. A clinical survey of gagging patients. *J Prosthet Dent* 1979;**42**:145–8.

85. Wilks CG, Marks IM. Reducing hypersensitive gagging. *Br Dent J* 1983;**155**:263–5.

86. Davies AE. Pharyngeal sensation and gag reflex in healthy subjects. *Lancet* 1995;**345**(8945):487–8.

87. Mayer E, Martory MD, Pegna AJ, et al. A pure case of Gerstmann syndrome with a subangular lesion. *Brain* 1999;**122**:1107–20.

88. Rusconi E. A disconnection account of Gerstmann syndrome: functional neuroanatomy evidence. *Ann Neurol* 2009;**66**(5):654–62.

89. Wingard EM, Barrett AM, Crucian GP, et al. The Gerstmann syndrome in Alzheimer's disease. *J Neurol Neurosurg Psychiatry* 2002;**72**:403–5.

90. Heimburger RF, Demyer W, Reitan RM. Implications of Gerstmann's syndrome. *J Neurol Neurosurg Psychiatry* 1964;**27**:52–7.

91. Futagi Y, Suzui Y. Neural mechanism and clinical significance of the plantar grasp reflex in infants. *Pediatr Neurol* 2010;**43**:81–6.

92. Vreeling FW, Houx PJ, Jolles J, et al. Primitive reflexes in Alzheimer's disease and vascular dementia. *J Geriatr Psychiatry Neurol* 1995;**8**:111–17.

93. Hogan DB, Ebly EM. Primitive reflexes and dementia: results from the Canadian study of health and aging. *Age Ageing* 1995;**24**:375–81.

5

94. Tremont-Lukats IW, Teixeira GM, Hernandez DE. Primitive reflexes in a case control study of patients with advanced human immunodeficiency virus type 1. *J Neurol* 1999;**246**:540–3.

95. Brown DL, Smith TL, Knepper LE. Evaluation of five primitive reflexes in 240 young adults. *Neurology* 1998;**51**:322.

96. von Keyserlingk AG, Naujokat C, Niemann K, et al. Global aphasia – with and without hemiparesis. A linguistic and CT scan study. *Eur Neurol* 1997;**38**(4):259–67.

97. Vreeling FW, Jolles J, Verchey FRJ, et al. Primitive reflexes in healthy, adult volunteers and neurological patients: methodological issues. *J Neurol* 1993;**240**:495–504.

98. De Renzi E, Barbieri C. The incidence of the grasp reflex following hemispheric lesion and its relation to frontal damage. *Brain* 1992;**115**:293–313.

99. Knecht S, Drager B, Bobe L, et al. Handedness and hemispheric language dominance in healthy humans. *Brain* 2000;**123**:2512–18.

100. Macphee GJA, Crowther JA, McApline CH. A simple screening test for hearing impairment in elderly patients. *Age Ageing* 1988;**17**:347–51.

101. Kerber KA, Baloh RW. Dizziness, vertigo, and hearing loss. In: Bradley WG, Daroff RB, Fenichel G, et al., editors. *Neurology in Clinical Practice*. 5th ed. Philadelphia: Butterworth-Heinemann; 2008.

102. Nadol JB. Hearing loss. *N Engl J Med* 1993;**329**:1092–102.

103. Cueva RA. Auditory brainstem response versus magnetic resonance imaging for the evaluation of asymmetric sensorineural hearing loss. *Laryngoscope* 2004;**114**:1686–92.

104. Milner D, McIntosh RD. The neurological basis of visual neglect. *Curr Opin Neurol* 2005;**18**:1–6.

105. Heilman KM, Watson RT, Valenstein E, et al. Localization of lesions in neglect. In: Kertesz A, editor. *Localization in Neuropsychology*. New York: Academic Press; 1983.

106. Vallar G, Perani D. The anatomy of unilateral neglect after right-hemisphere stroke lesions. A clinical/CT-scan correlation study in man. *Neuropsychologia* 1986;**24**:609–22.

107. Dobkin BH. Principles and practices of neurological rehabilitation. In: Bradley WG, Daroff RB, Fenichel G, et al., editors. *Neurology in Clinical Practice*. 5th ed. Philadelphia: Butterworth-Heinemann; 2008.

108. Goodale MA, Milner AD. *Sight Unseen: An Exploration of Conscious and Unconscious Vision*. Oxford: Oxford University Press; 2004.

109. Karnath H-O, Fruhman Berger M, Kuker W, et al. The anatomy of spatial neglect based on voxelwise statistical analysis: a study of 140 patients. *Cereb Cortex* 2004;**14**:1164–72.

110. Annema JT, Brahim JJ, Rabe KF. A rare cause of Ortner's syndrome (cardiovocal hoarseness). *Thorax* 2004;**59**:636.

111. Ortner NI. Recurrenslahmung bei Mitralstenose. *Wien Klin Wochenschr* 1897;**10**:753–5.

112. Chen JJ, Barton F, Branstetter IV, et al. Cricoarytenoid rheumaotoid arthritis: an important consideration in aggressive lesions in the larynx. *AJNR Am J Neuroradiol* 2005;**26**:970–2.

113. Kamanli A, Gok U, Sahin S, et al. Bilateral cricoarytenoid joint involvement in rheumatoid arthritis: a case report. *Rheumatology* 2001;**40**:593–4.

114. Czarnecki JSC, Pilley SFL, Thompson HS. The analysis of anisocoria: the use of photography in the clinical evaluation of unequal pupils. *Can J Ophthalmol* 1979;**14**:297–302.

115. Keane JR. Oculosympathetic paresis: analysis of 100 hospitalized patients. *Arch Neurol* 1979;**36**:13–16.

116. Giles CL, Henderson JW. Horner's syndrome: an analysis of 216 cases. *Am J Ophthalmol* 1958;**46**:289–96.

117. Biros MH, Heegaard WG. Head injury. In: Marx JA, Hockberger RS, Walls RM, et al., editors. *Rosen's Emergency Medicine*. 7th ed. Philadelphia: Mosby; 2010.

118. Zaal MJ, Volker-Dieben HJ, D'Amaro J. Prognostic value of Hutchinson's sign in acute herpes zoster ophthalmicus. *Graefes Arch Clin Exp Ophthalmol* 2003;**241**:187–91.

119. Teitelbaum JS, Eliasziw M, Garner M. Tests of motor function in patients suspected of having mild unilateral cerebral lesions. *Can J Neurol Sci* 2002;**29**:337–44.

120. Hallett M. NINDS myotactic reflex scale. *Neurology* 1993;**43**:2723.

121. Misulis KE. Sensory abnormalities of the limbs, trunk, and face. In: Bradley WG, Daroff RB, Fenichel G, et al., editors. *Neurology in Clinical Practice*. 5th ed. Philadelphia: Butterworth-Heinemann; 2008.

122. Impallomeni M, Fluynn MD, Kenny RA, et al. The elderly and their ankle jerks. *Lancet* 1984;**1**:670–2.

123. Bowditch MG, Sanderson P, Livesey JP. The significance of an absent ankle jerk reflex. *J Bone Joint Surg Br* 1996;**78B**:276–9.

124. Wartenberg R. Studies in reflexes: history, physiology, synthesis and nomenclature. I. *Arch Neurol Psychiatry* 1944;**51**:113–33.

125. Wartenberg R. Studies in reflexes: history, physiology, synthesis and nomenclature. II. *Arch Neurol Psychiatry* 1944;**51**:341–58.

126. Wartenberg R. Studies in reflexes: history, physiology, synthesis and nomenclature. III. *Arch Neurol Psychiatry* 1944;**51**:359–82.

127. Yoss RE, Corbin KB, MacCarty CS, et al. Significance of symptoms and signs in localization of involved root in cervical disk protrusion. *Neurology* 1957;**7**:673–83.

128. Lauder TD, Dillingham TR, Andary M, et al. Predicting electrodiagnostic outcome in patients with upper limb symptoms: are the history and physical examination helpful? *Arch Phys Med Rehabil* 2000;**81**:436–41.

129. Kortelainen P, Puranen J, Koivisto E, et al. Symptoms and signs of sciatica and their relation to the localization of the lumbar disc herniation. *Spine* 1985;**10**:88–92.

130. Lauder TD, Dillingham TR, Andary M, et al. Effect of history and exam in predicting electrodiagnostic outcome among patients with lumbosacral radiculopathy. *Am J Phys Med Rehabil* 2000;**79**:60–8.

131. Portnoy HD, Ahmad M. Value of the neurological examination, electromyography and myelography in herniated lumbar disc. *Mich Med* 1972;**71**:429–34.

132. Jensen OH. The level-diagnosis of a lower lumbar disc herniation: the value of sensibility and motor testing. *Clin Rheumatol* 1987;**6**:564–9.

133. Verma A. Infections of the nervous system. In: Bradley WG, Daroff RB, Fenichel G, et al., editors. *Neurology in Clinical Practice*. 5th ed. Philadelphia: Butterworth-Heinemann; 2008.

134. Lavin PJM, Morrison D. Neuro-ophthalmology: ocular motor system. In: Bradley WG, Daroff RB, Fenichel G, et al., editors. *Neurology in Clinical Practice*. 5th ed. Philadelphia: Butterworth-Heinemann; 2008.

135. Eggenberger E, Golnik K, Lee A, et al. Prognosis of ischemic internuclear ophthalmoplegia. *Ophthalmology* 2002;**109**:1676–8.

136. Keane J. Internuclear ophthalmoplegia; unusual causes in 114 of 410 patients. *Arch Neurol* 2005;**62**:714–17.

137. Kataoka S, Hori A, Shirakawa T, et al. Paramedian pontine infarction. Neurological/topographical correlation. *Stroke* 1997;**28**:809–15.

138. Lavin PJM, Donahue SP. Disorders of supranuclear control of ocular motility. In: Yanoff M, Duker JS, editors. *Ophthalmology*. 3rd ed. St Louis: Mosby; 2008.

139. Smith JL, Cogan DG. Internuclear ophthalmoplegia: a review of 58 cases. *Arch Ophthalmol* 1959;**61**:687–94.

140. Walker HK, Hall WD, Hurst JW. *Clinical Methods: The History, Physical, and Laboratory Examinations*. 3rd ed. Boston: Butterworth; 1990.

141. Nakao JH, Jafri FN, Shah K, Newman DH. Jolt accentuation of headache and other clinical signs: poor predictor of meningitis in adults. *Am J Emerg Med* 2014;**32**(1):24–8.

5

142. Leigh RJ, Zee DS. *The Neurology of Eye Movements*. 3rd ed. Philadelphia: FA Davis; 1999.

143. Kerchner GA, Lenz RA. Ptzcek RA. Channelopathies: episodic and electrical disorders of the nervous system. In: Bradley WG, Daroff RB, Fenichel G, et al., editors. *Neurology in Clinical Practice*. 5th ed. Philadelphia: Butterworth-Heinemann; 2008.

144. Amato AA, Brooke MH. Disorders of skeletal muscle. In: Bradley WG, Daroff RB, Fenichel G, et al., editors. *Neurology in Clinical Practice*. 5th ed. Philadelphia: Butterworth-Heinemann; 2008.

145. Mankodi A, Takahashi MP, Jiang H, et al. Expanded CUG repeats trigger aberrant splicing of ClC-1 chloride channel pre-mRNA and hyperexcitability of skeletal muscle in myotonic dystrophy. *Mol Cell* 2002;**10**:35–44.

146. Jacobson DM. Relative pupil-sparing third nerve palsy: etiology and clinical variables predictive of a mass. *Neurology* 2001;**56**:797–8.

147. Blake PY, Mark AS, Kattah J, et al. MR of oculomotor nerve palsy. *AJNR Am J Neuroradiol* 1995;**16**:1665–75.

148. Nistri M, Di Lorenzo PPN, Cellerini M, et al. Third-nerve palsy heralding aneurysm of posterior cerebral artery: digital subtraction angiography and magnetic resonance appearance. *J Neurol Neurosurg Psychiatry* 2007;**78**(2):197–8.

149. Olitsky SE, Hug D, Smith LP. Disorders of eye movement and alignment. In: Kliegman RM, Behrman RE, Jenson HB, Stanton BF, editors. *Nelson Textbook of Pediatrics*. 18th ed. Philadelphia: Saunders; 2007.

150. Rucker CW. Paralysis of the third, fourth, and sixth cranial nerves. *Am J Ophthalmol* 1958;**46**:787–94.

151. Rucker CW. The causes of paralysis of the third, fourth, and sixth cranial nerves. *Am J Ophthalmol* 1996;**61**:1293–8.

152. Green WR, Hackett ER, Schlezinger NS. Neuro-ophthalmologic evaluation of oculomotor paralysis. *Arch Ophthalmol* 1964;**72**:154–67.

153. Zorrilla E, Kozak GP. Ophthalmoplegia in diabetes mellitus. *Ann Intern Med* 1967;**67**:968–76.

154. Capo H, Warren F, Kupersmith MJ. Evolution of oculomotor nerve palsies. *J Clin Neuroophthalmol* 1992;**12**(1):12–15.

155. Hopf HC, Gutmann L. Diabetic 3rd nerve palsy: evidence for a mesencephalic lesion. *Neurology* 1990;**40**:1041–5.

156. Cogan DG, Mount HTJ. Intracranial aneurysms cause ophthalmoplegia. *Arch Ophthalmol* 1963;**70**:757–71.

157. Sanders S, Kawasaki A, Purvin VA. Patterns of extraocular muscle weakness in vasculopathic pupil-sparing, incomplete third nerve palsy. *J Neuroophthalmol* 2001;**21**:256–9.

158. Talley NJ, O'Connor S. Common short cases. In: Talley NJ, O'Connor S, editors. *Examination Medicine, A Guide to Physician Training*. 5th ed. Sydney: Churchill Livingstone; 2006. p. 226–322.

159. Isaacson RS. Optic atrophy. In: Ferri FF, editor. *Clinical Advisor 2011*. Philadelphia: Mosby; 2010.

160. Balcer LJ, Prasad S. Abnormalities of the optic nerve and retina. In: Bradley WG, Daroff RB, Fenichel G, et al., editors. *Neurology in Clinical Practice*. 5th ed. Philadelphia: Butterworth-Heinemann; 2008.

161. Owen G, Mulley GP. The palmomental reflex: a useful clinical sign? *J Neurol Neurosurg Psychiatry* 2002;**73**:113–15.

162. Gotkine M, Haggiag S, Abramsky O, et al. Lack of hemispheric localizing value of the palmomental reflex. *Neurology* 2005;**64**:1656.

163. De Noordhout AM, Delwaide PJ. The palmomental reflex in Parkinson's disease: comparison with normal subjects and clinical relevance. *Arch Neurol* 1988;**45**:425–7.

164. Kobayashi S, Yamaguchi S, Okada K, et al. Primitive reflexes and MRI findings, cerebral blood flow in normal elderly. *Gerontology* 1990;**36**:199–205.

165. Isakov E, Sazgon L, Costeff H, et al. The diagnostic value of three common primitive reflexes. *Eur Neurol* 1984;**23**:17–21.

166. Jacobs L, Gossman MD. Three primitive reflexes in normal adults. *Neurology* 1980;**30**:184–8.

167. Rodriguez MC, Guridi OJ, Alvarez L, et al. The subthalamic nucleus and tremor in Parkinson's disease. *Mov Disord* 1998;**13**(Suppl. 3):111–18.

168. Deuschl G, Raethjen J, Baron R, et al. The pathophysiology of parkinsonian tremor: a review. *J Neurol* 2000;**247**(5):V/33–48.

169. Stringham JM, Fuld K, Wenzel AJ. Spatial properties of photophobia. *Invest Ophthalmol Vis Sci* 2004;**45**:3838–48.

170. Brandt JD. Congenital glaucoma. In: Yanoff M, Duker JS, editors. *Ophthalmology*. 3rd ed. St Louis: Mosby; 2008.

171. Olesen J. Migraine: a neural pathway for photophobia in migraine. *Nat Rev Neurol* 2010;**6**:241–2.

172. Bradley WG, Daroff RB, Fenichel G, et al. *Neurology in Clinical Practice*. 5th ed. Philadelphia: Butterworth-Heinemann; 2008.

173. Flaherty AW. Movement disorders. In: Stern TA, Rosenbaum JF, Fava M, et al., editors. *Stern: Massachusetts general hospital comprehensive clinical psychiatry*. 1st ed. Philadelphia: Mosby; 2008.

174. Tremor Fact Sheet. National Institute of Neurological Disorders and Stroke. 2006. Available: http://www.ninds.nih.gov/disorders/tremor/detail_tremor.htm [9 Oct 2010].

175. Yip L, McGarbane B, Borron SW. Opioids. In: Shannon MW, Borron SW, Burns MJ, editors. *Haddad and Winchester's Clinical Management of Poisoning and Drug Overdose*. 4th ed. Philadelphia: Saunders; 2007.

176. Ghoneum MM, Dhanaraj J, Choi WW. Comparison of four opioid analgesics as supplements to nitrous anesthesia. *Clin Pharmacol Ther* 1984;**63**(4):405–12.

177. Crocco TJ, Tadros A, Kothari RU. Stroke. In: Marx JA, Hockberger RS, Walls RM, et al., editors. *Rosen's Emergency Medicine*. 7th ed. Philadelphia: Mosby; 2010.

178. Meehan TJ, Bryant SM, Aks SE. Drugs of abuse: the highs and lows of altered mental states in the emergency department. *Emerg Med Clin North Am* 2010;**28**:663–82.

179. Reid J. Alpha-adrenergic receptors and blood pressure control. *Am J Cardiol* 1986;**57**:6E–12E.

180. Van Zweiten PA. Overview of alpha-2-adrenoreceptor agonists with central action. *Am J Cardiol* 1986;**57**:3E–5E.

181. Hoffman BB, Lefkowitz RJ. Alpha-adrenergic receptor subtypes. *N Engl J Med* 1980;**302**:1390–6.

182. Greenberg M. *Handbook of Neurosurgery*. 5th ed. New York: Thieme; 2001.

183. Crouch ER Jr, Crouch ER, Grant T. Ophthalmology. In: Rakel RE, editor. *Textbook of Family Medicine*. 7th ed. Philadelphia: Saunders; 2007.

184. Whittaker RG, Schaefer AM, Taylor RW, Turnbull DM. Differential diagnosis in ptosis and opthalmoplegia: mitochondrial disease or myasthenia? *J Neurol* 2007;**254**:1138–9.

185. Iwamoto MA. Ptosis evaluation and management in the 21st century. *Curr Opin Ophthalmol* 1996;**7**:60–8.

186. Reddy AR, Backhouse OC. 'Ice-on-eyes', a simple test for myasthenia gravis presenting with ocular symptoms. *Pract Neurol* 2007;**7**:109–11.

187. Duong DK, Leo MM, Mitchell EL. Neuro-ophthalmology. *Emerg Med Clin North Am* 2008;**26**:137–80.

188. Newsome DA, Milton RC. Afferent pupillary defect in macular degeneration. *Am J Ophthalmol* 1981;**92**:396–402.

5

189. Girkin CA. Evaluation of the pupillary light response as an objective measure of visual function. *Ophthalmol Clin North Am* 2003;**16**:143–53.

190. Cox TA, Thompson HS, Hayreh SS, Snyder JE. Visual evoked potential and pupillary signs: a comparison in optic nerve disease. *Arch Ophthalmol* 1982;**100**:1603–6.

191. Cox TA, Thompson HS, Corbett JJ. Relative afferent pupillary defects in optic neuritis. *Am J Ophthalmol* 1981;**92**:685–90.

192. Notermans NC, van Dijk GW, van der Graff Y, et al. Measuring ataxia: quantification based on the standard neurological examination. *J Neurol Neurosurg Psychiatry* 1994;**57**:22–6.

193. Young RR. Spasticity: a review. *Neurology* 1994;**44**(Suppl. 9):S12–20.

194. Hewlett EL, Hughes MA. Toxins. In: Mandell GL, Bennett JE, Dolin R, editors. *Principles and Practice of Infectious Diseases*. 7th ed. Philadelphia: Churchill Livingstone; 2010.

195. Perry HE. Rodenticides. In: Shannon MW, Borron SW, Burns MJ, editors. *Haddad and Winchester's Clinical Management of Drug Overdose*. 4th ed. Philadelphia: Saunders; 2007.

196. Manon-Espaillat R, Ruff RL. Dissociated weakness of the sternocleidomastoid and trapezius muscle with lesions in the CNS. *Neurology* 1988;**38**:138–40.

197. Berry H, MacDonald EA, Mrazek AC. Accessory nerve palsy: a review of 23 cases. *Can J Neurol Sci* 1991;**18**:337–41.

198. Rigby WFC, Fan C-M, Mark EJ. Case 39-2002: a 35-year-old man with headache, deviation of the tongue, and unusual radiographic abnormalities. *N Eng J Med* 2002; **347**:2057–67.

199. Keane JR. Twelfth-nerve palsy. *Arch Neurol* 1996;**53**:561–6.

200. Scotti G, Melancon D, Olivier A. Hypoglossal paralysis due to compression by a tortuous internal carotid artery in the neck. *Neuroradiology* 1978;**14**:263–5.

201. Lemmering M, Crevits L, Defreyne L, Achten E, Kunnen M. Traumatic dissection of the internal carotid artery as unusual cause of hypoglossal nerve dysfunction. *Clin Neurol Neurosurg* 1996;**98**:52–4.

202. Massey EW, Heyman A, Utley C, Haynes C, Fuchs J. Cranial nerve paralysis following carotid endarterectomy. *Stroke* 1984;**15**:157–9.

203. Donahue SP. Nuclear and fascicular disorders of eye movement. In: Yanoff M, Duker JS, editors. *Ophthalmology*. 3rd ed. St Louis: Mosby; 2008.

204. Thomke F, Hopf HC. Isolated superior oblique palsies with electrophysiologically documented brainstem lesions. *Muscle Nerve* 2000;**23**:267–70.

205. Dhaliwal A, West AL, Trobe JD, et al. Third, fourth, and sixth cranial nerve palsies following closed head injury. *J Neuroophthalmol* 2006;**26**:4–10.

206. Khawam E, Scott AB, Jampolsky A. Acquired superior oblique palsy. *Arch Ophthalmol* 1967;**77**:761–8.

207. Urist MJ. Head tilt in vertical muscle paresis. *Am J Ophthalmol* 1970;**69**:440–2.

208. Younge BR, Sutula F. Analysis of trochlear nerve palsies: diagnosis, etiology, and treatment. *Mayo Clin Proc* 1977;**52**:11–18.

209. Miller D, Schor P, Magnante P. Optics of the normal eye. In: Yanoff M, Duker JS, editors. *Ophthalmology*. 3rd ed. St Louis: Mosby; 2008.

210. Katz G, Moseley M. Top Clinical Problems. Irving: Emergency Medicine Resident Association, 2008.

211. Rubin RM, Sadun AA, Piva A. Optic chiasm, parasellar region, and pituitary fossa. In: Yanoff M, Duker JS, editors. *Ophthalmology*. 3rd ed. St Louis: Mosby; 2008.

212. Ariyasu RG, Lee PP, LaBree LD, et al. Sensitivity, specificity, and predictive values of screening tests for eye conditions in the clinic-based population. *Ophthalmology* 1997; **104**(9):1369–70.

213. Rhee DJ, Pyfer MF. *The Wills Eye Manual*. 3rd ed. Philadelphia: Lippincott Williams & Wilkins; 1999.

214. Sieving PA, Caruso RC. Retinitis pigmentosa and related disorders. In: Yanoff M, Duker JS, editors. *Ophthalmology*. 3rd ed. St Louis: Mosby; 2008.

215. Johnson LN, Baloh FG. The accuracy of confrontation visual field test in comparison with automated perimetry. *J Natl Med Assoc* 1991;**83**:895–8.

216. Shainfar S, Johnson LN, Madsen RW. Confrontation visual field loss as a function of decibel sensitivity loss on automated static perimetry: implications on the accuracy of confrontation visual field testing. *Ophthalmology* 1995;**102**:872–7.

217. Trobe JD, Acosta PC, Krischer JP, et al. Confrontation visual field techniques in the detection of anterior visual field pathways lesions. *Ann Neurol* 1981;**10**:28–34.

218. Lee MS, Balcer LJ, Volpe NJ, et al. Laser pointer visual field screening. *J Neuroophthalmol* 2003;**23**:260–3.

219. Pandit RJ, Gales K, Griffiths PG. Effectiveness of testing visual fields by confrontation. *Lancet* 2001;**358**:1339–40.

220. Biller J, Love BB, Schneck MJ. Vascular diseases of the nervous system. In: Bradley WG, Daroff RB, Fenichel G, et al., editors. *Neurology in Clinical Practice*. 5th ed. Philadelphia: Butterworth-Heinemann; 2008.

221. Medical Research Council. *Aids to Examination of the Peripheral Nervous System*. London: Bailliere Tindall; 1986.

222. Gates P. The rule of 4 of the brainstem: a simplified method for understanding brainstem anatomy and brainstem vascular syndromes for the non-neurologist. *Intern Med J* 2005;**35**(4):263–6.

223. Griffin JW, Sheikh K. The Guillain–Barré syndromes. In: Dyck PJ, Thomas PK, editors. *Peripheral Neuropathy*. 4th ed. Philadelphia: Saunders; 2005.

224. Sanders DB, Howard JF Jr. Disorders of neuromuscular transmission. In: Bradley WG, Daroff RB, Fenichel G, et al., editors. *Neurology in Clinical Practice*. 5th ed. Philadelphia: Butterworth-Heinemann; 2008.

225. Gothe R, Kunze K, Hoogstraal H. The mechanisms of pathogenicity in the tick paralyses. *J Med Entomol* 1979;**16**:357.

226. Pascuzzi RM. Pearls and pitfalls in the diagnosis and management of neuromuscular junction disorders. *Semin Neurol* 2001;**21**:425.

227. Knepper LE, Biller J, Tranel D, et al. Etiology of stroke in patients with Wernicke's aphasia. *Stroke* 1989;**20**:1730–2.

5

CHAPTER 6

GASTROENTEROLOGICAL SIGNS

Ascites

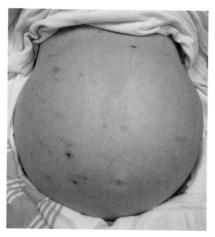

FIGURE 6.1
A person with massive ascites caused by portal hypertension due to cirrhosis
Copyright James Heilman MD.

Although itself not strictly a sign, a variety of clinical signs indicate the presence of ascites. Having an understanding of the different causes of ascites will assist with interpretation of additional signs present on physical examination.

Description
A pathological accumulation of fluid in the peritoneal cavity.

Condition/s associated with
As in oedema, variations in oncotic and hydrostatic pressure and vascular wall integrity are central to the development of ascites (see 'Peripheral oedema' in Chapter 3, 'Cardiovascular signs'). All the pathologies that create ascites effect one or more of these factors.

The causes of ascites can be broadly arranged into four categories according to mechanism (see Table 6.1).

Mechanism/s

Peripheral arterial vasodilatation theory
This hypothesis, shown in Figure 6.2, combines two premises: the 'underfill' and 'overflow' theories. Key initiating elements in both are *portal hypertension* and *nitric oxide-induced splanchnic vasodilatation*.

6

TABLE 6.1
Causes of ascites

Fluid imbalance (arterial vasodilatation theory)		Exudative
Cirrhosis – common		Exudate-secreting tumours (peritoneal carcinomatosis)
Congestive heart failure – common		Infections (e.g. TB)
Myxoedema		Inflammatory disease (e.g. SLE)
Budd–Chiari syndrome		
Chylous		Nephrogenic
Obstruction (e.g. malignant lymphoma)		Haemodialysis
Iatrogenic (e.g. transection of the lymphatics)		Nephrotic syndrome
Retroperitoneal lymph node dissection		

CLINICAL PEARL

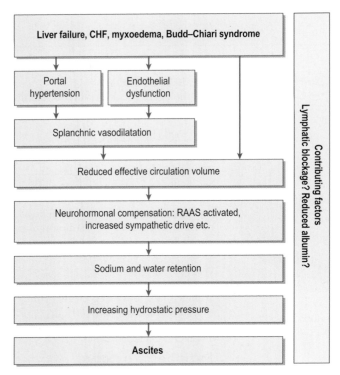

FIGURE 6.2
Mechanisms in the development of ascites

- *Underfill theory:* Imbalance in hydrostatic versus oncotic pressure causes the intravascular fluid to leak into the peritoneal cavity.[1] The resulting low blood volume activates the renin–angiotensin–aldosterone (RAA) pathway and the sympathetic nervous system to commence renal sodium and fluid retention, in an attempt to maintain volume.[1] As more volume is retained the hydrostatic pressure in the sinusoids causes fluid to be pushed out into the interstitial space. If the patient's lymphatic system is not robust enough to export the additional fluid away, it spills over into the peritoneal cavity to form ascites.

- *Overflow theory:* Primary renal sodium retention in patients with cirrhosis causes intravascular hypervolaemia. This increase in intravascular fluid, in turn, causes increased hydrostatic pressure that forces fluid to overflow into the peritoneal cavity.[2]

Further research following these two theories found that portal hypertension causes the release of nitric oxide and splanchnic bed vasodilatation, which reduces effective arterial blood flow to the kidneys. The RAAS is employed to increase plasma volume, further contributing to fluid overload and ascites.[3-5]

Contrary to popular belief, hypoalbuminaemia and low oncotic pressure have NOT been shown to play a substantial role in the development of ascites.[6]

Liver disease

In liver cirrhosis, destruction of the normal architecture, fibrosis and other structural changes contribute to increased sinusoidal pressure and raised *portal hypertension*. Exacerbating this is the presence of defective nitric oxide synthesis in the liver (responsible for vasodilatation) and the presence of vasoconstrictors, including endothelin,[6] angiotensin II, catecholamines and leukotrienes, all of which serve to favour sinusoidal constriction and the development of portal hypertension,[6] with the resultant driving hydrostatic force pushing fluid out into the peritoneal cavity.

Splanchnic vasodilatation, as mentioned above, is crucial to the development of ascites. It is thought that vasodilatation of the splanchnic bed is caused by the release of vasodilators, either due to sheer stress in the splanchnic circulation or as a result of neurohormonal signalling from the liver to the brain.[6-8] Nitric oxide, although decreased in the liver, is present and released in increased quantities from the systemic endothelium.[6] Other vasodilators, including calcitonin gene-related peptide (CGRP) and adrenomedullin, have also been implicated.[6]

As a result of this splanchnic vasodilatation, systemic vascular resistance falls, leading to decreased effective blood volume and, ultimately, the activation of the sympathetic and renin–aldosterone systems, and salt and water retention.

Finally, renal dysfunction is also seen in cirrhotic liver patients, with a reduction in GFR and salt and water excretion further contributing to the development of fluid retention and ascites.[6]

Congestive heart failure, Budd–Chiari syndrome

People with these conditions are thought to develop ascites because of reduced effective arterial volumes, leading to activation of the RAAS and salt and fluid retention (underfill theory).[3-5,9,10] Figure 6.3 shows the postulated mechanism of fluid retention and ascites in heart failure.

Nephrotic syndrome

Hypo-albuminaemia is universal in patients with nephrotic syndrome; however, the development of ascites in these patients is not solely caused by low albumin. Though not completely understood, ascites in this setting is likely to be much more complex and low albumin not the predominant mechanism.

Intra-renal pathology leading to *inadequate salt excretion* may play a role. Increased tubular reabsorption of salt has been demonstrated in animal models of nephrotic syndrome[3] and may also play a role in human pathology.

'Underfilling' may also play a role in some patients who have proteinuria and hypoalbuminaemia, contributing to a decreased circulating volume and activation of compensatory mechanisms, resulting in salt and water retention.[3]

These mechanisms have been summarised in Figure 6.4.

In a study looking at patients with nephrotic syndrome and ascites, concomitant liver disease and/or a degree of heart failure were also present and contributory to ascitic fluid development,[11] probably via a decrease in effective circulating volume and activation of RAAS and the sympathetic nervous system, with resulting salt and fluid retention.

6

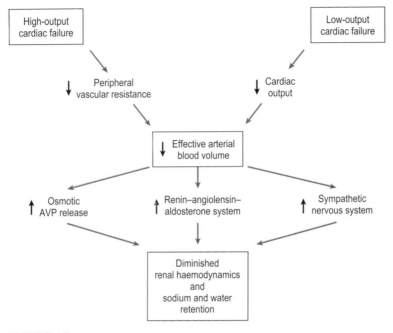

FIGURE 6.3

High-output and low-output cardiac failure
Although the initiating 'underfill' event differs in high- and low-output failure, the
subsequent pathways leading to renal sodium and water retention are similar. AVP = arginine
vasopressin.

*Schrier R. Pathogenesis of sodium and water retention in high output and low output cardiac failure,
nephrotic syndrome, cirrhosis and pregnancy. First of 2 parts. NEJM 1988; 319(16): Fig 1.*

Myxoedema mechanism/s

The mechanism of ascites in
hypothyroidism or myxoedema is
unclear. Previously two theories have
existed. Firstly, that low levels of
thyroid hormones cause *increased
extravasation* of *plasma proteins* due to
increased capillary permeability
combined with a lack of compensatory
lymphatic and protein flow return rate
to the plasma.[12,13]

The second theory suggested that
hyaluronic acid accumulates in the skin
and produces oedema through its
ability to absorb or adsorp water (i.e. its
ability to attract and hold water
molecules), although there is minimal
evidence for this direct effect.[12,14] The
hyaluronic acid is also thought to form
complexes with albumin which

prevents it from being picked up and
returned to the circulation via the
lymphatic system.[12]

In severe hypothyroidism, a variety
of changes occur in the cardiovascular
system and renal system including
decreased myocardial contractility and
renal dysfunction with inability to
excrete excess water (free water
clearance), which may also contribute
to fluid retention. Direct research on
these changes and ascites is lacking.

Exudative ascites

Exudative ascites may be caused by:

- increased intraperitoneal oncotic
  pressure (e.g. peritoneal
  carcinomatosis causes the tumour
  cells lining the peritoneum to
  produce exudates)

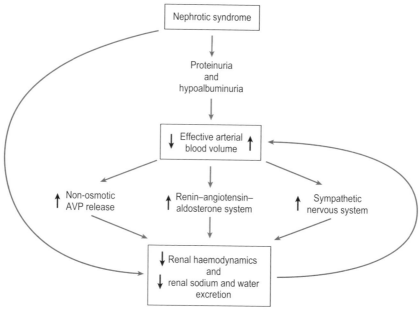

FIGURE 6.4

Nephrotic syndrome

The albuminuria and decrease in plasma oncotic pressure initiate the underfilling in nephrotic syndrome. Renal impairment and intra-renal factors may intervene, however, and in some circumstances restore or even expand effective blood volume. AVP = arginine vasopressin.

Schrier R. Pathogenesis of sodium and water retention in high output and low output cardiac failure, nephrotic syndrome, cirrhosis and pregnancy. First of 2 parts. NEJM 1988; 319(16): Fig 3.

- disruption of vessel wall integrity that allows fluid to leak through (e.g. patients with systemic lupus erythematosus can develop an inflammatory serositis, leading to exudate).[10,15]

Chylous ascites

Obstruction of lymphatic flow is the main underlying mechanism. This can be due to a pathological obstruction raising lymphatic pressures, resulting in fluid being pushed out and/or disrupting vessel integrity leading to leakage. Examples of these two scenarios are malignant lymphoma and surgical rupture of lymph nodes or vessels.[16,17]

Nephrogenic – haemodialysis

The causes of ascites in patients who receive haemodialysis are largely unknown. One possible explanation is that uraemia induces an inflammatory response that causes immune-complex formation and obstruction of lymphatic channels.[18,19]

Ascites clinical signs

Several clinical signs indicate the presence of ascites but none indicate the underlying cause. They are summarised in Table 6.2.

6

TABLE 6.2
Clinical signs of ascites

Sign	Description	PLR (95% CI)	NLR (95% CI)	Sensitivity (95% CI)	Specificity (95% CI)
Bulging flanks	Subjective bulging of the flanks	2.0 (1.5–2.6)	0.3 (0.2–0.6)	0.81 (0.69–0.93)	0.59 (0.50–0.68)
Flank dullness	Bilateral dullness to percussion of the abdomen accompanied by tympanic percussion centrally	2.0 (1.5–2.9)	0.3 (0.1–0.7)	0.84 (0.68–1.00)	0.59 (0.47–0.71)
Fluid wave/fluid thrill	Percussion on one side of the abdomen transmits a wave of fluid that is felt on the contralateral side	6.0 (3.3–11.1)	0.4 (0.3–0.6)	0.62 (0.47–0.77)	0.90 (0.84–0.96)
Puddle sign	With the patient resting on knees and elbows, the umbilical area is percussed for dullness to demonstrate fluid accumulation centrally due to gravity	1.6 (0.8–3.4)	0.8 (0.5–1.2)	0.45 (0.20–0.70)	0.73 (0.61–0.85)
Shifting dullness	With the patient supine, the examiner percusses the abdomen from the umbilicus towards him/herself. When dullness occurs, the location is noted and the patient is instructed to roll towards the examiner and assume the lateral decubitus position. The noted location is then percussed again and should become tympanic as fluid shifts laterally	2.7 (1.9–3.9)	0.3 (0.2–0.6)	0.77 (0.64–0.90)	0.63 (0.63–0.81)

Williams J, Simel D. Does this patient have ascites? JAMA 1991; 267(19): 2638–2644.

Sign value

The presence of ascites in a patient with liver disease suggests the presence of underlying cirrhosis with a PLR of 7.2 (CI 2.9–12),[20] and thus is helpful in understanding the extent and chronicity of disease.

Appreciating the mechanism behind ascites, and in particular cirrhosis-induced ascites, has substantial value in aiding understanding of the disease state and its sequelae, as well as insight into how therapeutic interventions act. In Figure 6.5, the pathogenesis of ascites is shown along with targets for various treatment opportunities.

In terms of the various signs that are used to detect the presence of ascites, there are variable sensitivities and specificities. A review[21] summarising available studies is shown in Tables 6.3 and 6.4. As seen in Table 6.2, all have

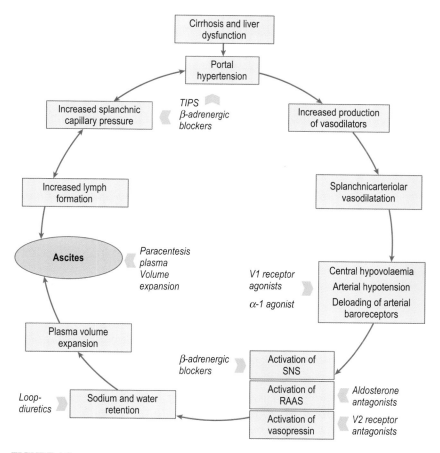

FIGURE 6.5

Pathophysiology of the development of ascites in cirrhosis and potential targets for treatment
SNS = sympathetic nervous system; RAAS = renin–angiotensin–aldosterone system; AVP = arginine vasopressin; TIPS = transjugular intrahepatic portosystemic shunt.

Moller S, Henriksen J, Bendtsen F. Ascites: pathogenesis and therapeutic principles. Scandinavian Journal of Gastroenterology 2009; 44: 902–911, Fig 1, Informa PLC.

TABLE 6.3
Accuracy of the clinical history*

Historical item or symptom	Positive likelihood ratio (LR+)	Negative likelihood ratio (LR−)	Sensitivity	Specificity
Increased girth	4.16	0.17	0.87	0.77
Recent weight gain	3.20	0.42	0.67	0.79
Hepatitis	3.20	0.80	0.27	0.92
Ankle swelling	2.80	0.10	0.93	0.66
Heart failure	2.04	0.73	0.47	0.73
Alcoholism	1.44	0.69	0.60	0.58
History of carcinoma	0.91	1.01	0.13	0.85

*Williams J, Simel D. Does this patient have ascites? JAMA 1991; 267(19): 2638–2644. Adapted from Simel DL, Halvorsen RA, Feussner JR. Quantitating bedside diagnosis: clinical evaluation of ascites. J Gen Intern Med. 1988; 3: 423–428.

value in clinical examination. In patients with abdominal distension, the sign with the best positive likelihood ratio (most likely to have ascites) is the fluid wave.[22] The best signs to exclude ascites are the absence of oedema (NLR 0.2) and absence of flank dullness.[22]

Serum albumin/ascitic gradient (SAAG) – a guide to pathophysiology and diagnosis of the sign

The serum albumin ascitic gradient (SAAG) is used to identify the presence of portal hypertension.

SAAG = serum albumin – ascitic fluid albumin

The theory is based on Starling's forces between the serum and ascitic fluid and the relationship between oncotic pressure, hydrostatic pressure and endothelial permeability.

In conditions when hydrostatic pressure is elevated (e.g. in portal hypertension), fluid is pushed out into the abdomen, and thus the serum albumin level becomes more concentrated compared to the ascitic fluid albumin, and the gap or gradient widens.

Conditions in which there is either low albumin in the serum (e.g. nephrotic syndrome) or protein leakage into the peritoneal cavity (e.g. inflammation, malignancy) result in higher protein and/or albumin content entering the peritoneal cavity, creating a low SAAG. Table 6.4 shows examples of causes of both high and low albumin gradients.

6

TABLE 6.4
Serum albumin ascitic gradient and pathologies

High albumin gradient (SAAG >11.1g/l)	Low albumin gradient (SAAG <11.1g/l)
Cirrhosis	Peritoneal carcinomatosis
Alcoholic hepatitis	Pancreatitis
Heart failure	Nephrotic syndrome
Budd–Chiari syndrome	Bacterial peritonitis
Portal vein thrombosis	

Asterixis (also hepatic flap)

See also 'Asterixis' in Chapter 2, 'Respiratory signs'.

Description

When the patient is asked to hold the arms extended with the hands dorsiflexed, a flapping hand movement that is brief, rhythmless and of low frequency (3–5 Hz) becomes apparent. Asterixis may be bilateral or unilateral.

Condition/s associated with

- Liver disease – most common
- Chronic obstructive pulmonary disease
- Stroke – rare

Hepatic mechanism/s

Little is known about the mechanism of asterixis induced by hepatic encephalopathy. Limited studies have suggested:

- Slowed oscillations in the primary motor cortex cause mini–asterixis, which may or may not be caused by problems in the motor cortex itself.[23]
- Dysfunction of the basal ganglia–thalamocortical loop may be involved.[24]

The net result of the pathology is the failure of the diencephalic motor centres in regulating tone between the agonist and antagonist muscles needed to maintain position and posture.[25]

Sign value

Asterixis is perhaps more valuable as a marker of severe disease, whatever the aetiology, rather than as a diagnostic tool.[26] One study used asterixis as a predictor of mortality in patients admitted with alcohol-related liver disease. It found that mortality rate was 56% in those with asterixis compared to 26% in those without.[27]

Bowel sounds

Bowel sounds are thought to occur as food or fluid is pushed through the intestines. As the intestines are hollow, the sounds made echo throughout the abdomen, and are often described as sounding like water through pipes. Bowel sounds may be heard 5–35 times per minute in a healthy person. It should be noted that to listen properly for bowel sounds the clinician would need to auscultate the abdomen for some time as, even in healthy people, sounds can be absent for up to 4 minutes.

Sign value

The variable amount and timing of bowel sounds makes the sign difficult to interpret and the evidence on their value is scarce and conflicting.

There is minimal evidence that hearing 'normal' bowel sounds argues against obstruction.[28] One study[29] of 600 acute abdomen patients found that only 24% of patients with small bowel obstruction had diminished or absent bowel sounds, while 48% of acute perforation patients had absent or decreased bowel sounds.

Another study[30] of greater than 1200 patients showed a sensitivity of 39.6%, specificity of 88.6%, with PPV 12.1% and NPV 97.4% of increased bowel sounds in the detection of intestinal obstruction, while decreased bowel sounds had a sensitivity of 25%, a specificity of 90.7%, PPV of 11.2% and NPV of 96.9%.

While normal bowel sounds may be of use in ruling out bowel pathology, their absence, increase or 'abnormality' could mean underlying pathology is present. It is crucial that other signs and symptoms be reviewed at the same time.

6

CLINICAL PEARL

Bowel sounds: absent

Description

As the name implies, the complete absence of bowel sounds on auscultation. How long one must listen before bowel sounds may be called absent is not clear, with times quoted anywhere from 1–5 minutes.

Condition/s associated with

More common

- Intestinal obstruction
- Paralytic ileus of any cause, e.g.:
  » Infection
  » Trauma
  » Bowel obstruction
  » Hypokalaemia
  » Vascular ischaemia
  » Side effect to drugs

Less common

- Mesenteric ischaemia
- Pseudo-obstruction (Ogilvie syndrome)

General mechanism/s

Absent bowel sounds may be caused by obstruction of an active intestine, resulting in an inability to push food or fluid through, or by an inactive bowel that is not undergoing peristalsis.

Bowel obstruction

In a mechanical obstruction due to any cause (hernia, volvulus, adhesion), the intestines are pushing against a fixed object. The normal oscillatory movement of food and water is not happening (as in a blocked pipe), so no sound is produced. If the obstruction continues, inflammation occurs and, if

vascular supply is compromised, normal peristalsis may also stop.

Infection

Although not entirely explained, there is evidence that the lipopolysaccharides (LPS) present on Gram-negative bacteria initiate an inflammatory response in the intestinal smooth muscle layer, which then reduces smooth muscle contractility, causing an ileus.[31]

Postoperative ileus

It is hypothesised that manipulation of the small intestine leads to postoperative ileus by promoting *inflammation of the smooth muscle layer*, which then causes a reduction in intestinal smooth muscle activity.[32]

There is also evidence to suggest that bacterial overgrowth occurs within the gut postoperatively and that the increased presence of bacteria and lipopolysaccharides contributes to inflammation caused by manipulation.[33]

The means by which inflammation causes ileus is likely to be related to the suppression of synaptic circuits of the

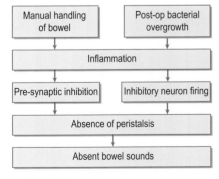

FIGURE 6.6
Possible postoperative ileus mechanism

enteric plexus, which organise normal propulsion of the intestines.[34] This suppression is caused by pre-synaptic inhibition of enteric motor neurons and/or continuous discharge of inhibitory neurons.

Hypokalaemia

Potassium is needed for normal polarisation and repolarisation of muscle cells. Hypokalaemia causes a *hyperpolarisation* of muscle cells, reducing excitability of the neurons and therefore smooth muscle activity, leading to ileus.

Pseudo-obstruction

The cause or mechanism of pseudo-obstruction, also known as Ogilvie syndrome, is not clear.

It is thought that an imbalance of autonomic innervation causes a functional bowel obstruction. Normal sacral parasympathetic tone is disrupted, causing an adynamic distal colon. Other studies suggest increased sympathetic tone is the cause – leading to decreased gut motility and sphincter closing. Peristalsis may be absent or impaired.

6

Bowel sounds: hyperactive (borborygmus)

Description

Frequent, loud, gurgling or 'rushing' bowel sounds that sometimes may be clearly heard even without a stethoscope.

Condition/s associated with:

More common

- Bowel obstruction
- Crohn's disease/ulcerative colitis
- Food hypersensitivity
- Gastroenteritis
- Normal

Less common

- Gastrointestinal haemorrhage

Mechanism/s

When obstruction is present, the bowel increases peristalsis in an attempt to overcome the blockage.

Bowel sounds: tinkling

Description

High-pitched 'tinkling' sound heard on auscultation of the abdomen that is often described as like pouring water into an empty glass.

Condition/s associated with

- Bowel obstruction

Mechanism/s

Evidence on the mechanism is limited. It is said to signify air or fluid accumulating and striking the bowel under pressure,[35] akin to rain falling on a tin roof.[36]

Sign value

There is very little evidence on tinkling bowel sounds as a sign.

6

Caput medusae

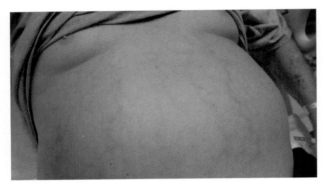

FIGURE 6.7
Caput medusae

Reproduced, with permission, from Saxena R, Practical Hepatic Pathology: A Diagnostic Approach, *Philadelphia: Saunders, 2011: Fig 6-4.*

Description

Dilated veins of the abdominal wall, named after the snakes that made up the hair of the goddess Medusa in Greek mythology.

Condition/s associated with

Any condition causing portal hypertension, e.g.:

- Cirrhosis of the liver
- Severe heart failure
- Inferior vena cava obstruction
- Budd–Chiari malformation

Mechanism/s

Portal hypertension causes backflow from the portal vein to the para-umbilical veins. The increased pressure and blood volume distend the veins.

Sign value

Caput medusae is a sign of advanced liver disease and portal hypertension. It is not common and would certainly be expected to be found with other clinical signs of portal hypertension.

To distinguish between inferior vena cava obstruction and portal hypertension with caput medusae, occlusion of the vein is required.

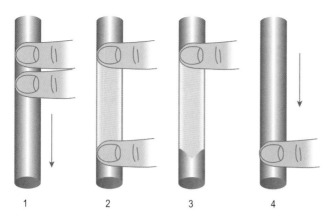

1   2   3   4

FIGURE 6.8
Measuring flow of a vein
Figuring out which way a prominent abdominal wall vein drains is a necessary skill for the clinician to determine where a blockage in the venous system is. Measure the flow of the vein below the umbilicus and use the following criteria:

- In severe portal hypertension, flow goes away from the umbilicus towards the feet.
- In inferior vena caval (IVC) obstruction, flow moves towards the head. Abdominal veins distend as they take blood back to the heart, bypassing the blocked IVC.

Based on Talley NJ, O'Connor S. Clinical Examination: A Systematic Guide to Physical Diagnosis, 5th edn, Marrickville, NSW: Churchill Livingstone Elsevier, 2006: Fig 5.20.

6

Cheilitis granulomatosa

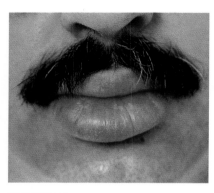

FIGURE 6.9
Cheilitis granulomatosa – diffuse swelling of the bottom lip

Reproduced, with permission, from Bolognia JL, Jorizzo JL, Rapini RP, Dermatology, 2nd edn, St Louis: Mosby, 2008: Fig 71-12.

Description

An uncommon painless enlargement of one or both lips. Histologically seen as non-necrotising granulomas with oedema and perivascular lymphocytic infiltration.

Condition/s associated with

- Idiopathic
- Crohn's disease – uncommon
- Sarcoidosis
- Melkersson–Rosenthal syndrome – rare

Mechanism/s

The cause and mechanism are unknown. Once thought to be a localised form of Crohn's disease or sarcoidosis, it can be seen either in association with or independent of these diseases.

With only limited research, theories as to the pathogenesis are based on hereditary/genetic, allergies, reaction to dental products, infective or immunological causes,[37] ultimately contributing to a delayed-type hypersensitivity response, resulting in an influx of inflammatory cells.

Having said that, there appears to be insufficient evidence to support genetic/ hereditary, infection or reaction to dental implants as possible causes.[37] Some studies[38] have shown up to 60% of patients with the disorder having atopy, and more recently in a review of over 100 patients an association with food was suspected in 30%.[39]

A Th1 immunological response has been demonstrated similar to that seen in Crohn's disease[37] but without a single antigen being found as the cause of the response.

Sign value

Possibly only seen in 0.5% of Crohn's disease patients, and most often after the diagnosis of Crohn's disease. However, some studies still suggest it may be an early manifestation of, or even predispose to, Crohn's disease.[40]

Coffee ground vomiting/ bloody vomitus/ haematemesis

Description

The vomiting of red blood or a coffee-ground-like substance. Haematemesis refers to the coughing up or vomiting of frank red blood.

Condition/s associated with

- Upper gastrointestinal bleeding[41]

More common

- Peptic ulcer disease
- Gastritis
- Oesophagitis
- Oesophageal varices

Less common

- Mallory–Weiss tear
- Vascular
- Tumour
- Vasculitis

General mechanism/s

Tearing or rupture of a blood vessel within the gastrointestinal tract, regardless of cause or aetiology, can precipitate haematemesis and/or coffee ground vomitus.

Coffee ground vomits owe their distinctive appearance to blood that has been oxidised by gastric acid, similar to malaena. It therefore indicates that the blood and/or bleeding has been present for some time, and potentially is higher up in the gastrointestinal tract (i.e. the duodenum or stomach).

Peptic ulcer disease

Inflammation and erosion of the normal mucosal surface into an underlying artery causes bleeding. Blood irritates the gut and is vomited back up.

Mallory–Weiss tear

Bleeding is due to longitudinal mucosal lacerations at the gastro-oesophageal junction or gastric cardia.

The mechanism behind Mallory–Weiss tears is not completely known but the theory is summarised in Figure 6.10. The sudden rise in abdominal/intragastric pressure from vomiting causes an increase in pressure across the gastro–oesophageal junction. This junction is relatively non-compliant and does not distend well with pressure. When the pressure gets high enough or is repeated (with multiple vomits), a mucosal laceration occurs, resulting in bleeding.

Oesophageal varices

In any cause of portal hypertension, the rise in portal vein pressure means blood is directed *away* into lower-pressure systems – collateral systems that include the oesophageal veins, abdominal veins and rectal veins. These veins become distended, thinner and more fragile. Rupturing of the thin-walled collateral veins/varices in the oesophagus causes pooling of blood and haematemesis. Gastric varices may also bleed in patients with portal hypertension.

6

CLINICAL PEARL

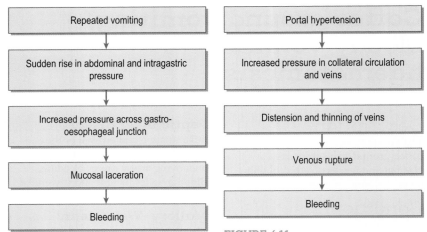

FIGURE 6.10
Mechanism of Mallory–Weiss tear

FIGURE 6.11
Mechanism of haematemesis in oesophageal varices

Sign value

There are a number of causes of upper gastrointestinal bleeding, and other sources of blood coming from the mouth need to be considered (e.g. nose, teeth, sinuses). However, both haematemesis and melaena are valuable signs and warrant immediate investigation, given the potential for catastrophic bleeding.

Courvoisier's sign

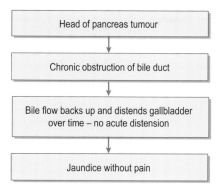

FIGURE 6.12
Possible mechanism of Courvoisier's sign

Description

Taught since 1890, the 'law' is that in a jaundiced patient the combination of a non-tender, distended gallbladder and obstructive jaundice is taken to indicate a non-calculus obstruction of the common bile duct.[42]

Despite many interpretations of Courvoisier's original finding, an accepted description is of a palpable, non-tender gallbladder in a patient with jaundice. It is commonly said to be a sign of obstruction to the biliary system by malignancy, although Courvoisier himself did not specifically associate it with malignancy.

Condition/s associated with

- Cholangiosarcoma
- Cancer of the head of the pancreas
- Cholelithiasis – uncommon

Mechanism/s

Dilatation of the gallbladder is the final pathway; however, the exact mechanism that gives rise to a painless, palpable gallbladder is unclear.

One explanation is that *chronic obstruction of the biliary system and/or gallbladder leads to higher biliary duct pressure* over a long period of time and does not provide the acute distension that usually causes inflammation and pain. Malignant causes of obstruction are more likely to provide chronic distension.[43]

For example, a cancer at the head of the pancreas causes sustained, unrelenting obstruction of bile flow, leading to distension of the gallbladder, whereas a gallstone will tend to cause intermittent obstruction with some bile still passing around the stone.

An alternative hypothesis (postulated originally by Courvoisier) is that chronic cholecystitis causes the gallbladder to become fibrotic and shrunken (i.e. it does not distend and therefore cannot cause pain). This has been shown to be somewhat inaccurate.[28]

Sign value

Given the many interpretations of Courvoisier's sign, evidence can be conflicting. However, assuming that a non-tender gallbladder in a patient with jaundice is the sign elicited, there is good evidence as to its value:

- In detecting obstructed bile ducts, sensitivity of 31%, specificity of 99%, PLR of 26.0.
- In detecting malignant obstruction in patients with obstructive jaundice, sensitivity of 26–55% and specificity of 83–90%.[28]

6

CLINICAL PEARL

More recently, a radiological study[44] validated Courvoisier's findings. MRCP was used to look at gallbladder volumes and did show a statistically significant difference, with less gallbladder distension from obstructive gallstones seen when compared to the volume present when neoplasms or strictures were the cause of obstruction.

Cullen's sign

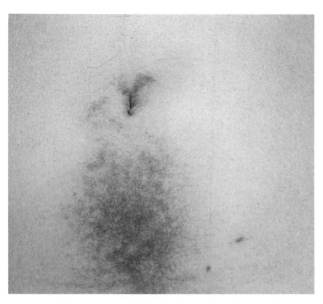

FIGURE 6.13
Cullen's sign
Reproduced, with permission, from Harris S, Naina HVK, Am J Med 2008; 121(8): 683.

Description
Periumbilical ecchymoses.

Condition/s associated with

More common
- Retroperitoneal bleeding
- Post surgery
- Iatrogenic – anticoagulation complication, postoperative
- Rectus sheath haematoma

Less common
- Ectopic pregnancy
- Intrahepatic haemorrhage
- Ischaemic bowel
- Ruptured abdominal aortic aneurysm
- Amoebic liver cyst
- Perforated duodenal ulcer
- Ruptured spleen
- Hepatocellular carcinoma

Mechanism/s
The final common pathway regardless of origin is *retroperitoneal bleeding*.

The retroperitoneum is connected to the gastro-hepatic ligament, then the falciform ligament, and finally to the round ligament (the obliterated umbilical vein), which tracks to the abdominal wall around the umbilicus. When a haemorrhage (from any cause) occurs, blood is able to move along these ligaments to the abdominal wall to produce ecchymoses.[45]

6

Sign value

Although often still taught as being a sign of pancreatitis, Cullen's sign is very non-specific. In fact, in a study of 770 cases of pancreatitis,[46] only 9 patients exhibited Cullen's sign. Similarly, its association with ectopic pregnancy is now very rare. In patients with acute pancreatitis, a mortality rate of 37% has been quoted in the presence of Cullen's sign.[46]

It is a relatively specific sign for retroperitoneal bleeding which will always warrant investigation. However, its absence does not exclude significant underlying pathology.

Erythema nodosum

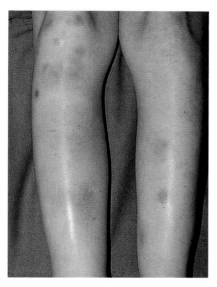

FIGURE 6.14
Erythema nodosum

Reproduced, with permission, from Kliegman RM et al., Nelson Textbook of Pediatrics, *18th edn, Philadelphia: Saunders, 2007: Fig 659-2.*

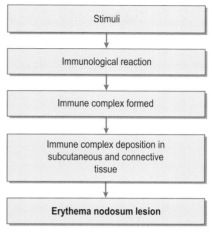

FIGURE 6.15
Erythema nodosum mechanism

Description

A skin disorder of acute onset with eruption of red, tender nodules and plaques, predominantly over the lower extremities, especially the extensor surfaces. It is a form of panniculitis.

Condition/s associated with

More common[47]

- Inflammatory bowel disease
- Infections – streptococcal, tuberculosis, URTIs, yersiniosis[48]
- Sarcoidosis
- Rheumatological disorders

- Drug reactions – usually sulfonamides and the oral contraceptive pill
- Malignancies
- Pregnancy

Mechanism/s

While up to 55% of erythema nodosum is thought to be idiopathic,[48] the predominant cause is assumed to be a *hypersensitivity reaction* to various stimuli.

In theory, immune complexes form after exposure to an antigen and are deposited in venules around areas of subcutaneous fat and connective tissue.[47] The subsequent inflammation causes the lesions. A number of immunological factors may be related:

- Reactive oxidative species have been found at lesion sites.[49]
- Delayed–type hypersensitivity histopathology has been found at mature lesion sites.[50]

6

- Complement activation has also been implicated.[51]

Why the lesions appear so frequently on the shins has not been explained. It has been suggested that a combination of a relatively meagre arterial supply, combined with a venous system that is subject to gravitational effects and has no mechanical pump and an inadequate lymphatic system, favour deposition in that area.[52]

Sign value

Erythema nodosum is not a sensitive or specific sign. However, if found, a review of the common causes is often performed. A recent study has found it to be present in approximately 4% of inflammatory bowel disorder patients.[53]

Grey Turner's sign

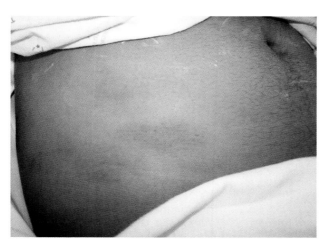

FIGURE 6.16
Grey Turner's sign
Reproduced, with permission, from Feldman M, Friedman LS, Brandt LJ, Sleisenger and Fordtran's Gastrointestinal and Liver Disease, 9th edn, Philadelphia: Saunders, 2010: Fig 58-3.

Description
Ecchymoses or purple discolouration of the flanks.

Condition/s associated with
- Any cause of retroperitoneal bleed
- Pancreatitis

Mechanism/s
A hole in the abdominal fascia. A defect in the transversalis fascia allows blood from the posterior pararenal space to move to the abdominal wall musculature and the subcutaneous tissue.[54]

Sign value
Seen in 14 of 770 patients with pancreatitis,[43] like Cullen's sign it is associated with increased severity of, but is not specific to, pancreatitis. Grey Turner's sign is non-specific but, if seen, the patient should be investigated for potential sources of retroperitoneal bleeding.

6

Guarding

Description

May be voluntary or involuntary in nature.

Voluntary guarding is the conscious contraction of the abdominal musculature, usually in response to fear of pain or anxiety.

Involuntary guarding is discussed under 'Rigidity and involuntary guarding' in this chapter.

Condition/s associated with

Any cause of peritonism:

- Inflammation of any visceral organ
- Abdominal infection
- Bleeding

Mechanism/s

In anticipation of pain the patient contracts the abdominal muscles as a protective response.

Sign value

Despite several studies, the sensitivity and specificity for guarding in the diagnosis of peritonitis is highly variable, ranging from 13–90% for sensitivity and 40–97% for specificity, with a PLR of 2.2 and NLR of 0.6.[22] While imaging modalities are often superior to physical examination in diagnosing specific disorders, the detection of guarding may help the clinician to consider appropriate tests.

Gynaecomastia

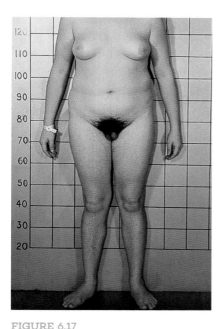

FIGURE 6.17
Gynaecomastia in an adolescent with a
congenital form of hypogonadism

*Reproduced, with permission, from Wales JKH,
Wit JM, Rogol AD,* Pediatric Endocrinology
and Growth, *2nd edn, Philadelphia: Elsevier/
Saunders, 2003: 165.*

Description

A benign proliferation of glandular
tissue in the male breast, clinically
presenting as a firm disc of tissue
underlying the nipple, which is at least
2 cm in diameter. Gynaecomastia
usually develops bilaterally. It can be
unilateral during the initial stages,
becoming bilateral after some months.
Only around 10% of cases are
unilateral.[55,56]

Gynaecomastia must be
differentiated from adipomastia/
lipomastia (pseudogynaecomastia),
which refers to fat deposition *without*
glandular proliferation (i.e. adipose
tissue rather than true breast tissue).

Condition/s associated with

More common

- Physiological
- Drugs, commonly:
  - » Cimetidine
  - » Digitalis
  - » Spironolactone
  - » Methyldopa
  - » Captopril
  - » Calcium channel blockers
  - » Chemotherapeutic agents
- Radiotherapy
- Hepatic cirrhosis
- Hypogonadism of any cause

Less common

- Hyperthyroidism
- Re-feeding syndrome
- Renal failure and dialysis
- Testicular tumours
- Congenital abnormalities (e.g.
  Kallmann's syndrome, Klinefelter's
  syndrome)

General mechanism/s

Gynaecomastia is principally caused by:

1. high levels of circulating
   oestrogen
2. increases in the oestrogen:
   testosterone ratio
3. androgen insensitivity.

All of these situations favour
increased oestrogen activity in the
glandular tissue of the breast, leading to
proliferation.

6

Physiological gynaecomastia

Most often occurs at puberty and middle age.

In males, important sources of oestrogen production are the testes via luteinising hormone (LH) and human chorionic gonadotropin (hCG) secretion, and peripheral tissue and fat (where aromatisation of androgens to oestrogens takes place).

- When present at puberty, gynaecomastia is believed to be caused by a faster than normal initial rise in oestrogen production.[57-59]
- Older males have decreased testicular function, increased weight and more fat storage. This leads to decreased testosterone production from the testes and increased androgen-to-oestrogen aromatisation peripherally.[57]

Drugs

There is increasing recognition of the mechanism/s induced by a number of common drugs. A summary of these is shown in Table 6.5.

Hepatic cirrhosis

In hepatic cirrhosis, the liver's normal metabolic functions are impaired, leading to a *reduced breakdown of androgens*. The increase in circulating androgens results in *increased aromatisation* in the periphery to oestrogens.[57,60]

TABLE 6.5
Drug-induced gynaecomastia mechanisms

Drug	Mechanism
Spironolactone	Multiple mechanisms:[61] 1. Increased aromatisation of testosterone to oestradiol 2. Decreased testosterone production from testes 3. Displacement of testosterone from steroid binding globulin, causing increased clearance 4. Binds to androgen receptors and prevents testosterone binding
Digoxin	Structurally similar to plant-derived oestrogens – can stimulate oestrogen receptor directly
Histamine 2 receptor blocker (e.g. cimetidine)	Several mechanisms proposed: 1. Blocks androgen receptors, causing increased oestrogen-to-androgen ratio 2. Alters prolactin level – negative feedback on gonadotropin hormone – less LH produced
Proton pump inhibitors	Inhibition of oestradiol metabolism – increases in oestrogen-to-androgen ratio
Anti-androgens (used in prostate cancer therapy or pre-sex change)	Decreased androgens – increased ratio of oestrogen to androgen
Testosterone replacement therapy	Increased testosterone leads to increased aromatisation of testosterone to oestrogen in peripheral tissues LH replacement also favours secretion of oestradiol from the Leydig cells of testes
Calcium channel blockers	Likely to be related to increased levels of prolactin

Hyperthyroidism
Few theories have been suggested for the relationship between gynaecomastia and hyperthyroidism. There may be increased adrenal androgen production and an increase in the rate of peripheral androgen aromatisation.[58,59]

Hypogonadism
As with ageing testes, primary failure of the testes leads to greater deficits in testosterone production compared to oestrogen. This imbalance may lead to gynaecomastia.

Re-feeding syndrome
It is believed that gonadal function is suppressed during starvation. When re-feeding occurs, the pituitary–adrenal axis is reactivated and increases testicular function. Gynaecomastia occurs as a result, via the same mechanism as in puberty.

Renal failure and dialysis
Similar to re-feeding after starvation, testicular function is suppressed during renal failure and then reactivated when the patient commences dialysis. Gynaecomastia is seen 1–7 months after dialysis initiation and usually resolves within a year.[62,63]

Testicular tumours
The Leydig cells of the testes produce both testosterone and oestrogen. Benign Leydig tumours produce an *abnormally high amount of oestrogen* compared to testosterone, and thus may give rise to gynaecomastia.[64]

Tumours that produce hCG also cause gynaecomastia. The increased *levels of hCG stimulate Leydig cells to produce more testosterone and oestrogen*. The testosterone is converted to oestrogen both physiologically in the periphery and pathologically by the tumour itself.[65]

Sign value
Although a non-specific finding, with up to 65% of pubertal boys and over 60% of 70 year olds displaying gynaecomastia, it is still a valuable sign,[66,67] especially if it is found in a patient with other clinical signs. Given that its mechanism is routed via either the gonads or peripheral fat, identifying gynaecomastia enables the underlying pathology to be localised more easily.

6

Haematuria

Description

The presence of red blood cells in the urine. It may be microscopic (i.e. only detected on urinalysis and/or microscopy) or be visible to the naked eye (i.e. macroscopic).

Condition/s associated with

Common

- Kidney stones
- Malignancy
- Trauma to the urinary tract (e.g. infection or instrumentation)

Less common

- Glomerulonephritis – nephritis syndrome
- IgA nephropathy
- Goodpasture's syndrome
- Vasculitis
- Interstitial nephritis
- Polycystic kidneys
- Papillary infarction

Mechanism/s

Bleeding from anywhere in the renal tract will result in haematuria. Figure 6.18 provides an overview of this.

Detailed pathophysiology of each cause of haematuria is outside the scope of this text. In short, disruption of the renal tract, either by an obstruction (stone), altered kidney structure (polycystic kidneys) or immunological deposition may cause destruction of architecture and bring blood into the urinary tract.

Sign value

While transient haematuria (particularly microscopic) is not uncommon and may be benign, persistent haematuria or haematuria with altered renal function and/or other concerning features requires immediate investigation. Painless macroscopic haematuria in an elderly person should be considered a malignancy until proven otherwise.

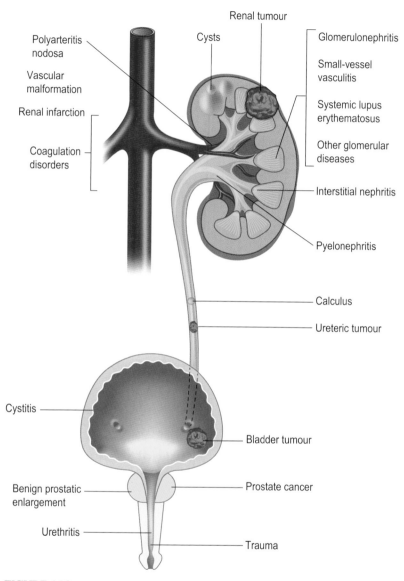

FIGURE 6.18
Causes of haematuria

Walker B, Davidson's Principles and Practice of Medicine, *22nd edn, London: Elsevier 2014: Fig 7.7.*

Hepatic encephalopathy

Description

Hepatic encephalopathy refers to an array of symptoms resulting from acute or chronic liver failure. Forgetfulness, decreased cognitive function, confusion, altered sleep–wake cycle, irritability, asterixis, decreased level of consciousness and even coma have all been reported.

Condition/s associated with

- Chronic liver failure
- Acute liver failure

Mechanism/s

Despite large amounts of research, the exact pathogenesis of hepatic encephalopathy has not been agreed upon.

Hepatic encephalopathy is most likely multi-factorial with neurotoxicity, oxidative stress, benzodiazepine-like ligands, astrocyte swelling, gamma-aminobutyric acid (GABA), abnormal histamine and serotonin transmission, and inflammation/oedema all playing some part.[68]

Some of the theories are discussed below. Of these, the ammonia theory is the most fully researched hypothesis at present.

Ammonia hypothesis

This is the most studied and currently most accepted explanation for hepatic encephalopathy. In this theory *decreased breakdown of ammonia* and the presence of *porto-systemic shunts* allow increased levels of ammonia to enter the systemic circulation and thence to the brain, disrupting normal CNS function. As a pathogen, ammonia may have the following effects:[69]

- In the brain increased ammonia levels result in swelling and dysfunction of the astrocytes to the point where they can no longer maintain the environment around the neurons, resulting in neuronal malfunction.

- Increased swelling of the astrocytes leads to oedema, an increase in resting membrane potential, altered chloride pumps[70] and disturbed neurotransmitters.

- In experimental studies, ammonia in high concentrations impairs neuronal transmission.

- Ammonia may alter the gene expression of proteins required for CNS function.

- High levels of ammonia result in physiological depression and a change of cerebral energy metabolism, leading to cell death through mitochrondrial dysfunction.[70,71]

Bacterial products

Bacteria have been shown to break down amino acids into products that can contribute to neurotoxicity and hepatic encephalopathy, such as *mercaptan and phenols*.[70] Produced in the intestines, they are shunted around the liver and enter the brain to ill effect. Bacteria are also possibly capable of producing GABA-like compounds and modulating inflammatory responses to cause or worsen encephalopathy.[70]

GABA-ergic hypothesis

In patients who present with hepatic encephalopathy, *increased levels of GABA*

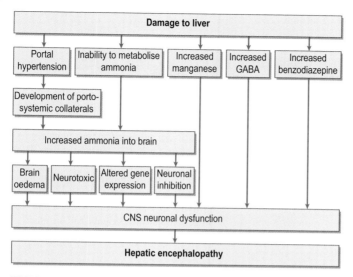

FIGURE 6.19
Mechanism/s involved in hepatic encephalopathy

(an inhibitory neurotransmitter) have been found. The proposed theory is that increased GABA levels result in inhibition of neuronal function and hepatic encephalopathy.[72] Why GABA levels are raised may be related to the increased synaptic availability of GABA through a *more permeable blood–brain barrier*, which is known to occur in hepatocellular failure.[71]

The inhibitory effects of higher levels of GABA may be further potentiated by *neurosteroids*, which are formed by mitochondria in response to increased levels of ammonia. Neurosteroids can bind to GABA receptors and potentiate further inhibitory signals.[70,71]

Benzodiazepine hypothesis

Increased levels of benzodiazepine-like substances have been reported in the brains of living people with hepatic encephalopathy.[73] As in the GABA-ergic hypothesis, this is thought to increase neuronal inhibition.

Manganese hypothesis

Manganese in chronically high levels is known to cause neuronal and basal ganglia damage. It is normally excreted via the hepatobiliary route. In liver failure, it is suggested that increased manganese levels damage the CNS and contribute to hepatic encephalopathy.

Neuroinflammation and TNF-α – a unifying theory?

More recently, an all-encompassing hypothesis involving tumour necrosis factor (TNF-α) has been proposed.[72] Under this premise, increased levels of TNF-α are responsible for neurotoxicity and hepatic encephalopathy. It is suggested that all of the stimuli that are mentioned in the other theories raise TNF-α levels and thus cause neurotoxicity. Increased levels of TNF-α have been shown to increase IL-1 and IL-6, leading to increased permeability of the blood–brain barrier and increased ammonia diffusion. Further treatment with

6

entaracept, a TNF-α inhibitor, has been shown to reduce severity of hepatic encephalopathy and prevent cerebral oedema. This theory is yet to be universally accepted.

Oxidative stress

It is proposed that after exposure to ammonia, benzodiazepenes, cytokines, hyponatremia or other stimulus, astrocyte metabolism is altered to promote the formation of reactive oxygen species (ROS), which may damage neurons and impair neuronal transmission.[70]

Sign value

Hepatic encephalopathy is specific to liver disease but needs to be differentiated from other pathologies that may produce a similar set of signs and symptoms. It is seen in 30–45% of patients with liver cirrhosis.[74]

In acute liver failure, the presence of hepatic encephalopathy has negative prognostic value.[75,76] In one study, 31% of patients in acute liver failure with encephalopathy required liver transplant or died,[75] and 71% of patients in another study of severely encephalopathic patients had similar outcomes.[76]

Hepatic foetor

Description

A sweet/musty odour emanating from the breath.

Condition/s associated with

• Hepatic failure

Mechanism/s

Due to the failing liver's inability to metabolise bacterially degraded methionine and mercaptan dimethyl sulfide, these substances pass through the lungs and are exhaled, producing a distinctive smell. Trimethylamine has also been implicated as a cause of the odour.[77]

Sign value

Although common in hepatic encephalopathy, it is detected infrequently. It can be mistaken for other odours, and therefore can be an inconsistent sign.[78]

6

Hepatic venous hum

Description

Low-pitched hum heard over the liver when auscultating with the bell of the stethoscope.

Condition/s associated with

- Portal hypertension
- Large haemangioma
- Hepatoma

Mechanism/s

A hepatic venous hum occurs with portal hypertension as the blood flows into the lower-pressure systemic system via collateral vessels from the higher-pressure portal system, creating a continuous and appreciable noise.[79]

Hepatomegaly

Description

An enlarged liver – usually larger than 13 cm in diameter from the superior to inferior border. Commonly found using percussion over the chest and abdomen with palpation of the lower liver border.

Condition/s associated with

There are many potential causes of hepatomegaly. Possible classifications include those given in Table 6.6.

Mechanism/s

The mechanisms involved in hepatomegaly are:

1. increased vascular engorgement
2. inflammation
3. deposition and expansion due to non-liver cells/materials
4. a combination of points 1–3.

Congestive heart failure

In congestive heart failure pressure backs up into the venous system due to ineffective filling or forward outflow, leading to a congested and engorged liver.

Infective

Inflammation and swelling of the liver is the principal mechanism in many of the infective pathologies (e.g. hepatitis, malaria, Epstein–Barr virus [EBV]). Inflammation may also contribute to other non-infective causes of hepatomegaly. Note that in hepatitis the liver may be enlarged or, over time, become scarred and shrunken.

Infiltrative

Infiltrative disorders such as sarcoidosis and haemochromatosis lead to the deposition of material in the liver, increasing its size. Similarly, primary or secondary malignancy enlarges the liver via tumour cell proliferation and inflammation.

Vascular

The Budd–Chiari syndrome involves an occlusion of veins draining the liver to the heart (i.e. from the hepatic venules, through the hepatic vein to the right atrium). The occlusion may be primary or secondary to an underlying procoagulant state (e.g. lupus anticoagulants, cancer, myeloproliferative disorders, drugs

6

TABLE 6.6
Causes of hepatomegaly

Infective	Infiltrative	Neoplastic	Metabolic	Vascular
Infective mononucleosis	Sarcoidosis	Hepatocellular carcinoma	Fatty liver	Heart failure
Hepatitis A and B	Haemochromatosis	Tumour metastases	Storage diseases	Budd–Chiari syndrome
Malaria	Amyloidosis	Haemangioma		
Liver cysts		Leukaemia		
Liver abscess		Lymphoma		
		Haematoma		

CLINICAL PEARL

etc.). The backup of pressure from the blockage back to the liver causes hepatic engorgement.

Sign value

Percussion of the liver span is highly operator-dependent and does not always provide an accurate estimation of liver size.[28] Studies[80,81] have shown mediocre sensitivity (61–92%) and poor specificity (30–43%) in using percussion to determine the size of the liver.[28] The reliability is therefore tenuous.

If the liver is palpated below the costal margin, it does have 100% specificity and a PLR of 233.7![82] However, this does not necessarily equal a big liver,[83] as normal-sized livers can be palpated below the costal margin. In two reviews of available studies,[22,83] in the presence of a palpable liver edge, PLR was moderate at 2.5[83] and 1.9.[22] If not palpable, the NLR was 0.45[83] and 0.6.[22] This suggests that the absence of a palpable liver in a low-probability patient is valuable and of more utility than finding a palpable liver edge.

The stiffness or firmness of the liver edge can also be assessed and a small recent study suggested that it may have some correlation with stiffness measured by transient elastography.[84]

In summary, percussing for size of the liver is unlikely to be accurate. However, if the liver is felt on deep palpation below the costal margin, it is more than likely enlarged.

Jaundice

Description
Yellowing of the skin, sclera and mucous membranes.

Condition/s associated with
There are many different causes of jaundice; they can be grouped as shown in Table 6.7.

Mechanism/s
Jaundice is caused by a build-up of *excess bilirubin which is deposited in the skin and mucous membranes*. Jaundice is not clinically evident until serum bilirubin exceeds 3 mg/L. Defects along the bilirubin pathway (shown in

Figure 6.20) lead to increased bilirubin and jaundice.

Pre-hepatic
Jaundice in this scenario is due to excessive breakdown of red blood cells and the release of unconjugated bilirubin. See 'Haemolytic/pre-hepatic jaundice' in Chapter 4, 'Haematological and oncological signs'.

Intrahepatic
In this case the liver's *ability to take up bilirubin, bind, conjugate and/or secrete it* into the bile canaliculi is impaired. This can be due to either acquired damage to or necrosis of liver cells or genetic deficiencies in the bilirubin pathway.

TABLE 6.7
Causes of jaundice

Pre-hepatic causes	Hepatic causes	Post-hepatic causes
See Chapter 4, 'Haematological and oncological signs'	More common	
	Alcohol	
	Malignancy	
	Viral hepatitis	
	Cirrhosis of the liver	Gallstones
	Cholestasis	
	Drug-induced (e.g. paracetamol)	
	Less common	
	Primary biliary cirrhosis	Pancreatic cancer
	Primary sclerosing cholangitis	Biliary atresia
	Gilbert's syndrome	Cholangiosarcoma
	Crigler–Najjar syndrome	
	Autoimmune hepatitis	

6

CLINICAL PEARL

Gilbert's syndrome is an example of a genetic deficiency in the bilirubin pathway. A genetic abnormality of the enzyme glucuronyltransferase reduces the liver's ability to conjugate bilirubin. As a result, unconjugated bilirubin cannot be excreted properly and hyperbilirubinaemia occurs to a level that eventually causes jaundice.

Similarly, in Dubin–Johnson syndrome, a genetic defect in a transporter (cMOAT) stops conjugated bilirubin from being secreted effectively, and bilirubin rises, resulting in jaundice.

There are many hepatic causes of jaundice. Any condition that can cause enough damage or destruction to the liver to prevent normal bilirubin processing can cause jaundice. More and less common causes are listed in Table 6.7.

Drug-induced liver injury

A huge number of drugs can cause liver injury and result in jaundice, among other things. A variety of mechanisms have been proposed and include:[85]

- formation of reactive metabolites
- bile salt export pump (BSEP) inhibition – leading to a build-up of bile salts in hepatocytes
- drug transporter/metabolising enzymes modulation
- mitochondrial toxicity[86]
- oxidative stress
- modulating adaptive/innate immune reactions
- biliary epithelial injury
- histone acetylation.

A small selection of pharmaceuticals that can cause jaundice via these pathways is shown in Table 6.8.

Post-hepatic

Post-hepatic jaundice is caused by a *blockage of bile ducts* preventing the excretion of conjugated bilirubin. Bilirubin backs up through the liver into the bloodstream.

Sign value

Jaundice is an important clinical sign and must be identified and investigated. If found, the clinician should attempt to identify other presenting features

TABLE 6.8
Mechanisms of common drug-induced liver injury

Drug	Mechanism/s
Augmentin (amoxicillin + clavulanic acid)	Stimulates an immune-driven response, especially in patients with genetic predisposition including: Class I & II HLA DQB1*0602, HLA DRB1*15014
Valproate	Mitochondrial injury Histone deacetylase inhibition
Cyclosporin	Bile salt pump inhibition
Flucloxacillin	Bile salt pump inhibition Immunological hypersensitivity reaction associated with patients with HLA B*5701
Paracetamol	Toxic doses saturate normal metabolism, more substrate is shunted down CYP2E1 metabolism resulting in excess NAPQI, glutathione is depleted and cannot neutralise NAPQI which is toxic to liver cell membranes

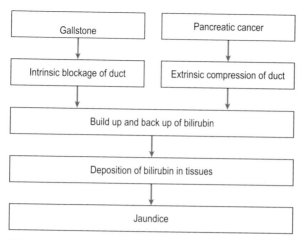

FIGURE 6.20
Example mechanism of post-hepatic jaundice

Dark-coloured urine/pale-coloured stools of biliary obstruction

Often associated with post-hepatic or obstructive jaundice is the sign of 'dark urine/pale stools'. In healthy people, unconjugated bilirubin is bound tightly to albumin and cannot be excreted in the urine (it cannot 'fit' through the glomerulus of the kidney). However, in patients with obstructive jaundice, conjugated bilirubin binds less tightly to albumin and may be excreted in the urine, giving it a dark tea colour.

Bile duct obstruction does not allow excretion of bilirubin into the intestines; therefore, the stool does not accumulate the bile pigments that normally make it dark in colour, and the patient will have a noticeably pale bowel motion.

---

which may point to the cause of jaundice (e.g. signs of chronic liver disease: palmar erythema, spider naevi, ascites, a palpable gallbladder, lymphadenopathy). In almost 80% of cases one can identify a hepatic versus post-hepatic cause of jaundice at the bedside, resulting in appropriate test ordering and a much shorter differential diagnosis list.[87]

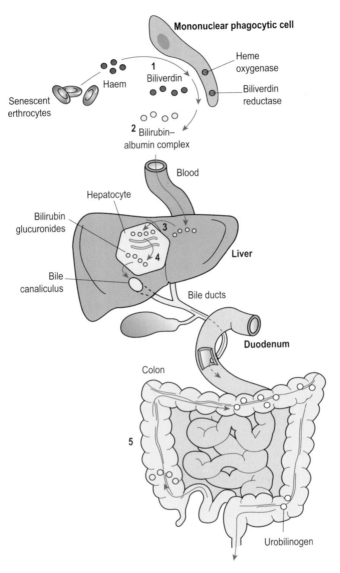

FIGURE 6.21

Bilirubin metabolism and elimination

1 Normal bilirubin production from haem (0.2–0.3 g/day) is derived primarily from the breakdown of senescent circulating erythrocytes.

2 Extrahepatic bilirubin is bound to serum albumin and delivered to the liver.

3 Hepatocellular uptake and **4** glucuronidation in the endoplasmic reticulum generate bilirubin, which is water-soluble and readily excreted into bile.

5 Gut bacteria deconjugate the bilirubin and degrade it to colourless urobilinogens. The urobilinogens and the residue of intact pigments are excreted in the faeces, with some reabsorption and excretion into urine.

Reproduced, with permission, from Kumar V, Abbas AK, Fausto N, Aster JC, Robbins and Cotran Pathologic Basis of Disease, Professional Edition, 8th edn, Philadelphia: Saunders, 2009: Fig 18-4.

Kayser–Fleischer rings

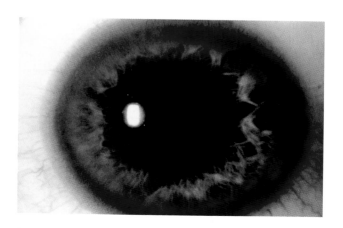

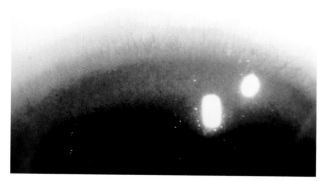

FIGURE 6.22
Kayser–Fleischer rings

Reproduced, with permission, from Liu M, Cohen EJ, Brewer GJ, Laibson PR, Am J Ophthalmol *2002; 133(6): 832–834.*

Description
Brown/blue rings at the periphery of the cornea.

Condition/s associated with

More common

- Wilson's disease

Less common

- Chronic active liver disease
- Primary biliary cirrhosis
- Multiple myeloma

Wilson's disease mechanism/s
Excess copper accumulation is the principal cause of this sign.

6

In Wilson's disease, copper is unable to be excreted into bile, leading to a toxic accumulation in the liver and the eventual cellular death of hepatocytes. Copper subsequently leaks into the systemic circulation[88] and copper chelates/granules are deposited in the inner portion of Descemet's membrane in the cornea.[89] The precise mechanism of entry of copper from the systemic circulation into this membrane is controversial. The two main theories are that copper is deposited via either the limbic system[90,91] or through the aqueous humour.[92]

Primary biliary cirrhosis mechanism/s

In primary biliary cirrhosis (PBC) there is reduced biliary tree outflow which in turn causes cholestasis. Copper that would normally be excreted into bile therefore accumulates in the liver, causing hepatotoxicity and leaking into the systemic circulation. As with Wilson's disease, copper is then able to be deposited in other tissues such as the cornea.[93]

Sign value

Kayser–Fleischer rings are present in 99% of patients with concomitant

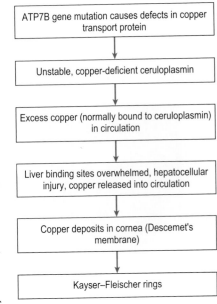

FIGURE 6.23
Mechanism of Kayser–Fleischer rings in Wilson's disease[94]

Adapted from Suvarna JC. Kayser-Fleischer ring. J Postgrad Med 2008; 54: 238–240.

neurological/psychiatric features of Wilson's disease, but in only 30–50% of patients without these features.[95] Therefore, in the absence of neurological/psychiatric features, other differential diagnoses should be considered.

Leuconychia

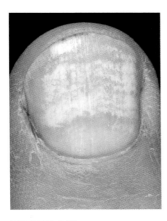

FIGURE 6.24
Leuconychia

Reproduced, with permission, from Habif TP, Clinical Dermatology, 5th edn, St Louis: Mosby, 2009: p. 964.

Description

Complete whitening of the nail plate.

Condition/s associated with

More common

- Hereditary
- Injury to nail base

Less common

- Hypoalbuminaemia
- Protein-losing enteropathies
- Hepatic cirrhosis
- Chronic renal failure
- Congestive heart failure
- Diabetes mellitus
- Hodgkin's lymphoma

Mechanism/s

The mechanism is unclear.

In hereditary leuconychia, it is thought that a defect in keratinisation of the cells of the nail plate and underlying matrix is the cause.[96] Instead of cornified cells with keratin forming in the nail matrix, large cells with a substance called keratohyaline are present. Keratohyaline reflects light and does not allow the underlying pink nail bed to be seen.

Liver disease

A form of leuconychia known as 'Terry's nails', where the nail is white proximally and brown distally, has been associated with liver disease, diabetes and congestive heart failure but not with hypoalbuminaemia.

How liver disease leads to this sign is not clear; however, the distal brown portion is thought to be caused by the deposition of melanin.[97]

Sign value

There is limited evidence on leuconychia's value as a sign and, given its wide array of causes, it is very non-specific. Of interest, Terry's nails is said to be present in 82% of liver cirrhosis patients; however, its significance is uncertain.[98]

6

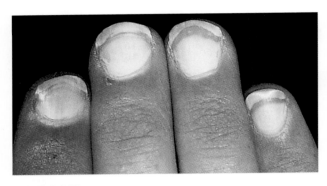

FIGURE 6.25
Terry's nails

Reproduced, with permission, from Habif TP, Clinical Dermatology, *5th edn, Philadelphia: Mosby, 2009: Fig 25-44.*

McBurney's point tenderness (Surgical sign)

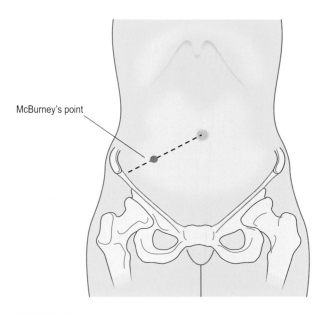

McBurney's point

FIGURE 6.26
McBurney's point
McGee S, Evidence Based Physical Diagnosis, *3rd edn, St Louis: Elsevier, 2012.*

Description

A point of maximum tenderness on palpation located one-third of the distance from the right anterior superior iliac spine to the umbilicus. The location is depicted in Figure 6.26.

Condition/s associated with

• Appendicitis

Mechanism/s

McBurney's point is said to be the most common surface location of the appendix.

When the appendix becomes inflamed such that it is no longer in the lumen of the bowel the peritoneum becomes locally irritated and tender.

Sign value

It is taught that McBurney's point tenderness suggests a later stage of appendicitis as inflammation would be expected to be severe if exacerbating surrounding structures. If present it does increase the likelihood (PLR 3.4) of appendicitis but it is not pathognomonic. It has variable sensitivity of 50–94% and specificity of 86%.[22]

Melaena

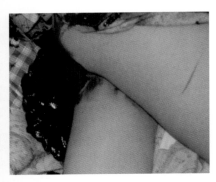

FIGURE 6.27
Melaena

Malik A et al. Dengue hemorrhagic fever outbreak in children in Port Sudan. Journal of Infection and Public Health *2010; 4(1): Fig 6.*

Description
Black, tarry, foul-smelling stools.

Condition/s associated with
- Gastrointestinal haemorrhage/bleed

More common
- Peptic ulcer disease
- Oesophageal varices
- Oesophagitis
- Gastritis

Less common
- Mallory–Weiss tear
- Neoplasm

Mechanism/s
Bleeding from any cause in the upper gastrointestinal tract can result in melaena. It is often said that bleeding must begin above the ligament of Treitz; however, this is not always the case. The black, foul-smelling nature of the stool is due to the *oxidation of iron from the haemoglobin*, as it passes through the gastrointestinal tract.

Sign value
If present, melaena requires complete investigation, bearing in mind that it is not necessarily specific to the location of the bleed.

Mouth ulcers (aphthous ulcer)

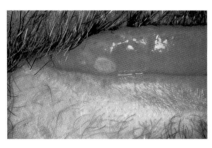

FIGURE 6.28
Mouth ulcer

Reproduced, with permission, from Kanski JJ, Clinical Diagnosis in Ophthalmology, 1st edn, Philadelphia: Mosby, 2006: Fig 10-45.

Description

A painful open lesion anywhere within the oral cavity.

Condition/s associated with

Numerous associations

More common

- Trauma
- Stress
- Toothpaste

Less common

- Iron deficiency
- Folate deficiency
- Vitamin B12 deficiency
- Food hypersensitivity
- Humoural/immunological
- Inflammatory bowel disease

- Behçet's disease
- SLE
- HIV/AIDS
- Nicorandil

Mechanism/s

The mechanism is unknown.

Regardless of cause, aphthous ulcers present with a breakage of the oral mucosa and infiltration of neutrophils.[99] It is likely that local, systemic, immunological and microbiological processes all play a role.[99-101]

More recently, toll-like receptors (TLR) have been causally implicated. A recent study suggests the superficial oral epithelium provides a barrier and is TLR 'free', and not responsive to pathogen-associated molecular pattern (PAMP). Increased permeability of this superficial epithelium through micronutrient deficiency, or trauma, may enable deeper TLRs to respond to oral microbial PAMPs and stimulate an inflammatory and immune response, leading to the development of an ulcer.[102]

Sign value

Given at least 10–25% of the population suffers from these ulcers, the value of the ulcers as a single sign is very limited.[103] It needs to be taken into context with other history and symptoms.

6

Muehrcke's lines

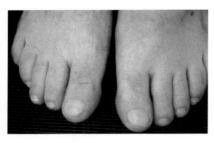

FIGURE 6.29
Muehrcke's lines

Reproduced, with permission, from James WD, Berger TG, Elston DM (eds), Andrews' Diseases of the Skin: Clinical Dermatology, 11th edn, Philadelphia: Saunders, 2011: Fig 7.

Description

Two white bands that run parallel to the lunula across the width of the nail. They are smooth and not raised. Normal-appearing pink nail-bed tissue is seen between the two white lines.

Condition/s associated with

- Hypoalbuminaemia
- Diseases causing serious metabolic stress
- Chemotherapy treatment
- Infection
- Trauma

Mechanism/s

The specific mechanism for each cause is unclear.

It is suspected to be due to abnormal amounts of stress on the body, *impeding protein formation.* Due to this low protein, oedema within the nail bed compresses underlying blood vessels and blanches the normal erythema of the nail bed, causing the characteristic lines.[104-107]

Sign value

Limited evidence is available on the value of Muehrcke's sign. It is associated with serum albumin levels of less than 22 g/L[98] and does disappear with correction of albumin deficiency.

Murphy's sign (Surgical sign)

VIDEO 6.1 ▶

Video 6.1 Access through Student Consult.

Description

As the examiner palpates the abdomen below the right subcostal margin, the patient is asked to take a deep breath in and, if on doing so, is caught by sudden pain, this is Murphy's sign.

Condition/s associated with

- Cholecystitis

Mechanism/s

On deep inspiration the lungs expand, pushing the liver downwards so the inflamed gallbladder is pushed onto the examiner's pressing hand, causing an unexpected sharp pain.

Sign value

While individual studies[108-110] have shown sensitivity of 48–97%, specificity of 48–79%, PLR of 1.9 and NLR of 0.6 for Murphy's sign, a systematic review[111] showed a PLR of 2.8 but could not rule out chance (95% CI, 0.8–8.6).

6

CLINICAL PEARL

Obturator sign (Surgical sign)

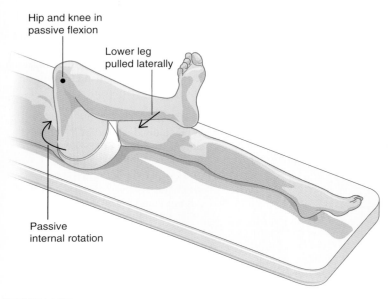

Hip and knee in passive flexion

Lower leg pulled laterally

Passive internal rotation

FIGURE 6.30
Eliciting the obturator sign

Description
Pain on internal rotation of the thigh.

Condition/s associated with
• Appendicitis

Mechanism/s
The inflamed appendix lies in contact with the obturator internus muscle.

When the leg is rotated, the obturator moves and the appendix is stretched and irritated.

Sign value
The obturator sign, if present, is valuable, with a specificity of 94%, but has a sensitivity of only 8%.[112]

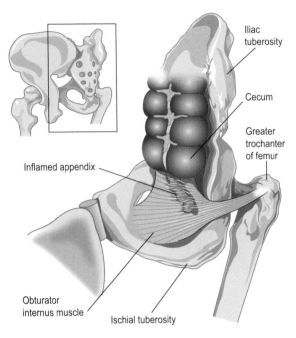

Iliac
tuberosity

Cecum

Greater
trochanter
of femur

Inflamed appendix

Obturator
internus muscle

Ischial tuberosity

FIGURE 6.31
Anatomy of the obturator sign in appendicitis

A note on appendicitis and clinical signs

Appendicitis has traditionally been taught to be a clinical diagnosis
with a variety of signs used to assist the clinician – the obturator,
psoas and Rovsing's signs and McBurney's point tenderness to name
a few. While both ultrasound and computer tomography (CT) are
better validated and offer significant diagnostic capabilities,
physical examination scores/algorithms taking in a variety of signs
and symptoms have been shown to have a sensitivity of 99% and a
specificity of 76%.[113] It is suggested that when patients present with
a series of signs and symptoms highly suggestive of appendicitis,
additional imaging *may be* unnecessary.[114] If there is any doubt of
the diagnosis imaging can assist.

6

Oliguria/anuria

Description

Although not easily observed as a sign, urine output can be enquired about and a routine fluid balance check is included in the review of many conditions. Oliguria is described as less than 400 mL urine output per day in adults and less than 0.5 mL/kg/hr in children. Anuria refers to urine output of less than 100 mL per day in adults.

Condition/s associated with

Like the classifications of acute renal failure, the conditions associated with oliguria can be split into 'Pre-renal', 'Renal' and 'Post-renal'.

Mechanisms/s

The aetiology of every condition that can result in low urine output is out of the scope of this text; however, brief mechanisms for groups of conditions are provided below.

Pre-renal

Oliguria resulting from pre-renal causes is principally due to *reduced renal perfusion*. Adequate perfusion of the kidneys is reliant on fluid (blood), adequate pipes (veins and arteries) and an adequate pump (heart). Problems with one or more of these three elements (e.g. dehydration [lack of fluid], sepsis [leaky pipes], heart failure [pump]) results in under-perfusion of the kidneys. The kidneys are exquisitely sensitive to decreased circulating volume or flow and have a number of compensatory mechanisms to activate (e.g. the renin–angiotensin II system), which ultimately results in retention of salt and water, and therefore less urine being passed.

Renal

Intrinsic renal impairment causing oliguria results from structural damage to the kidneys. If there is significant enough insult to the renal architecture, the kidneys cannot filter or function to produce urine.

Post-renal

Obstruction of the ureters, bladder or urethra will prevent urine from being passed. If this occurs for long enough it can cause intrinsic damage to the kidneys, further affecting urine production.

TABLE 6.9
Classifications of oliguria

Pre-renal	Renal	Post-renal
Dehydration	Acute tubular necrosis	Bladder outlet obstruction (e.g. stones/tumours)
Blood loss	Drugs	Bilateral ureteric obstruction
Sepsis	Toxins	
Cardiac failure	Glomerulonephritis	
Burns	Vascular (e.g. renal artery thrombosis)	
Drugs	Interstitial nephritis	
Anaphylaxis		

CLINICAL PEARL

Sign value

Oliguria is an essential sign to be aware of and can help guide therapy and also alert the clinician to developing pathology.

6

Palmar erythema

Description

A symmetrical and slightly warm reddened area on the thenar and hypothenar eminences of the palm.

- May have a mottled appearance or blanch when pressed.
- Not associated with pain, itch or scaling.
- May involve the palmar aspect of the fingers and proximal nail folds.[115,116]

Condition/s associated with

Documented in a large number of diseases; most common presentations include:

- Primary causes (where disease of pathological processes cannot be found)
  » Hereditary – rare
  » Pregnancy – common
  » Senile
- Secondary causes
  » Chronic liver disease
  » Autoimmune (e.g. rheumatoid arthritis)
  » Endocrinological – hyperthyroid
  » Neoplastic

General mechanism/s

Regardless of the initial cause, palmar erythema is the result of increased perfusion of the palms. Central to many mechanism/s that cause palmar erythema are increased oestrogen levels, increased oestrogen-to-testosterone ratios or raised circulating free oestrogens.

Oestrogen has a known proliferative effect on endometrial capillary density, and it is thought that this effect may have a similar effect on the palms.[117]

Other factors that may play a role include:

- disordered hepatic metabolism of bradykinin and other vasoactive substances[117]
- abnormal cutaneous vasoconstrictor/vasodilator reflexes.

Pregnancy

Most likely due to increased circulating oestrogens (as discussed previously) causing alterations to the structure and function of skin and microvasculature.[118]

Chronic liver disease

In cirrhotic patients there is decreased metabolism and clearance of androstenedione, which allows for greater peripheral conversion to oestrogen.[20] Raised circulating levels of oestrogens, oestradiol-to-testosterone ratio or free oestrogen lead to increased vascularity of the palms.

An alternative theory is that damaged local autonomic nerves and vasoconstrictor reflexes cause the erythema. The precipitating damage is caused by dysfunction of arteriovenous anastamoses which are present in cirrhotic patients.[119]

Rheumatoid arthritis

Palmar erythema is a common occurrence in rheumatoid arthritis, with over 60% of patients exhibiting the sign.[120] The pathogenesis remains largely unknown.[121]

Neoplastic

May arise from increased angiogenic factors and oestrogens from solid

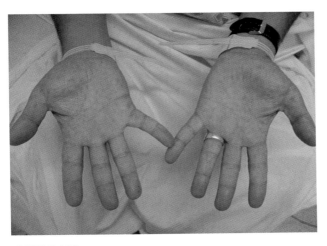

FIGURE 6.32
Palmar erythema in a patient with cirrhosis
Reproduced, with permission, from Goldman L, Ausiello D, Cecil Medicine, 23rd edn, Philadelphia: Saunders, 2007: Fig 149-5.

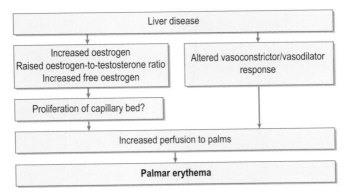

FIGURE 6.33
Mechanism of palmar erythema in liver disease

tumours.[117] In addition, if the liver is involved, raised oestrogen levels may contribute.

Hyperthyroid
Increased levels of oestradiol–17-beta are seen in some patients with hyperthyroidism and are the likely cause of the development of palmar erythema.[122]

Sign value
Palmar erythema, although non-specific, does have some value as a sign:

- It can vary according to the severity of the underlying disease.[117]
- In rheumatoid arthritis it is associated with a more favourable prognosis, fewer digital deformities and higher haemoglobin levels.[117]

6

- It is a frequent sign of liver cirrhosis, with as many as 23% of ultrasound-proven cirrhosis patients having concurrent palmar erythema.[118] It has some value in the diagnosis of cirrhosis in liver disease with sensitivity 46%, specificity 91%, PLR 5.0 and NLR 0.6.[20]
- Palmar erythema is present in 15% of patients with primary or metastatic brain malignancies.

Pruritic scratch marks/pruritus

Description

Scratch marks manifest as a sign related to an underlying symptom, pruritus, which is the sensation of itchiness. The absence of scratch marks in hard-to-reach places (e.g. between the shoulder blades) when they are present on the rest of the body may be an indication of severity of itch.

Condition/s associated with

Pruritus is associated with numerous skin conditions and systemic diseases. The systemic diseases that cause pruritus include, but are not limited to, those listed in Table 6.10.

General mechanism/s

The skin has many unmyelinated C-fibres that synapse with itch-specific secondary neurons. It is the irritation of the unmyelinated C-fibres by chemical mediators or 'pruritogens' that causes the sensation of itch.[123]

The main pruritogen is histamine. However, there are numerous others and more are being discovered each year. Potential mediators of pruritus are listed in Table 6.11.

These factors stimulate pruritus by:

- directly acting on epidermal nerve endings (e.g. histamine)
- liberating histamine from mast cells (e.g. neuropeptides)
- potentiating histamine (e.g. PGE_2, endogenous opioids).

Chronic renal failure

Many elements contribute to pruritus in chronic renal failure. The accumulation of *pruritogenic factors* due to the kidneys' inability to excrete them is thought to be the primary cause. Pathological features of chronic renal failure that contribute to pruritus include:[123,124]

- xerosis (dry skin)
- abnormal cutaneous mast cell proliferation
- secondary hyperparathyroidism
- increased pruritogenic cytokines
- increased vitamin A levels
- increased endogenous opioids
- impaired sweating
- peripheral neuropathy
- increased levels of magnesium, stimulating release of histamine
- increased levels of phosphate (cutaneous calcifications stimulating itch receptors).

Hepatobiliary

Like pruritus of chronic renal failure, the mechanism in hepatobiliary disorders is thought to be multi-factorial.

Accepted reasoning thus far has been that increased bile salts accumulate in blood and tissues, inducing pruritus. However, research now suggests that although bile salts may directly or indirectly play a part in pruritus, the evidence for them having a key role in the induction of pruritus in cholestasis is weak.[125] Steroids, steroid metabolites, histamine, serotonin, GABA and cannabinoids are just a few of the pruritogens thought to be involved in the development of itch in cholestasis.

6

TABLE 6.10
Causes of pruritus and pruritic scratch marks

Renal	Hepatobiliary	Haematological	Metabolic/endocrine	Neurological
		More common		
Chronic renal failure	Infectious hepatitis	Polycythaemia vera	Hyper/hypothyroid	
	Biliary obstruction	Leukaemia/lymphoma	Diabetes	
		Less common		
	Primary biliary cirrhosis	Iron deficiency anaemia	Multiple endocrine neoplasia (MEN) II	Multiple sclerosis
	Primary sclerosing cholangitis		Carcinoid syndrome	Cerebral tumour
	Drug-induced cholestasis			Stroke

TABLE 6.11
Potential chemical mediators of pruritus

Type of pruritogen	Examples
Amines	Histamine, serotonin, dopamine, adrenaline, noradrenaline, melatonin
Neuropeptides	Substance P, neurotensin, vasoactive intestinal peptide (VIP), somatostatin, α- and β-melanocyte-stimulating hormone (MSH), calcitonin gene-related peptide (CGRP), bradykinin, endothelin, neurokinin A and B, cholecystokinin (CCK), bombesin
Eicosanoids	PGE_1, PGE_2, PGH_2, LTB_4
Cytokines	IL-2, TNF-α and TNF-β, eosinophil products
Opioids	Met-enkephalin, leu-enkephalin, β-endorphin, morphine
Proteolytic enzymes	Tryptases, chymases, kallikrein, papain, carboxypeptidases

Based on Krajnik M, Zylicz Z, Netherlands J Med *2001; 58: 27–40; with permission.*

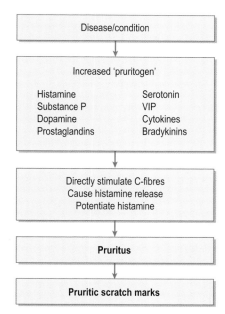

FIGURE 6.34
General mechanism of pruritus

One study[126] has found that lysophosphatidic acid may cause a rise in intracellular calcium that in turn activates itch–inducing nerve fibres in patients with cholestasis.

Haematopoietic
The mechanism is not clearly established.

- Histamine and serotonin have been associated with the pruritus of polycythaemia vera.[127]

In Hodgkin's lymphoma, some studies identify histamine as a central mediator,[124] whereas other studies[128] propose an autoimmune reaction to lymphoma cells inducing the liberation of bradykinins and leucopeptides.

Metabolic and endocrine
The mechanism is unclear.

Pruritus in hyperthyroidism is thought to be related to a decrease in the '*itch threshold*' due to increased body temperature, vasodilatation and activation of the kinin system by increased tissue activity and metabolism.[124]

In hypothyroidism, xerosis (dry skin) is the principal cause of itchiness.

Neurological disorders

The mechanism is unclear.

In multiple sclerosis, bouts of pruritus are attributed to the activation of artificial synapses between axons in partially demyelinated areas of the CNS.[123]

Sign value

Little research has been directed towards the value of pruritus as a symptom or sign. Given the wide variety of causes, specificity is low.

Prevalence in some conditions:

- 25–86% in uraemic patients with chronic renal failure[123,129]
- 20–25% in patients with jaundice; prevalent in 100% of primary biliary cirrhosis and a presenting symptom in 50%[130]
- 25–75% in polycythaemia vera[127]
- 4–11% in patients with thyrotoxicosis.[131]

Pruritus may precede the onset of disease by 5 years in Hodgkin's lymphoma.[132]

Psoas sign (Surgical sign)

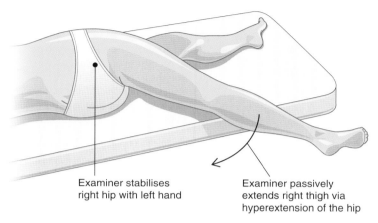

Examiner stabilises right hip with left hand

Examiner passively extends right thigh via hyperextension of the hip

FIGURE 6.35
Psoas sign

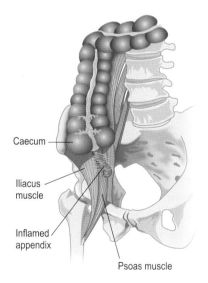

Caecum

Iliacus muscle

Inflamed appendix

Psoas muscle

FIGURE 6.36
Psoas sign anatomy

Description

The patient experiences pain on passive extension of the thigh.

Condition/s associated with

- Appendicitis
- Psoas abscess

Mechanism/s

If the appendix is in a retro-caecal position, it may be in contact with the psoas muscle. Therefore, movement of this muscle will irritate the inflamed appendix, causing pain. A similar process occurs with a psoas abscess.

Sign value

Sensitivity of 13–42%, specificity of 79–97%, PLR of 2.0.[22,133] See box 'A note on appendicitis' under 'Obturator sign' in this chapter.

6

Pyoderma gangrenosum

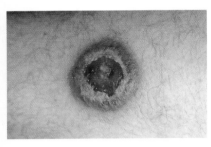

FIGURE 6.37
Pyoderma gangrenosum

Reproduced, with permission, from Weston WL, Lane AT, Morelli JG, Color Textbook of Pediatric Dermatology, *4th edn, London: Mosby, 2007: Fig 14-46.*

Description

A rare, chronic, often destructive, inflammatory skin condition in which a painful nodule or pustule breaks down to form a progressively enlarging ulcer with a raised, tender, undermined border.[134]

Condition/s associated with

- Idiopathic: 25–50% of cases
- Inflammatory bowel disease: up to 50% of cases
- Rheumatological disease
- Paraproteinaemia
- Haematological malignancy

Mechanism/s

The mechanisms of both idiopathic and secondary causes of pyoderma gangrenosum are not clear. It is thought to be related to a loss of *innate immune regulation* and *altered neutrophil chemotaxis*,[135] but how and why this occurs is still to be explained.

Sign value

There is little evidence regarding the value of pyoderma gangrenosum (PG) as a sign. However, given it has been associated with some form of systemic disease in up to 50% of cases,[135] its presence in an otherwise healthy individual warrants suspicion and investigation.

- Its association with inflammatory bowel disease may be overstated, with one case series showing PG occurred in 0.48% of patients with UC and 0.33% of patients with Crohn's disease.[136] Similarly, a prospective cohort study of 2402 French patients with IBD found PG in 0.75% of their patients, with no association between severity of IBD and presence of PG.[53]
- 7% of PG have been associated with haematological malignancy.
- Arthritis has been associated in 37% of cases.[136]

Rebound tenderness (Surgical sign)

Description

The clinician presses hard on the abdomen and then quickly removes their hand (i.e. the pressure). The patient feels sudden *pain on the release of pressure* rather than the preceding palpation.

Condition/s associated with

- Any cause of peritonitis

Mechanism/s

When the abdomen is pushed down and then quickly released, the peritoneum rebounds and, if it is inflamed, the rebound movement will activate pain sensory fibres.

Sign value

Originally said to be one of the cardinal signs of peritonitis; however, recent evidence has found little value as a sign. Studies have shown a wide variation in sensitivity (40–95%) and specificity (20–89%) and PLR 2.0.[28]

6

Rigidity and involuntary guarding (Surgical sign)

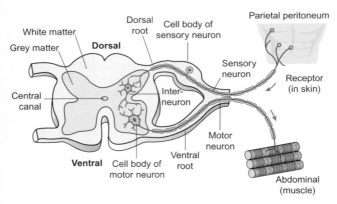

FIGURE 6.38
Example of reflex arc in rigidity/involuntary guarding

Description
A constant involuntary contraction of the abdominal musculature where the abdomen is literally 'rigid' to palpation. There will also be tenderness present.

Condition/s associated with
• Causes of peritonism

Mechanism/s
Inflammation of the peritoneum stimulates a *reflex arc* resulting in the contraction of the abdominal muscles.

The parietal peritoneum is innervated by somatic nerve fibres that produce sharp localised pain (unlike the visceral peritoneum). When a pathological process (e.g. appendicitis) occurs and affects the parietal peritoneum, somatic sensory neurons are stimulated. These neurons travel via the spinal nerves and synapse in the dorsal horn of the spinal cord. Here they interconnect with a motor neuron in the ventral horn of the spinal cord which in turn stimulates a localised area of abdominal muscle to contract, forming a reflex arc (see Figure 6.38). As the initial reflex bypasses the brain, the patient has little control over it (i.e. it is involuntary).

Sign value
Rigidity, if present, is a valuable sign, with a sensitivity of 6–40%, a specificity of 86–100% and a PLR of 3.6.[28]

Rovsing's sign (Surgical sign)

Description
When the left lower quadrant is palpated, the patient feels pain in the right lower quadrant.

Condition/s associated with
Traditionally appendicitis; although theoretically inflammation of any organ in the right lower quadrant may elicit Rovsing's sign.

Mechanism/s
When the left side of the abdomen is pressed upon, the peritoneum is stretched tight over the inflamed appendix, causing irritation to the appendix and peritoneum and thus localising the pain felt.

Sign value
Sensitivity of 7–68% and specificity of 58–96%, PLR of 2.3 and NLR of 0.7.[22]

6

CLINICAL PEARL

Scleral icterus

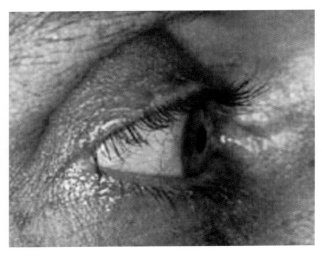

FIGURE 6.39
Scleral icterus

Reproduced, with permission, from Stern TA, Rosenbaum JF, Fava M, Biederman J, Rauch SL, Massachusetts General Hospital Comprehensive Clinical Psychiatry, 1st edn, Philadelphia: Mosby, 2008: Fig 21-17.

Description

Yellow discolouration of the sclera.

Condition/s associated with

See 'Jaundice' in this chapter.

Mechanism/s

Hyperbilirubinaemia leads to bilirubin deposition in the sclera. For full details see 'Jaundice' in this chapter.

Sign value

The difficulty with scleral icterus as a sign lies in the ability of the examiner to identify it! In one study,[137] 58% of examiners detected scleral icterus in patients with total serum bilirubin of 2.5 mg/dL, whereas 68% of examiners detected scleral icterus in patients with total serum bilirubin of 3.1 mg/dL.

Sialadenosis

Description

A persistent enlargement of the parotid gland (and occasionally submandibular salivary glands). It is neither inflammatory nor neoplastic in origin. Clinically, sialadenosis is palpable as a soft, bilateral, symmetrical and non-tender enlargement of the parotid glands.

Condition/s associated with

- Diabetes mellitus – rare
- Malnutrition
- Alcoholism

Alcoholism mechanism/s

There is debate surrounding the precise origin of sialadenosis in chronic alcoholism. Cellular hypertrophy and disturbed fat metabolism are the two main causes proposed. The former involves autonomic nerve dysregulation and, thus, accumulation of intracellular zymogen (a precursor to amylase) granules, either via increased production or reduced secretion from the cell. Zymogen excess leads to cellular hypertrophy. Fatty infiltration of the gland owing to altered fat metabolism has also been implicated, particularly in the later stages.[138-140]

Sign value

Sialadenosis is a valuable indicator of possible chronic liver disease, as it occurs in 30–80% of patients with alcohol-related cirrhosis.[141]

6

Sister Mary Joseph nodule (Surgical sign)

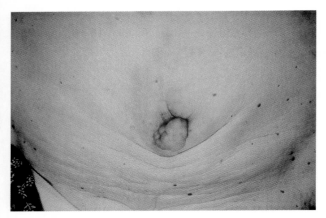

FIGURE 6.40
Periumbilical nodule and erythema – Sister Mary Joseph nodule

Reproduced, with permission, from Brenner S, Tamir E, Maharshak N, Shapira J, Clinics Dermatol *2001; 19(3): 290–297.*

Description

A firm, metastatic tumour nodule located at the umbilicus.

Condition/s associated with

- Adenocarcinoma of abdominal organs, including:
  - » Stomach
  - » Large bowel
  - » Pancreas
  - » Ovary
  - » Colorectal

Mechanism/s

It is possible that the vascular and lymphatic systems provide the conduit to the umbilicus. *Direct spread* from the peritoneum is thought to be the most common route for the metastases and nodule.

Different cancers may have a predilection to differing routes of metastases. Ovarian cancer can spread via the peritoneum and extend directly through the abdominal wall, whereas pancreatic cancer often disseminates via the lymphatics.[142]

Sign value

There are few studies on the sensitivity and specificity of the Sister Mary Joseph nodule and reviews are often limited to case studies or series.

If present the nodule warrants immediate investigation. It has a negative prognostic value, with most patients dying within a few months of diagnosis[143,144] and less than 15% of patients alive at two years.[145] In developing countries the nodule is more common, possibly representing a delay in cancer identification.[146]

In up to 10–15% of cases presenting with a Sister Mary Joseph nodule, the primary site of cancer will not be found.[147]

Spider naevus

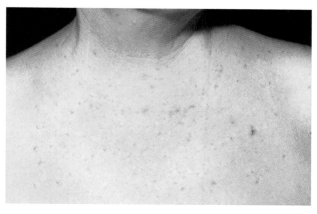

FIGURE 6.41
Spider naevi

Reproduced, with permission, from Talley NJ, O'Connor S, Clinical Examination, 6th edn, Sydney: Churchill Livingstone, 2009: Fig 6-10.

Description

Skin lesion consisting of a central arteriole with thread–like vessels (said to resemble a spider's legs) radiating outwards. Blanching occurs when the spider naevus is compressed by hand, and refilling occurs from the central arteriole outwards when released. Naevi can vary in size from a pinhead to 5 mm in diameter.[148]

Condition/s associated with

More common

- 10–15% of healthy adults and young children
- Alcohol-related liver disease
- Hepatitis B and C
- Pregnancy
- Oral contraceptive pill and other oestrogen formulations

Less common

- Thyrotoxicosis

Mechanism/s

Evidence regarding the pathophysiology is lacking. Of the few studies, increased plasma oestrogen and substance P have been identified as causative with regard to vasodilatation and neo-vascularisation.[149] Furthermore, the ratio of serum oestradiol to free testosterone is raised in male cirrhotic patients compared to the general population.[150]

Sign value

The presence of spider naevi is an important tool in predicting the degree of liver cirrhosis.

A study by Romagnuolo et al. used the presence of spider naevi, platelet count, splenomegaly and albumin level as variables to calculate the likelihood

6

CLINICAL PEARL

ratio of cirrhosis to fibrosis.[151] This study found:

- The presence of spider naevi was significantly associated with moderate to severe inflammation, significant fibrosis and cirrhosis of the liver.
- The presence of spider naevi and elevated ferritin was a good predictor of inflammation.

- Spider naevi with either splenomegaly or thrombocytopenia were good predictors of fibrosis.

More recently, a meta-analysis of 86 studies[20] found a positive likelihood ratio of 4.3 (CI 2.4-6.2) for the diagnosis of liver cirrhosis if spider naevi were present, with a sensitivity and specificity of 46% and 89% respectively. It was noted to be one of the most reliable signs in the study.

Splenomegaly

Description

The 'gold standard' definition of splenomegaly is splenic weight (post-splenectomy) of 50–250 g, decreasing with age.[152] In practice, splenomegaly is detected through palpation of the abdomen during physical examination and/or by imaging.

Condition/s associated with

There are many different organ systems and pathological processes that may give rise to splenomegaly. Table 6.12 summarises the possible aetiologies.[153]

TABLE 6.12
Diseases causing splenomegaly

Category	Group	Examples
Infection	Acute	Infectious mononucleosis, viral hepatitis, septicaemia, typhoid, cytomegalovirus (CMV), toxoplasmosis
	Subacute/chronic	Tuberculosis, subacute bacterial endocarditis, brucellosis, syphilis, HIV
	Tropical/parasitic	Malaria, leishmaniasis, schistosomiasis
Haematological	Myeloproliferative	Myelofibrosis, chronic myeloid leukaemia (CML), polycythaemia vera, essential thrombocytosis
	Lymphoma	Non-Hodgkin lymphoma (NHL), Hodgkin lymphoma
	Leukaemia	Acute leukaemia, chronic lymphocytic leukaemia (CLL), hairy cell leukaemia, prolymphocytic leukaemia
	Congenital	Hereditary spherocytosis, thalassaemia, HbSC disease
	Others	Autoimmune haemolysis, megaloblastic anaemia
Congestive		Cirrhosis, splenic/portal/hepatic vein thrombosis or obstruction, congestive cardiac failure
Inflammatory	Collagen diseases	SLE, rheumatoid arthritis (Felty's)
	Granulomatous	Sarcoidosis
Neoplastic		Haemangioma, metastases (lung, breast carcinoma, melanoma)
Infiltrative		Gaucher's disease, amyloidosis
Miscellaneous		Cysts

Based on Pozo AL, Godfrey EM, Bowles KM, Blood Rev 2009; 23(3): 105–111; with permission.

Mechanism/s

The mechanism/s for most causes of splenomegaly can be broken down into the following groups:

- increased or excessive immunological response causing hypertrophy
- hypertrophy in response to increased red cell destruction
- congestive engorgement in response to increased pooling of blood
- primary myeloproliferative disorders
- infiltrative disorders depositing non-splenic material within the spleen
- neoplastic disorders.

Hypertrophy from immunological response

Associated with infectious mononucleosis, bacterial endocarditis, cytomegalovirus (CMV), HIV and other infections. When there is an increased immunological response, such as occurs in infection, the *spleen increases in size and function to accommodate additional white cell proliferation/maturation.*

Increased red blood cell destruction

Can occur in hereditary spherocytosis, glucose-6-phosphate dehydrogenase deficiency (G6PD deficiency or favism) and beta-thalassaemia.

If there is increased red blood cell destruction, there is also increased activity in maturing lymphocytes attacking the red blood cells, leading to hypertrophy. Additionally, in order to cope with the increased destruction of red blood cells, hyperplasia of the splenic sinus cells also occurs.[154]

Congestive engorgement

Regardless of the cause of portal hypertension, when it is present there is an increase in blood backing up into

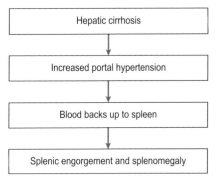

FIGURE 6.42
Mechanism of splenomegaly in liver cirrhosis

downstream vessels, including the splenic vein and so the spleen. Increased pooling of blood back into the spleen results in engorgement and hypersplenism.

There is also evidence that impaired venous return leads to increased intra-splenic destruction of red blood cells and increased phagocytic cell activity in the spleen, contributing to hypersplenism.[155]

Myeloproliferative disorders

A number of factors contribute to the splenic enlargement seen in myeloproliferative disorders:[155-158]

1. an increase in pooling of red blood cells in the spleen
2. greater splenic vascularity
3. increased cellularity in the spleen (e.g. increased cells transiting and caught in the spleen)
4. reticular element expansion
5. expansion of lymphoid components of the spleen.

These factors are dependent, to some extent, on the lineage of the cells proliferating. In one study[158] of patients with primary proliferative polycythaemia (polycythaemia vera), the increase in spleen size was attributed mainly to the increase in splenic vascularity; in myelofibrosis and in hairy cell leukaemia, it was associated with an increase in both splenic vascularity and cellularity; whereas in chronic granulocytic leukaemia (CGL) and CLL, the increase was attributed more to cellularity than to vascularity.

Sign value
A palpable spleen and/or splenomegaly is pathological until proven otherwise and requires immediate investigation.

Although sometimes difficult to palpate, if the spleen is definitely felt it is strongly associated with splenomegaly, with a sensitivity of 18–78%, specificity of 89–99% and PLR of 8.5.[28] A summary of the value of various manoeuvres that can be used to assess splenomegaly is presented in Table 6.13.[159,160]

TABLE 6.13
Relative value of signs to elicit splenomegaly

Manoeuvre	Sensitivity	Specificity	PLR	NLR
Supine palpation	78.6	92.1	91.7	79.5
Middelton's manoeuvre	85.7	86.8	87.7	84.6
Traube's space percussion	62–76.2	63.2–72	69.6	70.6
Castell's manoeuvre	82–85.7	31.6–83	58.1	66.7
Nixon's manoeuvre	59–66.7	81.6–94	80	68.9

What is the cause of the splenomegaly?

This is a frequently asked question and in truth there are many causes of splenomegaly. However, even though further investigations are required for formal diagnosis, several other clinical signs can help prioritise differential diagnoses when splenomegaly is present:
- splenomegaly and lymphadenopathy → infection (e.g. HIV) and malignancy
- splenomegaly and spider naevi, hepatomegaly, jaundice → liver disease
- splenomegaly and fever → consider infectious causes
- splenomegaly and conjunctival pallor, petechiae, ecchymoses → cell line and haematological issues
- splenomegaly, peripheral oedema, raised JVP → vascular congestion
- massive splenomegaly → myelofibrosis, haematological malignancies and some infections.

Steatorrhoea

Description

Stools that are foul-smelling, soapy, bulky and oily in appearance. Quantitatively defined as stool fat greater than 7 g of fat per day. Patients may describe the faeces as difficult to flush down the toilet and very foul-smelling.

Condition/s associated with

- Typically, malabsorption syndromes including, but not limited to:

More common

- Thyrotoxicosis
- Coeliac disease
- Inflammatory bowel disease
- Drugs (e.g. lipase inhibitors)
- Alteration of anatomy of upper GI tract post surgery
- Cirrhosis of the liver
- *Giardia lamblia* infection

Less common

- Blocked bile ducts
- Lymphatic obstruction
- Whipple's disease
- Biliary tree disease (e.g. primary sclerosing cholangitis, primary biliary cirrhosis)

Mechanism/s

An inability *to break down* (**luminal**), *absorb* (**mucosal**) *or transport* (**post-absorptive/lymphatic**) fats cause steatorrhoea. The increased fat load in the faeces causes diarrhoea by an osmotic effect.

Pancreatic insufficiency (luminal)

When more than 90% of pancreatic function is lost, the enzymes that break down fats in the intestinal lumen (e.g. pancreatic lipase) are not produced in sufficient quantities. This means fats are unable to be broken down and, therefore, cannot be absorbed.

Cirrhosis and biliary obstruction (luminal)

In cirrhosis, bile acids sufficient to break down fats are not produced by the ailing liver. Similarly, in biliary obstruction, bile is unable to be secreted into the intestine; therefore fats are not metabolised and are excreted in the stool.

Coeliac disease (mucosal)

Damage to the intestinal mucosa prevents the normal absorption of lipid molecules so more remain in the intestine and are eventually excreted.

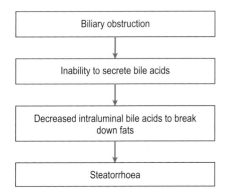

FIGURE 6.43
Mechanism of steatorrhoea

Lymphatic obstruction (post-absorptive)

In rare congenital disorders (e.g. congenital intestinal lymphangiectasia) or after trauma, the lymphatic system may become blocked or compromised. The reassembled lipids are not able to be transported away from the bowel and are excreted in the stool.[161]

6

Striae

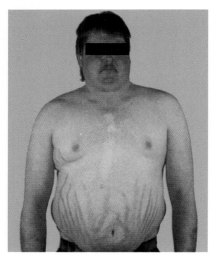

FIGURE 6.44
Abdominal striae
(Also note moon facies and central
adiposity.) This patient had Cushing's
syndrome.

*Reproduced, with permission, from Kumar V,
Abbas AK, Fausto N, Aster JC, Robbins and
Cotran Pathologic Basis of Disease,
Professional Edition, 8th edn, Philadelphia:
Saunders, 2009: Fig 24-43.*

Description
Areas of skin with irregular bluish/
purple bands or stripes. The colour of
striae may change over time and fade.

Condition/s
associated with
- Obesity and weight gain
- Cushing's syndrome

- Pregnancy
- Puberty
- Steroid therapy

Mechanism/s
The mechanism of striae is still not
clear. Several theories have been
proposed for its pathogenesis:

- Infection leading to the release of
  striatoxin that damages tissues[161]
- Mechanical effect of stretching,
  which leads to rupture of the
  connective tissue framework (e.g.
  pregnancy, obesity,
  weightlifting).[162]
- Normal growth, as seen in
  adolescence and the pubertal spurt,
  which leads to an increase in the
  size of some body regions.[163]

Cushing's syndrome
In Cushing's syndrome, there is an
increase in hormones thought to have a
catabolic effect on fibroblasts (essential to
form the collagen and elastin needed to
keep skin taut), leading to dermal and
epidermal tearing.[164]

Sign value
A relatively non-specific sign. Striae
has been shown to be prevalent in
14–56% of patients with confirmed
Cushing's syndrome.[165] Despite this
low prevalence some researchers have
suggested that the presence of red striae
in an obese patient may warrant
screening for Cushing's syndrome.[165]

Uveitis/iritis

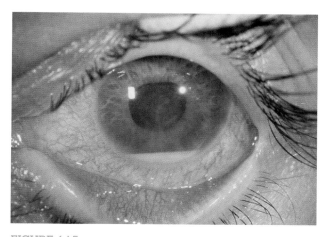

FIGURE 6.45
Severe anterior uveitis associated with HLA-B27

Reproduced, with permission, from Yanoff M, Duker JS, Ophthalmology, *3rd edn, St Louis: Mosby, 2008: Fig 7-32.*

Description

The uveal tract is comprised of the iris, ciliary body and choroids. When this area becomes inflamed and reddened, it is described as uveitis. If only the iris becomes inflamed, it is simply iritis.

Condition/s associated with

More common

- Eye trauma
- Infection

Less common

- Inflammatory bowel disease (IBD)
- Vasculitis

General mechanism/s

The pathogenesis of uveitis is poorly understood.

Trauma

- Initially, the mechanism in trauma was thought to be due to foreign antigens becoming sequestered in the uvea.
- Recently, it has been suggested that *microbiological contamination (which accompanies the trauma) and foreign antigens and necrotic products promote pro-inflammatory processes.* Inflammation then causes reddening of the eye.[166]

Infection

Molecular mimicry and non-antigen-specific stimulation of the immune response are the two mechanism/s of uveitis in infection.[166]

In molecular mimicry, self-antigens cross-react with pathogens. The immune system then mounts a response against the self-antigen,

6

thinking that it is foreign, resulting in inflammation.

It is also believed that the innate immune system can recognise microbial products such as endotoxin, ligands and RNA. If these are located in the eye, they will stimulate inflammation.

Non-infectious causes

Non-infectious uveitis is thought to be an autoimmune phenomenon, the underlying mechanism of which is a loss of immune tolerance to retinal proteins and tyrosine products.[167]

In some conditions (e.g. Behçet's syndrome), natural regulatory T cells or nTreg (which suppress autoreactive T cells) have been shown to be depleted after ocular attacks or bouts of uveitis.[167]

There is also evidence that in certain conditions the innate immune system is activated in response to antigens or non-antigen stimulus, contributing to inflammation.

Inflammatory bowel disease

No clear mechanism.

It is likely that uveitis in IBD requires a genetic predisposition and an abnormal immune response that damages the involved tissues.[168] Studies[169] have found associations between uveitis and HLA-B27, –B58 and –DRB1*0103. The triggering of the actual inflammation is still being investigated.

References

1. Sherlock S, Shaldon S. The aetiology and management of ascites in patients with hepatic cirrhosis: a review. *Gut* 1963;**4**:95–105.

2. Lieberman FL, Denison EK, Reynolds TB. The relationship of plasma volume, portal hypertension, ascites, and renal sodium retention in cirrhosis: the overflow theory of ascites formation. *Ann NY Acad Sci* 1970;**70**:202–12.

3. Schrier RW. Pathogenesis of sodium and water retention in high-output and low-output cardiac failure, nephrotic syndrome, cirrhosis, and pregnancy: first of two parts. *N Engl J Med* 1988;**319**:1065–72.

4. Schrier RW. Pathogenesis of sodium and water retention in high-output and low-output cardiac failure, nephrotic syndrome, cirrhosis, and pregnancy: second of two parts. *N Engl J Med* 1988;**319**:1127–32.

5. Chiprut RO, Knudsen KB, Liebermann TR, et al. Myxedema ascites. *Am J Digest Dis* 1976;**21**:807–8.

6. Moller S, Henriksen J, Bendtsen F. Ascites: pathogenesis and therapeutic principles. *Scand J Gastroenterol* 2009;**44**:902–11.

7. Moller S, Henriksen JH. The systemic circulation in cirrhosis. In: Gines P, Arroyo V, Rodes J, Schrier RW, editors. *Ascites and renal dysfunction in liver disease*. Malden: Blackwell; 2005. p. 139–55.

8. Wiest R. Splanchnic and systemic vasodilatation: the experimental models. *J Clinc Gastroenterol* 2007;**41**:S272–87.

9. De Castro F, Bonacini M, Walden JM, et al. Myxedema ascites: report of two cases and review of the literature. *J Clin Gastroenterol* 1991;**13**:411–14.

10. Yu AS, Hu KQ. Management of ascites. *Clin Liver Dis* 2001;**5**(2):541–68.

11. Ackerman Z. Ascites in nephrotic syndrome: incidence, patients' characteristics and complications. *J Clin Gastroenterol* 1996;**22**(1):31–4.

12. Jeong-Seon J, et al. Myxedema ascites: case report and literature review. *J Korean Med Sci* 2006;**21**:761–4.

13. Parving H-H, et al. Mechanisms of edema formation in myxedema increased protein extravasation and relatively slow lymphatic drainage. *NEJM* 1979;**301**:460–5.

14. Bonvalet JP. Myxedema with inappropriate antidiuresis and hyperaldosteronism. *Ann Med Interne* 1970;**121**:949–55.

15. Pockros PJ, Esrason KT, Nguyen C, et al. Mobilization of malignant ascites with diuretics is dependent on ascitic fluid characteristics. *Gastroenterology* 1992;**103**:1302–6.

16. Brown MW, Burk RF. Development of intractable ascites following upper abdominal surgery in patients with cirrhosis. *Am J Med* 1986;**80**:879–83.

17. Miedema EB, Bissada NK, Finkbeiner AE, et al. Chylous ascites complicating retroperitoneal lymphadenectomy for testis tumors: management with peritoneovenous shunting. *J Urol* 1978;**120**:377–82.

18. Bichler T, Dudley DA. Nephrogenous ascites. *Am J Gastroenterol* 1983;**77**:73–4.

19. Han SHB, Reynolds TB, Fong TL. Nephrogenic ascites: analysis of 16 cases and review of the literature. *Medicine* 1998;**77**:233–45.

20. Udell JA, et al. Does this patient with liver disease have cirrhosis? *JAMA* 2012;**307**(8):832–42.

21. Williams J, Simel D. Does this patient have ascites? *JAMA* 1992;**267**(19):2638–44.

22. McGee S. *Evidence Based Physical Diagnosis*. 3rd ed. St Louis: Elsevier; 2012.

23. Timmermann L, Gross J, Kircheis G, Häussinger D, Schnitzler A. Cortical origin of mini-asterixis in hepatic encephalopathy. *Neurology* 2002;**58**(2):295–8.

24. Timmermann L, Gross J, Butz M, Kircheis G, Häussinger D, Schnitzler A. Mini-asterixis in hepatic encephalopathy induced by pathologic thalamo-motor-cortical coupling. *Neurology* 2003;**61**(5):689–92.

6

25. Mendizabal M, Silva MO. Asterixis. *N Engl J Med* 2010;**363**:e14. doi: 10.1056/NEJMicm0911157.

26. Gokula RM, Khasnis A. Asterixis. *J Postgrad Med* 2003;**49**(3):272–5.

27. Hardison WG, Lee FI. Prognosis in acute liver disease of the alcoholic patient. *N Engl J Med* 1966;**275**:61–6.

28. McGee S. *Evidence Based Physical Diagnosis*. 2nd ed. St Louis: Elsevier; 2007.

29. Staniland JR, Ditchburn J, De Dombal FT. Clinical presentation of acute abdomen: study of 600 patients. *BMJ* 1972;**3**:393–8.

30. Bohner H, et al. Simple data from history and physical examination help to exclude bowel obstruction and to avoid radiographic studies in patients with acute abdominal pain. *Eur J Surg* 1998;**164**:777–84.

31. Eskandari MK, Kalff JC, Billiar TR, et al. Lipopolysaccharide activates the muscularis macrophage network and suppresses circular smooth muscle activity. *Am J Physiol* 1997;**273**:G727–34.

32. Kalff JC, Schraut WH, Simmons RL, Bauer AJ. Surgical manipulation of the gut elicits an intestinal muscularis inflammatory response resulting in paralytic ileus. *Ann Surg* 1998;**228**:625–53.

33. Schwarz NT, Simmons RL, Bauer AJ. Minor intraabdominal injury followed by low dose LPS administration act synergistically to induce ileus. *Neurogastroenterol Motil* 2000;**11**(2):288.

34. Wood J. Chapter 26: Neurogastroenterology and gastrointestinal motility. In: Rhoades RA, Tanner GA, editors. *Medical Physiology*. 2nd ed. Philadelphia: Lippincott Williams & Wilkins; 2003.

35. Kirton CA. Assessing bowel sounds. *Nursing* 1997;**27**(3):64.

36. Epstein O. The abdomen. In: Epstein O, Perkin GD, Cookson J, et al., editors. *Clinical Examination*. 4th ed. Edinburgh: Mosby Elsevier; 2008.

37. Grave B, et al. Orofacial granulomatosis – a 20 year review. *Oral Dis* 2009;**15**:46–51.

38. James J, et al. Orofacial-granulomatosis and clinical atopy. *J Oral Med* 1986;**41**(1):29–30.

39. McCartan BE, et al. Characteristics of patients with orofacial granulomatosis. *Oral Dis* 2011;**17**:696–704.

40. van der Waal RI, Schulten EA, van de Scheur MR, Wauters IM, Starink TM, van der Waal I. Cheilitis granulomatosa. *J Eur Acad Dermatol Venereol* 2001;**15**(6):519–23.

41. Palmer K. Management of haematemesis and melaena. *Postgrad Med J* 2004;**80**:399–404.

42. Courvoisier LJ. *Casuistisch-statistische Beitrage zur Pathologic and Chirurgie der Gallenweger*. Leipzig: Vogel; 1890.

43. Chung RS. Pathogenesis of the 'Courvoisier Gallbladder'. *Dig Dis Sci* 1983;**28**(l):33–8.

44. Murphy K, et al. Does Courvoisier's sign stand the test of time? *Clin Radiol* 2012;**67**:e27–30.

45. Harris S, Harris HV. Cullen's sign revisited. *Am J Med* 2008;**121**(8):682–3.

46. Dickson AP, Imrie CW. The incidence and prognosis of body wall ecchymosis in acute pancreatitis. *Surg Gynecol Obstet* 1984;**159**:343–7.

47. Requena L, Sanchez E. Erythema nodosum. *Dermatol Clin* 2008;**26**:524–38.

48. Blake T, Manahan M, Rodins K. Erythema nodosum – a review of an uncommon panniculitis. *Dermatol Online J* 2014;**20**(4). Available: https://escholarship.org/uc/item/2dt0z3mz.

49. Kunz M, Beutel S, Brocker E. Leucocyte activation in erythema nodosum. *Clin Exp Dermatol* 1999;**24**:396–401.

50. Winkelmann RK, Fostrom L. New observations in the histopathology of erythema nodosum. *J Invest Dermatol* 1975;**65**:441–6.

51. Jones JV, Cumming RH, Asplin CM. Evidence for circulating immune complexes in erythema nodosum and early sarcoidosis. *Ann NY Acad Sci* 1976;**278**:212–19.

52. Ryan TJ. Cutaneous vasculitis. In: Champion RH, Burton JL, Burns DA, et al., editors. *Textbook of Dermatology*. 6th ed. Oxford: Blackwell Scientific Publications; 1998. pp. 2155–225.

53. Farhi D, Cosnes J, Zizi N, et al. Significance of erythema nodosum and pyoderma gangrenosum in inflammatory bowel diseases. *Medicine* 2008;**87**(5):281–93.

54. Bem J, Bradley EL 3rd. Subcutaneous manifestations of severe acute pancreatitis. *Pancreas* 1998;**16**:551–5.

55. Lucas LM, Kumar KL, Smith DL. Gynecomastia. A worrisome problem for the patient. *Postgrad Med* 1987;**82**:73–81.

56. Nuttall FQ. Gynecomastia as a physical finding in normal men. *J Clin Endocrinol Metab* 1979;**48**:338–40.

57. Niewoehner CB, Nuttall FQ. Gynecomastia in a hospitalized male population. *Am J Med* 1984;**77**:633–8.

58. Olivo J, Gordon GG, Rafi F, Southren AL. Estrogen metabolism in hyperthyroidism and in cirrhosis of the liver. *Steroids* 1975;**26**:41.

59. Southren A, Olivo J, Gordon GG, et al. The conversion of androgens to estrogens in hyperthyroidism. *J Clin Endocrinol Metab* 1974;**38**(2):207–14.

60. Gordon GG, Olivo J, Rafi F, Southren AL. Conversion of androgens to estrogens in cirrhosis of the liver. *J Clin Endocrinol Metab* 1975;**40**:1018.

61. Eckman A, Dobs A. Drug induced gynecomastia. *Expert Opin Drug Saf* 2008;**7**(6): 691–702.

62. Schmitt GW, Shehadeh I, Sawin CT. Transient gynecomastia in chronic renal failure during chronic intermittent hemodialysis. *Ann Int Med* 1968;**69**:73–9.

63. Morley JE, Melmed S. Gonadal dysfunction in systemic disorders. *Metabolism* 1979;**28**: 1051–73.

64. Gabrilove JL, Nicolis GL, Mitty HA, Sohval AR. Feminising interstitial cell tumour of the testis: personal observations and a review of the literature. *Cancer* 1975;**35**: 1184–202.

65. Tseng A, Horning SJ, Freiha FS, Resser KJ, Hannigen JF, Torti FM. Gynecomastia in testicular cancer patients. *Cancer* 1985;**56**:2534–8.

66. Nydick M, Bustos J, Dale JH, Rawson RW. Gynecomastia in adolescent boys. *JAMA* 1961;**178**:109–14.

67. Bannayan GA, Hajdu SI. Gynecomastia: clinicopathological study of 351 cases. *Am J Clin Pathol* 1972;**57**:431.

68. Eroglu Y, Byrne WJ. Hepatic encephalopathy. *Emerg Med Clin North Am* 2009; 401–14.

69. Jalan R, Shawcross D, Davies N. The molecular pathogenesis of hepatic encephalopathy. *Int J Biochem Cell Biol* 2003;**35**:1175–81.

70. Cichoz-Lach H, Michalak A. Current pathogenetic aspects of hepatic encephalopathy and noncirrhotic hyperammonemic encephalopathy. *World J Gastroenterol* 2013;**19**(1): 26–34.

71. Jones A, Mullen K. Theories of the pathogenesis of hepatic encephalopathy. *Clin Liver Dis* 2012;**16**:7–26.

72. Odeh M. Pathogenesis of hepatic encephalopathy: the tumour necrosis factor-α theory. *Eur J Clin Invest* 2007;**37**:291–304.

73. Mullen K, Dasarathy S. Hepatic encephalopathy. In: Schiff ER, Sorrell MF, Maddrey WC, editors. *Schiff's Diseases of the Liver*. 8th ed. Philadelphia: Lippincott-Raven; 1999. pp. 545–81.

74. Poordad FF. Review article: the burden of hepatic encephalopathy. *Aliment Pharmacol Ther* 2006;**25**(1):3–9.

6

75. Vaquero J, Polson J, Chung C, et al. Infection and the progression of hepatic encephalopathy in acute liver failure. *Gastroenterology* 2003;**125**:755–64.

76. Bernal W, Hall C, Karvellas CJ, et al. Arterial ammonia and clinical risk factors for encephalopathy and intracranial hypertension in acute liver failure. *Hepatology* 2007; **46**(6):1844–52.

77. Mitchell S, Ayesh R, Barrett T, Smith R. Trimethylamine and foetor hepaticus. *Scand J Gastroenterol* 1999;**34**(5):524–8.

78. Sandhir S, Weber FL Jr. Portal-systemic encephalopathy. *Curr Practice Med* 1999;**2**: 103–8.

79. Talley NJ, O'Connor S. *Clinical Examination: A Systematic Guide to Physical Diagnosis*. 5th ed. Sydney: Churchill Livingstone Elsevier; 2006.

80. Sapira JD, Williamson DL. How big is the normal liver? *Arch Intern Med* 1979;**139**: 971–3.

81. Rajnish J, Amandeep S, Namita J, et al. Accuracy and reliability of palpation and percussion in detecting hepatomegaly: a rural based study. *Indian J Gastroenterol* 2004; **23**:171–4.

82. Ariel IM, Briceno M. The disparity of the size of the liver as determined by physical examination and by hepatic gamma scanning in 504 patients. *Med Ped Oncology* 1976; **2**:69–73.

83. Naylor DC. Physical examination of the liver. *JAMA* 1994;**271**(23):1859–65.

84. Lenci B. Physical examination of the liver: does it make sense in the third millennium. *Liver Int* 2013;**33**:806–7.

85. Yuan L. Mechanisms of drug induced liver injury. *Clin Liver Dis* 2013;**17**(4):507–18.

86. Aleo MD, et al. Human drug-induced liver injury severity is highly associated with dual inhibition of liver mitochondrial function and bile salt export pump. *Hepatology* 2014;**60**(3):1015–22.

87. O'Connor KW, Snodgrass PJ, Swonder JE, et al. A blinded prospective study comparing four current noninvasive approaches in the differential diagnosis of medical versus surgical jaundice. *Gastroenterology* 1983;**84**(6):1498–504.

88. Aoki T. Genetic disorders of copper transport – diagnosis and new treatment for the patients of Wilson's disease. *No to Hattatsu* 2005;**37**(2):99–109.

89. Innes JR, Strachan IM, Triger DR. Unilateral Kayser–Fleischer rings. *Br J Ophthalmol* 1986;**70**:469–70.

90. Cairns JE, Walshe JM. The Kayser–Fleischer ring. *Trans Ophthalmol Soc UK* 1970;**40**: 187–90.

91. Tso MOM, Fine BS, Thorpe HE. Kayser–Fleischer ring and associated cataract and Wilson's disease. *Am J Ophthalmol* 1975;**79**:479–88.

92. Ellis PP. Ocular deposition of copper in hypercupremia. *Am J Ophthalmol* 1969;**68**: 423–7.

93. Tauber JJ. Pseudo-Kayser–Fleischer ring of the cornea associated with non-Wilsonian liver disease. A case report and literature review. *Cornea* 1993;**12**(1):74.

94. Suvarna JC. Kayser-Fleischer ring. *J Postgrad Med* 2008;**54**:238–40.

95. Kasper D, Braunwald E, Fauci A, Hauser S, Longo D, Jameson J. *Harrison's Principles of Internal Medicine*, vol. 2. 16th ed. New York: McGraw-Hill; 2005 [Ch 339].

96. Kates SL, Harris GD, Nagle DJ. Leukonychia totalis. *J Hand Surg* 1986;**11B**(3): 465–6.

97. Grossman M, Scher RK. Leukonychia. Review and classification. *Int J Dermatol* 1990;**29**(8):535–41.

98. Tosti A, Iorizzo M, Piraccini BM, Starace M. The nail in systemic diseases. *Dermatol Clin* 2006;**24**(3):341–7.

99. Lingyong J, Bing F, Lina H, Chao W. Calcium regulating the polarity: a new pathogenesis of aphthous ulcer. *Med Hypotheses* 2009;**73**:933–4.

100. Rhee SH, Kim YB, Lee ES. Comparison of Behçet's disease and recurrent aphthous ulcer according to characteristics of gastrointestinal symptoms. *J Korean Med Sci* 2005;**20**:971–6.

101. Messady D, Younai F. Apthous ulcers. *Dermatol Ther* 2010;**23**:281–90.

102. Hietanen J, et al. Recurrent aphthous ulcers – a toll like receptor–mediated disease? *J Oral Pathol Med* 2012;**41**:158–64.

103. Jurge S, Kuffer R, Scully C, Porter SR. Mucosal disease series number VI. Recurrent aphthous stomatitis. *Oral Dis* 2006;**12**:1–21.

104. Baran R, Tosti A. Nails. In: Freedberg IM, Eisen AZ, Wolff K, et al., editors. *Dermatology in General Medicine*. 5th ed. New York: McGraw-Hill; 1999. pp. 752–68.

105. Unamuno P, Fernandez-Lopez E, Santos C. Leukonychia due to cytostatic agents. *Clin Exp Dermatol* 1992;**17**:273–4.

106. Bianchi L, Iraci S, Tomassoli M, Carrozzo AM, Ninni G. Coexistence of apparent transverse leukonychia (Muehrcke's lines type) and longitudinal melanonychia after 5-fluorouracil/adriamycin/cyclophosphamide chemotherapy. *Dermatology* 1992;**185**: 216–17.

107. Schwartz RA, Vickerman CE. Muehrcke's lines of the fingernails (abstract). *Arch Intern Med* 1979;**139**:242.

108. Adedji OA, McAdam WAF. Murphy's sign, acute cholecystitis and elderly people. *J R Coll Surg Engl* 1996;**28**:88–9.

109. Singer AJ, McCracken G, Henry MC, et al. Correlation of clinical laboratory and hepatobiliary scanning findings in patients with suspected cholecystitis. *Ann Emerg Med* 1996;**28**:267–72.

110. Mills LD, Mills T, Foster B. Association of clinical and laboratory variables with ultrasound findings in right upper quadrant abdominal pain. *South Med J* 2005;**98**: 155–61.

111. Trowbridge RL, Rutkowski NK, Shojania KG. Does this patient have acute cholecystitis? *JAMA* 2001;**289**(1):80.

112. Berry J, Malt RA. Appendicitis near its centenary. *Ann Surg* 1984;**200**:567–75.

113. Park JS, Jeong JH, Lee JI, et al. Accuracies of diagnostic methods for acute appendicitis. *Am Surg* 2013;**79**:101.

114. Nelson DW, et al. Examining the relevance of the physician's clinical assessment and the reliance on computed tomography in diagnosing acute appendicitis. *Am J Surg* 2013;**205**:452–6.

115. Perera GA. A note on palmar erythema (so-called liver palms). *JAMA* 1942;**119**(17): 1417–18.

116. Bean W. Acquired palmar erythema and cutaneous vascular 'spiders'. *Am Heart J* 1943;**25**:463–77.

117. Serrao R, Zirwas M, English JC. Palmar erythema. *Am J Clin Dermatol* 2007;**8**(6): 347–56.

118. Nadeem M, Yousof MA, Zakaria M, et al. The value of clinical signs in diagnosis of cirrhosis. *Pak J Med Sci* 2005;**21**(2):121–4.

119. Leonardo G, Arpaia MR, Del Guercio R, Coltorti M. Local deterioration of the cutaneous venoarterial reflex of the hand in cirrhosis. *Scand J Gastroenterol* 1992;**27**: 326–32.

120. Bland JH, O'Brien R, Bouchard RE. Palmar erythema and spider angiomata in rheumatoid arthritis. *Ann Intern Med* 1958;**48**(5):1026–31.

121. Saario R, Kalliomaki JL. Palmar erythema in rheumatoid arthritis. *Clin Rheumatol* 1985;**4**(4):449–51.

122. Chopra IJ, Abraham GE, Chopra U, et al. Alterations in circulating estradiol-17 in male patients with Grave's disease. *N Engl J Med* 1972;**286**(3):124–9.

123. Etter L, Myers S. Pruritus in systemic disease: mechanisms and management. *Dermatol Clin* 2002;**20**:459–72.

6

124. Kranjik M, Zylicz Z. Understanding pruritus in systemic disease. *J Pain Symptom Manage* 2001;**21**(2):151–68.

125. Kremer AE, Beuers U, Oude Elferink RPJ, Pusl T. Pathogenesis and treatment of pruritus in cholestasis. *Drugs* 2008;**68**(15):2163–87.

126. Kremer AE, et al. Lysophosphatidic acid is a potential mediator of cholestatic pruritus. *Gastroenterology* 2010;**139**:1008.

127. Fjellner B, Hägermark Ö. Pruritus in polycythaemia vera: treatment with aspirin and possibility of platelet involvement. *Acta Dermatovenerol* 1979;**59**:505–12.

128. Albert HS, Warner RR, Wasserman LR. A study of histamine in myeloproliferative disease. *Blood* 1966;**28**:796–806.

129. Murphy M, Carmichael A. Renal itch. *Clin Exp Dermatol* 2000;**25**:103–6.

130. Botero F. Pruritus as a manifestation of systemic disorders. *Cutis* 1978;**21**:873–80.

131. Caravati C, Richardson D, Wood B, et al. Cutaneous manifestations of hyperthyroidism. *South Med J* 1969;**62**:1127–30.

132. Lober CW. Should the patient with generalized pruritus be evaluated for malignancy? *J Am Acad Dermatol* 1988;**19**:350–2.

133. Wagner JM, McKinney WP, Carpenter JL. Does this patient have appendicitis? *JAMA* 1996;**276**:1589–94.

134. Ruocco E, Sangiuliano S, Gravina AG, Miranda A, Nicoletti G. Pyoderma gangrenosum: an updated review. *JEADV* 2009;**23**:1008–17.

135. Ahronowitz I, Harp J, Shinkai K. Etiology and management of pyoderma gangrenosum a comprehensive review. *Am J Clin Dermatol* 2012;**13**(3):191–211.

136. Powell FC, Schroeter AL, Su WP, et al. Pyoderma gangrenosum: a review of 86 patients. *Q J Med* 1985;**55**(217):173–86.

137. Ruiz MA, Saab S, Rickman LS. The clinical detection of scleral icterus: observations of multiple examiners. *Mil Med* 1997;**162**(8):560–3.

138. Bohl L, Merlo C, Carda C, Gómez de Ferraris ME, Carranza M. Morphometric analysis of the parotid gland affected by alcoholic sialosis. *J Oral Pathol Med* 2008;**37**(8):499–503. [Epub 2008 Feb 19].

139. Mandel L, Hamele-Bena D. Alcoholic parotid sialadenosis. *J Am Dent Assoc* 1997;**128**(10):1411–15.

140. Mandel L, Vakkas J, Saqi A. Alcoholic (beer) sialosis. *J Oral Maxillofac Surg* 2005;**63**(3):402–5.

141. Proctor GB, Shori DK. The effects of ethanol on salivary glands. In: Preedy VR, Watson PR, editors. *Alcohol and the Gastrointestinal Tract*. Boca Raton: CRC Press; 1996. pp. 111–22.

142. Ullery BW, Wachtel H, Raper SE. Sister Mary Joseph's nodule presenting as large bowel obstruction: a case report and brief review of the literature. *J Gastrointest Surg* 2013;**17**:1832–5.

143. Chen P, Middlebrook MR, Goldman SM, Sandler CM. Sister Mary Joseph nodule from metastatic renal cell carcinoma. *J Comput Assist Tomogr* 1998;**22**:756.

144. Dubreuil A, Compmartin A, Barjot P, Louvet S, Leroy D. Umbilical metastasis or Sister Mary Joseph's nodule. *Int J Dermatol* 1998;**37**:7.

145. Powell FC, Cooper AJ, Massa MC, et al. Sister Mary Joseph's nodule: a clinical and histologic study. *J Am Acad Dermatol* 1984;**10**:610–15.

146. Chalya PL, et al. Sister Mary Joseph's nodule at a university teaching hospital in northwestern Tanzania: a retrospective review of 34 cases. *World J Surg Oncol* 2013;**11**:151.

147. Falchi M, Cecchini G, Derchi LE. Umbilical metastasis as first sign of cecal carcinoma in a cirrhotic patient (Sister Mary Joseph nodule). Report of a case. *Radiol Med* 1999;**98**:84–96.

148. Khasnis A, Gokula RM. Spider nevus. *J Postgrad Med* 2002;**48**(4):307–9.

149. Li CP, Lee FY, Hwang SJ, et al. Role of substance P in the pathogenesis of spider angiomas in patients with nonalcoholic liver cirrhosis. *Am J Gastroenterol* 1999;**94**: 502–7.

150. Pirovino M, Linder R, Boss C, Kochli HP, Mahler F. Cutaneous spider nevi in liver cirrhosis: capillary microscopical and hormonal investigations. *Klin Wochenschr* 1988;**66**: 298–302.

151. Romagnuolo J, Jhangri GS, Jewall LD, Bain VG. Predicting the liver histology in chronic hepatitis C: how good is the clinician? *Am J Gastroenterol* 2001;**96**:3165–74.

152. Neiman RS, Orazi A. *Disorders of the Spleen*. 2nd ed. Philadelphia: Saunders; 1999.

153. Pozo AL, Godfrey EM, Bowles KM. Splenomegaly: investigation, diagnosis and management. *Blood Rev* 2009;**23**(3):105–11.

154. Stutte HJ, Heusermann U. Splenomegaly and red blood cell destruction: a morphometric study on the human spleen. *Virchows Arch Abt B Zellpath* 1972;**12**:1–21.

155. Pettit JE, Williams ED, Glass HI, Lewis SM, Szur L, Wicks CJ. Studies of splenic function in the myeloproliferative disorders and generalised malignant lymphomas. *Br J Haematol* 1971;**20**:575–86.

156. Lewis SM, Catovsky D, Hows JM, Ardalan B. Splenic red cell pooling in hairy cell leukaemia. *Br J Haematol* 1977;**35**:351–7.

157. Witte CL, Witte MH. Circulatory dynamics of spleen. *Lymphology* 1983;**16**:60–71.

158. Zhang B, Lewis SM. The splenomegaly of myeloproliferative and lymphoproliferative disorders: splenic cellularity and vascularity. *Eur J Haematol* 1989;**43**:63–6.

159. Grover S. Does this patient have splenomegaly? *JAMA* 1993;**270**:2218–21.

160. Chongtham DS. Accuracy of palpation and percussion maneuvers in the diagnosis of splenomegaly. *Indian J Med Sci* 1997;**51**:409–16.

161. Kogoj F. Seitrag zur atiologie und pathogenese der stria cutis distensae. *Arch Dermatol Syphilol* 1925;**149**:667.

162. Agache P, Ovide MT, Kienzler JL, et al. Mechanical factors in striae distensae. In: Moretti G, Rebora A, editors. *Striae Distensae*. Milan: Brocades; 1976. pp. 87–96.

163. Osman H, Rubeiz N, Tamim H, et al. Risk factors for the development of striae gravidarum. *Am J Obstet Gynecol* 2007;**196**:62.e1–5.

164. Stevanovic DV. Corticosteroid induced atrophy of the skin with telangiectasia: a clinical and experimental study. *Br J Dermatol* 1972;**87**:548–56.

165. Schneider HJ, et al. Discriminatory value of signs and symptoms in Cushing's syndrome revisited: what has changed in 30 years? *Clin Endocrinol (Oxf)* 2013;**78**: 152–4.

166. Gery I, Chan CC. Chapter 7.2: Mechanism/s of uveitis. In: Yanoff M, Duker JS, editors. *Ophthalmology*. 3rd ed. St Louis: Mosby; 2008.

167. Lee RWJ, Dick AD. Current concepts and future directions in the pathogenesis and treatment of non-infectious intraocular inflammation. *Eye* 2012;**26**:17–28.

168. Singleton EM, Hutson SE. Anterior uveitis, inflammatory bowel disease, and ankylosing spondylitis in a HLA-B27-positive woman. *South Med J* 2006;**99**(5):531–3.

169. Orchard TR, Chua CN, Ahmad T, Cheng H, Welsh KI, Jewell DP. Uveitis and erythema nodosum in inflammatory bowel disease: clinical features and the role of HLA genes. *Gastroenterology* 2002;**123**(3):714–18.

6

CHAPTER 7

ENDOCRINOLOGICAL SIGNS

Acanthosis nigricans (AN)

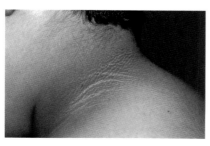

FIGURE 7.1
Acanthosis nigricans
Reproduced, with permission, from Weston WL, Lane AT, Morelli JG, Color Textbook of Pediatric Dermatology, 4th edn, London: Mosby, 2007: Fig 17-62.

Description

A grey-black, papillomatous thickening of the skin at the flexor areas. It is usually symmetrical and feels akin to velvet. Acanthosis nigricans (AN) is most common around the posterolateral neck, axillae, groin and abdominal folds.

Condition/s associated with

More common

- Type 2 diabetes
- Obesity

Less common

- Cushing's syndrome
- Acromegaly
- Malignancy
- PCOS
- Other states of hyperinsulinaemia

General mechanism/s

The mechanism is complex, with most cases occurring in the presence of *insulin resistance.* This leads to *hyperinsulinaemia,* which in turn stimulates the *proliferation of keratinocytes* (which contain melanin) *and fibroblasts.*

Detailed mechanism/s

Keratinocytes normally multiply to form a thickened keratin (a fibrous structural protein) layer of the skin. Melanin is taken up and deposited within the nuclei. Further proliferation of keratinocytes, stimulated by hyperinsulinaemia, leads to a thicker keratin layer with darker pigmentation, due to the melanin present.

Similarly, fibroblasts produce collagen. Excess proliferation leads to additional collagen deposition, which when combined with the additional keratin layer, may contribute to the distinctive 'velvet' feel of acanthosis nigricans.

Hyperinsulinaemia stimulates proliferation by:

- directly stimulating insulin-like growth factor-1 (IGF-1) receptors on fibroblasts and keratinocytes, causing proliferation
- decreasing levels of some IGF-1-binding proteins. This causes an increased level of free IGF-1 in circulation, which stimulates the IGF-1 receptor on fibroblasts and keratinocytes leading to proliferation.[1]

Other mediators may include:

- epidermal growth factor receptor (EGFR)
- fibroblast growth factor receptor (FGFR)
- androgens.

Three types of insulin resistance have been described:[2]

1 type A – dysfunction of insulin receptors
2 type B – caused by antibodies against insulin receptors
3 type C – post-insulin receptor defects.

Any of these pathways may cause hyperinsulinaemia and result in acanthosis nigricans.

There is evidence that obesity is associated with dysfunction of insulin receptors, leading to a compensatory rise in insulin levels. The high levels of insulin activate IGF-1 receptors on keratinocytes, leading to excess proliferation.

In the case of acromegaly there are two contributory pathways. Firstly, excess of growth hormone causes increased production of IGF-1, which stimulates the IGF-1 receptor on keratinocytes. Secondly, insulin resistance may be present, leading to hyperinsulinaemia and insulin–based stimulation of keratinocytes and fibroblasts.[3]

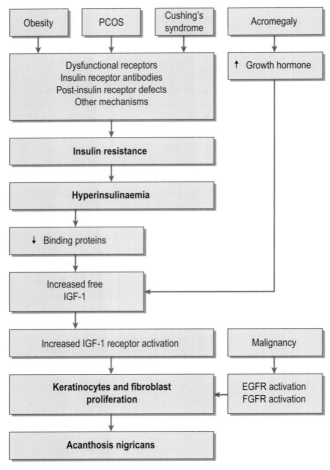

FIGURE 7.2
Mechanisms of acanthosis nigricans

Some malignancies can cause AN, such as those which produce insulin receptor antibodies (stimulating secretion of insulin) or epidermal growth factor,[4] which can also contribute to this sign.

Sign value

The exact prevalence of AN is unclear and varies with different population groups. AN has been shown to be a valuable indicator of hyperinsulinism and insulin resistance in adults and children.[5-7] Further, AN has been strongly associated with multiple risk factors for type 2 diabetes[8-10] and the development of metabolic syndrome,[5] and is strongly correlated with the level of obesity. It has also been suggested that it is an independent risk factor for the development of diabetes.[11] Research is still ongoing regarding its utility as a prognostic indicator for the development of diabetes in children. Recent research has shown that, in patients aged 8–12 years who have AN, more than 25% had altered glucose metabolism.[5] In a study of middle school students in the USA, acanthosis nigricans was present in 28% of the cohort and was associated with a 50–100% increased likelihood of dysglycemia, even after consideration of established diabetes risk factors.[12]

7

Angioid streaks

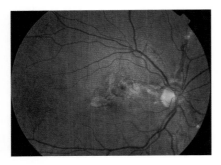

FIGURE 7.3
Angioid streaks
Reproduced, with permission, from Kanski JJ,
Clinical Diagnosis in Ophthalmology,
1st edn, Philadelphia: Mosby, 2006: Fig 13-78.

Description

Angioid streaks appear as irregular, jagged, tapering lines radiating from the peri-papillary retina into the macula and peripheral fundus.[13]

Condition/s associated with

More common

- Pseudoxanthoma elasticum
- Paget's disease of bone
- Haemoglobinopathies

Less common

- Ehlers–Danlos syndrome
- Acromegaly
- Neurofibromatosis

Mechanism/s

Angioid streaks are believed to result from *small breaks within a brittle or calcified Bruch's membrane*. The specific mechanism for the abnormality in Bruch's membrane has not been established and calcification is not significant in some disease associations. Suggested contributing factors include:

- elastic degeneration of the membrane
- iron deposition in elastic fibres from haemolysis with secondary mineralisation[14]
- nutritional impairment due to sickling, stasis and small vessel occlusion.

It is thought that lines of force from intra- and extraocular eye muscles cause cracking of the brittle membrane.

Sign value

Nearly 50% of patients with angioid streaks have an underlying disease, so further investigation is warranted. Some studies have demonstrated associations with the following disease states:

- Present in 80–87% of patients with pseudoxanthoma elasticum.[14]
- Present in 2–15% of patients with Paget's disease.[14]
- 0–6% of patients with haemoglobinopathy will develop angioid streaks.[15]
- It is not a valuable sign for acromegaly.

Atrophic testicles

Description

The mean volume of the adult testis is said to be 18.6 ± 4.8 mL.[2] Testicles with a smaller volume than this can be described as atrophic. Testicles are often measured by using an ellipsoid orchidometer – by this method most adults have a volume >15 mL per testicle.[2]

Condition/s associated with

More common

- Trauma
- Cirrhosis of the liver
- Varicocoele

Less common

- Klinefelter's syndrome
- Prader–Willi syndrome
- Hypopituitarism
- Infection
- Anabolic steroid use

Mechanism/s

70–80% of testicular volume is made up of seminiferous tubules, so any damage or dysfunction to these may cause atrophy.

Normal development of the testicles requires adequate blood flow and appropriate amounts of luteinising and follicular stimulating hormones. Testicular atrophy can be caused by *ischaemia*, *trauma*, lack of *hormonal* stimulation (*as primary or secondary hypogonadism*) or a primary *genetic* abnormality.

Klinefelter's syndrome (47XXY)

In Klinefelter's syndrome, a genetic abnormality results in an extra X chromosome. As a consequence, as gonadotropins (LH and FSH) rise during puberty, the seminiferous tubules fibrose and shrink and may become obliterated. Hence, the volume of the testicle is reduced. Why this occurs is unclear.

Prader–Willi syndrome

A genetic abnormality on chromosome 15 leads to decreased production of GnRH, which leads to low or altered FSH/LH levels and less stimulation of the testicles to produce testosterone and sperm. As a result of 'under-utilisation', the testicles atrophy.

Anabolic steroid use

Exogenous steroids cause suppression of the hypothalamic axis, in particular LH production, and therefore suppression of testosterone production, ultimately leading to atrophy.

Varicocoele

Varicocoeles cause testicular dysfunction and in some cases, atrophy, through a number of factors, including increased scrotal temperature, altered blood flow, increased oxidative stress and decreased testosterone production.

Cirrhosis of the liver

The damaged liver is unable to break down androgens, making more available for peripheral conversion to oestrogen. The liver is also unable to break down normally produced oestrogens. High levels of oestrogen cause reduced testosterone and sperm production and decreased seminiferous tubule size, resulting in testicular atrophy.

Alcohol

Alcohol causes atrophy of the testicle through direct and indirect mechanisms.

7

- Direct – alcohol and some of its breakdown products are toxic to Lleydig cells and decrease spermatogenesis.
- Indirect – alcohol can suppress hypothalamic and pituitary function. Studies have shown reduced LH levels with alcohol use.[16,17]

Sign value

Although it is a non-specific sign, if testicular atrophy is present, investigations for other underlying hormonal symptoms, signs and causes should be carried out.

Ballotable kidney

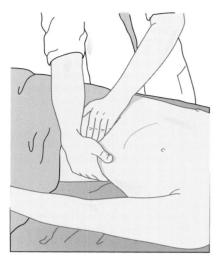

FIGURE 7.4
Balloting the kidneys

Description
With the patient supine, one hand is placed over the flank, and the other on the anterior aspect of the costophrenic angle. The hand underneath 'ballots' (from the French 'to toss') the kidney upwards. The kidney is ballotable if felt by the anterior hand during this manoeuvre.

Condition/s associated with

More common
• Polycystic kidney disease

Less common
• Renal cell carcinoma
• Wilm's tumour
• Amyloidosis
• Lymphoma
• Ureteric obstruction
  – hydronephrosis

Mechanism/s
An enlarged kidney, from whatever cause (e.g. tumour, amyloid infiltration or aberrant cystic expansion), is closer in proximity to the anterior abdominal wall and is more likely to be palpable when pushed upwards.

Unilateral causes
• Polycystic kidney disease – either asymmetrical or following unilateral nephrectomy
• Renal cell carcinoma
• Hydronephrosis
• Hypertrophy of solitary kidney
• Renal vein thrombosis
• You are feeling the liver

Bilateral causes
• Polycystic kidney disease
• Bilateral renal cell carcinoma
• Bilateral hydronephrosis
• Infiltrative disease (e.g. haematological malignancy)
• Acromegaly
• You are feeling the liver and spleen

Sign value
There is little or no evidence as to the value of the ballotable kidney. In general, they are not usually palpable, so if they are felt, investigation is needed. However, a non-ballotable kidney by no means excludes pathology in the kidneys.

7

Bruising

Description

This refers to bruising caused by minimal trauma (i.e. an insult that would not normally result in a bruise).

Condition/s associated with

- Cushing's syndrome
- Renal failure with uraemia

See 'Ecchymoses, purpura and petechiae' in Chapter 4, 'Haematological/oncological signs', for further causes.

Mechanism/s

Cushing's syndrome

Loss of subcutaneous connective tissue, due to the catabolic effects of glucocorticoids, exposes underlying vessels prone to rupture. It is a similar mechanism to that of striae.

Renal failure with uraemia

The mechanism is complex and unclear.

It is thought that uraemic blood alters *platelet function, causing ineffective activation, aggregation and attachment* to blood vessel endothelium[18] rather than thrombocytopenia.

The major elements involved in this clotting dysfunction are shown in Figure 7.5.

- *Platelet function.* Defects in secretion of pro–aggregation factors, an imbalance between platelet agonists and inhibitors, excess parathyroid hormone (which inhibits platelet aggregation) and decreased thromboxane A2 all contribute to either ineffective activation or aggregation.[18]

- *Vessel wall attachment.* Normally, platelets have certain proteins that are responsible for attachment to both other platelets and vessel endothelium – helping clot formation and stopping bleeding. Uraemic toxins cause drops in glycoprotein[19,20] GP 1b and dysfunction in other receptors ($\alpha_{IIb}\beta_3$) that are necessary for platelet attachment to blood vessel walls, as well as normal interaction with vWF and fibrinogen, thus inhibiting effective platelet clotting as well as attachment. Rises in other inhibitors, such as NO and PGI_2, are also present in uraemic patients, contributing to defective platelet clotting and thus easy bruising.[18]

- *Anaemia.* Red blood cells are integral to normal platelet activation and the clotting process. In ordinary quantities, they 'push' platelets towards the vascular endothelium and increase ADP-enhancing platelet activation. Uraemic patients are often anaemic and these regular processes are often diminished or absent, leading to prolonged bleeding time. Some studies have suggested that anaemia is the primary reason for prolonged bleeding time in uraemic patients.[21]

- *Other factors.* Drugs, including cephalosporins and aspirin, have been shown to affect platelet function.

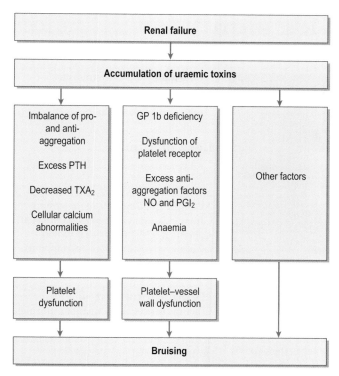

FIGURE 7.5
Mechanism of bruising in renal failure

Chvostek's sign

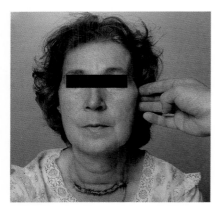

FIGURE 7.6
Clinical signs of hypocalcaemia
Chvostek's sign is elicited by tapping over
the facial nerve, producing a contraction of
the upper lip muscle.
From Besser CM, Thorner MO,
Comprehensive Clinical Endocrinology, *3rd
edn, St Louis: Mosby, 2002.*

See also 'Trousseau's sign' in this
chapter.

Description

Tapping on the patient's cheek at a
point anterior to the ear and just below
the zygomatic bone to stimulate the
facial nerve results in twitching of the
ipsilateral facial muscles. It is suggestive
of latent tetany and increased
neuromuscular excitability.

Condition/s associated with

More common

Hypocalcaemia of any cause:

- Hypoparathyroidism
- Low vitamin D

- Pseudohypoparathyroidism
- Pancreatitis
- Hyperventilation/respiratory
  alkalosis

Less common

- Hypomagnesaemia

Mechanism/s

All of the conditions associated with
Chvostek's sign cause *increased neuronal
excitability*. This means that, when the
facial nerve is stimulated (by tapping),
it is *more* likely to fire and stimulate
muscle contraction.

Hypocalcaemia

Calcium is needed to maintain normal
neuronal membrane permeability by
acting on and blocking *sodium channels*
on the neuronal membrane.[22] If
extracellular calcium is low and/or not
available, the *sodium channels are more
permeable*. As more sodium enters the
cell, the cell becomes less polarised and
is more easily stimulated to reach
action potential.

Respiratory alkalosis/ hyperventilation

Respiratory alkalosis and
hyperventilation result in less active
ionised calcium – as opposed to total
calcium. It is the decrease in *ionised
calcium* that causes increased
excitability.

Respiratory alkalosis most often
occurs due to hyperventilation. When
a patient hyperventilates, they blow off
carbon dioxide, CO_2. The alteration in
CO_2 shifts the Henderson–Hasselbach
equation in favour of CO_2 production
in order to replace losses.

The end result of this is a drop in circulating hydrogen ions (i.e. alkalosis). The amount of calcium that is free and ionised (or unbound to proteins) is heavily dependent on serum pH. When the pH is high (alkalotic), more calcium binds to proteins, making less active calcium available in the extracellular fluid for regular processes, such as blocking sodium channels and maintaining membrane stability.

Hypomagnesaemia

How hypomagnesaemia causes tetany is not well understood. It is clear that magnesium is essential *for maintaining ion channels and transporters in excitable tissues.*

Magnesium influences a number of cellular processes including:

- Na^+/ATPase activity – low magnesium decreases Na^+/ATPase activity
- blocking potassium channels on cells – low magnesium allows greater loss of potassium from cells
- low magnesium inhibits parathyroid hormone and can lead to hypocalcaemia – which can contribute to tetany
- calcium ion channel activity.

Sign value

There is little evidence for the value of examining for a positive Chvostek's sign. Nonetheless, it is accepted as a crude test for hypocalcaemia and neuronal excitability. It is suggested

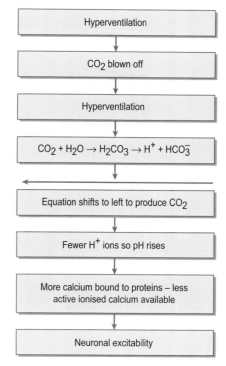

FIGURE 7.7
Mechanisms of Chvostek's sign in hyperventilation

that the specificity of the test is low, as up to 25% of patients with normal calcium levels may exhibit the sign.[23] Further, 29% of patients with hypocalcaemia did not exhibit it.[24] More recently, six out of 11 medical students and residents had the sign.[25] Its value as a sign is limited, especially given the availability of pathology testing.

7

Cushingoid habitus

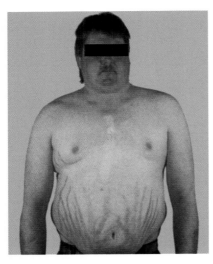

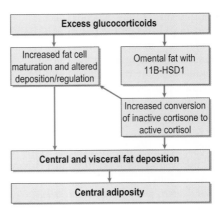

FIGURE 7.9
Mechanism of central adiposity in Cushing's syndrome

FIGURE 7.8
Central adiposity, moon facies; striae are also present

Reproduced, with permission, from Kumar V, Abbas AK, Fausto N, Aster JC, Robbins and Cotran Pathologic Basis of Disease, Professional Edition, 8th edn, Philadelphia: Saunders, 2009: Fig 24-43.

Condition/s associated with

- Cushing's syndrome

Central adiposity mechanism/s

Central adiposity represents deposition of intra-abdominal visceral fat, NOT subcutaneous fat.

Glucocorticoids regulate adipose tissue differentiation, function and distribution. They are potent activators of adipose stromal cells to become mature adipocytes or fat cells.

Studies have shown that certain types of fat, including omental (but *not* subcutaneous), are able to convert inactive cortisone to cortisol via an enzyme, 11B-HSD1.[22] Exposure to insulin and cortisol further increases the levels of this enzyme, increasing production of active cortisol.

Chronic exposure to glucocorticoids can increase omental generation of cortisol, which stimulates more adipocytes into differentiating into

Description

Central adiposity
Progressive central obesity commonly involving the face, neck, chest and abdomen. Internal structures and organs are also affected.

Moon facies
An erythematous, rounded facial appearance as a result of fat deposition in the bitemporal regions.

Buffalo hump
Fat deposition between the scapulae and behind the neck.

Supraclavicular fat pads also indicate central adiposity.

mature fat cells, causing central adiposity.[26]

Glucocorticoid modulation of a metabolic enzyme, adenosine monophosphate-activated protein kinase (AMPK), has been suggested to contribute to central obesity in Cushing's syndrome.[27] Glucocorticoids have been shown to decrease AMPK levels in visceral adipose tissues, leading to increased lipogenesis, increased lipolysis and increased lipid stores. Glucocorticoids have been shown to increase AMPK in the hypothalamus and possibly stimulate appetite,[27] both of which can contribute to central adiposity.

The cause of the characteristic preferential deposition in the face (moon facies) and posterior neck (buffalo hump) is not clear.

Sign value

- Central obesity is said to be the most common initial sign, present in over 90% of patients according to some texts,[6] while others suggest frequency between 44% and 93%[28] with a LR of 3.0 if present.

- Moon facies is seen in 67–100% of patients,[2] with sensitivity of 98% and specificity of 41% for Cushing's syndrome.[29]

- A buffalo hump may also be seen in other conditions, including AIDS and generalised obesity, and is not specific to Cushing's syndrome.

7

Diabetic amyotrophy (lumbar plexopathy)

Description

Diabetic neuropathy associated with painful muscle wasting, particularly affecting the thighs, legs and buttocks, with reduced reflexes and power in the lower limbs. Marked weight loss is common. Typically resolves after 12 or more months.

Condition/s associated with

- Diabetes

Mechanism/s

The mechanism is uncertain; possibly a form of lumbosacral plexopathy. Ischaemic injury, metabolic derangement and inflammation have all been suggested as causes.[30]

Studies have shown inflammatory infiltrates, immunoglobulin and complement depositions in the small blood vessels,[31-34] suggesting an *immune-mediated vasculitis* may be involved.

Diabetic retinopathy

Description

Diabetic retinopathy is an umbrella term used to describe a number of characteristic ophthalmological pathologies in the presence of diabetes. Some of the terms and causes overlap with hypertensive retinopathy and have common final pathways. See 'Hypertensive retinopathy' in Chapter 3, 'Cardiovascular signs'. Broadly speaking, diabetic retinopathy can be broken down into the categories shown in Table 7.1.

Condition/s associated with

- Diabetes
- Hypertensive retinopathy can also display similar changes

Mechanism/s

The mechanism behind diabetic retinopathy has not been well established.

Chronic hyperglycaemia is thought to be the main reason for diabetic retinopathy,[35] via a series of changes that ultimately lead to two key pathological states:

1 *altered vascular permeability* – disrupted or leaky vessels
2 *ischaemia of the retina* with associated *neovascularisation*.

These changes are present in the vision-threatening forms of macular oedema and proliferative diabetic retinopathy.

There are many additional processes that also contribute to the development of these two states. Table 7.2 lists some of the proposed mechanisms.

Sign value

Diabetic retinopathy is an important sign and must be monitored regularly. The greater the extent of retinopathy at diagnosis, the higher the risk of progression; this reinforces the importance of tight blood glucose

TABLE 7.1
Diabetic retinopathy

Non-proliferative retinopathy	
Cotton wool spots	Ischaemic swelling of the optic nerve layer causes a white, round or patchy appearance
Dot and blot haemorrhages	Larger red dots with distinct (dot) or indistinct (blot) borders
Hard exudates	Lipids deposited within the retina create white or yellowish deposits with a waxy appearance
Microaneurysms	Distinct round red dots
Proliferative retinopathy	
Neovascularisation arising from the optic disc or vessels	
Macular oedema	
Thickening and oedema involving the macula (may occur at any stage of proliferative or non-proliferative diabetic retinopathy)	

7

CLINICAL PEARL

TABLE 7.2
Mechanism/s and effects that contribute to diabetic retinopathy

Proposed mechanism	Effect
Endothelial dysfunction	The retinal endothelium is more than a barrier for blood vessels. It mediates vascular tone and releases factors involved in haemostasis, vessel growth and inflammation. Endothelial dysfunction may be precipitated by hyperglycaemia, insulin resistance and hyperinsulinemia, either independently or as a group.[36] Studies have shown endothelial dysfunction is present and crucial in all stages of diabetic retinopathy[1]
BMP (bone metalloproteinases)	BMPs have been shown to be upregulated in patients with diabetic retinopathy.[36] They have been implicated in the promotion of VEGF and inflammation
Chronic hyperglycaemia	Hyperglycaemia impairs retinal blood flow autoregulation[37] causing increased flow, leading to shear stress on retinal blood vessels. This leads to the release of vasoactive substances, which results in vascular leakage and *macular oedema*. It also contributes to sorbitol production – see below
Sorbitol	Sorbitol is formed in the breakdown of glucose. Excess sorbitol can cause osmotic damage to cells and alter other proteins – leading to altered vascular permeability
Advanced glycated end products	Excess glucose combines with amino acids and proteins, inactivates key enzymes, alters cellular proteins,[35] induces reactive oxygen species and contributes to inflammation. This results in vascular damage and ischaemia. Glucose may also link with collagen and cause microvascular complications
Vascular endothelial growth factor (VEGF)	VEGF is induced by retinal hypoxia[35] and can cause breakdown of the blood–retina barrier, leading to macular oedema. VEGF is also associated with the new blood vessels seen in proliferative retinopathy
Inflammation	Increased adhesion of leukocytes to capillary walls decreases blood flow and increases hypoxia. This can contribute to breakdown of the blood–retina barrier and development of macular oedema[35] A chronic inflammatory state has also been shown to release cytokines that induce insulin resistance, worsening glycemic control and endothelial dysfunction[38]
Microthrombosis	Leads to occlusion of retinal capillaries, ischaemia and capillary leakage. Leakage stimulates growth factors including VEGF
Other factors	Pigment – epithelial-derived factors
	Growth factors and IGF-1
	Reactive oxidative species

Based on Frank RN, New England Journal of Medicine *2004; 350: 48–58; with permission.*

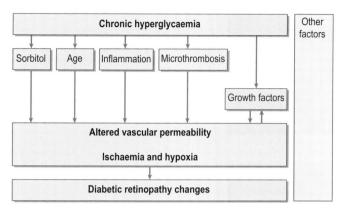

FIGURE 7.10
Simplified mechanism of diabetic retinopathy

control in a person with the condition.[39] As proliferative retinopathy and macular oedema can be treated with success in most cases, preventing blindness, both screening and detection in any setting is essential.

Changes associated with diabetic retinopathy are seen in:

- almost all patients who have had type 1 diabetes mellitus for 20 years
- 80% of patients who have had type 2 diabetes mellitus for 20 years.

After 10 years, proliferative retinopathy is seen in 50% of patients with type 1 diabetes[40] and 10% of patients with type 2 diabetes.[39]

The ability of clinicians to diagnose *sight-threatening* retinopathy has also been assessed.[28] Key findings were:

- Macular oedema is rarely ever identified by non-specialists.
- Use of an ophthalmoscope by non-specialists with the patient's pupils dilated yielded sensitivity of 53–69% and specificity of 91–96% with a PLR of 10.2.

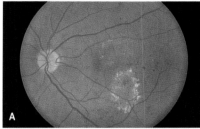

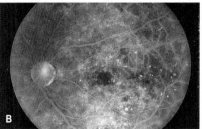

FIGURE 7.11
Non-proliferative diabetic retinopathy with microaneurysms
A Small dot haemorrhages, microaneurysms, hard (lipid) exudates, circinate retinopathy, an intraretinal microvascular abnormality and macular oedema. **B** Fluorescein angiography of the eye shown in **A**. Microaneurysms are seen as multiple dots of hyperfluorescence, but the dot haemorrhages do not fluoresce. The foveal avascular zone is minimally enlarged.

Reproduced, with permission, from Yanoff M, Duker JS, Ophthalmology, 3rd edn, London: Mosby, 2008: Fig 6-19-1.

7

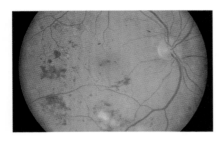

FIGURE 7.12

Non-proliferative retinopathy with some blot haemorrhages, splinter haemorrhages and cotton wool spots

Reproduced, with permission, from Yanoff M, Duker JS, Ophthalmology, 3rd edn, London: Mosby, 2008: Fig 6-19-2.

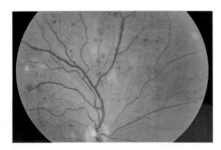

FIGURE 7.13

Severe proliferative diabetic retinopathy with cotton wool spots, intraretinal microvascular abnormalities and venous bleeding

Reproduced, with permission, from Goldman L, Ausiello D, Cecil Medicine, 23rd edn, Philadelphia: Saunders, 2007: Fig 449-16.

Frontal bossing

Description

A pathological prominence of the forehead.

Condition/s associated with

More common

- Acromegaly – commonly associated but acromegaly itself is a rare hormonal condition
- Fragile X syndrome – a common cause of intellectual disability in males, associated with a large cranium, including a prominent forehead
- Extramedullary haematopoiesis – see the description under 'Chipmunk facies' in Chapter 4, 'Haematological/oncological signs'

Less common

- Basal cell naevus syndrome
- Congenital syphilis
- Cleidocranial dysostosis
- Crouzon syndrome
- Hurler syndrome
- Pfeiffer syndrome
- Rubinstein–Taybi syndrome
- Russell–Silver syndrome

Mechanism/s

In acromegaly, excess circulating growth hormone causes overgrowth of the cranium, in particular the bones of the forehead.

7

Galactorrhoea

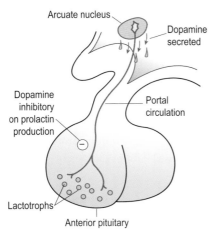

FIGURE 7.14
Dopamine–prolactin inhibition

Description

Lactation occurring in non-breastfeeding females. It is always pathological in males.

Condition/s associated with

- Hyperprolactinaemia (see Table 7.3)
- Idiopathic
  » Liver disease – rare
  » Hypogonadism

General mechanism/s

Prolactin stimulates breast and milk gland development as well as (with

TABLE 7.3
Causes of hyperprolactinaemia

Physiological	Pharmacological	Pathological
More common		
Exercise	Dopamine antagonists • atypical and typical antipsychotics • metaclopramide	Prolactin-secreting adenoma
Pregnancy	H_2 antagonists (e.g. cimetidine)	Pituitary stalk compression
Puerperium	Methyldopa	Chest wall stimulation
Sleep	Oestrogens	Hypothyroidism
Nipple stimulation	Phenothiazines	
Less common		
Seizures	Opiates	Acromegaly
Newborns	SSRIs	Hypoglycaemia
	Verapamil	Renal failure
	Tricyclic antidepressants	Multiple sclerosis
	MAOIs	Spinal cord lesions
	Oral contraceptive pill	

oxytocin) stimulating lactation in the post-partum period. Oestrogen and progesterone are also needed for breast development.

Normally, prolactin (unlike other pituitary hormones) is tonically *inhibited* by dopamine, which is persistently secreted by the arcuate nucleus, travels down the pituitary stalk (on the tuberoinfundibular axis) and stops cells in the anterior pituitary (lactotrophs) from producing prolactin (see Figure 7.14).

Therefore, hyperprolactinaemia and galactorrhoea may be caused by:

- excess prolactin secretion
- disruption of the normal inhibitory process of dopamine
- failed excretion of prolactin.

Note: Having hyperprolactinaemia does not necessarily mean galactorrhoea will follow.

Selected pharmaceutical mechanism/s

The galactorrhoea caused by commonly used antipsychotics (e.g. olanzapine, risperidone) and anti-nausea drugs (metaclopramide) is due to blocking of dopamine. This causes the inhibitory effect of dopamine on prolactin to be reduced, producing hyperprolactinaemia.

Methyldopa depletes dopamine stores and competitively inhibits L-dopa conversion to dopamine, thereby reducing dopamine and inhibition of prolactin.

Verapamil directly stimulates lactotrophs,[41] producing more prolactin.

Selective serotonin reuptake inhibitors (SSRIs) increase the level of serotonin available, which has a stimulating effect on prolactin secretion.

Prolactinomas

Prolactinomas are a type of pituitary adenoma, a neoplastic growth of pituitary lactotroph tissue. Prolactinomas secrete prolactin in large quantities and are not effectively inhibited by normal levels of dopamine.

Pituitary stalk compression

Stalk compression by any cause (e.g. craniopharyngioma, trauma, pituitary adenoma) disrupts or destroys the normal tuberoinfundibular pathway that allows dopamine to travel from the arcuate nucleus, via the portal circulation, to the lactotrophs to inhibit prolactin secretion. Hyperprolactinaemia follows.

Hypothyroidism

In hypothyroidism, thyrotrophin-releasing hormone (TRH) is elevated as a compensatory response to low thyroxine. TRH is a potent prolactin-releasing factor.

Chest wall stimulation

Chest wall stimulation due to any cause (e.g. breast surgery, mechanical trauma, herpes zoster) can produce a neurogenic reflex to stimulate the production of prolactin[2] via the suppression of dopamine.

It is thought that stimuli are passed via the intercostal nerves to the posterior column of the spinal cord, to the brainstem and then the hypothalamus where dopamine secretion is decreased.[41]

Acromegaly

Hyperprolactinaemia and galactorrhoea may result from:

- mass effect of the pituitary adenoma causing stalk compression
- excess growth hormone that has a stimulatory effect on prolactin
- in very rare cases, a pituitary adenoma may produce both growth hormone and prolactin.

7

Renal failure

Thought to be due to decreased clearance of prolactin.

Newborn galactorrhoea

High maternal oestrogen levels pass through the placenta, causing development of foetal breast tissue.

Sign value

Galactorrhoea in any male, and in a non-breastfeeding female, requires attention. It is a non-specific sign that, if present, requires a thorough history and examination to find more localising signs.

- Galactorrhoea will occur in a majority of women with prolactinomas but is much less common in males.[2]

- 13% of patients with acromegaly may display galactorrhoea[2] and 10% of patients with primary hypothyroidism will have high levels of prolactin.[42]

- Less than 10% of cases of galactorrhoea are caused by systemic diseases;[43] drug-induced, idiopathic, physiological and neoplastic (e.g. prolactinoma) causes are more common.

Goitre

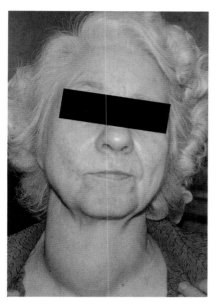

FIGURE 7.15
Large goitre
*Reproduced, with permission, from Little JW,
Falace DA, Miller CS, Rhodus NL,* Dental
Management of the Medically
Compromised Patient, *7th edn, St Louis:
Mosby, 2008: Fig 1-12.*

Description

An enlargement of the thyroid gland
causing distension in the front of the
neck,[44] which is often both visible and
palpable on examination.

Condition/s associated with

- Graves' disease
- Hashimoto's disease
- Congenital
- Adenomatous (thyroid adenoma)
- Iodine deficiency
- Toxic multinodular goitre
- Thyroid carcinoma

Mechanism/s

The mechanism of development
depends on the underlying cause.
However, the final common pathway
for most goitres will involve one or
more of the following:

- primary TSH stimulation (or
  TSHR stimulation by an antibody
  in Graves' disease) of thyroid cells
  causing cellular hyperplasia
- TSH activation of thyroid cells
  causing cellular hyperplasia
  secondary to low levels of thyroid
  hormone (can be due to problems
  with thyroid hormone production
  or secretion)
- autonomous hyperfunction.

Table 7.4 summarises the various
causes of goitres and the relevant
mechanism/s.

Sign value

Goitre (regardless of type) is found in
70–93%[45-47] of patients with
hyperthyroidism. It therefore has
relatively good sensitivity. However, up
to 30% of elderly patients have been
found to have a goitre without
underlying thyroid disease, so it is less
valuable as a specific sign[10] for
hormonal disturbance. A review of
studies looking at detection of a goitre
by physical examination found a
sensitivity of 70% and specificity of
82% with a positive likelihood ratio of
3.8. If a goitre was not palpated the
negative likelihood ratio was 0.37.[48]

A goitre with a focal nodule in the
thyroid should always be investigated
to exclude thyroid cancer, especially in
the euthyroid patient.

7

TABLE 7.4

Mechanisms of goitre development

Hyperthyroid goitres	Mechanism
Graves' disease	*Thyroid receptor antibodies stimulate TSH receptors* on the thyroid gland, causing cellular hyperplasia and thyroid gland hypertrophy Infiltration of immune cells may also contribute to enlargement
Toxic multinodular goitre	*Autonomous hyperfunction.* Goitres can change from TSH–dependent hyperplasia to autonomous hyperfunction. Oxygen reactive species and other processes may precipitate gene mutations, leading to chronic activation of the Gs and/or other proteins, which causes chronic proliferation of thyroid cells[2,49]
Single toxic adenoma	*Autonomous hyperfunction* as described above
Iodine deficiency	In iodine deficiency, the cause of the goitre is *still TSH over-stimulation and cellular hyperplasia* but it is secondary to *impaired hormone synthesis* An iodine level of less than 0.01 mg (10 µg) per day impedes thyroid hormone synthesis. In response to low levels of thyroid hormones, more TSH is produced and secreted via feedback mechanisms, causing cellular hyperplasia
Iodine excess	Excess iodine *can block the secretion of thyroid hormones, leading to low levels* and a compensatory rise in TSH, and therefore *TSH-related cellular hyperplasia*[50]
Congenital disorders	Defects in hormone synthesis result in a compensatory rise in TSH and, consequently, TSH–stimulated cellular hyperplasia
Adenomatous	Mutations in the TSH pathway, most often the TSH receptor and Gs unit, lead to excess cAMP and the production of a few 'highly growth-prone cells' that, when stimulated by TSH, grow exponentially more than the homogenous surrounding tissue, producing an adenoma[51]
Goitrogens (e.g. cabbage, turnips, lithium, sulfonylureas)	Block secretion of thyroid hormone[50]
Hypothyroid/ euthyroid goitres	
Hashimoto thyroiditis	*Secondary rises in TSH and lymphocytic invasion* are responsible for goitre formation in Hashimoto's disease In Hashimoto thyroiditis, lymphocytes are sensitised to the thyroid gland and destroy normal architecture. This destruction in the gland causes a drop in T_3 and T_4, and a compensatory rise in TSH, which causes goitre development through cellular hyperplasia. Heavy lymphocytic infiltration also adds to the formation of the goitre

Granuloma annulare

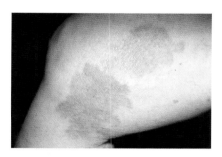

FIGURE 7.16
Granuloma annulare

Reproduced, with permission, from Rakel RE, Textbook of Family Medicine, *7th edn, Philadelphia: Saunders, 2007: Fig 44-27.*

Description

A ring of small, firm, flesh-coloured or red papules, often found on the dorsal surfaces of hands and feet.[52] A rolled border with central clearing can develop over time.

The lesion may be localised or disseminated across the body, subcutaneous or perforating (reaching deeper into subcutaneous tissue).

Condition/s associated with

More common

- Infections and immunisations (e.g. herpes zoster; hepatitis B, C)
- Trauma
- Diabetes mellitus (historically, type 1 DM)

Less common

- Drugs (e.g. gold therapy, allopurinol, amlodipine)
- Malignancy (e.g. Hodgkin's and non-Hodgkin's lymphoma, leukaemia)
- Rheumatoid arthritis

Mechanism/s

The mechanism behind the development of connective tissue surrounded by inflammatory infiltrate is not clear.

Suggested theories include:[53]

- primary degeneration of connective tissue initiating granulomatous inflammation
- lymphocyte-mediated immune reaction leading to macrocyte and cytokine activation and destruction of connective tissue
- a vasculitis or other microangiopathy causing tissue injury.

Sign value

Limited evidence exists on the true value of the sign.

Historically, granuloma annulare has been associated with type 1 diabetes. The degree of association has been reviewed multiple times, without a definite link established. Some of the evidence regarding this is as follows:

- Cases have been reported with type 2 DM.[54]
- Granuloma annulare rarely pre-dates the development of diabetes.[54]
- In one study of 100 patients with granuloma annulare, 21% of patients with the generalised disease had diabetes.[55]
- Another study found a higher incidence of diabetes in localised granuloma.[56]

7

Graves' ophthalmopathy (orbitopathy)

Description

Graves' ophthalmopathy encompasses a number of eye signs present in Graves' disease. The progression in severity of these is classified in Table 7.5.

Condition/s associated with

- Graves' disease

Mechanism/s

Much progress has been made towards identifying specific mechanisms in Graves' disease; however, a genetic predisposition is yet to be found.[57] Integral to many of the signs is *immunoreactivity against the thyrotropin receptor, including autoantibodies*, and the *dysregulation of normal orbital fibroblast function by this autoimmune immunoreactivity.*[58] Through a variety of processes this results in ocular muscle swelling and fibrosis.

In Graves' disease, anti-thyroid receptor antibodies are produced as part of the pathological process. These antibodies act on the thyroid, receptors in orbital tissue[59] and orbital fibroblasts. When stimulated by thyroid autoantibodies and cytokines, fibroblasts proliferate and produce large amounts of *hydrophilic* hyaluronan, a type of glycoaminoglycan that *attracts and sequesters fluid.*[57,58] At the same time, a *subgroup of fibroblasts differentiates into mature adipocytes.* It is these two changes (with associated lymphocytic infiltration) that result in the enlarged ocular muscles and orbital fat pads seen in patients with Graves' ophthalmopathy.

In addition to this, stimulation of *insulin-like growth factor receptor* on orbital fibroblasts results in the recruitment of more activated T cells and immune cells. This further stimulates existing fibroblasts to produce prostaglandin E2 and hyaluronan,[1] which accumulate between muscle fibres, making them larger.

Activated immune cells also produce *proadipogenic substances* that stimulate the maturation of more adipocytes, which expands tissue volume even further.

With the increase in size of soft tissue and muscles involved with the orbit (due to the combination of adipocytes, hyaluronan and inflammatory cell infiltrates), pressure within the orbital cavity is increased – ultimately affecting eye function.

TABLE 7.5

Classification of eye changes seen in Graves' disease

Class	Definition
0	No signs or symptoms
1	Only signs (e.g. lid lag, upper lid retraction, stare)
2	Soft tissue involvement: periorbital oedema, congestion/redness of the conjunctiva, chemosis
3	Proptosis
4	Extraocular involvement: upward gaze limitation, lateral gaze limitation
5	Corneal involvement: keratitis
6	Sight loss: optic nerve involvement

Based on Werner SC, Journal of Clinical Endocrinology and Metabolism *1969; 29: 782 and 1977; 44: 203; with permission.*

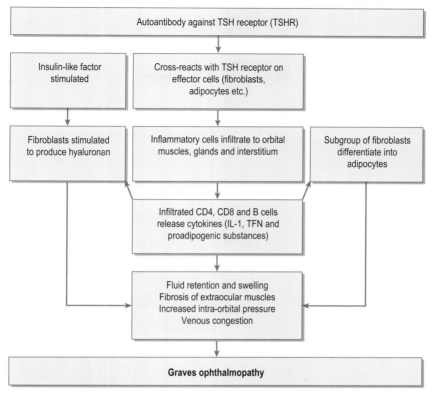

FIGURE 7.17
Simplified mechanism of Graves' ophthalmopathy

7

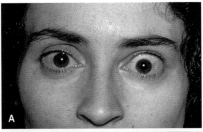
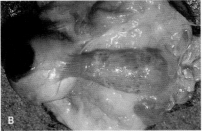
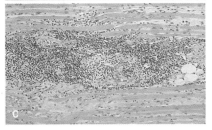

FIGURE 7.18
Graves' disease
A In Graves' disease, exophthalmos often looks more pronounced than it actually is because of the extreme lid retraction that may occur. This patient, for instance, had minimal proptosis of the left eye but marked lid retraction. **B** The orbital contents obtained post mortem from a patient with Graves' disease. Note the enormously thickened extraocular muscle. **C** Both fluid and inflammatory cells separating the muscle bundle may be seen. The inflammatory cells are predominantly lymphocytes, plus plasma cells.
Reproduced, with permission, from Yanoff M, Duker JS, Opthalmology, 3rd edn, London: Mosby, 2008: Fig 12-12-15.

Summary of mechanism/s

There are a large number of eye signs associated with Graves' disease. Some are similar and almost overlap, and underlying mechanisms can contribute to the development of multiple signs. Table 7.6 summarises a collection of signs that may be seen on physical examination.

Sign value

Graves' orbitopathy or ophthalmopathy is common. Approximately 25–50% of patients with Graves' disease suffer from one or more eye-related features,[58,60,61] 3–5% of patients suffer from severe eye disease,[62] and up to 70% of patients have subclinical eye disease identified on imaging. Many of the signs are very specific for underlying Graves' disease. Quantifying the value of each individual sign is difficult; however, there is some evidence for the following:

- Lid retraction has a sensitivity of 34% and specificity of 99% and LR of 31.5 for Graves' disease.[45]
- Lid lag has a sensitivity of 19% and specificity of 99% and LR of 17.6 for Graves' disease.[45]

TABLE 7.6
Summary of eye signs in thyrotoxicosis and mechanism/s

Name	Description	Mechanism
Upper lid retraction	The upper eyelid is noticeably retracted, exposing a larger amount of the upper sclera. It may produce Dalrymple's sign (described below)	Contributing factors include:[58] • Excess thyroid hormone causes increased sympathetic stimulation of the superior tarsal muscle (aka Mueller's muscle – a sympathetically innervated smooth muscle that assists in elevating the eyelid) • Over-activation of the levator muscle as it contracts against a tight inferior rectus muscle • Scarring between levator and surrounding tissues does not allow for normal closure
Von Graefe's sign	A dynamic sign; as the eye moves down, the eyelid does not follow smoothly but at a slower rate, exposing the superior limbus[63]	The specific mechanism has not been found. Likely a combination of factors contributing to upper lid retraction (see above)
Lagophthalmus	Inability to close the eyes	The specific mechanism is not known. Likely a combination of factors contributing to upper lid retraction (see above)
Abadie's sign	*Spasm* of the levator palpebrae when retracting the upper eyelid	The specific mechanism is not known. Likely a combination of factors contributing to upper lid retraction (see above)
Dalrymple's sign	*Widening of the palpebral fissure* Retraction of the *eyelids* on outward stare so that the palpebral opening is unusually wide	A combination of: 1) proptosis, making it more difficult for the eyelid to cover all of the eye; and 2) hypertonicity/over-activation of the levator and Mueller's muscle, resulting in upper lid retraction and hence widening of the palpebral fissure
Griffith's sign	Lower lid lag on upward gaze	Most likely over-activity/sympathetic stimulation of nerves supplying the lower eyelid, with or without mechanical restriction of muscles involved in eyelid closure
Stellwag's sign	Infrequent and incomplete blinking, often accompanied by Dalrymple's sign	Normal blinking is mainly controlled by the obicularis oculi (closing the eye) and levator palpebrae (opening the eye) with Mueller's muscle to assist in eye widening. Excess stimulation and over-activation of Mueller's muscle and levator palpebrae due to high levels of thyroid hormone causes the opening element of blinking to be accentuated

7

TABLE 7.6

Summary of eye signs in thyrotoxicosis and mechanism/s—cont'd

Name	Description	Mechanism
Diplopia	'Double vision'	Inflammation, swelling and eventually fibrosis of the extraocular muscles do not allow efficient conjugate eye movements, which normally maintain corresponding visual objects on the retinas of both eyes
Ballet's sign	Restriction of one or more extraocular muscles	Lymphocytic invasion, inflammation and oedema lead to fibrosis and scarring of the ocular muscles. Restriction of the range of movement follows
Chemosis	Swelling or oedema of the conjunctiva	Venous compression and decreased venous drainage are likely to contribute. Inflammatory cell infiltrate may also play a role. Chemosis is also seen in reactions to allergies and foreign bodies
Gaze limitation	The normal range or field of vision is decreased	Inflammation, swelling and eventually fibrosis restrict the range of movement and contraction of the extraocular muscles. The eyeball cannot move as much and vision becomes limited
Sight loss	Decreased vision	Progressive swelling of surrounding tissues raises the orbital bony cavity pressure to a point at which the optic nerve is compressed and/or damaged and vision is impaired or lost
Periorbital fullness	Swelling around the orbit	Primarily due to decreased venous drainage from venous compression in the orbital space, leading to swelling of veins and capillaries and oedema[58]
Proptosis (exophthalmos)	Forward displacement of the eyes	Swelling of the ocular muscles, fat pads and tissues within the bony cavity 'push' the eyeball forward
Riesman's sign	Bruit heard over the closed eye with a stethoscope	Increased blood flow through the orbit caused by hyperdynamic state

Hirsutism

Description

Excessive hair growth on the face and body, in particular associated with a male-type pattern of hair growth in women.

Condition/s associated with

More common

- Polycystic ovary syndrome (PCOS) – most common cause
- Cushing's disease
- Idiopathic

Less common

- Congenital adrenal hyperplasia
- Ovarian tumours
- Adrenal tumours
- Hyperthecosis – very rare

Mechanism/s

While there are a number of causes, the common pathway resulting in hirsutism is androgen excess. Androgens increase hair follicle size and hair fibre diameter and lengthen the growth phase. The most common androgens are testosterone, DHEA-S and androstenedione.

Polycystic ovary syndrome

PCOS results in *excess androgen production*. The means by which this occurs is still under investigation, as is the pathogenesis of the syndrome itself. In healthy ovaries, luteinising hormone (LH) stimulates theca cells to produce androgen precursors and androgens by means of a number of enzymes. In patients with PCOS, theca cells are simply more efficient at producing androgens.[64,65] The excess androgens, in turn, increase hair follicle size and diameter and lengthen the growth phase.

Factors contributing to the increased production of androgens in PCOS include:

- increased frequency of GnRH pulses and, therefore, LH pulses
- insulin (increased in PCOS) acts synergistically with LH to increase androgen production
- insulin also inhibits sex-binding hormone globulin, which binds to testosterone, thus increasing free or active testosterone.

Cushing's syndrome

The mechanism is not clear. Excess ACTH has been shown to cause hyperstimulation of the zona fasciculata and zona glomerulosa, producing cortisol, androgens and potentially hirsutism.[2]

Congenital adrenal hyperplasia

In the most common form of congenital adrenal hyperplasia, there is a deficiency of the enzyme 21-hydroxylase. This enzyme is essential in the pathway that produces aldosterone and mineralocorticoids from cholesterol. When it is insufficiently present, the pathway is shunted away from the production of mineralocorticoids to the production of androgens. The androgens then act on hair follicles as previously described.

Adrenal tumours

A rare cause of androgen excess.

Some tumours may secrete testosterone but most secrete DHEA, DHEA-S and cortisol, which then act on hair follicles as discussed above. In such cases, patients may be virilised

7

and may have severe hirsutism in terms of the body sites (e.g. chest and back) and area affected.

Sign value

Seen in 60–70% of Cushing's syndrome and 42–90% of Caucasian patients with PCOS.[2,66] It is not specific to any pathology, and most cases of hirsutism are idiopathic and benign. Rapid onset of new onset significant hirsutism should raise the suspicion of an androgen-secreting tumour.

Hypercarotinaemia/ carotenoderma

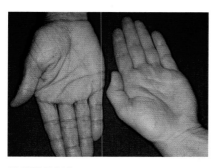

FIGURE 7.19
Carotenoderma (left) and normal hand (right)

Reproduced, with permission, from Haught JM, Patel S, English JC, Journal of American Academy of Dermatology 2007; 57(6): 1051–1058.

Description

A yellow/orange discolouration of the skin that, unlike jaundice, does not often affect the sclerae. Often found over nasolabial folds, palms and soles.

Condition/s associated with

More common

• Excess vegetable intake

Less common

• Nephrotic syndrome
• Diabetes mellitus

• Hypothyroidism
• Hyperlipidaemia
• Porphyria
• Anorexia nervosa
• Liver disease

Mechanism/s

Results from carotene deposition in the stratum corneum.[67] This can occur through three main mechanism/s:

• excess intake of foods rich in beta-carotene
• hyperlipidaemia
• failure to convert carotene into vitamin A in the liver.

Carotene is found in many fruits and vegetables. It is absorbed and eventually converted to vitamin A. Carotene absorption is enhanced by lipids (beta lipoprotein in particular), bile acids and pancreatic lipase.[67] Thus, anything that increases absorption or decreases conversion to vitamin A may lead to hypercarotinaemia and carotenoderma (see Table 7.7).

Sign value

Carotenoderma is considered harmless and finding the underlying cause is valuable only to avoid complications of that disease. For instance, carotenoderma may be the initial presentation of an eating disorder.

7

TABLE 7.7

Summary of mechanisms of carotenoderma/hypercarotinaemia

Condition	Mechanism
Nephrotic syndrome	Raised lipids in nephrotic syndrome enhance beta-carotene absorption
Diabetes	Hyperlipidaemia and impaired conversion of beta-carotene to vitamin A raises levels
Hypothyroidism	Hyperlipidaemia and impaired conversion of beta-carotene to vitamin A raises levels
Anorexia	Multiple suggested mechanism/s • Diet heavy in beta-carotene foods (e.g. carrots) • Acquired defect in metabolism of vitamin A[67] • Decreased catabolism of beta-lipoprotein[68]
Liver disease	Failure to convert beta-carotene to vitamin A

Hyperpigmentation and bronzing

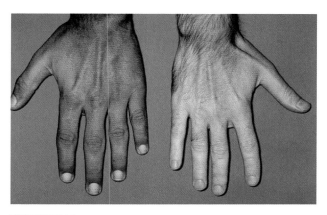

FIGURE 7.20
Hyperpigmentation seen in Addison's disease
Reproduced, with permission, from James WD, Berger TG, Elston DM (eds), Andrews' Diseases of the Skin: Clinical Dermatology, *11th edn, Philadelphia: Saunders, 2011: Fig 24-3.*

Description

Two different terms with similar presentations and classically associated with different pathologies.

Haemochromatosis sign

Hyperpigmentation of the skin, often described as a *bronzed and/or blue hue or slate grey*. Generally diffuse but the colour may be more pronounced on the face, neck and extensor surfaces.

Addison's disease sign

Diffuse 'tanning' of the body – especially sun-exposed areas, bony prominences, skin folds, scars and extensor surfaces.

Condition/s associated with

- Addison's disease (ACTH-dependent causes) – very common
- Cushing's disease (ACTH-dependent causes) – less common
- Haemochromatosis

Mechanism/s

Addison's disease

ACTH activates melanocyte-stimulating hormone (MSH) receptors on melanocytes, which secrete melanin, giving the skin a tanned appearance.

Pro-opiomelanocortin (POMC) is a precursor molecule from which two forms of MSH and ACTH are synthesised. One form of MSH, α-MSH, which is responsible for skin tanning, is identical to ACTH in the first 13 amino acids. Owing to this similarity, it is thought that ACTH is able to stimulate melanocytes to produce melanin, which is then taken up by skin cells to produce the characteristic darkening.

Cushing's disease

In Cushing's disease, where ACTH is secreted by pituitary tumours, 'tanning' may occur by stimulation of

7

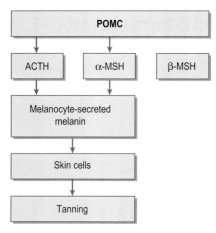

FIGURE 7.21
Mechanism of hyperpigmentation seen in Addison's disease

melanocytes in a similar process to Addison's disease.

Haemochromatosis

Two separate mechanisms contribute to hyperpigmentation in haemochromatosis. These are:

1 *haemosiderin deposition in the skin* and

2 *increased melanin production.*

Haemochromatosis is a state of excess iron absorption. The excess iron can be deposited in a variety of organs, including the skin. When deposited in the skin, haemosiderin changes the pigment, giving it a blue hue.

The change in pigmentation is also due to excess iron irritating dermal tissue and inducing inflammation, which stimulates melanin production.

Sign value

Hyperpigmentation is a valuable sign. It is seen in 92% of patients with chronic primary adrenocortical insufficiency and is one of the earliest manifestations of the condition.[2] It is also valuable in differentiating between primary and secondary adrenocortical insufficiency. In secondary adrenocortical insufficiency (caused by damage to the pituitary gland), ACTH is not secreted and, therefore, hyperpigmentation does not occur.

In Cushing's disease, it is seen less regularly (4–16% of patients),[69] so the negative predictive value is low. If present, it is valuable in localising the pathology in the hypothalamic axis. As in Addison's disease, hyperpigmentation is ACTH-dependent so, if present, the causes of Cushing's syndrome are narrowed to those that produce ACTH (see the box below).

Using hyperpigmentation to help localise the problem in endocrinological disorders

As explained above, hyperpigmentation is a sign that can help the clinician localise the cause of both Addison's disease and Cushing's syndrome. Hyperpigmentation helps identify whether excess ACTH is present or not.

Suspected Addison's + hyperpigmentation?

Cause: damage to the adrenal gland (primary adrenocortical insufficiency)
- Autoimmune – most common in developed countries
- Metastatic malignancy
- Adrenal haemorrhage
- Infectious – TB (most common in developing countries), CMV, HIV
- Adrenoleukodystrophy
- Congenital adrenal hyperplasia
- Drugs (e.g. ketoconazole)

Suspected Cushing's syndrome + hyperpigmentation?

Cause: ACTH-dependent excess cortisol
- Pituitary adenoma
- Ectopic ACTH (non-pituitary neoplasm)
- Ectopic CRH secretion (rare)

7

Hyperreflexia

Description
Used to describe exaggeration of normal reflexes.

Condition/s associated with

- Hyperthyroidism
- Upper motor neuron lesions (see Chapter 5, 'Neurological signs')

Hyperthyroid mechanism/s
The mechanism is not understood. *Increased conduction velocity and amplitude of nerves* in patients with elevated levels of thyroid hormones has been suggested. How this is brought about by thyroid hormones, directly or indirectly, is not clear. Thyroid hormones are thought to have a number of possible effects which may contribute to the development of hyperreflexia, including:

- ability to increase *the presence* of receptors for adrenaline and noradrenaline and, therefore, *responsiveness* to any circulating adrenaline or noradrenaline. It was once thought that thyroid hormone contributed to increased circulating catecholamines; however, this has been called into question since normal levels of catecholamines have been found in hyper and hypothyroid patients[70]
- decreasing inhibitory g-protein receptors and increasing stimulatory g-protein receptors[71]
- up-regulation of beta receptors in skeletal muscle[72]
- amplification of catecholamine action at post-receptor sites, with increased catecholamine sensitivity[2]
- T3-mediated increased Ca^{2+}ATPase and Na^+/K^+ ATPase pump concentration, which may affect speed and amplitude of skeletal muscle contraction on stimulation.[73]

Hyperthyroid tremor

VIDEO 7.2 ▶

Video 7.2 Access through Student Consult.

Description

A high-frequency, low-amplitude tremor seen in the hands, face and head that worsens on movement. It is a fine tremor which is supra-physiological.

Condition/s associated with

- Hyperthyroidism

Mechanism/s

The tremor is thought to be a result of increased sympathetic activity due to excess thyroid hormone inducing a boost in beta–adrenergic sensitivity and activity.[74]

Sign value

Tremor is seen in up to 69–76%[45,75] of patients with hyperthyroidism, with a specificity of 94%[45] and PLR of 11.4. If present in a patient with suspected hyperthyroidism, it is a valuable sign.

7

Hyporeflexia/delayed ankle jerks (Woltman's sign)

Description

Delayed or slower-than-normal reflexes, in particular a slow relaxation phase of the reflex.

Condition/s associated with

- Hypothyroidism
- Multiple neurological conditions (see Chapter 5, 'Neurological signs')
- Anorexia nervosa
- Advanced age
- Drugs (especially beta-blockers)
- Hypothermia

Mechanism/s

In hypothyroidism, hyporeflexia is thought to be related to decreased muscle levels of myosin ATPase, causing a delay in muscle contraction[76] and a slowing in the rate of calcium re-accumulation in the sarcoplasmic endoplasmic reticulum,[77] which is needed for normal muscle contraction and relaxation.

Thyroid hormones are intimately involved in a variety of other processes that may ultimately influence reflexes (as described in hyperreflexia in this chapter), as well as influencing myelin production, axonal transportation,[78] adrenoreceptor presence/sensitivity and ATPase channel expression. They may also influence conduction of neuronal impulses and muscle stimulation.

Sign value

There are mixed reports on the value of hyporeflexia (in particular the Achilles reflex) as a diagnostic sign for hypothyroidism and for hyperthyroidism.

The half-relaxation time in well people is approximately 240 to 320 ms.[79]

- One study found 75% of hypothyroid patients had a delayed relaxation phase, with a PPV of 72.
- Another study found 91% of patients with hyperthyroidism and 100% of hypothyroid patients had a half-relaxation time outside the normal range, suggesting a very high sensitivity of the test.[80]
- Other studies[81] found up to 35% of hyperthyroid and 12% of hypothyroid patients were in the normal range.

All of these studies were completed using specialised recording devices that would not be routinely used day-to-day. Having readily available thyroid function testing makes this sign less momentous in today's practice in isolation from other signs or symptoms.

The thyroid and the skin

Thyroid hormone is vital in the development and maintenance of normal skin function, structure and appearance, via direct influences on fibroblasts and keratinocytes, as well as impacting on oxygen consumption, protein synthesis and mitosis.[82]

It is no surprise that changes in the skin's appearance often accompany the presence of a thyroid abnormality.

Hypothyroidism

In a hypothyroid patient, the skin may be 'cold, xerotic and pale'[82] and hair condition dry, coarse, and brittle.[83] The mechanism/s which cause this are shown in Table 7.8.

The changes in hyperthyroidism include warm, moist, soft skin and are less easily explained. They are shown in Table 7.9.

TABLE 7.8
Basic mechanisms of skin changes in hypothyroidism

Coldness	Reduction in core temperature and cutaneous vasoconstriction to compensate for reduced thermogenesis and core temperature[82]
Dryness	Reduction in gland secretion Atrophic glands
Xerosis	Poor hydration of stratum corneum[82] Affected development of Odland bodies
Pale	Increased dermal mucopolysaccharides and dermal water content[82,83] alter refraction of light
Dry, brittle hair	T3 has been shown to cause proliferation of outer keratinocytes and dermal papilla cells;[84] therefore, a lack of T3 affects the structure and appearance of the hair Reduced cell proliferation has been noted in hypothyroid patients[3] Decreased sebum secretion contributes to dry appearance[82]

TABLE 7.9
Basic mechanisms for skin changes in hyperthyroidism

Warmth	Increased cutaneous blood flow
Moisture	Secondary to underlying hypermetabolic state,[82] vasodilatation owing to this and gland activity

7

Hypotension

Description

Abnormally low blood pressure, usually less than 100 mmHg systolic.

Condition/s associated with

- Addison's disease
- Hypothyroidism

Mechanism/s

Numerous causes, see Chapter 3, 'Cardiovascular signs'.

Addison's disease

Dehydration and volume loss is the primary cause of hypotension in Addison's disease.

Mineralocorticoids regulate sodium retention and potassium excretion in the urine, sweat, saliva and GI tract. A deficiency of mineralocorticoids and, to a much lesser extent, corticosteroids leads to *salt wasting* and *failure to concentrate urine*, thus producing *decreased circulatory volume, dehydration* and *hypotension*.

Deficiency of glucocorticoids (adrenaline) may also lower the basal tone of the vasculature and, therefore, resting systolic blood pressure.

Hypothyroidism

Thyroid hormones have multiple effects on the cardiovascular system (see 'Thyroid hormone and the cardiovascular system' box and Figure 7.22).

Sign value

A common sign in acute primary adrenal insufficiency – up to 88% of patients exhibit hypotension.[2] However, given the myriad causes of hypotension, its value as an isolated sign is limited. Conversely, the presence of *hyper*tension is a strong negative predictor of a diagnosis of Addison's disease.[85,86]

Thyroid hormone and the cardiovascular system

Thyroid hormones have myriad effects on different peripheral tissues and systems. The cardiovascular system is no different and understanding the role of thyroid hormones (in particular T3) will help the clinician identify and interpret signs related to either excess or deficit.

T3 enters the myocyte and binds to nuclear receptors, which then attach to thyroid response elements in target genes. These in turn bind to DNA and regulate gene expression, which has a variety of effects including:[87]

- altered myosin heavy chain expression
- expression of myofibrillin proteins that make up thick filaments
- increased Ca^{2+} ATPase (required for myocardial contraction and relaxation)
- increased beta-adrenergic receptor expression
- altered ion transporter expression.

T3 also has direct effects on peripheral vascular resistance, lowering it when present in excess and vice versa.[87] Increased tissue thermogenesis also contributes to decreased peripheral resistance.

Further, T3 can increase EPO, circulating blood volume and preload.

In summary
- increased heart rate, contractility and blood pressure in hyperthyroidism
- in general, the opposite in hypothyroidism

7

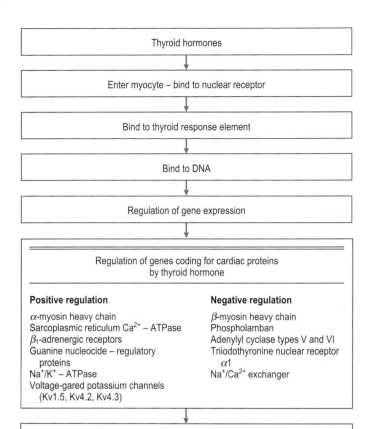

Regulation of genes coding for cardiac proteins
by thyroid hormone

Positive regulation

α-myosin heavy chain
Sarcoplasmic reticulum Ca^{2+} – ATPase
β_1-adrenergic receptors
Guanine nucleocide – regulatory
  proteins
Na^+/K^+ – ATPase
Voltage-gared potassium channels
  (Kv1.5, Kv4.2, Kv4.3)

Negative regulation

β-myosin heavy chain
Phospholamban
Adenylyl cyclase types V and VI
Triiodothyronine nuclear receptor
  $\alpha1$
Na^+/Ca^{2+} exchanger

Changes in cardiovascular function
associated with thyroid disease

Measure	Normal Range	Values in hyper-thyroidism	Values in hypo-thyroidism
Systemic vascular resistance (dyn·sec·cm^{-4})	1700	700–1200	2100–2700
Heart rate (beats/min)	72–84	88–130	60–80
Ejection fraction (%)	50–60	>60	≤60
Cardiac output (hours/min)	4.0–6.0	>7.0	<4.5
Isovolumic relaxation time (msec)	60–80	25–40	>80
Blood volume (% of normal value)	100	105.5	84.5

FIGURE 7.22

Mechanisms of action of thyroid hormones and the cardiovascular system

Adapted from Klein I, Ojamaa K. Thyroid hormone and the cardiovascular system. New England Journal of Medicine *2001; 344(7): 501–509, Tables 1 and 2.*

Macroglossia

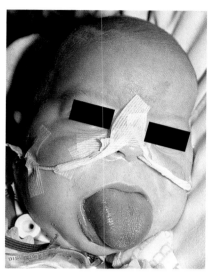

FIGURE 7.23
Macroglossia in an infant
Reproduced, with permission, from Eichenfield LF et al., Neonatal Dermatology, *2nd edn, Philadelphia: Saunders, 2008: Fig 27-11.*

Description
Enlargement of the tongue disproportionate to jaw and oral cavity size; also described as a resting tongue that protrudes beyond the teeth or alveolar ridge.

True macroglossia is defined as macroglossia with characteristic hypertrophied or hyperplastic histological findings. Pseudomacroglossia is said to be tongue enlargement seen in relation to a small mandible but also with histological abnormalities.[88]

Condition/s associated with
There is a plethora of conditions that may cause apparent or actual macroglossia. These include, but are not limited to:

More common
- Hypothyroidism – in children
- Beckwith–Wiedemann syndrome – in children
- Down syndrome
- Lymphangioma – in children
- Haemangioma – in children
- Idiopathic hyperplasia – in children
- Metabolic disorders – in children
- Amyloidosis (both primary and secondary disorders) – most common cause in adults
- Acromegaly
- Traumatic

Less common
- Triploid syndrome
- Neurofibromatosis
- Syphilis
- Tuberculosis

Mechanism/s
Most of the individual mechanisms for each condition are unclear. In brief, macroglossia can be the result of *deposition of abnormal proteins/tissue* into the tongue, *overgrowth/hypertrophy* of normal tongue tissue, and inflammation and swelling of the tongue. A summary of the causes and basic mechanisms can be seen in Table 7.10 and is discussed below.

7

TABLE 7.10
Causes of macroglossia by mechanism

Tissue overgrowth
Beckwith–Wiedemann syndrome Acromegaly Hypothyroidism
Abnormal deposition/ infiltration
Lymphatic malformations Hypothyroidism Neoplasms Storage diseases Amyloidosis Syphilis Tuberculosis
Inflammation
Hereditary angio-oedema Anaphylactic reaction Direct trauma
Relative/ pseudomacroglossia
Down syndrome

Beckwith–Wiedemann syndrome

An abnormality on chromosome 11 leading to excess growth of normal structures and tissue, including tongue tissue.

Hypothyroidism

Thought to be as a result of *myocyte hypertrophy and deposition of myxoedema*, which leads to accumulation of fluid.[89,90]

Amyloidosis

In primary or secondary amyloidosis, there is excess production of an abnormal protein (amyloid). This protein can be *deposited in the tongue tissue*, leading to macroglossia.

Acromegaly

Acromegaly is a disorder of excess growth hormone, which stimulates a further excess of insulin growth factor. It is thought that these growth factors stimulate hypertrophy of various tissues, including the tongue, leading to hypertrophy and macroglossia.

Lymphangioma

Lymphangioma is a malformation and hyperplasia of the lymphatic system. When this occurs near or results in *deposition into the tongue* tissue, macroglossia is possible.

Sign value

There are few evidence-based reviews on the value of macroglossia as a sign. However, if it is seen, it will almost always be pathological and should be investigated.

Necrobiosis lipoidica diabeticorum (NLD)

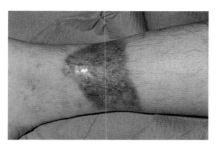

FIGURE 7.24
Necrobiosis lipoidica diabeticorum

Reproduced, with permission, from Swartz MH, Textbook of Physical Diagnosis, *6th edn, Philadelphia: Saunders, 2009: Fig 15-15.*

Description
One or more sharply demarcated yellow-brown plaques on the anterior pretibial region.

Condition/s associated with
• Diabetes

Mechanism/s
The mechanism has not been identified.

What is known is that NLD is a chronic granulomatous inflammatory disorder, with connective tissue degeneration; however, its relationship to glucose level and the pathological process have not been established.[91]
Theories include:[92]

• a form of immune-mediated vasculitis

• abnormal collagen deposition

• microangiopathy

• impaired neutrophil migration.

Sign value
One study showed a strong association with autoimmune (type 1) diabetes, in which almost two-thirds of patients with lesions had diabetes and 5–10% had glucose tolerance abnormalities.[93]

On the other hand, a more recent study showed only 11% of patients with NLD had diabetes,[17] and the prevalence of NLD in patients with diabetes was only 0.3–3.0%.[93]

In 25% of patients with the condition, the lesion develops prior to diabetes.[94]

7

Onycholysis (Plummer's nail)

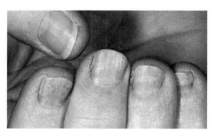

FIGURE 7.25
Onycholysis – separation of the distal nail bed

Reproduced, with permission, from Habif TP, Clinical Dermatology, *5th edn, Philadelphia: Mosby, 2009: Fig 25-29.*

Description
Separation of the nail plate from the nail bed.

Condition/s associated with

More common
- Trauma
- Infection
- Psoriasis
- Drug related

Less common
- Hyperthyroidism
- Sarcoidosis
- Connective tissue disorders

Mechanism/s
The mechanism, aside from trauma, is unclear. With respect to hyperthyroidism, one theory proposes that rapid nail growth and thyrotoxic catabolism results in nail separation.[95]

It is possible that any process which disturbs the nail bed may cause oncholysis. In psoriasis, the formation of a granular nail bed layer may precipitate the disrupted nail plate.[96]

Drug related
Most drug-related causes of nail pathology are a result of either:

- direct toxic effect on the epithelium of the nail bed with epidermolysis[97]

or

- excretion and accumulation of the drug within the nail bed and destruction of the epithelium, resulting in formation of a haemorrhagic blister (taxanes, anthracyclines, rituximab are examples).[97]

Sign value
There is little evidence of the prevalence of onycholysis in hyperthyroid patients. It can be seen in 5% of hyperthyroid patients.[95] Other signs and symptoms are likely to present themselves prior to onycholysis.

Pemberton's sign

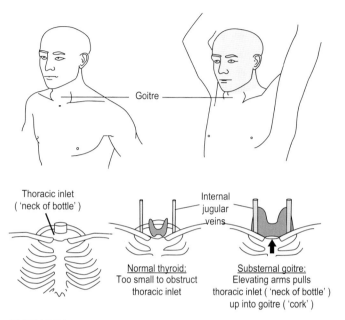

FIGURE 7.26
Pemberton's sign

Reproduced, with permission, from McGee S, Evidence-Based Physical Diagnosis, 2nd edn, Philadelphia: Saunders, 2007: Fig 22-6.

Description

The development of facial flushing, neck distension, engorged neck veins, stridor and raised JVP when a patient raises and holds the arms above the head.

Condition/s associated with

- Retrosternal/substernal goitre – common
- Tumour

Mechanism/s

A prevailing theory is that when the arms are raised, the ring of the thoracic inlet is brought upwards and gets stuck on the goitre. The goitre is said to 'cork' the thoracic inlet and, in doing so, compress the adjacent internal jugular veins. Blood backs up, causing distension of the neck veins and facial plethora. Stridor occurs with pressure on the upper airway from any mass, be it tumour or goitre.

However, recently[98] an MRI review of a patient with a positive Pemberton's sign demonstrated that there was no craniocaudal movement of the goitre relative to the thoracic inlet. It was found that the movement of the clavicles obstructing the neck vessels (in particular the right external jugular and subclavian vein confluence) caused the characteristic sign. This new case report might suggest an alternative mechanism to the 'cork' hypothesis.

7

Sign value

The frequency of Pemberton's sign is unknown in patients with substernal goitres.[28]

Periodic paralysis

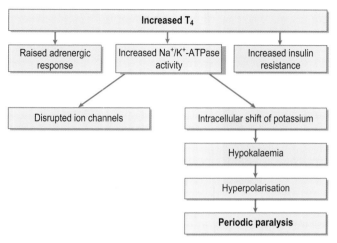

FIGURE 7.27
Mechanism of periodic paralysis in hyperthyroidism
Based on Radulescu D, Parv A, Pripon S et al., Endocrinologist *2010; 20(2): 72–74.*

Description

Periodic paralysis presents as episodes of painless muscle weakness that are often sudden and associated with preserved consciousness. Proximal muscles are affected more than distal muscles, and reflexes are decreased or absent. Periodic paralysis is associated with *hypokalaemia*.

Condition/s associated with

- Hyperthyroidism
- Congenital – most forms

Mechanism/s

Defects in muscle ion channels are the main cause of thyrotoxic periodic paralysis, although the how or why is unclear.[99] Hyperthyroidism increases the activity of the Na^+/K^+ pumps on muscle cells, producing a large and rapid shift of potassium intracellularly and leading to hyperpolarisation and absent muscle cell depolarisation.

Sign value

It is a rare event affecting between 2% and 20%, and 0.1% and 0.2%, in Asian and American populations, respectively. There is no correlation between severity of hyperthyroidism and the manifestation of paralysis.[100]

7

Plethora

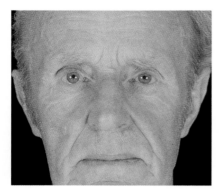

FIGURE 7.28
Polycythemia vera
Facial plethora in a 65-year-old man (Hb,
22 g/dl; WBC, 17 × 10 9/L; platelets,
550 × 10 9/L; total RCV, 65 ml/kg).

Hoffbrand V, Pettit JE, Vyas P, Color Atlas of
Clinical Hematology, *4th edn, Philadelphia:
Elsevier, 2010: Fig 15.3.*

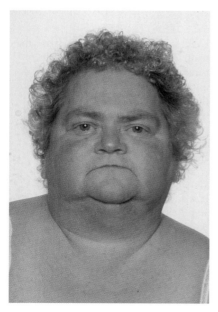

FIGURE 7.29
Moon face and plethora in Cushing's
syndrome

Lennard TWJ, Endocrine Surgery, *5th edn,
Philadelphia: Elsevier, 2014: Fig 3.14.*

Description

An excess of blood in a body part,
usually used to describe a red, florid
complexion.[44]

Condition/s associated with

More common

- Chronic alcoholism
- Cushing's disease
- Parenchymal lung disease
- Menopause
- Hyperthyroidism

Less common

- Polycythaemia
- Hypernephroma
- SVC obstruction
- Mitral stenosis
- Carcinoid syndrome

General mechanism/s

Plethora can be caused by an increased
volume of blood flow to the face, any
factor that may dilate the blood vessels
in the area or blood vessels being closer
to the skin's surface.

Cushing's disease

In Cushing's disease, excess cortisol
causes degradation and atrophy of the
epidermis and underlying connective
tissue. This leads to apparent thinning
of the skin and the appearance of facial
plethora.[2]

Carcinoid syndrome

Excess serotonin release seen in
carcinoid syndrome causes the
dilatation of skin vessels and the
appearance of plethora.

Mitral stenosis

Mitral stenosis leads to increased pressure from the left side of the heart. This leads to increased venule and venous pressure, engorging small capillaries and causing plethora.

Parenchymal lung disease

Parenchymal lung disease may cause raised pulmonary artery pressure and, therefore, pressure back to the right side of the heart and into the venous system. This, in turn, can increase venous pressure, causing engorgement of blood vessels in the face.

Sign value

Seen in 70% of patients with Cushing's syndrome,[2] plethora has only limited specificity given its many possible aetiologies.

7

Polydipsia

Description

Although strictly more a symptom than a sign, excessive drinking can be witnessed and is often linked to polyuria. Polydipsia is the chronic and excessive sensation of thirst and intake of fluid.[44] Differentiation should be made between true thirst due to dehydration-causing polyuria and that due to a dry mouth alone (due to effects of medicines or local factors).

Condition/s associated with

More common

- Diabetes mellitus
- Diabetes insipidus
- Anticholinergics

Less common

- Hypercalcaemia
- Psychogenic polydipsia
- Sjögren's syndrome
- Primary hyperaldosteronism

Mechanism/s

Often secondary to polyuria and as a response to dehydration (from diabetes mellitus, diabetes insipidus, hypercalcaemia). See 'Polyuria' in this chapter.

Sjögren's syndrome

In Sjögren's syndrome, an autoimmune disorder stops the production of saliva (and affects lacrimal glands). The result of this is a dry mouth, and the patient continues to drink in order to alleviate the discomfort.

Psychogenic polydipsia

This is thought to be a multi-factorial malfunction of the hypothalamic thirst centre, involving the chronic intake of excessive amounts of water, which reset the thirst and ADH cue points. In other words, patients need to drink more to satisfy their feeling of thirst and/or ADH is inappropriately suppressed.

Positive symptoms of schizophrenia, compulsive behaviour, stress reactions, drinking to counteract anticholinergic side effects to drugs and elevated dopamine responses stimulating the thirst centre have all been suggested as possible triggers.

Primary hyperaldosteronism

Excess aldosterone leads to hypokalaemia which, in turn, causes a decrease in aquaporin water tubules in the cortical collecting ducts of the kidneys. With less water able to be reabsorbed, more is excreted, leading to polyuria.

Polyuria

Description

Passing of a large volume of urine within a defined period of time.[44] Although not truly a sign, it is important in a number of endocrinological and renal conditions, and in some settings can be measured.

Condition/s associated with

More common

- Diabetes mellitus
- Diabetes insipidus
- Excess IV fluids
- Osmotic mannitol infusion, radiocontrast media, high-protein tube feeds
- Drugs (e.g. diuretics, lithium)
- Caffeine
- Post-obstructive diuresis

Less common

- Hypokalaemia
- Hypercalcaemia
- Psychogenic polydipsia (e.g. schizophrenia)
- Excess IV fluids
- Cushing's syndrome
- Primary hyperaldosteronism
- Inability to concentrate urine: sickle cell trait or disease, chronic pyelonephritis, amyloidosis

Mechanism/s

Polyuria usually develops via two basic mechanisms: osmotic load and excretion of free water.

1 In some conditions, there is a high 'osmotic load' of the serum being filtered through the kidney due to the *excretion of non-absorbable solutes (e.g. glucose)*. This leads to an *osmotic diuresis*. Put simply, this means large quantities of bigger solutes in the renal tubules of the kidney hold water 'in', rather than allowing it to be reabsorbed. In addition, the concentration gradient in the proximal tubules is altered, affecting sodium reabsorption and urine concentration.

2 The second main pathway is an *inappropriate excretion of free water*,[101] which is usually due to abnormalities in vasopressin production or in response to vasopressin plus an inability to concentrate urine.

Diabetes mellitus

Polyuria in diabetes mellitus is due to *osmotic diuresis* from excretion of excess glucose. The high levels of glucose present exceed the kidney's ability for reabsorption and it is 'lost' in the urine. Water is drawn out by osmosis in the tubule of the kidney. Polyuria in this setting indicates symptomatic hyperglycaemia.

Diabetes insipidus

Diabetes insipidus (DI) can be categorised as either central or peripheral. Nephrogenic DI can be further classified as either congenital or acquired. The basic mechanisms are shown in Table 7.11.

Post-obstructive diuresis

Seen in bilateral urinary tract obstruction, the mechanism behind post-obstructive diuresis/polyuria is complex and is conceptualised in Figure 7.30.

7

CLINICAL PEARL

TABLE 7.11
Mechanisms of diabetes insipidus (DI)

	Abnormality	Mechanism
Central DI	Idiopathic or secondary to any disorder that leads to damage to the vasopressin (ADH)-secreting neurons in the posterior pituitary	Inadequate excretion of ADH from the pituitary → inadequate activation of the V2 receptors and aquaporins → water is not reabsorbed and is lost in urine
Congenital nephrogenic DI	Mutation of V2 receptor on distal tubule of the kidney	V2 receptor is not responsive to ADH stimulation → failed activation of aquaporin channels → water not appropriately retained and so lost in urine
	Mutation of aquaporin water channel	Mutation of aquaporin water channel does not allow for adequate reuptake of water when the V2 receptor is stimulated by ADH. The water is excreted in urine
Acquired nephrogenic DI	Hypokalaemia	Hypokalaemia leads to decreased expression of aquaporin 2 channels → decreased water uptake and therefore increased diuresis
	Hypercalcaemia	Hypercalcaemia leads to decreased expression of aquaporin 2 channels → decreased water uptake and therefore increased diuresis

Glucose in the urine and drugs for glycaemic control

Knowing the mechanism of reabsorption of glucose in the kidney and the mechanism of polyuria in diabetes helps to understand some of the new therapeutic agents targeting glucose control.

A new class of drugs has been developed to further enhance loss of glucose in the urine to try to improve glycaemic control. The SGLT2 inhibitors inhibit the key sodium–glucose transporter which reabsorbs glucose from the tubules back into the blood. By blocking these, less glucose is reabsorbed; more is lost in the urine and hopefully blood sugar levels fall. Trials have shown reasonable success, with an obvious side effect of mild increase in polyuria.

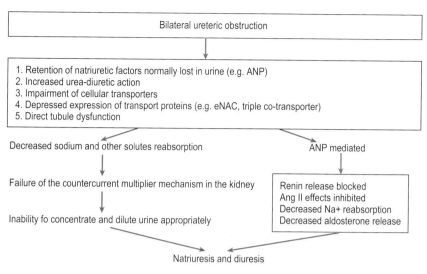

FIGURE 7.30
Mechanisms involved in post-obstructive diuresis

Some research has shown that natriuretic factors[102] such as ANP, which are normally lost in the urine, are retained during the obstructive phase and therefore still exert their effect after the obstruction is relieved. ANP has several actions that facilitate diuresis including blocking the release of renin at the macula densa, blocking the effects of angiotensin 2, and effecting sodium reabsorption and aldosterone release.[103]

Urinary tract obstruction has also been shown to directly damage tubular function of the kidney and alter the expression of transporter proteins required for the normal handling of solutes and electrolytes. The net result is failure of the countercurrent multiplier mechanism of the kidney, failure of sodium reabsorption and, ultimately, ineffective urinary dilution and concentration. All of these processes contribute to salt and water wasting, resulting in a post-obstructive diuresis.

Lithium

Lithium has a number of effects on the kidney. The relationship between lithium and polyuria is hypothesised to be impairment of the stimulatory effect of ADH on adenylate cyclase[104] which, when present, normally leads to the production of water channels in the cortical collecting duct.

Other influences lithium may have include:

- partial inhibition of aldosterone's capacity to increase eNAC expression and salt reabsorption; as a consequence, salt is lost in the urine and water follows it out[105]

- potentially inhibiting sodium reabsorption in the cortical collecting channel. Decreased sodium reabsorption leads to salt wasting and water follows sodium out in the urine.[106]

7

Polyuria: Cushing's syndrome

Excess glucocorticoids have been shown to inhibit osmosis–stimulated ADH secretion as well as directly enhancing free water clearance,[44] thus producing polyuria.

Hyperglycaemia causing osmotic diuresis is rarely the cause of polyuria in Cushing's syndrome.

Psychogenic polyuria mechanism/s

Seen in concert with psychogenic polydipsia; see 'Psychogenic polydipsia mechanism/s' under 'Polydipsia' in this chapter.

Pre-tibial myxoedema (thyroid dermopathy)

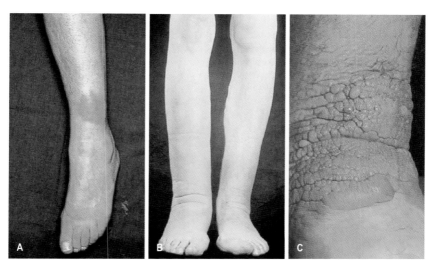

FIGURE 7.31
Thyroid dermopathy
A Localised plaque on the outer aspect of the skin. **B** Sheet-like involvement of the lower leg, with coarse skin, thickened hair and non-pitting oedema. **C** Horny form over shin and dorsum of the foot.

In Ferri F, Ferri's Color Atlas and Text of Clinical Medicine, *Philadelphia: Elsevier, 2009: Fig 268-3. (From Besser CM, Thorner MO,* Comprehensive Clinical Endocrinology, *3rd edn, St Louis: Mosby, 2002.)*

Description
Thickening of the skin limited to the pre-tibial area. However, as the thickening may occur in other parts of the body, the term 'thyroid dermopathy' is more correct.

Condition/s associated with
- Graves' disease

Mechanism/s
The mechanism behind pre-tibial myxoedema is similar to (or an extension of) that seen in Graves' ophthalmopathy. *Immunological, cellular and mechanical factors contribute* to the production and localisation of glycoaminoglycans and the sequestration of fluid to produce the characteristic skin changes.

In Graves' disease, lymphocytes infiltrate the dermal tissues around the pre-tibia.[107] It is also hypothesised that there is an over-expression of TSH receptors at certain sites, including the pre-tibial area. These receptors are stimulated by antibodies produced by local immune cells, which lead to fibroblast secretion of glycoaminoglycans and the sequestration of fluid. Similar to Graves' orbitopathy, TSH receptor antibodies stimulate an immunological

7

response which also causes the activation and proliferation of fibroblasts, and subsequent mucin production.[57]

Mechanical forces play a role in the localisation of the skin changes.[108-110] Dependent oedema, produced by reduced lymphatic return, increases the pooling of disease-related cytokines and chemokines and other factors that increase the effect[111] in the immediate area.

Sign value

Pre-tibial myxoedema is a rare sign clinically and is almost always preceded by the more common eye signs of Graves' disease. It is seen in 0.5–4.3% of patients with a history of thyrotoxicosis and in up to 13% of patients with Graves' ophthalmopathy.[57,107,112] Interestingly, forearm changes of so-called pre-tibial myxoedema are commonly present in cases of clinically definite Graves' disease, and can be detected by ultrasound as skin thickening. If pre-tibial myxoedema is found, look for thyroid acropachy (clubbing) as it will be present in 20% of cases.[57]

Prognathism

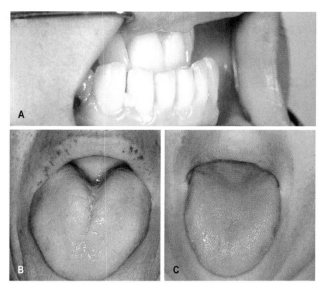

FIGURE 7.32
Prognathism (**A**) and macroglossia (**B**) in acromegaly
These are shown with a tongue of normal size (**C**) for comparison.
In Ferri F, Ferri's Color Atlas and Text of Clinical Medicine, *Philadelphia: Elsevier, 2009: Fig 264-8. (From Besser CM, Thorner MO,* Comprehensive Clinical Endocrinology, *3rd edn, St Louis: Mosby, 2002.)*

Description

Abnormal protrusion of one or both jaws, particularly the mandible, relative to the broader facial skeleton.[44]

Condition/s associated with

- Congenital defects
- Acromegaly

Mechanism/s

The final mechanism of prognathism in acromegaly is likely related to the excess production of *growth hormone and insulin-like growth factor-1, causing excess bone growth in the jaw.*

Acromegalic patients have an *overproduction of growth hormone* (GH) from the anterior pituitary gland. GH has effects on body tissues, both directly and indirectly, through the stimulation of insulin-like growth factor-1 (IGF-1). IGF-1, in particular, has growth-promoting effects on a variety of body systems including bone, resulting in excess growth in a variety of locations including the mandible.

Sign value

Prognathism virtually never occurs in acromegaly in isolation, so its value as a diagnostic sign is limited. Conversely, if no other signs associated with acromegaly are present, congenital abnormality is the most likely cause.

7

Proximal myopathy

Description

Weakness of the proximal muscles of the girdle including the quadriceps and biceps. Can be easily demonstrated by asking the patient to rise from a seated position and/or to pretend to be brushing their hair or hanging out washing.

Condition/s associated with

Many potential causes including, but not limited to:

More common

- Hyperthyroidism
- Hypothyroidism
- Cushing's syndrome
- Peripheral neuropathies
- Polymyalgia rheumatica

Less common

- Addison's disease
- Hyperparathyroidism
- Sarcoidosis
- Coeliac disease
- Polymyositis
- Dermatomyositis
- Genetic muscular dystrophies

Mechanism/s

Hyperthyroid

The mechanism is uncertain. Possible causes include:[113-116]

- increased cellular metabolism and energy utilisation
- increased catabolism and protein degradation
- inefficient energy utilisation

- disturbance of the function of muscle fibres due to increased mitochondrial respiration
- accelerated protein degradation and lipid oxidation
- enhanced beta-adrenergic sensitivity
- insulin resistance.

It is thought that an accelerated metabolism combined with insulin resistance results in muscle glycogen depletion, reductions in ATP and creatine phosphate concentrations. These changes and a reduction in muscle creatinine contribute to weakness.[117]

Hypothyroidism

Lack of thyroid hormone slows normal metabolic function, including protein-turnover-impaired carbohydrate metabolism.[118,119] Hypothyroidism also reduces muscle enzyme activity, glucose uptake, mitochrondrial oxidation capacity and muscle glycogenolysis. All of these elements are causal in muscle cells neither possessing nor utilising energy as efficiently, resulting in weakness.

Hyperparathyroidism

The mechanism is unclear.

It is known that PTH does impact on skeletal muscle but given that it alters calcium, phosphate and vitamin D, it is difficult to pinpoint an exact cause of the proximal muscle weakness.[112] Potential theories are shown in Table 7.12.

Cushing's syndrome

The catabolic effects of glucocorticoids *break down proteins in the muscle fibres*, causing weakness. Additional factors

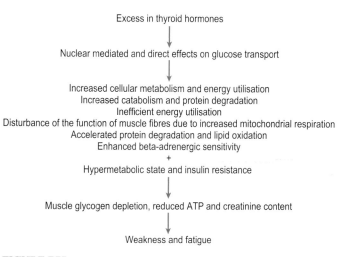

Excess in thyroid hormones

↓

Nuclear mediated and direct effects on glucose transport

↓

Increased cellular metabolism and energy utilisation
Increased catabolism and protein degradation
Inefficient energy utilisation
Disturbance of the function of muscle fibres due to increased mitochondrial respiration
Accelerated protein degradation and lipid oxidation
Enhanced beta-adrenergic sensitivity
+
Hypermetabolic state and insulin resistance

↓

Muscle glycogen depletion, reduced ATP and creatinine content

↓

Weakness and fatigue

FIGURE 7.33
Mechanisms of proximal myopathy in hyperthyroidism

TABLE 7.12
Possible causes of proximal muscle weakness in hyperparathyroidism

PTH-mediated changes	PTH-stimulated protein breakdown of skeletal muscle, which may be mediated by:[117] <ul><li>PTH activating cAMP and inducing an increase in mitochrondial calcium permeability which then activates intracellular proteases[120]</li><li>PTH, also via activation of cAMP dependent phosphorylation, may reduce the sensitivity of calcium to troponin and the activity of myofibrillar proteins needed for effective functioning.[117]</li></ul>
Vitamin D	Impaired activation of vitamin D to the active form of $1,25(OH_2)D_3$ results in an inability of the sarcoplasmic reticulum to maintain appropriate levels of calcium, which affects myofibrillar functioning.[117]

induced by excess steroids include hypokalaemia, depressed protein synthesis, decreased sarcolemmal activity and increased myosin degeneration.[117] Patients with Cushing's syndrome often have low levels of physical activity which may also play a role.

In some cases *hypokalaemia*, from excess mineralocorticoids causing potassium excretion via the kidney, may exacerbate the situation. This is due to an imbalance in the electrochemical gradient between the intracellular and extracellular spaces. Simply put, a potassium gradient is required between the two spaces in order for cells to effectively 'fire' (i.e. depolarise and repolarise). Decreasing the potassium outside a cell causes *hyper-polarisation of the cell*, making it *harder* for the cells (in this case proximal skeletal muscle fibres) to fire.

In patients with secondary Cushing's syndrome, excess ACTH may also contribute to weakness[117] and impair muscular transmission via decreasing the endpoint potential.[117]

7

Addison's disease

Normal levels of steroid hormones are required for the function of a variety of systems which impact muscle power. Adrenal insufficiency has been shown to:

- impair muscle carbohydrate metabolism
- cause electrolyte imbalances – e.g. hyperkalaemia
- alter muscle blood flow and even adrenergic sensitivity.[117]

These issues can all contribute to the development of proximal myopathy.

Hyperkalaemia, from a loss of mineralocorticoid activity (which normally facilitates renal wasting of potassium) is coupled with a depletion of muscle intracellular potassium and depressed Na^+/K^+ ATPase activity, further affecting muscle function.[117]

Sign value

Seen in 60–80% of patients with hyperthyroidism, but also seen in numerous other endocrinological and other disorders. It is not common for proximal myopathy to be an initial presentation of hyperthyroidism.

In hypothyroidism, it is seen in 30–80% of patients and, therefore, has only moderate sensitivity and low specificity.

Skin tags (acrochordon)

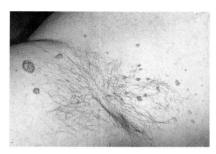

FIGURE 7.34
Skin tags

Reproduced, with permission, from Habif TP,
Clinical Dermatology, *5th edn, Philadelphia:*
Mosby, 2009: Fig 20-17.

Description

Pedunculated papules or nodules that
are most commonly located on the
eyelids, neck and axillae.[121]

Condition/s associated with

- Normal variant
- Diabetes
- Acromegaly

Mechanism/s

The mechanism is unclear.
Theories have included:

- Frequent irritation
- Normal ageing process
- Hormone levels (e.g. high levels of
growth hormone in acromegaly).

Sign value

Of limited value, as skin tags are very
common in the general population. It
has been claimed that the incidence is
greater in diabetic, obese patients as
well as those with acromegaly.
Interestingly, recent studies have shown
an association between the presence of
skin tags and insulin resistance.[122,123] In
addition, one small study has suggested
that skin tags are increased in patients
with metabolic derangements and
may present as a risk marker of
cardiovascular disease and
atherosclerosis.[124]

7

Steroid acne

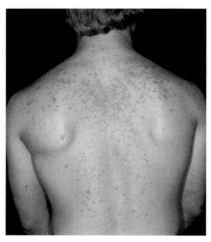

FIGURE 7.35
Steroid-induced acne

Reproduced, with permission, from Habif TP, Clinical Dermatology, 5th edn, Philadelphia: Mosby, 2009: Fig 7-33.

Description

Steroid acne differs from normal acne vulgaris in that it is of uniform size and symmetric distribution and usually present on the neck, chest and back. It is typically flesh or pink-to-red coloured, with dome-shaped papules and pustules.

Condition/s associated with

More common
- Endogenous and exogenous androgen sources
- Diabetes
- Drug therapy

Less common
- Hodgkin's disease
- HIV infection

Mechanism/s

Steroid excess in Cushing's syndrome may exacerbate existing acne; however, it may more often be an acne-like condition called malassezia (pityrosporum) folliculitis.[125] This is characterised by an alteration in normal skin conditions, including changes to immunity, sebum production and the growth of normal skin flora.[126] The end result is plugging of the hair follicle and an environment that allows a particular yeast (*Malassezia furfur*) to proliferate.

In Cushing's disease, it is possible that alterations of immunity caused by corticosteroid excess will allow fungal proliferation.

High levels of androgens and sebum production may also contribute.

Trousseau's sign

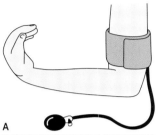

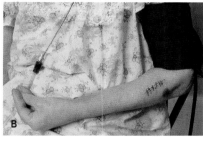

A

B

FIGURE 7.36
Trousseau's sign
A Trousseau's sign is produced when a sphygmomanometer cuff is inflated to above systolic pressure for up to 3 minutes. **B** This patient had four-gland hyperplasia and developed transient postoperative hypocalcaemia. All four glands were removed, and pieces from one were autotransplanted into the forearm. The site of the transplantation can be seen clearly.

B From Besser CM, Thorner MO, Comprehensive Clinical Endocrinology, *3rd edn, St Louis: Mosby, 2002.*

VIDEO 7.4 ▶

Video 7.4 Access through Student Consult.

Description
After inflating a cuff above the patient's systolic blood pressure and leaving it inflated for 3 minutes, muscular contraction – including flexion of the wrist and MCP joints, hyperextension of the fingers and flexion of the thumb on the palm – occurs (see Figure 7.36).

Condition/s associated with
More common
- Hypocalcaemia of any cause:
  » Hypoparathyroidism
  » Low vitamin D
  » Pseudohypoparathyroidism
  » Pancreatitis
- Hyperventilation/respiratory alkalosis

Less common
- Hypomagnesaemia

Mechanism/s
See 'Chvostek's sign' in this chapter for an explanation of the increased neuronal excitation or tetany seen in conditions associated with the sign. By inducing ischaemia in the arm through the cuff, neuronal excitation (and hence muscular contraction) is exaggerated, producing the characteristic sign.

Sign value
1–4% of normal patients will have a positive Trousseau's sign; however, it is more specific than Chvostek's sign for latent tetany and hypocalcaemia, said to be present in 94% of patients with hypocalcemia and in only 1% of persons with normal calcium levels.[127]

7

Uraemic frost

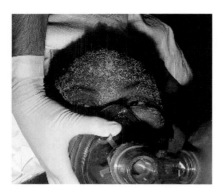

FIGURE 7.37
Uraemic frost

Reproduced, with permission, from Marx JA, Hockberger RS, Walls RM et al. (eds), Rosen's Emergency Medicine, 7th edn, Philadelphia: Mosby, 2009: Fig 95-4.

Description
Fine white or yellowish frosting on the skin.

Condition/s associated with
• Renal failure

Mechanism/s
In untreated renal failure, blood urea levels rise to such an extent that the urea content in sweat also mounts. Normal evaporation of sweat plus high urea concentration results in crystallisation and deposition of the urea on the skin.

Sign value
With early dialysis, uraemic frost is a very rare occurrence in countries with adequate medical care available.

Vitiligo

Description

A chronic disorder of the skin, usually progressive, consisting of depigmented white patches which are often surrounded by a hyperpigmented border.[44]

Condition/s associated with

Autoimmune diseases including:

- Graves' disease
- Addison's disease
- Hashimoto's thyroiditis
- Pernicious anaemia
- SLE
- Inflammatory bowel disease

Mechanism/s

The mechanism is not yet fully understood.

Destruction of dermal melanocytes occurs but how or why this happens is not definitely known. The many theories include autoimmune, cytotoxic, biochemical, oxidant–antioxidant, neural and viral mechanisms. Several studies also point to a significant role of genetic susceptibility to vitiligo.[128]

Research has demonstrated circulating antibodies to melanocytes in patients with vitiligo, and the levels of antibodies have been correlated with disease severity.[129] Similarly, auto-reactive cytologic T cells and certain inflammatory cytokines are seen at increased levels in patients with vitiligo and may play a role in their destruction.[130]

Other factors present with vitiligo that might lead to destruction of melanocytes include: oxidative stress,[128,130,131] neural disruption and increased levels of CMV and other viruses.[37]

Sign value

Seen in 20% of patients with primary adrenocortical insufficiency (Addison's disease).[132] It also clusters with pernicious anaemia.

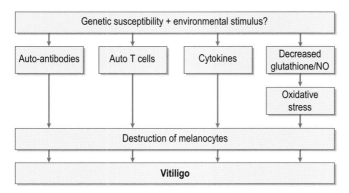

FIGURE 7.38
Mechanism of vitiligo

7

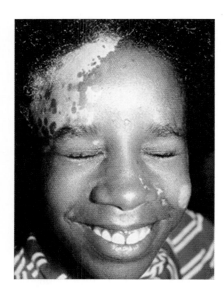

FIGURE 7.39
Vitiligo

Reproduced, with permission, from Anderson DM, Dorland's Dictionary, 30th edn, Philadelphia: Elsevier, 2003.

Webbed neck (pterygium colli deformity)

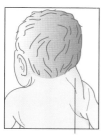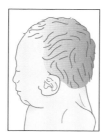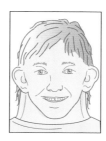

Webbed neck

FIGURE 7.40
Webbed neck

Description

An accentuated skin fold that runs along the side of the neck to the shoulders.

Condition/s associated with

- Turner syndrome
- Noonan syndrome

Mechanism/s

The mechanism is unclear. In Turner syndrome, there is an absence of all or part of one sex chromosome; it is not known how this leads to a webbed neck.

In Noonan syndrome, nearly 50% of patients have a genetic mutation of a gene on chromosome 12 that modulates cellular differentiation and proliferation.[6]

Sign value

An uncommon sign and, if truly present, a webbed neck is almost always pathological.

In Turner syndrome, up to 40% of females will have a webbed neck.[6]

7

References

1. Nam SY, Lee EJ, Kim KR, et al. Effect of obesity on total and free insulin-like growth factor (IGF)-1, and their relationship to IGF-binding protein (BP)-1, IGFBP-2, IGFBP-3, insulin, and growth hormone. *Int J Obes Relat Metab Disord* 1997;**21**:355–9.

2. Gardner DG, Shoback D. *Greenspan's Basic and Clinical Endocrinology*. 8th ed. New York: McGraw-Hill; 2007.

3. Centurion SA, Schwartz RA. Cutaneous signs of acromegaly. *Int J Dermatol* 2002; **41**(10):631–4.

4. Ellis DL, Kafka SP, Chow JC, et al. Melanoma, growth factors, acanthosis nigricans, the sign of Leser–Trelat, and multiple acrochordons. A possible role for alpha-transforming growth factor in cutaneous paraneoplastic syndromes. *N Engl J Med* 1987;**317**:1582–7.

5. Guran T, Turan S, Akcay T, Bereket A. Significance of acanthosis nigricans in childhood obesity. *J Paediatr Child Health* 2008;**44**:338–41.

6. Sadeghian G, Ziaie H, Amini M, Ali Nilfroushzadeh M. Evaluation of insulin resistance in obese women with and without acanthosis nigricans. *J Dermatol* 2009; **36**:209–12.

7. Hud JA, Cohen JB, Wagner JM, Cruz PD Jr. Prevalence and significance of acanthosis nigricans in an adult obese population. *Arch Dermatol* 1992;**128**(7):941–4.

8. Kong AS, Williams RL, Smith M, et al. Acanthosis nigricans and diabetes risk factors: prevalence in young persons seen in southwestern US primary care practices. *Ann Fam Med* 2007;**5**(3):202–8.

9. Katz AS, Goff DC, Feldman SR. Acanthosis nigricans in obese patients: presentations and implications for prevention of atherosclerotic vascular disease. *Dermatol Online J* 2000;**6**:1.

10. Nguyen TT, Kell MF. Relation of acanthosis nigricans by hyperinsulinemia and insulin sensitivity in overweight African American and white children. *J Pediatr* 2001;**138**:453–4.

11. Stuart CA, Gilkinson CR, Smith MM, Bosma AN, Keenan BS, Nagamani M. Acanthosis nigricans as a risk factor for non-insulin dependent diabetes mellitus. *Clin Pediatr (Phila)* 1998;**37**:73–80.

12. Rafalson L, et al. The association between acanthosis nigricans and dysglycemia in an ethnically diverse group of eighth grade students. *Obesity (Sliver Spring)* 2013;**21**(3): E328–33.

13. Fletcher EC, Chong NHV, Shetlar DJ. Chapter 10: Retina. In: Riordan-Eva P, Whitcher JP, editors. *Vaughan and Asbury's General Ophthalmology*. 17th ed. 2007. Available: http://proxy14.use.hcn.com.au/content.aspx?aID=3088798 [28 Oct 2010].

14. Clarkson JG, Altman RD. Angioid streaks. *Surv Ophthalmol* 1982;**26**:235–46.

15. Vander JF. Chapter 6.35: Angioid streaks. In: Yanoff M, Duker JS, editors. *Ophthalmology*. 3rd ed. St Louis: Mosby; 2008.

16. Gordon GG, Altman K, Southern AL, Rubin E, Lieber CS. Effects of alcohol (ethanol) administration on sex hormone metabolism in normal men. *N Engl J Med* 1976;**295**(15):793–7.

17. van Thiel DH. Ethanol: its adverse effects upon the hypothalamic–pituitary–gonadal axis. *J Lab Clin Med* 1983;**101**(1):21–33.

18. Boccardo P, Remuzzi G, Galbusera M. Platelet dysfunction in renal failure. *Semin Thromb Hemost* 2004;**30**(5):579–89.

19. Mezzano D, Tagle R, Panes O, et al. Hemostatic disorder of uraemia; the platelet defect, main determinant of the prolonged bleeding time, is correlated with indices of activation of coagulation and fibrinolysis. *Thromb Haemost* 1996;**76**:312–21.

20. Sloand EM, Sloand JA, Prodouz K, et al. Reduction of platelet glycoprotein 1B in uraemia. *Br J Haematol* 1991;**77**:375–81.

21. Fernandez F, Goudable C, Sie P, et al. Low haematocrit and prolonged bleeding time in uraemic patients: effect of red cell transfusions. *Br J Haematol* 1985;**59**:139–48.

22. Alan SL. Disorders of magnesium and phosphorus. In: Goldman L, Ausiello D, editors. *Cecil Medicine*. 23rd ed. Philadelphia: Saunders; 2007.

23. Hoffman E. The Chvostek sign: a clinical study. *Am J Surg* 1958;**96**:33–7.

24. Fonseca OA, Calverley JR. Neurological manifestations of hypoparathyroidism. *Arch Intern Med* 1967;**120**:202–6.

25. Méneret A. Chvostek sign, frequently found in healthy subjects, is not a useful clinical sign. *Neurology* 2013;**80**(11):1067.

26. Bujalska IJ, Kumar S, Stewart P. Does central obesity reflect Cushing's disease of the omentum. *Lancet* 1997;**349**:1210–13.

27. Christ-Grain M. AMP-activated protein kinase mediates glucocorticoid induced metabolic changes: a novel mechanism in Cushing's Syndrome. *FASEB J* 2008; **22**(6):1672–83.

28. McGee S. *Evidence Based Physical Diagnosis*. 2nd ed. St Louis: Elsevier; 2007.

29. Streeten DHP, Stevenson CT, Dalakos TG, et al. The diagnosis of hypercortisolism. Biochemical criteria for differentiating patients from lean and obese normal subjects and from females on oral contraceptives. *J Clin Endocrinol* 1969;**29**:1191–211.

30. Chan YC, Lo YL, Chan ESY. Immunotherapy for diabetic amyotrophy. *Cochrane Database Syst Rev* 2009;(3):Art. No.: CD006521, doi:10.1002/14651858.CD006521. pub2.

31. Dyck PJ, Norell JE, Dyck PJ. Microvasculitis and ischemia in diabetic lumbosacral radiculoplexus neuropathy. *Neurology* 1999;**53**(9):2113–21.

32. Said G, Goulon-Goeau C, Lacroix C, Moulonguet A. Nerve biopsy findings in different patterns of proximal diabetic neuropathy. *Ann Neurol* 1994;**35**(5):559–69.

33. Llewelyn JG, Thomas PK, King RH. Epineural microvasculitis in proximal diabetic neuropathy. *J Neurol* 1998;**245**(3):159–65.

34. Kelkar P, Masood M, Parry GJ. Distinctive pathologic findings in proximal diabetic neuropathy (diabetic amyotrophy). *Neurology* 2000;**55**(1):83–8.

35. Frank RN. Diabetic retinopathy. *N Engl J Med* 2004;**350**:48–58.

36. Hussein KA. Bone morphogenetic protein 2: a potential new player in the pathogenesis of diabetic retinopathy. *Exp Eye Res* 2014;**125**:79–88.

37. Kohner EM, Patel V, Rassam MB. Role of blood flow and impaired autoregulation in the pathogenesis of diabetic retinopathy. *JAMA* 2002;**288**:2579.

38. Tomic M, et al. Inflammation, haemostatic disturbance, and obesity: possible link to pathogenesis of diabetic retinopathy in type 2 diabetes. *Mediators Inflamm* 2013;**818671**. doi:10.1155/2013/818671.

39. Klein R, Klein BE, Moss SE, Davis MD, DeMets DL. The Wisconsin Epidemiologic Study of Diabetic Retinopathy. III. Prevalence and risk of diabetic retinopathy when age at diagnosis is 30 or more years. *Arch Ophthalmol* 1984;**102**:527–32.

40. Klein R, Klein BBK, Moss SE, Davis MD, Demets DL. The Wisconsin Epidemiologic Study of Diabetic Retinopathy. III. Prevalence and risk of diabetic retinopathy when age at diagnosis is less than 30 years. *Arch Ophthalmol* 1984;**102**: 520–6.

41. Leung AKC, Pacaud D. Diagnosis and management of galactorrhea. *Am Fam Physician* 2004;**70**(3):543–50, 553–554.

42. Tyrrell JB, Wilson CB. Pituitary syndromes. In: Friesen SE, editor. *Surgical Endocrinology: Clinical Syndromes*. Philadelphia: Lippincott; 1978.

43. Pena KS, Rosenfeld JA. Evaluation and treatment of galactorrhea. *Am Fam Physician* 2001;**63**(9):1763–70.

44. *Dorland's Medical Dictionary*. 30th ed. Philadelphia: Elsevier; 2003.

45. Nordyke RA, Gilbert FI, Harada ASM. Graves' disease: influence of age on clinical findings. *Arch Intern Med* 1988;**148**:626–31.

7

46. Hegedus L, Hansen JM, Karstrup S. High incidence of normal thyroid gland volume in patients with Graves' disease. *Clin Endocrinol (Oxf)* 1983;**19**:603–7.

47. Hegedus L, Hansen JM, Veiergang D, Karstrup S. Thyroid size and goitre frequency in hyperthyroidism. *Dan Med Bull* 1987;**34**:121–3.

48. Sminoski K. Does this patient have a goiter? *JAMA* 1995;**273**(10):813–17.

49. Krohn K, et al. Molecular pathogenesis of euthyroid and toxic multinodular goitre. *Endocr Rev* 2005;**26**:504–24.

50. Bauer DC, McPhee SJ. Chapter 20: Thyroid disease. In: McPhee SJ, Hammer GD, editors. *Pathophysiology of Disease*. 6th ed. 2009. Available: http://proxy14.use.hcn.com.au/content.aspx?aID=5371499 [22 Oct 2010].

51. Kumar V, Abbas A, Fausto N. In: Robbins SL, Cotran RS, editors. *Pathologic Basis of Disease*. 7th ed. Philadelphia: Elsevier; 2005.

52. Habif TP. *Clinical Dermatology*. 5th ed. Philadelphia: Mosby; 2009.

53. Prendiville JS. Chapter 43: Granuloma annulare. In: Wolff K, Goldsmith LA, Katz SI, Gilchrest B, Paller AS, Leffell DJ, editors. *Fitzpatrick's Dermatology in General Medicine*. 7th ed. 2007. Available http://proxy14.use.hcn.com.au/content.aspx?aID=2959059 [22 Oct 2010].

54. Choudry K, Charles-Holmes R. Are patients with localised nodular granuloma annulare more likely to have diabetes mellitus? *Clin Exp Dermatol* 2000;**25**:451.

55. Dabsky K, Winkelmann RK. Generalised granuloma annulare: clinical and laboratory findings in 100 patients. *J Am Acad Dermatol* 1989;**20**:39–47.

56. Veraldi S, Bencini PL, Drudi E, et al. Laboratory abnormalities in granuloma annulare: a case control study. *Br J Dermatol* 1997;**126**:652–3.

57. Bartalena L, Fatourechi V. Extrathyroidal manifestations of Graves' disease: a 2014 update. *J Endocrinol Invest* 2014;**37**:691–700.

58. Bahn RS. Graves' ophthalmopathy. *N Engl J Med* 2010;**362**:726–38.

59. Smith TJ. Pathogenesis of Graves' orbitopathy: a 2010 update. *J Endocrinol Invest* 2010;**33**:414–21.

60. von Arx GF. Editorial. *Orbit* 2009;**28**(4):209–13.

61. Tanda ML, et al. Prevalence and natural history of Graves' orbitopathy in a large series of patients with newly diagnosed Graves' hyperthyroidism seen at a single center. *J Clin Endocrinol Metab* 2013;**98**(4):1443–9.

62. Bartalena L, et al. Consensus statement of the European Group on Graves' Orbitopathy on the management of Graves' orbitopathy. *Thyroid* 2008;**18**(3):273–85.

63. Gaddipati RV, Meyer DR. Eyelid retraction, lid lag, lagophthalmos, and von Graefe's sign quantifying the eyelid features of Graves' ophthalmopathy. *Ophthalmology* 2008;**115**(6):1083–8.

64. Nelson VL, Legro RS, Strauss JF III, McAllister JM. Augmented androgen production is a stable steroidogenic phenotype of propagated theca cells from polycystic ovaries. *Mol Endocrinol* 1999;**13**:946–57.

65. Nelson VL, Qin KN, Rosenfield RL, et al. The biochemical basis for increased testosterone production in theca cells propagated from patients with polycystic ovary syndrome. *J Clin Endocrinol Metab* 2001;**86**:5925–33.

66. Kopera D. Endocrinology of hirsutism. *Int J Trichology* 2010;**2**(1):30–5.

67. Maharshak N, Shapiro J, Trau H. Carotenoderma – a review of the current literature. *Int J Dermatol* 2003;**42**:178–81.

68. Schwabe AD. Hypercarotenaemia in anorexia nervosa. *JAMA* 1968;**205**:533–4.

69. Duyff RF, van den Bosch J, Laman DM, van Loon BJP, Linssen WHJP. Neuromuscular findings of thyroid dysfunction: a prospective clinical and electrodiagnostic study. *J Neurol Neurosurg Psychiatry* 2000;**68**:750.

70. Nilsson OR, Karlberg BE. Thyroid hormones and the adrenergic nervous system. *Acta Med Scand Suppl* 1983;**672**:27–32.

71. Goodman M. *Basic Medical Endocrinology*. 4th ed. Massachusetts: Elsevier; 2008.

72. Gardner DG, Shoback D. *Greenspan's Basic and Clinical Endocrinology*. 9th ed. China: McGraw-Hill Medical; 2011.

73. Everts ME. Effects of thyroid hormones on contractility and cation transport in skeletal muscle. *Acta Physiol Scand* 1996;**156**(3):325–33.

74. Nieman LK. Clinical manifestations of Cushing's syndrome. In: Martyn KA, editor. *UpToDate*. Waltham, MA: UpToDate; 2010.

75. Henderson JM, Portmann L, Van Melle G, Haller E, Ghika JA. Propranolol as an adjunct therapy for hyperthyroid tremor. *Eur Neurol* 1997;**37**(3):182–5.

76. Adams RD, Victor M. *Principles of Neurology*. 4th ed. New York: McGraw-Hill; 1989. pp. 1133–9.

77. Ianuzzo D, Patel P, Chen V, et al. Thyroidal trophic influence on skeletal muscle myosin. *Nature* 1977;**270**:74–6.

78. Pawar S, et al. Usefulness of blink reflex in hypothyroid patients with or without polyneuropathy. A case control study. *Indian J Physiol Pharmacol* 2014;**1**(58):56–60.

79. Reinfrank RF, Kaufmann RP, Wetstone HJ, Glennon JA. Observations of the Achilles reflex test. *JAMA* 1967;**199**:1–4.

80. Cheah JS, Tan BY. The Achilles tendon reflex time as a parameter of thyroid function. *Singapore Med J* 1969;**10**(4):272–9.

81. Gupta SP, Kumar V, Ahuja MMS. Evaluation of Achilles reflex time as a test of thyroid function. *South Med J* 1973;**66**(7):754–8.

82. Kasumagic-Halilovic E, Begovic B. Thyroid autoimmunity in patients with skin disorders. In: Agrawal NK, editor. *Thyroid Hormone*. Chapter 11. doi:10.5772/45980.

83. Safer J. Thyroid hormone action on skin. *Curr Opin Endocrinol Diabetes Obes* 2012;**19**(5):388–93.

84. Schell H, et al. Cell cycle kinetics of human anagen scalp hair bulbs in thyroid disorders determined by DNA flow cytometry. *Dermatologica* 1991;**182**:23–6.

85. Dunlop D. Eighty-six cases of Addison's disease. *BMJ* 1963;**2**:887.

86. Irvine WJ, Barnes EW. Adrenocortical insufficiency. *Clin Endocrinol Metab* 1972;**1**:549.

87. Klein I, Ojamaa K. Thyroid hormone and the cardiovascular system. *NEJM* 2001;**344**(7):501–9.

88. Weiss LS, White JAJ. Macroglossia: a review. *J la State Med Soc* 1990;**142**:13–16.

89. Rizer FM, Schechter GL, Richardson MA. Macroglossia: etiological considerations and management techniques. *Int J Pediatr Otorhinolaryngol* 1985;**8**:225–36.

90. Wittmann AL. Macroglossia in acromegaly and hypothyroidism. *Virchows Archiv A, Pathol Anat Histol* 1977;**373**(4):353–60.

91. Peyrí J, Moreno A, Marcoval J. Necrobiosis lipoidica. *Semin Cutan Med Surg* 2007;**26**(2):87–9.

92. Kota SK, et al. Necrobiosis lipoidica diabeticorum: a case-based review of literature. *Indian J Endocrinol Metab* 2012;**16**(4):614–20.

93. Gordon GG, Altman K, Southern AL, Rubin E, Lieber CS. Effects of alcohol (ethanol) administration on sex hormone metabolism in normal men. *N Engl J Med* 1976;**295**(15):793–7.

94. Joachim Dissemond J. Images in clinical medicine. Necrobiosis lipoidica diabeticorum. *N Engl J Med* 2012;**366**:2502.

95. Anoop T, Jabbar P, Sujathan P. Plummer's nails. *N Z Med J* 2008;**121**(1280):66–7.

96. Jadhav VM, Mahajan PM, Mhaske CB. Nail pitting and onycholysis. *Indian J Dermatol Venereol Leprol* 2009;**75**:631–3.

97. Piraccini BM, Alessandrini A. Drug related nail disease. *Clin Dermatol* 2013;**31**:618–26.

98. De Fillipis EA, et al. Pemberton's sign: explained nearly 70 years later. *J Clin Endocrinol Metab* 2014;**99**(6):1949–54.

7

99. Radulescu D, Parv A, Pripon S, Radulescu ML, Gulei I, Buzoianu A. Hypokalemic periodic paralysis in hyperthyroidism-rare event: case presentation and review of literature. *Endocrinologist* 2010;**20**(2):72–4.

100. Denker BM, Brenner BM. Chapter 45: Azotemia and urinary abnormalities. In: Fauci AS, Braunwald E, Kasper DL, et al., editors. *Harrison's Principles of Internal Medicine.* 17th ed. 2008. Available: http://proxy14.use.hcn.com.au/content.aspx?aID=2868002 [25 Oct 2010].

101. Walker RJ, Weggery S, Bedford JJ, et al. Lithium-induced reduction in urinary concentrating ability and urinary aquaporin 2 (AQP2) excretion in healthy volunteers. *Kidney Int* 2005;**67**(1):291–4.

102. Harris R, Yarger W. The pathogenesis of post-obstructive diuresis. The role of circulating natriueritc and diuretic factors, including urea. *J Clin Invest* 1975;**56**:880–7.

103. Frokiaer J, Zeidel ML, et al. Chapter 37. Urinary tract obstruction. In: Taal MW, et al., editors. *Brenner and Rector's The Kidney.* 9th ed. Philadelphia: Elsevier; 2011. pp. 1383–410.

104. Garofeanu CG, Weir M, Rosas-Arellano MP, et al. Causes of reversible nephrogenic diabetes insipidus: a systematic review. *Am J Kidney Dis* 2005;**45**(4):626–37.

105. Nielsen J, Kwon TH, Christensen BM, et al. Dysregulation of renal aquaporins and epithelial sodium channel in lithium-induced nephrogenic diabetes insipidus. *Semin Nephrol* 2008;**28**(3):227–44.

106. Bartley GB, Fatourechi V, Kadrmas EF, et al. The incidence of Graves' ophthalmopathy in Olmstead County, Minnesota. *Am J Ophthalmol* 1995; **120**(4):511–17.

107. Rapoport B, Alsabeh R, Aftergood D, et al. Elephantiasic pretibial myxoedema: insight into and a hypothesis regarding the pathogenesis of the extrathyroidal manifestation of Graves' disease. *Thyroid* 2000;**10**(8):685–92.

108. Davis TF. Trauma and pressure explain the clinical presentation of Graves' disease triad. *Thyroid* 2000;**10**(8):629–30.

109. Bahn RS. Clinical review 157; pathophysiology of Grave's ophthalmopathy: the cycle of disease. *J Clin Endocrinol Metab* 2003;**88**(5):1936–46.

110. Fatourechi V. Pretibial myxoedema pathophysiology and treatment options. *Am J Clin Dermatol* 2005;**6**(5):295–306.

111. Fatourechi V, Garrity JA, Bartley GB, et al. Orbital decompression in Graves' ophthalmopathy associated with pretibial myxoedema. *J Endocrinol Invest* 1993; **16**(6):433–7.

112. Horak HA, Pourmand R. Metabolic myopathies. *Neurol Clin* 2000;**18**(1):204–14.

113. Kissel JT, Mendell JR. The endocrine myopathies. In: Rowland LP, Dimauro S, editors. *Handbook of Clinical Neurology Myopathies.* New York: McGraw-Hill; 1994. p. 527.

114. Kaminski HJ, Ruff RL. Endocrine myopathies (hyper and hypo function of adrenal, thyroid, pituitary and parathyroid glands and iastrogenic corticosteroid myopathy). In: Engel AG, Franzini-Armstrong C, editors. *Myology.* 2nd ed. New York: McGraw-Hill; 1994. p. 1726.

115. Erkintalo M, Bendahan D, Mattei JP, et al. Reduced metabolic efficiency of skeletal muscle energetics in hyperthyroid patients evidenced quantitatively by in vivo phosphorus-31 magnetic resonance spectroscopy. *Metabolism* 1998;**47**:769.

116. Anderson W, Xu L Endocrine Myopathies. Emedicine. Available: http://emedicine.medscape.com/article/1170469 [26 Oct 2010].

117. Anagnos A. Endocrine neuromyopathies. *Neurology Clin* 1997;**15**(3):673–96.

118. Kissel JT, Mendell JR. The endocrine myopathies. In: Rowland LP, Di Mauro S, editors. *Myopathies.* In: Vinken PJ, Bruyn, Klawans HL, *Handbook of Clinical Neurology* (vol 62, revised series 18) Amsterdam: Elsevier; 1992. p. 527.

119. Harting M, Hicks MJ, Levy ML. Chapter 64: Dermal hypertrophies. In: Wolff K, Goldsmith LA, Katz SI, Gilchrest B, Paller AS, Leffell DJ, editors. *Fitzpatrick's*

Dermatology in General Medicine. 7th ed. 2007. Available: http://proxy14.use.hcn.com.au/content.aspx?aID=2968331 [22 Oct 2010].

120. Bazcynski R, Ernst S, Herrick R, et al. Effect of parathyroid hormone on energy metabolism of skeletal muscle. *Kidney Int* 1985;**28**:722.

121. Tamega AA, Aranha AM, Guiotoku MM, Miot LD, Miot HA. Association between skin tags and insulin resistance. *An Bras Dermatol* 2010;**85**(1):25–31.

122. Agarwal JK, Nigam PK. Acrochordon: a cutaneous sign of carbohydrate intolerance. *Australas J Dermatol* 1987;**28**:132–3.

123. Sari R, Akman A, Alpsoy E, Balci MK. The metabolic profile in patients with skin tags. *Clin Exp Med* 2009;**10**(3):193–7.

124. Dermatological Society of New Zealand. Steroid acne. Available: http://dermnetnz.org/acne/steroid-acne.html [21 Oct 2010].

125. Bower S, Hogan DJ, Mason S Malassezia (pityrosporum) folliculitis. Emedicine. Available: http://emedicine.medscape.com/article/1091037-overview [1 Mar 2010].

126. Halder RM, Taliaferro SJ. Chapter 72: Vitiligo. In: Wolff K, Goldsmith LA, Katz SI, Gilchrest B, Paller AS, Leffell DJ, editors. *Fitzpatrick's Dermatology in General Medicine*. 7th ed. 2007. Available: http://proxy14.use.hcn.com.au/content.aspx?aID=2972969 [19 Sep 2010].

127. Jesus JE, Landry A. Images in clinical medicine. Chvostek's and Trousseau's signs. *N Engl J Med* 2012;**367**:e15.

128. Bystryn J-C. Immune mechanisms in vitiligo. *Clin Dermatol* 1997;**15**:853.

129. Palermo B, et al. Specific cytotoxic T lymphocyte responses against Melan-A/MART1, tyrosinase and gp100 in vitiligo by the use of major histocompatibility complex/peptide tetramers: the role of cellular immunity in the etiopathogenesis of vitiligo. *J Invest Dermatol* 2001;**117**(2):326–32.

130. Hazneci E, et al. A comparative study of superoxide dismutase, catalase, and glutathione peroxidase activities and nitrate levels in vitiligo patients. *Int J Dermatol* 2005;**44**:636.

131. Rocha IM, et al. Lipopolysaccharide and cytokines induce nitric oxide synthase and produce nitric oxide in cultured normal human melanocytes. *Arch Dermatol Res* 2001;**293**:245.

132. Nieman LK. Clinical manifestations of adrenal insufficiency in adults. In: Martyn KA, editor. *UpToDate*. Waltham, MA: UpToDate; 2010.

7

Figure Credits

Figure 1.3 Based on Woodward T, Best TM, The painful shoulder: part 1, clinical evaluation. *Am Fam Phys* 2000; 61(10): 3079–3088.

Figures 1.4, 1.10 Based on Firestein GS, Budd RC, Harris ED et al., *Kelley's Textbook of Rheumatology*, 8th edn, Philadelphia: WB Saunders, 2008; Figs 42-24, 35-9A and B.

Figures 1.21, 1.33, 1.36, 1.38, 1.54 Firestein GS, Budd RC, Harris ED et al., *Kelley's Textbook of Rheumatology*, 8th edn, Philadelphia: WB Saunders, 2008; Figs 47-10, 72-3, 82-5, 47-12, 66-5.

Figure 1.7 Based on Ferri FF, *Ferri's Clinical Advisor*, Philadelphia: Elsevier, 2011; Fig 1-223.

Figures 1.8, 1.9 Based on DeLee JC, Drez D, Miller MD, *DeLee and Drez's Orthopaedic Sports Medicine*, 3rd edn, Philadelphia: Saunders, 2009; Figs 20B2-27, 20B2-28.

Figures 1.11, 1.44 Goldman L, Ausiello D, *Cecil Medicine*, 23rd edn, Philadelphia: Saunders, 2007: Figs 287-3, 285-9.

Figure 1.13 James WD, Berger T, Elston D, *Andrews' Diseases of the Skin: Clinical Dermatology*, 11th edn, Philadelphia: Saunders, 2011: Fig 26-12.

Figure 1.14 Mann JA, Ross SD, Chou LB, Foot and ankle surgery. In: Skinner HB, *Current Diagnosis & Treatment in Orthopedics*, 4th edn, Fig 9-8.

Figure 1.15 Based on Jeffcoate WJ, Game F, Cavanagh PR, *Lancet* 2005; 366: 2058–2061.

Figure 1.16 Based on Multimedia Group LLC, Occupation Orthopedics. Available: http://www.eorthopod.com/eorthopodV2/index.php?ID=7244790dd ace6ee8ea5da6f0a57f8b45&disp_type= topic_detail&area=6&topic_id= 4357b9903d317fcb3ff32f72b24cb6b6 [28 Feb 2011].

Figure 1.17 Based on Frontera WR, Silver JK, Rizzo Jr TD, *Essentials of Physical Medicine and Rehabilitation*, 2nd edn, Philadelphia: Saunders, 2008: Fig 24-2.

Figures 1.18, 1.34, 1.49 Habif TP, *Clinical Dermatology*, 5th edn, Philadelphia:

Mosby, 2009: Figs 17-20, 17-21, 8-23, 17-30.

Figure 1.24 Floege J et al., *Comprehensive Clinical Nephrology*, 4th edn, Philadelphia: Saunders, 2010: Fig 64-13.

Figures 1.28, 1.45 DeLee JC, Drez D, Miller MD, *DeLee and Drez's Orthopaedic Sports Medicine*, 3rd edn, Philadelphia: Saunders, 2009: Figs 22C1-5, 17H2-16.

Figure 1.35 Kumar V, Abbas AK, Fausto N, Aster J, *Robbins and Cotran Pathologic Basis of Disease, Professional Edition*, 8th edn, Philadelphia: Saunders, 2009: Fig 11-28.

Figure 1.37 Tyring SK, Lupi O, Hengge UR, *Tropical Dermatology*, 1st edn, London: Churchill Livingstone, 2005: Fig 11-16.

Figure 1.40 Hochberg MC et al., *Rheumatology*, 5th edn, Philadelphia: Mosby, 2010: Fig 144-7.

Figures 1.47, 1.48 Jupiter JB, Arthritic hand. In: Canale TS, Beaty JH, *Campbell's Operative Orthopaedics*, 11th edn, Philadelphia: Elsevier, 2007: Figs 70-13, 70-14.

Figure 1.53 Goldstein B, Chavez F, *Phys Med Rehabil State Art Rev* 1996; 10: 601–630.

Figure 1.55 Shields HM et al., *Clin Gastroenterol Hepatol* 2007; 5(9): 1010–1017.

Figure 1.58 Harish HS, Purushottam GA, Wells L, Torsional and angular deformities. In: Kliegman RM et al., *Nelson Textbook of Pediatrics*, 18th edn, Philadelphia: Saunders, 2007: Fig 674-8.

Figure 1.59 Adam A, Dixon AK (eds), *Grainger & Allison's Diagnostic Radiology*, 5th edn, New York: Churchill Livingstone, 2008: Fig 67.13.

Figure 1.61 Based on Pettit RW et al., *Athletic Training Edu J* 2008; 3(4): 143–147.

Figure 2.1 Based on West JB, *West's Respiratory Physiology*, 7th edn, Philadelphia: Lippincott Williams & Wilkins, 2005: Fig 8-1.

Figures 2.3, 2.12 http://what-when-how. com/acp-medicine/ventilatory-control- during-wakefulness-and-sleep-part-2/.

Figure 2.5 Khayat R et al., Sleep-disordered breathing in heart failure: identifying and treating an important but often unrecognized comorbidity in heart failure patients. *Journal of Cardiac Failure* 2013; 19(6): Fig 4. Elsevier 2013.

Figure 2.6 Goodman CC, Snyder TE. *Differential Diagnosis for Physical Therapists: Screening for Referral*, 4th edn, Philadelphia, PA: WB Saunders/Elsevier, 2007. In: Goodman CC, Screening for gastrointestinal, hepatic/biliary, and renal/urologic disease. *Journal of Hand Therapy* 2010; 23(2): 140–157. © 2010.

Figure 2.7 Accuracy of the physical examination in evaluating pleural effusion. *Cleveland Clinic Journal of Medicine* 2008; 75(4).

Figure 2.9 Based on Aggarwal R, Hunter A, *BMJ*. Available: http://archive.student. bmj.com/issues/07/02/education/52.php [28 Feb 2011].

Figures 2.11, 2.16 McGee S. *Evidence Based Physical Diagnosis*, 3rd edn, St Louis: Elsevier, 2012: p. 151, Figs 18-2, 28-2.

Figure 2.13 Casas-Mendez LF et al., Biot's breathing in a woman with fatal familial insomnia: is there a role for noninvasive ventilation? *J Clin Sleep Med* 2011; 7(1): 89–91.

Figure 2.14 Swartz MH, *Textbook of Physical Diagnosis: History and Examination*, 6th edn, St Louis: Mosby, 2004.

Figure 2.17 Kanchan Ganda, http://ocw.tufts.edu/Content/24/lecturenotes/311144/312054_medium.jpg. © 2006.

Figure 2.20 Chung KF, Management of cough. In: Chung KF, Widdicombe JG, Boushey HA (eds), *Cough: Causes, Mechanisms and Therapy*. Oxford: Blackwell, 2003: 283–297.

Figure 2.21 Rebick G, Morin S, The thinker's sign. *Canadian Medical Association Journal* 2008; 179(6): 611, Fig 1A. © 2008.

Figure 2.22 Based on Manning HL, Schwartzstein RM, *N Engl J Med* 1995; 333(23): 1547–1553.

Figure 2.24 Sun X-G et al., Exercise physiology in patients with primary pulmonary hypertension. *Circulation* 2001; 104: 429–435; Fig 4. AHA 2001.

Figure 2.25 Shamberger RC, Hendren WH III, Congenital deformities of the chest wall and sternum. In: Pearson FG, Cooper JD et al. (eds), *Thoracic Surgery*, 2nd edn, Philadelphia: Churchill Livingstone, 2002: 1352.

Figure 2.27 Douglas G, Nicol F, Robertson C, *Macleod's Clinical Examination*, 13th edn, Edinburgh: Elsevier, 2013: Fig 7.14C.

Figure 2.28 Kliegman RM, Behrman RE, Jenson HB, Stanton BF: *Nelson Textbook of Pediatrics*, 18th edn, Philadelphia: Elsevier, 2004: Fig 195-1.

Figure 2.29 Johnston C, Krishnaswamy N, Krishnaswamy G, The Hoover's sign of pulmonary disease: molecular basis and clinical relevance. *Clin Mol Allergy* 2008; 6: 8.

Figure 2.30 Goldman L, Ausiello D, *Cecil Medicine*, 23rd edn, Philadelphia: Saunders, 2007: Fig 189-2.

Figure 2.32 Based on Gardner WN, *Chest* 1996; 109: 516–534.

Figure 2.36 Parrillo JE, Dellinger RP, *Critical Care Medicine: Principles of Diagnosis and Management in the Adult*, 4th edn, St Louis: Elsevier 2014: Fig 64.1.

Figures 2.38, 2.39 Cheng TO. Platypnea-orthodeoxia syndrome: etiology, differential diagnosis and management. *Catheterization and Cardiovascular Interventions* 1999; 47: 64–66.

Figure 2.41 Roberts JR, Hedges JR, *Clinical Procedures in Emergency Medicine*, 5th edn, Philadelphia: Saunders, 2009: Fig 10-12.

Figure 2.42 Girnius AK, Ortega R, Chin LS. Subcutaneous emphysema of the eyelid on emergence from general anesthesia after a craniotomy. *Journal of Clinical Anesthesia* 2010; 22(5): Fig 1. Elsevier.

Figure 3.2 Based on Chatterjee K, Bedside evaluation of the heart: the physical examination. In: Chatterjee K et al. (eds), *Cardiology. An Illustrated Text/Reference*, Philadelphia: JB Lippincott, 1991: Fig 48.5.

Figure 3.3 Based on Vender JS, Clemency MV, Oxygen delivery systems, inhalation therapy, and respiratory care. In: Benumof JL [ed], *Clinical Procedures in Anesthesia and Intensive Care*, Philadelphia: JB Lippincott, 1992: Fig 13-3.

Figure 3.4 Surawicz B, Knilans TK, *Chou's Electrocardiography in Clinical Practice*, 6th edn, Elsevier 2008, Fig 17.1.

Figure 3.5A Ragosta M, *Cardiac Catheterization*, Philadelphia: Saunders, 2010; Ch 6, 58–74. © 2010 Saunders.

Figure 3.5B Mark JB, *Atlas of Cardiovascular Monitoring*. New York: Churchill Livingstone, 1998: Figs 3-3, 18-10.

Figure 3.7 Andreoli TE, Benjamin IJ, Griggs RC, Wing EJ. In: *Andreoli and Carpenter's Cecil Essentials of Medicine*, 8th edn, Philadelphia: Elsevier, 2011: Ch 4, 32–45, Fig 4.2.

Figure 3.8 Stephens NA, Fearon KCH. Anorexia, cachexia and nutrition, *Medicine* 2007; 36(2): Fig 3.

Figure 3.12 Marx JA, Hockberger RS, Walls RM et al. (eds), *Rosen's Emergency Medicine*, 7th edn, Philadelphia: Mosby, 2009: Fig 29.2.

Figure 3.15 Williams RC, Autoimmune disease etiology – a perplexing paradox or a turning leaf? *Autoimmun Rev* 2007-03-01Z, 6(4): 204–208, Fig 2. Copyright © 2006.

Figure 3.16 Douglas G, Nicol F, Robertson C, *Macleod's Clinical Examination*, 13th edn, Fig 3.6.

Figures 3.17, 3.18 McMullen SM, Ward P. Cyanosis. *The American Journal of Medicine* 2013; 126(3): 210–212, Figs B, A.

Figures 3.21, 3.23 Based on Yanoff M, Duker JS (eds),*Ophthalmology*, 3rd edn, St Louis: Mosby, 2008: Figs 6-15-2, 6-20-2.

Figure 3.22 Effron D, Forcier BC, Wyszynski RE, Chapter 3: Funduscopic findings. In: Knoop KJ, Stack LB, Storrow AB, Thurman RJ, *The Atlas of Emergency Medicine*, 3rd edn, McGraw-Hill.

Figure 3.27 Based on Mandell GL, Bennett JA, Dolin R, *Mandell, Douglas, and Bennett's Principles and Practice of Infectious Diseases*, 7th edn, Philadelphia: Churchill Livingston, 2009: Fig 195-15.

Figure 3.31 Chiaco C, The jugular venous pressure revisited. *Cleveland Clinic Journal of Medicine* 2013; 80(10): 641, Fig 2.

Figure 3.33 Ragosta M, *Cardiac Catheterisation an Atlas and DVD*, Saunders, 2009: Fig 6-30.

Figure 3.34 Abrams J, *Synopsis of Cardiac Physical Diagnosis*, 2nd edn, Butterworth-Heinemann, 2001: 25–35. In: *Braunwald's Heart Disease: A Textbook of Cardiovascular Medicine*, 10th edn, Philadelphia: Elsevier, 2015.

Figure 3.35 Modified from Lorell BH, Grossman W, Profiles in constrictive pericarditis, restrictive cardiomyopathy and cardiac tamponade. In: Baim DS, Grossman W (eds), *Grossman's Cardiac Catheterization, Angiography, and Intervention*, 6th edn, Philadelphia: Lippincott Williams & Wilkins, 2000: 832.

Figures 3.36, 3.55 Goldman L, Ausiello D, *Cecil Medicine*, 23rd edn, Philadelphia: Saunders, 2007: Figs 77-11, 76-2.

Figure 3.37 Mann DL et al., *Braunwald's Heart Disease: A Textbook of Cardiovascular Medicine*, 10th edn, Philadelphia: Elsevier 2015, Fig 63.40. (Modified from O'Rourke RA, Crawford MH, The systolic click-murmur syndrome: clinical recognition and management. *Curr Probl Cardiol* 1976; 1: 9.)

Figure 3.38 Ait-Oufell H. Mottling score predicts survival in septic shock. *Intensive Care Medicine* 2011; 37: 803.

Figures 3.39, 3.41, 3.71 Talley N, O'Connor S, *Clinical Examination*, 6th edn, Sydney: Elsevier Australia, 2009: Figs 4.48A, 4.46A, 4-42.

Figures 3.43, 3.48, 3.53 Keane JF et al. (eds), *Nadas' Pediatric Cardiology*, 2nd edn, Philadelphia: Saunders, 2006: Figs 31-6, 33-20, 35-3.

Figure 3.44 Libby P et al., *Braunwald's Heart Disease: A Textbook of Cardiovascular Medicine*, 8th edn, Philadelphia: Saunders, 2007: Fig 11.9B.

Figure 3.45 Based on Pennathur A, Anyanwu AC (eds), *Seminars in Thoracic and Cardiovascular Surgery* 2010; 22(1): 79–83.

Figure 3.46 Adapted from Avery ME, First LP (eds), *Pediatric Medicine*, Baltimore: Williams & Wilkins, 1989.

Figure 3.51 Based on Talley N, O'Connor S, *Clinical Examination*, 6th edn, Sydney: Elsevier Australia, 2009: Fig 4.45A.

Figure 3.52 Blaustein AS, Ramanathan A, Tricuspid valve disease. *Cardiology Clinics* 1998; 16(3): 551–572.

Figure 3.54 Adsllc_commonswiki, https://en.wikipedia.org/wiki/Patent_ductus_arteriosus#/media/File:Patent_ductus_arteriosus.svg.

Figures 3.56, 3.64 Marik et al. Surviving sepsis: going beyond the guidelines. *Annals of Intensive Care* 2011; 1(1): Figs 4, 1.

Figure 3.58 Rangaprasad L et al., Itraconazole associated quadriparesis and edema: a case report. *Journal of Medical Case Reports* 2011; 5: 140.

Figures 3.63, 3.66 Gunn SR, Pinsky MR, Implications of arterial pressure variation in patients in the intensive care unit, MD. *Current Opinion in Critical Care* 2001; 7: 212–217, Fig 4.

Figure 3.65 Marik et al. Hemodynamic parameters to guide fluid therapy. *Annals of Intensive care* 2011, 1: 2. Critical Care/Current Science Ltd.

Figure 3.68 Based on Lip GYH, Hall JE, *Comprehensive Hypertension*, 1st edn, Elsevier, 2007: Fig 11-3.

Figure 3.69 Wu LA, Nishimura RA. Pulsus paradoxus. *New England Journal of Medicine* 2003; 349: 666.

Figure 3.74 Sack DA, Sack RB, Nair GB, et al., Cholera. *Lancet* 2004; 363: 223–233. Kleigman et al., *Nelson Textbook of Pediatrics*, Chapter 201, 1400–1403.e1: Fig 201.2. © 2016 Elsevier.

Figure 3.75 Adams JG, Wallace CA, *Emergency Medicine*, Elsevier 2013. Courtesy Marc E. Grossman, MD, FACP.

Figure 3.77 Based on McGee S, *Evidence Based Physical Diagnosis*, 2nd edn, St Louis: Science Direct, 2007: Fig 36.1.

Figure 3.80 Rakel RE, *Textbook of Family Medicine*, 7th edn, Philadelphia: Saunders, 2007: Fig 44-66.

Figure 4.1 Forbes CD, Jackson WF, *Color Atlas and Text of Clinical Medicine*, 3rd edn, London: Mosby, 2003.

Figure 4.3 Adapted from Falk S, Dickensen AH. Pain and nociception: mechanisms of cancer-induced bone pain. *Journal of Clinical Oncology* 2014; 32(16): Fig 2. American Society of Clinical Oncology.

Figure 4.4 Based on Swanson TA, Kim SI, Flomin OE, *Underground Clinical Vignettes Step 1: Pathophysiology I, Pulmonary, Ob/Gyn, ENT, Hem/Onc*, 5th edn, Lippincott, Williams & Wilkins, 2007; Fig 95-1.

Figure 4.5 Talley N, O'Connor S, *Clinical Examination* 7th edn, Elsevier, 2013: Fig 38.4B.

Figures 4.6, 4.7, 4.14 Little JW, Falace DA, Miller CS, Rhodus NL, *Dental Management of the Medically Compromised Patient*, 7th edn, St Louis: Mosby Elsevier, 2008: Figs 25-9, 25-16, 24-6.

Figure 4.8 Libby P, Bonow R, Zipes R, Mann D, *Braunwald's Heart Disease: A Textbook of Cardiovascular Medicine*, 8th edn, Philadelphia: Saunders, 2007: Fig 84-1.

Figure 4.9 Sidwell RU et al., *J Am Acad Dermatol* 2004; 50(2, Suppl 1): 53–56.

Figure 4.10 Stern TA, Rosenbaum JF, Fava M, Biederman J, Rauch SL, *Massachusetts General Hospital Comprehensive Clinical Psychiatry*, 1st edn, Philadelphia: Mosby, 2008: Fig 21-17.

Figure 4.11 Grandinetti LM, Tomecki KJ, Nail abnormalities and systemic disease. In: Carey WD, *Cleveland Clinic: Current Clinical Medicine*, 2nd edn, Philadelphia: Saunders, 2010: Fig 4.

Figure 4.12 Ho ML, Girardi PA, Williams D, Lord RVN, *J Gastroenterol Hepatol* 2008; 23(4): 672.

Figure 4.13 World Articles in Ear, Nose and Throat website. Available: http://www.entusa.com/oral_photos.htm [9 Feb 2011].

Figure 4.16 Katz JW, Falace DA, Miller CS, Rhodus NL, *Comprehensive Gynecology*, 5th edn, Philadelphia: Mosby, 2007: Fig 15-13B.

Figures 5.1, 5.12, 5.17, 5.18, 5.20, 5.33, 5.36, 5.38, 5.41, 5.50, 5.69, 5.70, 5.71, 5.78, 5.80, 5.83, 5.96, 5.98, 5.106, 5.117, 5.135, 5.196 Daroff RB, Bradley WG et al., *Neurology in Clinical Practice*, 5th edn, Philadelphia: Butterworth-Heinemann, 2008: Figs 74-7, 78-4, 12A-1, 12A-3, 54C-8, 74–9, 12A-1, 6-3, 17-6, 74-1, 15-9, 15–11, 82-4, 39-3, 30-3, 74-13, 74-16, 39-1, 14-3, 12A-1, 12A-4.

Figures 5.2, 5.3, 5.4, 5.6, 5.22, 5.47, 5.61, 5.62, 5.64, 5.65, 5.68, 5.73, 5.77, 5.99, 5.100, 5.103, 5.104, 5.115, 5.116 Yanoff M, Duker JS, *Ophthalmology*, 3rd edn, St Louis: Mosby, 2008: Figs 9-14-4, 9-15-1, 9-19-5, 11-10-2, 9-11-3, 12-5-4, 11-10-2, 11-10-1, 9-15-1, 9-14-2, 9-23-1, 9-19-5, 9-17-4, 11-10-4, 9-15-1, 9-13-4, 2-6-7, 6-16-6, 9-2-3.

Figure Credits

Figure 5.5 Based on Dyck PJ, Thomas PK, *Peripheral Neuropathy*, 4th edn. Philadelphia: Saunders, 2005: Fig 9-1.

Figures 5.7, 5.8 Bromley SM, *Am Fam Physician* 2000; 61(2): 427–436: Figs 2A, 2B.

Figure 5.9 Aziz TA, Holman RP, *Am J Med* 2010; 123(2): 120–121.

Figures 5.10, 5.23, 5.48, 5.59, 5.63, 5.81, 5.105, 5.121 Goldman L, Ausiello D, *Cecil Medicine*, 23rd edn, Philadelphia: Saunders, 2007: Figs 450-2, 430-6, 450-5, 450-2, 449-2, 430-3.

Figures 5.11, 5.27, 5.29, 5.31, 5.55, 5.101 Barrett KE, Barman SM, Boitano S et al., *Ganong's Review of Medical Physiology*, 23rd edn. Modified from Kandel ER, Schwartz JH, Jessell TM (eds), *Principles of Neural Science*, 4th edn, McGraw Hill, 2000.

Figure 5.13 Bertorini TE, *Neuro-muscular Case Studies*, 1st edn, Philadelphia: Butterworth-Heinemann, 2007: Fig 76-1.

Figure 5.14 Benzon H et al., *Raj's Practical Management of Pain*, 4th edn, Philadelphia: Mosby, 2008: Fig 10-1.

Figures 5.15, 5.16, 5.24, 5.82 Rodriguez-Oroz MC, Jahanshahi M, Krack P et al., Initial clinical manifestations of Parkinson's disease: features and pathophysiological mechanisms. *Lancet Neurol* 2009; 8: 1128–1139: Figs 2, 3.

Figure 5.19 Purves D, Augustine GJ, Fitzpatrick D et al. (eds), *Neuroscience*, 2nd edn, Sunderland (MA): Sinauer Associates, 2001: Fig 10.4.

Figure 5.21 Browner BD, *Skeletal Trauma*, 4th edn, Philadelphia: Saunders, 2008: Fig 25-7.

Figure 5.25 University of California, San Diego, A Practical Guide to Clinical Medicine. Available: http://meded.ucsd.edu/clinicalmed/neuro2.htm

Figure 5.26 O'Rahilly R, Muller F, Carpenter F, *Basic Human Anatomy: A Study of Human Structure*, Philadelphia: Saunders, 1983: Fig 46-8.

Figure 5.28 LeBlond RF, DeGowin RL, Brown DD, *DeGowin's Diagnostic Examination*, 10th edn, Fig 14.13.

Figure 5.30 Townsend CM, Beauchamp RD, Evers BM, Mattox K, *Sabiston Textbook of Surgery*, 18th edn, Philadelphia: Saunders, 2008: Fig 41-13.

Figure 5.32 Stern TA et al., *Massachusetts General Hospital Comprehensive Clinical Psychiatry*, 1st edn, Elsevier Health Sciences, 2008: Fig 72-7.

Figures 5.34, 5.74 Dyck PJ, Thomas PK, *Peripheral Neuropathy*, 4th edn, Philadelphia: Saunders, 2005: Figs 50-4, 9-5.

Figure 5.35 Timestra JD, Khatkhate N, *Am Fam Phys* 2007; 76(7): 997–1002.

Figures 5.39, 5.40, 5.49, 5.79, 5.119 Flint PW et al., *Cummings Otolaryngology: Head and Neck Surgery*, 5th edn, Mosby, 2010: Figs 128-6, 163-1, 122-8, 30-9, 166-4.

Figure 5.42 Albert ML, Articles, *Neurology* 1973; 23(6): 658. doi:10.1212/WNL.23.6.658; doi:10.1212/WNL.23.6.658 1526-632X.

Figure 5.43 Based on Neurocenter. Available: http://neurocenter.gr/N-S.html [5 Apr 2011].

Figures 5.44, 5.118 Canale ST, Beaty JH, *Campbell's Operative Orthopaedics*, 11th edn, St Louis: Mosby, 2007: Figs 59-39, 32-5.

Figure 5.45 Drake R, Vogl AW, Mitchell AWM, *Gray's Anatomy for Students*, 2nd edn, Philadelphia: Churchill Livingstone, 2009: Fig 8-164.

Figure 5.46 Fernandez-de-las-Penas C, Cleland J, Huijbregts P (eds), *Neck and Arm Pain Syndromes*, 1st edn, London: Churchill Livingstone, 2011: Fig 9-1.

Figure 5.51 Duong DK, Leo MM, Mitchell EL, *Emerg Med Clin N Am* 2008; 26: 137–180, Fig 3.

Figures 5.52, 5.66 Marx JA, Hockberger RS, Walls RM et al., *Rosen's Emergency Medicine*, 7th edn, Philadelphia: Mosby, 2010: Fig 38-5.

Figure 5.53 Palay D, Krachmer J, *Primary Care Ophthalmology*, 2nd edn, Philadelphia: Mosby, 2005: Fig 6-9.

Figures 5.54, 5.76, 5.95, 5.122 Clark RG, *Manter and Gatz's Essential Neuroanatomy and Neurophysiology*, 5th edn, Philadelphia: FA Davis Co, 1975.

Figure 5.56 Miley JT, Rodriguez GJ, Hernandez EM et al., *Neurology* 2008; 70(1): e3–e4: Fig 1.

Figure 5.57 Adapted from Medscape, Overview of vertebrobasilar stroke. Available: http://emedicine.medscape.com/article/323409-media [5 Apr 2011]. Courtesy B D Decker Inc.

Figure 5.58 Walker HK, Hall WD, Hurst JW, *Clinical Methods: The History, Physical, and Laboratory Examinations*, 3rd edn, Boston: Butterworths, 1990: Fig 50.2.

Figure 5.60 Libby P, Bonow RO, Mann DL, Zipes DP, *Braunwald's Heart Disease: A Textbook of Cardiovascular Medicine*, 8th edn, Philadelphia: Saunders, 2007: Fig 87-7.

Figure 5.67 Isaacson RS, Optic atrophy. In: Ferri FF, *Clinical Advisor* 2011. Philadelphia: Mosby, 2011: Fig 1-220.

Figure 5.72 Murphy SM et al., *Neuromuscular Disorders* 2011; 21(3): 223–226, Copyright © 2010 Elsevier B.V.

Figure 5.75 Based on McGee S, *Evidence Based Physical Diagnosis*, 2nd edn, Philadelphia: Saunders, 2007: Fig 57.1

Figure 5.94 Based on http://virtual.yosemite.cc.ca.us/rdroual/Course%20Materials/Physiology%20101/Chapter%20Notes/Fall%202007/chapter_10%20Fall%202007.htm [5 Apr 2011].

Figure 5.97 Rué, V. et al., Delayed hypoglossal nerve palsy following unnoticed occipital condyle fracture. *Neurochirurgie* 2013; 59(6): 221–223. Copyright © 2013 Elsevier Masson SAS.

Figure 5.102 Based on Scollard DM, Skinsnes OK, Oropharyngeal leprosy in art, history, and medicine. *Oral Surg, Oral Med, Oral Pathol, Oral Radiol, Endodontol* 1999; 87(4): 463–470.

Figure 5.107 Based on the Scottish Sensory Centre, Functional assessment of vision. Available: http://www.ssc.education.ed.ac.uk/courses/vi&multi/vmay06c.html [5 Apr 2011].

Figure 5.120 Lewandowski CA, Rao CPV, Silver B, Transient ischemic attack: definitions and clinical presentations. *Ann Emerg Med* 2008; 52(2): S7–S16: Fig 7.

Figure 6.1 James Heilman, MD (2011). CC BY-SA 3.0.

Figures 6.3, 6.4 Schrier R, Pathogenesis of sodium and water retention in high output and low output cardiac failure, nephrotic syndrome, cirrhosis and pregnancy. First of 2 parts. *NEJM* 1988; 319(16), Figs 1, 3.

Figure 6.5 Moller S et al., Ascites: pathogenesis and therapeutic principles. *Scandinavian Journal of Gastroenterology* 2009; 44: 901–911, Fig 1. Informa PLC.

Figure 6.7 Saxena R, *Practical Hepatic Pathology: A Diagnostic Approach*, Philadelphia: Saunders, 2011: Fig 6-4.

Figure 6.8 Based on Talley NJ, O'Connor S, *Clinical Examination: A Systematic Guide to Physical Diagnosis*, 5th edn, Marrickville, NSW: Churchill Livingstone Elsevier, 2006: Fig 5.20.

Figure 6.9 Bolognia JL, Jorizzo JL, Rapini RP, *Dermatology*, 2nd edn, St Louis: Mosby, 2008: Fig 71-12.

Figure 6.13 Harris S, Naina HVK, *Am J Med* 2008; 121(8): 683.

Figure 6.14 Kliegman RM et al., *Nelson Textbook of Pediatrics*, 18th edn, Philadelphia: Saunders, 2007: Fig 659-2.

Figure 6.16 Feldman M, Friedman LS, Brandt LJ, *Sleisenger and Fordtran's Gastrointestinal and Liver Disease*, 9th edn, Philadelphia: Saunders, 2010: Fig 58-3.

Figure 6.17 Wales JKH, Wit JM, Rogol AD, *Pediatric Endocrinology and Growth*, 2nd edn, Philadelphia: Elsevier/Saunders, 2003: 165.

Figure 6.18 Walker B, *Davidson's Principles and Practice of Medicine*, 22nd edn, Elsevier 2014: Fig 7.7.

Figures 6.21, 6.44 Kumar V, Abbas AK, Fausto N, Aster JC, *Robbins and Cotran Pathologic Basis of Disease, Professional Edition*, 8th edn, Philadelphia: Saunders, 2009: Figs 18-4, 24-43.

Figure 6.22 Liu M, Cohen EJ, Brewer GJ, Laibson PR, *Am J Ophthalmol* 2002; 133(6): 832–834.

Figure 6.23 Adapted from Suvarna JC, Kayser-Fleischer ring. *J Postgrad Med* 2008; 54: 238–240.

Figures 6.24, 6.25 Habif TP, *Clinical Dermatology*, 5th edn, St Louis: Mosby, 2009: 964, Fig 25-44.

Figure 6.26 McGee S, *Evidence Based Physical Diagnosis*, 3rd edn, St Louis: Elsevier, 2012.

Figure 6.27 Malik A et al., Dengue hemorrhagic fever outbreak in children in Port Sudan. *Journal of Infection and Public Health* 2010; 4(1): Fig 6.

Figure 6.28 Kanski JJ, *Clinical Diagnosis in Ophthalmology*, 1st edn, Philadelphia: Mosby, 2006: Fig 10-45.

Figure 6.29 James WD, Berger TG, Elston DM (eds), *Andrews' Diseases of the Skin: Clinical Dermatology*, 11th edn, Philadelphia: Saunders, 2011: Fig 7.

Figure 6.32 Goldman L, Ausiello D, *Cecil Medicine*, 23rd edn, Philadelphia: Saunders, 2007: Fig 149-5.

Figure 6.37 Weston WL, Lane AT, Morelli JG, *Color Textbook of Pediatric Dermatology*, 4th edn, London: Mosby, 2007: Fig 14-46.

Figure 6.39 Stern TA, Rosenbaum JF, Fava M, Biederman J, Rauch SL, *Massachusetts General Hospital Comprehensive Clinical Psychiatry*, 1st edn, Philadelphia: Mosby, 2008: Fig 21-17.

Figure 6.40 Brenner S, Tamir E, Maharshak N, Shapira J, *Clinics Dermatol* 2001; 19(3): 290–297.

Figure 6.41 Talley NJ, O'Connor S, *Clinical Examination*, 6th edn, Sydney: Churchill Livingstone, 2009: Fig 6-10.

Figure 6.45 Yanoff M, Duker JS, *Ophthalmology*, 3rd edn, St Louis: Mosby, 2008: Fig 7-32.

Figure 7.1 Weston WL, Lane AT, Morelli JG, *Color Textbook of Pediatric Dermatology*, 4th edn, London: Mosby, 2007: Fig 17-62.

Figure 7.3 Kanski JJ, *Clinical Diagnosis in Ophthalmology*, 1st edn, Philadelphia: Mosby, 2006: Fig 13-78.

Figures 7.6, 7.36B Besser CM, Thorner MO, *Comprehensive Clinical Endocrinology*, 3rd edn St Louis, Mosby, 2002.

Figure 7.8 Kumar V, Abbas AK, Fausto N, Aster JC, *Robbins and Cotran Pathologic Basis of Disease, Professional Edition*, 8th edn, Philadelphia: Saunders, 2009: Fig 24-43.

Figures 7.11, 7.12, 7.18 Yanoff M, Duker JS, *Ophthalmology*, 3rd edn, London: Mosby, 2008: Figs 6-19-1, 6-19-2, 12-12-15.

Figure 7.13 Goldman L, Ausiello D, *Cecil Medicine*, 23rd edn, Philadelphia: Saunders, 2007: Fig 449-16.

Figure 7.15 Little JW, Falace DA, Miller CS, Rhodus NL, *Dental Management of the Medically Compromised Patient*, 7th edn, St Louis: Mosby, 2008: Fig 1-12.

Figure 7.16 Rakel RE, *Textbook of Family Medicine*, 7th edn, Philadelphia: Saunders, 2007: Fig 44-27.

Figure 7.19 Haught JM, Patel S, English JC, *J Am Acad Dermatol* 2007; 57(6): 1051–1058.

Figure 7.20 James WD, Berger TG, Elston DM (eds), *Andrews' Diseases of the Skin: Clinical Dermatology*, 11th edn, Philadelphia: Saunders, 2011: Fig 24-3.

Figure 7.22 Adapted from Klein I, Ojamaa K. Thyroid hormone and the cardiovascular system. *New England Journal of Medicine* 2001; 344(7): 501–509, Tables 1 and 2.

Figure 7.23 Eichenfield LF et al., *Neonatal Dermatology*, 2nd edn, Philadelphia: Saunders, 2008: Fig 27-11.

Figure 7.24 Swartz MH, *Textbook of Physical Diagnosis*, 6th edn, Philadelphia: Saunders, 2009: Fig 15-15.

Figures 7.25, 7.34, 7.35 Habif TP, *Clinical Dermatology*, 5th edn, Philadelphia: Mosby, 2009: Figs 25-29, 20-17, 7-33.

Figure 7.26 McGee S, *Evidence Based Physical Diagnosis*, 2nd edn, Philadelphia: Saunders, 2007: Fig 22-6.

Figure 7.27 Based on Radulescu D, Parv A, Pripon S et al., *Endocrinologist* 2010; 20(2): 72–74.

Figure 7.28 Hoffbrand V, Pettit JE, Vyas P, *Color Atlas of Clinical Hematology*, 4th edn, Philadelphia: Elsevier, 2010: Fig 15.3.

Figure 7.29 Lennard TWJ, *Endocrine Surgery*, 5th edn, Philadelphia: Elsevier, 2014: Fig 3.14.

Figures 7.31, 7.32 Besser CM, Thorner MO, *Comprehensive Clinical Endocrinology*, 3rd edn, St Louis, Mosby, 2002. In: Ferri FF, *Ferri's Color Atlas and Text of Clinical Medicine*, Saunders, 2009.

Figure 7.37 Marx JA, Hockberger RS, Walls RM et al. (eds), *Rosen's Emergency Medicine*, 7th edn, Philadelphia: Mosby, 2009: Fig 95-4.

Figure 7.39 Anderson DM, *Dorland's Dictionary*, 30th edn, Philadelphia: Elsevier, 2003.

Index

X

xanthelasmata, 303–304, 303*f*
    hyperlipidaemic, 303
    normolipidaemic, 303
x-descent
    absent, 227
    prominent, 228

Y

y-descent
    absent, 229–230, 229*f*
    prominent, 231–232, 231*f*, 232*b*
Yergason's sign, 70–71, 70*f*